BIOLOGICAL EFFECTS AND MEDICAL APPLICATIONS OF ELECTROMAGNETIC ENERGY

Prentice Hall Advanced Reference Series

Physical and Life Sciences

PRENTICE HALL
Biophysics and Bioengineering Series
Abraham Noordergraaf, Editor

AGNEW AND MCCREERY, EDS. *Neural Prostheses: Fundamental Studies*
GANDHI, ED. *Biological Effects and Medical Applications of Electromagnetic Energy*

FORTHCOMING BOOKS IN THIS SERIES (*tentative titles*)

ALPEN *Radiation Biophysics*
COLEMAN *Integrative Human Physiology: A Quantitative View of Homeostasis*
DAWSON *Engineering Design of the Cardiovascular System*
HUANG *Principles of Biomedical Image Processing*
JOU AND LLEBOT *Introduction to the Thermodynamics of Biological Processes*
MAYROVITZ *Analysis of Microcirculation*
SCHERER *Respiratory Fluid Mechanics*
VAIDHYANATHAN *Regulation and Control in Biological Systems*
WAAG *Theory and Measurement of Ultrasound Scattering* . . .

BIOLOGICAL EFFECTS AND MEDICAL APPLICATIONS OF ELECTROMAGNETIC ENERGY

Om P. Gandhi, Editor

PRENTICE HALL
Englewood Cliffs, New Jersey 07632

Library of Congress Cataloging-in-Publication Data

Biological effects and medical applications of electromagnetic energy
/ Om P. Gandhi, editor.
       p. cm. — (Prentice Hall biophysics and bioengineering
series)
    Includes bibliographical references.
    ISBN 0-13-082728-2
    1. Electromagnetic fields—Physiological effect.
2. Electromagnetic fields—Health aspects. 3. Electromagnetic
fields—Therapeutic use. I. Gandhi, Om P., 1935–   . II. Series:
Prentice Hall biophysics and bioengineering.
    [DNLM: 1. Electromagnetics. 2. Radiobiology. WN 610 B6154]
QP82.2.E43B548   1990
612'.014—dc20
DNLM/DLC
for Library of Congress   90–6850
                                                                  CIP

Editorial/production supervision
  and interior design: Mary Espenschied
Cover design: Wanda Lubelska Design
Manufacturing buyer: Kelly Behr

Prentice Hall Advanced Reference Series

Prentice Hall Biophysics and Bioengineering Series

 ©1990 by Prentice-Hall, Inc.
A Division of Simon & Schuster
Englewood Cliffs, New Jersey 07632

The publisher offers discounts on this book when ordered
in bulk quantities. For more information, write:

        Special Sales/College Marketing
        Prentice Hall
        College Technical and Reference Division
        Englewood Cliffs, NJ 07632

Printed in the United States of America
10 9 8 7 6 5 4 3 2 1

ISBN   0-13-082728-2

Prentice-Hall International (UK) Limited, *London*
Prentice-Hall of Australia Pty. Limited, *Sydney*
Prentice-Hall Canada Inc., *Toronto*
Prentice-Hall Hispanoamericana, S.A., *Mexico*
Prentice-Hall of India Private Limited, *New Delhi*
Prentice-Hall of Japan, Inc., *Tokyo*
Simon & Schuster Asia Pte. Ltd., *Singapore*
Editora Prentice-Hall do Brasil, Ltda., *Rio de Janeiro*

TO

*The pioneers who by their brilliant
and careful research have put this
field on a solid scientific footing*

Contents

Foreword

Originally in the form of a collection of clay tablets, then as a papyrus roll, and eventually as bound sheets of paper, the book has served to record events and ideas uppermost in the contemporary human mind for the last 45 to 50 centuries.

In one familiar classic role it continues as a teaching aid in the instruction of the next generation: the textbook. The noble textbook may have several precursors.

In the last few centuries, as new research areas are discovered or older ones become accessible owing to the creation of new methods, the professional journals have become the initial repositories of reports that treat the various aspects in excruciating detail. As the number of publications multiplies, it tends to become a challenge to find and especially to digest such a collection of papers owing to real or apparent contradictions in measurement results or promulgated interpretations. A well-organized and critical collection in book form tends to crystallize the issues and purify the interpretation, thereby facilitating further progress in that research area.

Once the proper methodology or the governing principle has been identified, a book can serve to set forth the solution, thus reducing the volume of current literature by a significant factor.

Eventually, a book tracing the generation and growth of ideas in a broader field can serve to expose guiding philosophical convictions over a more extended period of research, often resulting in striking insights.

The Biophysics and Bioengineering Series is intended to serve these several purposes in the broad field defined in its name by providing monographs prepared by expert investigators. Originally published by Academic Press, the series is continued by Prentice Hall.

The following volumes have appeared thus far: *Circulatory System Dynamics*, by Abraham Noordergraaf, 1978; *An Introduction to Microcirculation*, by Mary P. Wiedeman, Ronald F. Tuma, and Harvey N. Mayrovitz, 1978; *Physiology and Electrochemistry of Nerve Fibers*, by Ichiji Tasaki, 1982; *Biomaterials*, by L. L. Hench and E. C. Ethridge, 1982; *Neural Prostheses*: *Fundamental Studies*, edited by William F. Agnew and Douglas B. McCreery, 1990.

Abraham Noordergraaf
Series Editor

Preface

With the expanding use of electromagnetic (EM) energy, the public is becoming increasingly aware of and concerned about the potential biohazards of EM fields. Continuing disparity in the safety standards worldwide and the lack of knowledge of EM field's nonthermal mechanisms of interaction with biological systems have contributed to the confusion that presently exists in the public mind. In addition to the myriad present-day applications from electric power lines to radio, television, communications, and a variety of industrial and medical devices, several future applications are anticipated. An example of this is the use of EM hyperthermia as an adjuvant for cancer therapy.

Different chapters in this book represent the state of the knowledge in the various aspects of the field as reviewed by the recognized leaders in the respective areas. Part 1 of the book, consisting of three chapters, deals with the nomenclature and the radio frequency (RF) field exposure standards in the various countries and some of their problems. Part 2 of the book deals with the bioengineering aspects of EM fields. Discussed in this part are the environmental and professionally encountered fields, electrical properties of biological tissues, and experimental and numerical techniques for determination of EM absorption and its distribution in man and animals. Biological effects and health implications of EM fields from ELF (extremely low frequency) to millimeter-wave frequencies are discussed in Part 3, Chapters 9 to 17. In view of the reported links between EM fields and cancer, several chapters have commented on this issue. Chapter 17, Epidemiologic Studies of Cancer and EM Fields, by Charlotte Silverman, is of particular interest in this regard. Medical applications of EM fields are discussed in Part 4. The last chapter of the book is devoted to some common misconceptions about this field.

I wish to express my sincere thanks to Professor Abraham Noorder-graaf of the University of Pennsylvania for inviting me to undertake this task. He has been most cooperative and understanding of the delays in the completion of the book. Without his help this book would not have been completed. I have also benefitted from prior experience as a guest editor of a couple of special issues in this field by *Proceedings of the IEEE* (Institute of Electrical and Electronics Engineers) and by *IEEE Engineering in Medicine and Biology* magazine, where I had the opportunity to work with many of the authors who have contributed to this book. I am grateful to several of these authors for suggestions on the contents of the book. Special gratitude must also be expressed to Frances Lingle on our secretarial staff for her capable typing of several of the chapters.

Om P. Gandhi

About the Editor

Dr. Om P. Gandhi is a professor of Electrical Engineering at the University of Utah, Salt Lake City. He is an author or coauthor of one technical book and over 200 journal articles on microwave tubes, solid-state devices, and electromagnetic dosimetry and has recently written the textbook *Microwave Engineering and Applications* published by Pergamon Press. He has been a principal investigator on numerous industrially and federally funded research projects since 1974, and serves or has served as a consultant to several government agencies and private industries.

Dr. Gandhi was elected Fellow of the Institute of Electrical and Electronics Engineers "for contributions to the understanding of nonionizing radiation effects, to the development of electron devices, and to engineering education." He received the Distinguished Research award of the University of Utah for 1979–1980 and a special award for "Outstanding Technical Achievement" from the Institute of Electrical and Electronics Engineers, Utah Section, in 1975. He edited a *Proceedings of the IEEE* Special Issue (January 1980) on Biological Effects and Medical Applications of Electromagnetic Energy, and a Special Issue (March 1987) of the *IEEE Engineering in Medicine and Biology* magazine on Effects of Electromagnetic Radiation. He is Cochairman of the Subcommittee ANSI C95.4 and a past Chairman of the IEEE Committee on Man and Radiation (COMAR). His name is listed in *Who's Who in the World*, *Who's Who in America*, *Who's Who in Engineering*, and *Who's Who in Technology Today*.

Contributors

Eleanor R. Adair
John B. Pierce Foundation Laboratory
and Yale University
New Haven, Connecticut

L. E. Anderson
Bioelectromagnetics Section
Pacific Northwest Laboratory
Richland, Washington

Tadeusz M. Babij
Electrical Engineering Department
Florida International University
Miami, Florida

Howard I. Bassen
Walter Reed Army Institute of
Research
Washington, D.C.

Douglas A. Christensen
Departments of Electrical
Engineering and Bioengineering
University of Utah
Salt Lake City, Utah

Stephen F. Cleary
Physiology Department

Medical College of Virginia
Virginia Commonwealth University
Richmond, Virginia

John A. D'Andrea
Bioenvironmental Assessment
Department
Naval Aerospace Medical Research
Laboratory
Pensacola, Florida

John O. de Lorge
Bioenvironmental Assessment
Department
Naval Aerospace Medical Research
Laboratory
Pensacola, Florida

Carl H. Durney
Departments of Electrical
Engineering and Bioengineering
University of Utah
Salt Lake City, Utah

Om P. Gandhi
Department of Electrical Engineering
University of Utah
Salt Lake City, Utah

Magdy F. Iskander
Department of Electrical Engineering
University of Utah
Salt Lake City, Utah

James C. Lin
Department of Bioengineering
University of Illinois
Chicago, Illinois

K. G. Lövstrand
High Voltage Research Institute
Uppsala University
Uppsala, Sweden

K. Hansson Mild
National Institute of Occupational
  Health
Umeå, Sweden

Shirley M. Motzkin
Life Sciences/Chemistry
Polytechnic University
Brooklyn, New York

Mary Ellen O'Connor
Department of Psychology
The University of Tulsa
Tulsa, Oklahoma

John M. Osepchuk
Research Division
Raytheon Company
Lexington, Massachusetts

Michael H. Repacholi
Royal Adelaide Hospital
Adelaide, South Australia

Charlotte Silverman
Office of Science and Technology
Center for Devices and Radiological
  Health
Food and Drug Administration
Rockville, Maryland

Maria A. Stuchly
Radiation Protection Bureau
Health and Welfare Canada
Ottawa, Ontario, Canada

Stanislaw S. Stuchly
Department of Electrical
  Engineering
University of Ottawa
Ottawa, Ontario, Canada

Part 1

GENERAL

1

Introduction to Electromagnetic Fields

OM P. GANDHI

ELECTROMAGNETIC SPECTRUM

This book focuses on the biological effects of electromagnetic (EM) fields for the frequency range of 50/60 Hz to 10^{11} Hz or from power line frequencies to millimeter waves. The EM spectrum and some of its typical applications are illustrated in Figure 1-1. As shown in Figure 1-1, the radiofrequency (RF) part of the EM spectrum (0 to 300 GHz) is useful for a variety of applications that have been expanding rapidly in recent decades. Some present and potential applications of RF energy are discussed in an article by Gandhi (1982). Some of the well-known applications are electrical power lines, radio and television, point-to-point communication systems for long-distance telephone and television and for commercial applications such as data links; public safety; remote control; airborne, marine, and ground radars; aircraft altimeter and guidance systems; microwave ovens; industrial applications such as RF sealers; and a variety of medical devices.

The various frequency bands of the RF part of the spectrum are given in Table 1-1 (ITT Handbook, 1968). The frequency range from 300 MHz to 300 GHz is also loosely called the microwave part of the spectrum.

ELECTROMAGNETIC FIELDS

EM waves are marked by *electric* (**E**) and *magnetic* (**H**) fields (hence the name "electromagnetic") that, having been emitted from a transmitting source or an *antenna*, are propagating through space at the velocity of light. The number of times the electric or the magnetic field pulsates per second at a given point is called *frequency* (f) of the wave. This is expressed in cycles per second or *hertz* (Hz) in honor of the early German radiophysicist Heinrich Hertz. For a variety of applications, such as heating or Doppler radar, a *continuous wave* (CW) or a wave that is constant in frequency and amplitude (of **E** and **H**) with time is used. For most applications, however, a wave that is modulated in amplitude (amplitude modulation, or AM) or frequency (frequency modulation, or FM) is used

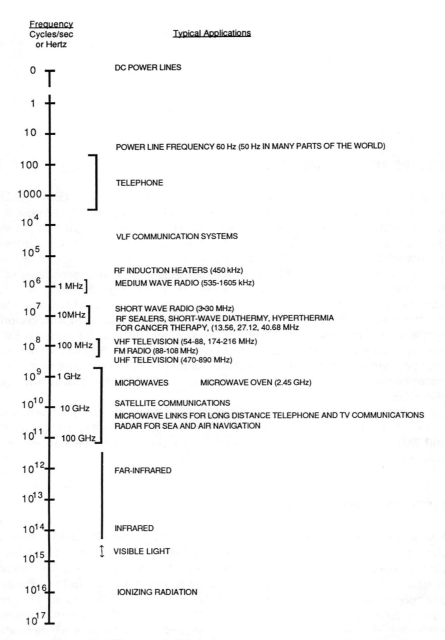

Figure 1-1 Electromagnetic spectrum and some typical applications.

TABLE 1-1   **Frequency Bands of Radiofrequency Part
of Electromagnetic Spectrum**

Frequency range	Band	Abbreviation
0–30 Hz		
30–300 Hz	Extremely low frequency	ELF
0.3–3 kHz	Voice frequency	VF
3–30 kHz	Very low frequency	VLF
30–300 kHz	Low frequency	LF
0.3–3 MHz	Medium frequency	MF
3–30 MHz	High frequency	HF
30–300 MHz	Very high frequency	VHF
0.3–3 GHz	Ultra-high frequency	UHF
3–30 GHz	Super-high frequency	SHF
30–300 GHz	Extremely high frequency	EHF

to transfer speech, picture, or data information from one point to another. For several applications, most notably radar, pulses or bursts of waves are used. For such waves in addition to frequency (during each of the bursts), the pulse duration (in microseconds or μ s) and the pulse repetition rate (in hertz) are also prescribed.

The *wavelength* of EM waves (λ) is the distance the wave travels in a time corresponding to one period ($1/f$) of the wave. In free space therefore

$$\lambda = c/f \qquad (1)$$

where c is the velocity of light in air (approximately 3×10^8 m/s). For RF waves the wavelength may vary from several hundred meters ($\lambda = 300$ m for $f = 1$ MHz) to a fraction of a centimeter. By comparison the wavelengths for visible light vary from approximately 4×10^{-5} cm for violet light to 7.2×10^{-5} cm for red light because of the very high frequencies (on the order of 10^{15} Hz) involved.

FAR AND NEAR FIELDS: PLANE WAVES

At distances from the source larger than $2 D^2/\lambda$, where D is the maximum dimension of the radiating antenna, and in the absence of obstacles, the electric and magnetic fields may typically be at right angles to one another (**E** $\perp$ **H**) and perpendicular to the direction of propagation (k) of the wave. Furthermore, in such a case the time-averaged magnitudes of **E** and **H** at any given point are proportional to one another such that $E/H = 120\pi$ or 377. The EM waves under these conditions are said to be in the *far-field* region of the source. If the distance to the source of radiation is considerable (as for EM fields because of distant radio and television antennas), these waves are also called *plane waves*, since the field at all points in a plane normal to the direction of propagation is identical in both magnitude and variation with time.

Many of the real-life exposures are in the far-field region of the antennas. In the absence of nearby objects, the EM fields incident upon the body would be those of plane waves; that is, **E, H,** and k that are mutually perpendicular and $E/H = 377$ ohms. Since proximity to scattering objects is often the case, the nature of the incident fields is quite complex and exposure may in fact be from several directions on account of scattering of EM waves from these objects.

Another class of exposures that often involve somewhat higher-intensity EM fields affects maintenance personnel and operators of RF equipment. Such exposures are invariably in the near-field regions of the devices, which implies that, as mentioned earlier, electric and magnetic fields are not related in any simple fashion, either for direction or for the relative magnitudes. Environmental and professionally encountered EM fields are discussed in Chapter 4.

POLARIZATION, POWER DENSITY, AND SPECIFIC ABSORPTION RATE

The polarization of an EM wave is the direction of the electric field. Vertically and horizontally polarized waves are used, for example, for AM radio and for television, respectively, which simply implies that the E fields are vertical or horizontal, respectively, for these two types of broadcast communications. As discussed in Chapter 8, absorption of EM energy varies not only with the frequency but also rather drastically with polarization, particularly in the resonant range of frequencies. Circularly and elliptically polarized waves are also used for special applications. For these waves the electric field rotates with time as though to trace either a circle or an ellipse. Instantaneous power density p is the product of vectors **E** and **H**. Because sinusoidally varying signals in time are often used, a time-average power density that is one half of the peak values is encountered.

For electrically conducting media such as the biological tissues, the rate of energy dissipated per unit volume at a given point is given by $\sigma E^2/2$ in watts per cubic meter, where σ is the electrical conductivity of the medium. If specific absorption rate (SAR) or power dissipated per unit mass is required, the quantity $\sigma E^2/2$ needs to be divided by the mass density of the tissue. The SAR in watts per kilogram is thus given by

$$\text{SAR} = \frac{\sigma E^2}{2\rho} \qquad (2)$$

where ρ is the mass density of the tissue in kilograms per cubic meter. The values for the mass densities of the various tissues are given in Table 6-1.

UNITS, COMMONLY USED PREFIXES, AND PHYSICAL CONSTANTS

The units for the various quantities associated with EM waves in the metric system of units are given in Table 1-2. Some commonly used prefixes are given in Table 1-3. Some physical constants are given in Table 1-4.

TABLE 1-2   Quantities and Their Units

Quantity	Common symbol	Name of unit	Symbol of unit
Current density	J	Amperes per square meter	A/m^2
Dielectric constant	ϵ_r	Ratio ϵ/ϵ_0; dimensionless	—
Electric energy density	w_E	Joules per cubic meter	J/m^3
Electric field	E	Volts per meter	V/m
Electric flux density	D	Coulombs per square meter	C/m^2
Electrical conductivity	σ	Siemens per meter	S/m
Energy	W	Joule	J
Frequency	f	Hertz	Hz
Magnetic energy density	w_H	Joules per cubic meter	J/m^3
Magnetic field	H	Amperes per meter	A/m
Magnetic flux density	B	Tesla	T
Permeability	μ	Henrys per meter	H/m
Permittivity	ϵ	Farads per meter	F/m
Power	P	Watt	W
Power density	p	Watts per square meter	W/m^{2*}
Voltage	V	Volt	V

* 1 W/m^2 = 0.1 mW/cm^2.

8

General   Part 1

TABLE 1-3   Prefixes and Their Abbreviations

Prefix	Abbreviation	Unit
Pico	p	10^{-12}
Nano	n	10^{-9}
Micro	μ	10^{-6}
Milli	m	10^{-3}
Centi	c	10^{-2}
Kilo	k	10^{3}
Mega	M	10^{6}
Giga	G	10^{9}

TABLE 1-4   Physical Constants

Physical constant	Magnitude
Velocity of light c	2.998×10^8 m/s
Permittivity of free space ϵ_0	8.854×10^{-12} F/m
Permeability of free space and biological tissues μ_0	$4\pi \times 10^{-7}$ H/m
Intrinsic impedance of free space $\sqrt{\mu_0/\epsilon_0}$	120π or 377 ohms
Charge of an electron	1.6×10^{-19} C
Mass of an electron	9.1×10^{-31} kg
Planck's constant h	6.624×10^{-34} J-s
Boltzmann's constant k_B	1.3805×10^{-23} J/degree Kelvin

REFERENCES

GANDHI, O.P. (1982). Present and future benefits: applications of radiofrequency and microwave energy. *In*: Steneck, N.H. (ed.). Risk/benefit analysis: the microwave case. San Francisco, San Francisco Press, Inc.

International Telephone and Telegraph Corporation (ITT) handbook (1968): Reference data for radio engineers, 5th ed. Indianapolis, Howard W. Sams & Co.

2

Radiofrequency Field Exposure Standards: Current Limits and Relevant Bioeffects Data

MICHAEL H. REPACHOLI

Concern among the general population and workers about nonionizing radiation has arisen partly from fears that a radiofrequency (RF) field, especially in the microwave region, is capable of producing a range of biological effects that could be hazardous to human health. Many believe that, although acute effects have been studied and largely characterized, chronic, low-level exposures have received little attention and thus the possibility that long-term exposure could cause cancer, Down's syndrome, or cataracts has not been resolved.

In an attempt to assess the many and varied biological effects reported in the literature and to identify effects pertinent to a health risk assessment, a number of national and international agencies have provided detailed literature reviews that could form a data base for the development of human RF exposure standards.

Reviews of the RF bioeffects literature have been produced by the World Health Organization (WHO, 1981; Suess, 1982; Suess and Benwell, 1987); American National Standards Institute (ANSI, 1982), Environmental Protection Agency (Elder and Cahill, 1984); National Council on Radio Protection and Measurement (NCRP, 1986), and International Radiational Protection Association (IRPA, 1988). The WHO (1981), ANSI (1982), and other reviews and literature were used to develop the IRPA (1984) guidelines, and more recent literature and other national standards were used to draft the updated IRPA (1988) guidelines.

SCIENTIFIC LITERATURE

When guidelines or standards on human exposure limits are issued, some people may become concerned that more recent reports were not taken into account. These publications are generally in the form of preliminary unconfirmed results or data from in-vitro experiments. It must be understood that exposure limits can be drafted only on the basis of the established literature containing proven results, since to base standards on preliminary data or unproven hypotheses means that the limit values could change significantly with further research. Using established literature allows exposure limits to be determined with a higher degree of confidence about their protective level.

Certain criteria must be met if claims of positive or negative effects are to be accepted into the body of established scientific literature. These include the following (Repacholi, 1988):

1. The experimental techniques, methods, and conditions should be as completely objective as possible.

2. All data analyses should be fully and completely objective, with no relevant data deleted from consideration and with uniform analytical methods used.

3. The published description of the methods should be given in sufficient detail that a critical reader would be convinced that all reasonable precautions have been taken to meet requirements 1 and 2.

4. The results should demonstrate an effect of the relevant variable at a high level of statistical significance using appropriate tests. The effects of interest should ordinarily be shown by a majority of test organisms, and the responses found should be consistent.

5. The results should be quantifiable and susceptible to confirmation by independent researchers. Preferably the experiments should be repeated and the data confirmed independently, or the claimed effects should be consistent with results of similar experiments in which the biological systems involved were comparable.

6. The results should be viewed with respect to previously accepted scientific principles before new ones are ascribed to them.

From the body of established literature, a distinction must be made between in vitro and in vivo studies. Some serious researchers believe that the results of their in vitro studies should be used to derive or significantly affect the value of limits for human RF exposure standards. In vitro studies are conducted to elucidate mechanisms of interaction or to identify biological effects that need to be researched to determine whether they occur in in vivo systems. Standards-setting organizations can place only limited value on the results of in vitro experiments unless they have been clearly established for particular effects (such as mutagenicity of drugs). Standards based on unsubstantiated reports or unproven hypotheses or speculations have no valid rationale.

RADIOFREQUENCY STANDARDS

There have been a number of recent reviews of current RF standards (Polk and Postow, 1986; Mild, 1987; Repacholi, 1987; Stuchly, 1987; Sliney, 1988), so this review covers only major standards or recent proposals. Early standards addressed mainly the microwave region (300 MHz to 300 GHz) because of the introduction and proliferation of radar, telecommunications, and radio and television broadcasting. Later standards recognized the vastly expanded use of the EM spectrum, especially at lower frequencies where concerns were raised about high exposures received from RF induction heaters and heat sealers and other industrial applications of RF energy.

Recently some organizations have expanded their standards to provide guidance on the whole spectrum (FRG, 1986; NRPB, 1986) or at least to develop exposure criteria that would cover the concerns of video display terminal operators (ACGIH, 1987). The latest ANSI standard redrafting committee is considering expansion of its scope to include frequencies from 3 kHz to 300 GHz (ANSI, 1988).

With the increasing knowledge about RF dosimetry (absorption and distribution of RF energy in the human body and the differing absorption of the electric and magnetic fields), standards are becoming more sophisticated. Gone are the days when a standard was merely one power density value over the frequency range of interest. Modern standards have frequency ranges that take account of the differences in RF absorption in humans.

The basic premise of modern standards is that the severity of an effect is directly related to the rate of RF energy absorbed and hence the introduction of the concept of specific absorption rate (SAR). SAR, measured in watts per kilogram, has the advantage of providing a reasonable basis on which to physically scale the exposure parameters that produced results of in vivo experiments in various biological systems to the equivalent RF exposure parameters that could be predicted to produce the same effects in humans.

The international (IRPA, 1988) and most Western RF standards have accepted, on the basis of reviews of all appropriate scientific literature, a threshold RF exposure of 4 W/kg as necessary under normal environmental conditions to produce behavioral changes in animals. In high temperatures this threshold is reduced to above 1 W/kg (Elder and Cahill, 1984). These behavioral changes (decreased endurance, work decrement, work stoppage, etc.) found in carefully controlled repeated experiments on rodents and subhuman primates are the most sensitive of the effects of RF exposure. Standards have generally required that limits of RF absorption be set that do not allow more than one tenth of the threshold SAR value (that is, 0.4 W/kg) to be exceeded.

In many countries, drafting of exposure standards is carried out by committees representing employers, employees, and government. Thus, although scientific analysis may suggest certain limits, committee compromises may prevent a uniform factor of safety from being obtained in the final values over the whole frequency range.

INTERNATIONAL GUIDELINES

The International Non-Ionizing Radiation Committee of IRPA recently published a revision, shown in Tables 2-1 and 2-2, of its 1984 guideline (IRPA, 1988). This revision, based on research data obtained over the preceding 4 years, did not alter the threshold exposures on which the basic limit was derived: whole-body exposure to RF fields should not exceed 0.4 W/kg. The IRPA revision was essentially a fine-tuning that included the following:

1. Although the whole body average SAR could not exceed 0.4 W/kg, reports from Gandhi (1985), Gandhi et al. (1985), Guy and Chou (1985), M. Stuchly et al. (1985, 1986), and S. Stuchly et al. (1986), indicated that under certain conditions the local peak SAR in the extremities (particularly wrists and ankles) could exceed 0.4 W/kg by a factor of up to 300 at certain frequencies. Because of this an additional recommendation was introduced for frequencies above 10 MHz where in the extremities a local SAR of 2 W/0.1 kg is not to be exceeded and that 1 W/0.1 kg should not be exceeded in any other body part.

2. The IRPA (1984) guidelines on peak pulsed fields were based on few bioeffects data, and values recommended were imprecise and unnecessarily restrictive. The IRPA (1988) has addressed this problem by suggesting that the equivalent plane-wave power density

TABLE 2-1   IRPA Occupational Exposure Limits to Radiofrequency Fields*

Frequency (MHz)	Unperturbed RMS field strength		Equivalent plane-wave power density (P_{eq})	
	Electric E(V/m)	Magnetic H(A/m)	W/m^2	mW/cm^2
0.1–1	614	1.6/f	—	—
>1–10	614/f	1.6/f	—	—
>10–400	61	0.16	10	1
>400–2000	3 $f^{1/2}$	0.008 $f^{1/2}$	f/40	f/400
>2000–300,000	137	0.36	50	5

Reprinted with permission from International Radiational Protection Association (1988). Guidelines on limits of exposure to radiofrequency electromagnetic fields in the frequency range from 100 MHz to 300 GHz. *Health Phys.* 54:115–123. Copyright 1988, Pergamon Press.

* Hazards of RF burns should be eliminated by limiting currents from contact with metal objects. In most situations this can be achieved by reducing the *E* values from 614 to 194 V/m in the range from 0.1 to 1 MHz and from 614/f to 194/f$^{1/2}$ in the range from >1 to 10 MHz.

TABLE 2-2   IRPA General Public Exposure Limits to Radiofrequency Fields*

Frequency (MHz)	Unperturbed RMS field strength		Equivalent plane-wave power density (P_{eq})	
	Electric E(V/m)	Magnetic H(A/m)	W/m²	mW/cm²
0.01	87	$0.23/f^{1/2}$	—	—
>1–10	$87/f^{1/2}$	$0.23/f^{1/2}$	—	—
>10–400	27.5	0.073	2	0.2
>400–2000	$1.375\ f^{1/2}$	$0.0037\ f^{1/2}$	f/200	f/2000
>2000–300,000	61	0.16	10	1

Reprinted with permission from International Radiational Protection Association (1988). Guidelines on limits of exposure to radiofrequency electromagnetic fields in the frequency range from 100 MHz to 300 GHz. *Health Phys.* 54:115–123. Copyright 1988, Pergamon Press.

f, Frequency in megahertz.

(P_{eq}) averaged over the pulsed width not exceed 1000 times the P_{eq} for frequencies above 10 MHz, or equivalently 32 times the electric or magnetic field limits below 10 MHz.

Canada

RF exposure limits were proposed in Canada (Repacholi, 1978) and issued in 1979 as a safety code by the Federal Department of Health and Welfare (Health and Welfare Canada, 1979). A revision of these Canadian recommendations has recently been proposed by Stuchly (1987). The proposed limits for occupational exposure are shown in Table 2-3 and for the general public in Table 2-4.

Although the proposed limits are similar to the IRPA (1988) values, a different approach has been taken to restrict the high local SARs that can occur, particularly to the extremities. The occupational proposal limits the local SAR to 8 W/kg over any 1 g of tissue, except at the body surface or in the limbs where the limit is 25 W/kg. In addition, the standards recommend that the local SAR to the eye not exceed 0.4 W/kg. The proposal for the general public limits the SAR averaged over any 20 percent of the body mass to 0.2 W/kg, the local SAR in the eye to no more than 0.4 W/kg, and the local SAR over any 1 g of tissue to no more than 4 W/kg except on the body surface or in the arms and legs, where the maximum SAR is 12 W/kg.

TABLE 2-3   Proposed Canadian Occupational Exposure Limits

Frequency (MHz)	Electric field strength E(V/m)	Magnetic field strength H(A/m)	Power density (W/m^2)
0.01–1.2	600	4.0	—
1.2–3	600	4.8/f	—
3–30	1800/f or 3120/f$^{3/2}$*	4.8/f	—
30–100	60 or 20*	0.16	—
100–300	60 or 0.2 f	0.16	10
300–1500	3.45 f$^{1/2}$	0.0093 f$^{1/2}$	
1500–300,000	140	0.36	50

Reprinted with permission from Stuchly, M.A. (1987). Proposed revision of the Canadian recommendations on radiofrequency-exposure protection. *Health Phys.* *53*:649–665. Copyright 1987, Pergamon Press.

f, Frequency in megahertz.

* The lower limits apply when the exposed person is separated less than 0.1 m from what can be considered electrical ground; in all other cases the higher limits apply.

TABLE 2-4   Proposed Canadian General Population Exposure Limits

Frequency (MHz)	Electric field strength E(V/m)	Magnetic field strength H(A/m)	Power density (W/m^2)
0.01–1.2	280	1.8	—
1.2–3	280	2.1/f	—
3–30	849/f or 1600/f$^{3/2}$*	2.1/f	—
30–100	28 or 10*	0.07	—
100–300	28 or 0.1 f	0.07	2
300–1500	1.61 f$^{1/2}$	0.004 f$^{1/2}$	
1500–300,000	60	0.16	10

Reprinted with permission from Stuchly, M.A. (1987). Proposed revision of the Canadian recommendations on radiofrequency-exposure protection. *Health Phys.* *53*:649–665. Copyright 1987, Pergamon Press.

f, Frequency in megahertz.

* The lower limits apply when the exposed person is separated less than 0.1 m from electrical ground; in all other cases the higher limits apply.

The rationale for the Canadian proposal can be summarized as follows:

1. The threshold for adverse health effects is 3 to 4 W/kg, so the electric field, magnetic field, and power density limits for occupational exposure were based on restricting the whole-body-averaged SAR value to 0.4 W/kg, and for the general public the whole-body-averaged SAR is limited to 0.08 W/kg. The lower limit for the general public is based on the same rationale as the WHO (1981), IRPA (1984), and NCRP (1986) guidelines: that duration of the public's RF exposure is potentially 24 hours a day for 7 days a week, compared with 8 hours a day, 5 days a week for workers, and that the aged, infants, and chronically ill may be more susceptible to RF effects. Hence an extra safety factor of 5 is incorporated into the exposure limits to allow for these possibilities.

2. Lower limits are proposed for a grounded person (less than 10 cm from electrical ground) exposed to RF fields in the frequency range 3 to 300 MHz, since higher RF absorption occurs in people grounded for these frequencies.

3. Local SAR limits are proposed to take account of the high values that could occur at the body surface and the extremities (Gandhi et al., 1986).

4. Below 30 MHz, the limits take account of RF shocks and burns, and different electric and magnetic field strengths are recommended because of the differences in absorption in the human body by these two fields.

Sweden

The National Board of Occupational Safety and Health (NBOSH) sets the RF occupational exposure limits in Sweden. In 1977 these limits, averaged over 6 minutes, were 5 mW/cm^2 for frequencies of 10 to 300 MHz and 1 mW/cm^2 for frequencies of 300 MHz to 300 GHz, with a ceiling value of 25 mW/cm^2 averaged over 1 second for the whole frequency range.

Using the IRPA (1984) and ANSI (1982) standards as a basis (Mild, 1987), the Board has issued a new RF exposure standard, which took effect January 1, 1988 (NBOSH, 1987). The new limits are shown in Table 2-5. Ceiling values, never to be exceeded, are 300 V/m and 0.8 A/m in the frequency range 3 to 300 MHz and 300 V/m in the frequency range 0.3 to 300 GHz. If a worker is closer than 10 cm to electrical ground, the ceiling limits are 100 V/m and 0.27 A/m in the frequency range 3 to 60 MHz.

TABLE 2-5   Occupational RF Exposure Limits in Sweden

Frequency range (MHz)	Exposure limits	
	E(V/m)	H(A/m)
3–30	140 or 47*	0.4 or 0.13*
30–300	60 or 20*	0.16 or 0.05*
	(up to 60 MHz)	
300–300,000	60	—

Data from National Board of Occupational Safety and Health (1987). High frequency electromagnetic fields. Stockholm, NBOSH.

* Lower limit applies only if worker is closer than 10 cm to electrical ground.

The limits were based on thermal considerations (Mild, 1987), but the fundamental quantities restricted are the electric and magnetic field strengths. For frequencies greater than 300 MHz, the standard is similar to the Australian standard for occupational exposure (Australia, 1985).

The Swedish National Institute of Radiation Protection issues general public exposure limits. In 1978 the Institute recommended that the power density be kept below 1 mW/cm^2, and if possible below 0.1 mW/cm^2 over the long term. According to Mild (1987), the Institute will issue new guidelines shortly.

Federal Republic of Germany

In July 1984 the Federal Republic of Germany published its RF exposure standard, which covers the range 10 kHz to 3000 GHz (upper frequencies into the infrared region). This standard (Table 2-6) is applicable for occupational and general public exposure.

The German standard has two parts, which derive from different sources, one for high frequencies and the other for low frequencies. The low-frequency section is based on the work of Bernhardt (1979, 1985). With the premise that induced electric current within tissues is the decisive factor for producing biological effects, threshold values of field strength or current density required to cause biological effects were compiled from experimental and theoretical studies. These data were used to determine "safe," "dangerous," and "hazardous" current density curves as a function of frequency. The exposure limits were set by reducing the electric and magnetic field strengths necessary to cause a specific effect (ventricular fibrillation) by a factor of about 300 to arrive at the final values.

The high-frequency section of the standard is based on the SAR concept (ANSI, 1982; IRPA, 1984). However, a factor of 4 below the whole-

TABLE 2-6   Electromagnetic Radiation Protection Standard for Occupational
and General Public Exposure in the Federal Republic of Germany

Frequency range (MHz)	Exposure limits		
	E(V/m)	H(A/m)	mW/cm^2
0.01–0.03	2000 (peak)	500 (peak)	—
0.01–0.03	1500	350	—
0.03–2	1500	7.5/f	—
2–30	3000/f	7.5/f	—
30–3000	100	0.25	2.5
3000–12,000	1.83 f$^{1/2}$	0.005 f$^{1/2}$	0.0008 f
12,000–3,000,000	200	0.5	10

Data from Federal Republic of Germany, Deutsches Institut fur Normen (DIN) (1984).
Hazards for electromagnetic fields: protection of persons in the frequency range from
10 kHz to 300 GHz. DIN 578.848, Teil 2, Berlin, DIN.
f, Frequency in megahertz.

body SAR of 4 W/kg was considered sufficient for safety. The limits for
frequencies between 0.3 and 3 GHz were not raised because such high-
intensity fields may cause hot spots in the brain.

To provide protection limits in the EM spectrum down to static
electric and magnetic fields, the Federal Republic of Germany issued a
proposal to cover the frequency range 0 to 3000 GHz. This proposal
applies to occupational and general public exposure. For the frequency
range up to 30 kHz, the proposal is based on the work of Bernhardt
(1985), who calculated the maximum current density induced in humans
exposed to electric and magnetic fields of varying frequencies. The proposal aims to keep induced current densities below 1 mA/m^2, the value
of current densities naturally occurring in the body and hence not considered hazardous. Above 30 kHz the proposed limits are derived purely
on a thermal basis in which SAR values are kept at a sufficient safety
margin below 4 W/kg (FRG, 1986).

United States

In 1982 the American National Standards Institute (ANSI) issued
its radiation protection guide, a voluntary standard for occupational and
general public exposure for frequencies in the range 300 kHz to 100
GHz. This guide, shown in Table 2-7, is based on limiting the whole-
body-averaged SAR to 0.4 W/kg, a factor of 10 lower than the threshold
for observing the most sensitive RF bioeffects.

There has been some criticism (Gandhi, 1985; Gandhi et al., 1985)
of the ANSI guide, particularly at the lower frequencies. Gandhi (1985)

TABLE 2-7   American National Standards Institute Standard for Occupational
and General Public Exposure

Frequency range (MHz)	Exposure limits		
	E(V/m)	H(A/m)	mW/cm^2
0.3–3	632	1.6	100
3–30	1897/f	4.74/f	900/f^2
30–300	63.2	0.16	1.0
300–1500	3.65 f$^{1/2}$	0.009 f$^{1/2}$	f/300
1500–100,000	141	0.35	5.0

Data from American National Standards Institute. American national standard C95.1, Safety levels with electromagnetic fields (300 kHz–100 GHz). New York, Institute of Electrical and Electronic Engineers, Inc.

f, Frequency in megahertz.

pointed out that potentially large RF-induced currents and high local SARs could occur in the legs and ankles and that hazards could result from contact with commonly encountered ungrounded objects in the ANSI-recommended E fields for the frequency band 0.3 to 62.5 MHz. Gandhi (1988) has suggested the following modifications of the ANSI standard to overcome these problems (Table 2-8):

1. For ungrounded individuals, induced RF current should be <100 mA as measured through both feet or <50 mA through each foot. For frequencies less than 100 kHz, the allowable induced current

TABLE 2-8   Proposed Radiofrequency Limits for Occupational Exposure

Frequency range (MHz)	Exposure limits		
	E(V/m)	H(A/m)	mW/cm^2
0.003–0.1	614*	163	—
0.1–3	614*	16.3/f	—
3–30	1842/f*	16.3/f	—
100–300	61.4*	16.3/f	—
300–3000	61.4(f/300)$^{1/2}$	0.163(f/300)$^{1/2}$	f/300
3000–300,000	194	0.05	10

Data from Gandhi, O.P. (1988). Advances in dosimetry of radiofrequency radiation and their past and projected impact on the safety standards. Presented to the IEEE Instrumentation and Technology Conference, San Diego, Apr. 19–22, 1988.

f, Frequency in megahertz.

I (in milliamperes) should not exceed $I = f_{kHz}$. These limits ensure that local SARs do not exceed about 10 W/kg for adults.

2. For contact with electrical ground, the maximum RF current as measured with a contact current meter should not exceed $I = 0.5$ f_{kHz}mA for $3 < f < 100$ kHz, or $I = 50$ mA for $f > 100$ kHz.

These values should keep the RF currents below the perception threshold for grasping contact with metal objects. The RF current limits suggested by Gandhi (1988) are similar, although more complex, than the limit of 50 mA suggest by IRPA (1988).

In its latest draft revision, ANSI (1988) is proposing a number of changes:

1. Its frequency range to include 3 kHz to 300 GHz
2. Limits on induced body currents to prevent RF shocks and burns
3. Relaxation of limits on exposure to magnetic fields at low frequencies
4. Relaxation of exposure limits at high frequencies to be compatible at 300 GHz with existing infrared exposure limits
5. Relaxation of limits for partial-body exposure
6. Introduction of lower exposure limits for the general public

At its meeting in June 1988 the ANSI Committee decided to delay final decisions on the exposure limits until their subcommittee on risk assessment presented its report.

In his recent review, Sliney (1988) suggested that, although sometimes disputed, occupational limits for RF exposure in the United States are promulgated by the American Conference of Governmental and Industrial Hygienists (ACGIH, 1987).

Both the ANSI and ACGIH guides are voluntary standards. Since they are advisory, they are not legally enforceable. Legally enforceable standards exist at the state and local government levels.

The Environmental Protection Agency (Elder and Cahill, 1984) completed an excellent review that was to be used as a scientific rationale for developing general public exposure limits. Four alternative approaches for limiting exposure were proposed (EPA, 1986); three were regulatory and suggested limits of 0.04, 0.08, and 0.4 W/kg on whole-body SAR. The fourth proposal was nonregulatory and included information and technical assistance programs. To date no action has been taken on any of the proposals.

The National Council on Radiation Protection and Measurements devoted a chapter of its text (NCRP, 1986) to RF exposure criteria and rationales. This is an excellent text and is currently being used by the ANSI committee to revise its guide.

United Kingdom

In May 1986 the National Radiological Protection Board (NRPB, 1986) published its recommendations on protection of workers and the general public from possible hazards from exposure to electric and magnetic fields with frequencies below 300 GHz. Like the FRG (1986) proposal, the NRPB consultative document covers the electromagnetic spectrum down to static (0 Hz) fields. The exposure limits have differing durations as shown in Tables 2-9 to 2-11.

The NRPB (1986) limits are basically consistent with the WHO (1981, 1987; Suess, 1982; Suess and Benwell, 1987), IRPA (1984), and ANSI (1982) guidelines. Some differences in detail exist, particularly with regard to the translation of basic limits (such as 0.4 W/kg SAR) into electric and magnetic field strengths and power densities at various frequencies.

Soviet Union

The Soviet Union in 1958 was the first country to issue a standard limiting exposure to RF fields in the microwave region (300 MHz to 300 GHz). The occupational standard specified the power density and exposure duration in three maximum permissible limits: up to 10 μW/cm^2 for an 8-hour period, 100 μW/cm^2 for up to 2 hours, and 1000 μW/cm^2 for up to 20 minutes during the work day. This standard remained in force for 23 years until changed to the standard shown in Table

---

TABLE 2-9   Limits for Occupational Radiofrequency Exposure up to 2 Hours a Day

Frequency range (MHz)	Exposure limits		
	E(V/m)	H(A/m)	mW/cm^2
0.05–0.3	2000	5/f	—
0.3–10	$6 \times 10^2/f$	5/f	—
10–30	60	5/f	—
30–100	60	0.16	1
100–500	$6\,f^{1/2}$	$0.016\,f^{1/2}$	f/100
500–300,000	135	0.36	5

Data from National Radiological Protection Board (1986). Advice on the protection of workers and members of the general public from the possible hazards of electric and magnetic fields with frequencies below 300 GHz: a consultative document. Didcot, U.K., Harwell.

f, Frequency in megahertz.

TABLE 2-10   Limits for General Public Radiofrequency Exposure for 5 Hours a Day

Frequency range (MHz)	Exposure limits		
	E(V/m)	H(A/m)	mW/cm^2
0.05–0.365	800	2/f	—
0.365–0.475	800	5.5	—
0.475–0.580	$3.8 \times 10^2/f$	5.5	—
0.580–10	$3.8 \times 10^2/f$	3.2/f	—
10–30	38	3.2/f	—
30–300	38	0.1	0.4
300–1500	$2.2\ f^{1/2}$	$0.006\ f^{1/2}$	f/750
1500–300,000	85	0.23	2.0

Data from National Radiological Protection Board (1986). Advice on the protection of workers and members of the general public from the possible hazards of electric and magnetic fields with frequencies below 300 GHz: a consultative document. Didcot, U.K., Harwell.

f, Frequency in megahertz.

TABLE 2-11   Limits for Continuous Radiofrequency in Residential Areas

Frequency range (MHz)	Exposure limits		
	E(V/m)	H(A/m)	mW/cm^2
0.05–1	170	0.46/f	—
1–10	170/f	0.46/f	8/f^2
10–300	17	0.046	0.08
300–1500	$f^{1/2}$	$2.6 \times 10^{-3} f^{1/2}$	f/3750
1500–300,000	40	0.1	0.4

Data from National Radiological Protection Board (1986). Advice on the protection of workers and members of the general public from the possible hazards of electric and magnetic fields with frequencies below 300 GHz: a consultative document. Didcot, U.K., Harwell.

f, Frequency in megahertz.

2-12. Occupational exposure limits for the submicrowave region were introduced in 1976 and updated in 1984 (U.S.S.R., 1984a).

The occupational standard was based on laboratory studies and health surveys of workers. These studies suggested that adverse health effects could occur at exposures above 1 mW/cm^2 in the microwave region. One tenth of this threshold value was recommended as safe for exposure of healthy adults, but an extra safety factor of 10 was incorporated to

TABLE 2-12   Occupational Exposure Limits in the Soviet Union

Frequency range (MHz)	Electric field strength (V/m)	Magnetic field strength (A/m)	Power density (mW/cm^2)
0.06–3	50	5 (up to 1.5 MHz)	
3–30	20	—	
30–50	10	0.3	
50–300	5	0.15	
300–300,000	—	—	0.2/t*

Data from Savin, B.N., et al. (1983). *Gig. Tr. Prof. Zabol.* 3:1–4; and U.S.S.R. State Committee or Standards (GOST) (1984). Occupational safety standards system: electromagnetic fields of radiofrequencies; permissible levels on work-places and requirements for control. (In Russian.) GOST 12, 1,006–84. Moscow, Standards Publishers.

t, Exposure time in hours.

* Standard for stationary antennas. For rotating antennas the limit is 2/t mW/cm^2.

allow for individual variation in sensitivity as identified in the human studies. This resulted in a limit of 10 μW/cm^2 for continuous occupational exposure. Increases in exposure were allowed for shorter exposure times (0.1 mW/cm^2 for 2 hours and 1 mW/cm^2 for 20 minutes per day).

Changes in the occupational microwave standard explained by Savin et al. (1983) suggest that the 1976 microwave standard set too high an energy load for short-term, high-power density exposures (for example, 10 μW/cm^2 for 8 hours = 80 μWh/cm^2, but 1000 μW/cm^2 for 20 minutes = 333 μWh/cm^2). Studies on workers exposed for 15 to 20 years to levels of 0.01 to 0.1 mW/cm^2 were found to have no adverse effects. Analysis of data suggested a time-dependent threshold of effects of 1 mW/cm^2 for 2 hours per day, so a safety factor of 10 was incorporated to ensure that no cumulative effects could occur, setting the basic limit at 0.1 mW/cm^2 for 2 hours per day. The rest of the standard was then derived from this basic limit.

The rationale for the Soviet standards is described in greater detail in Minin (1975) and more recently by Davydov et al. (1984), Davydov (1985), and Czerski (1985).

The general public exposure standard (U.S.S.R., 1984b) (Table 2-13) is a result of relaxing the 1978 standard by raising the power density limit for continuous exposure from 0.005 to 0.01 mW/cm^2. Although the reason for this change has not been published, Savin et al. (1983) suggest that both the new general public and occupational limits were influenced by practical engineering and economic considerations. An English translation of the Soviet standard has been provided in *Microwave News* (New Soviet, 1985).

TABLE 2-13   General Public Exposure Limits in the Soviet Union

Frequency (MHz)	Electric field strength (V/m)	Magnetic field strength (A/m)	Power density (mW/cm^2)
0.03–0.3	25	—	—
0.3–3	15	—	—
3–30	10	—	—
30–300	3	—	—
300–30,000	—	—	0.01

Data from U.S.S.R. Ministry of Health Protection (1984). Temporary health standards and regulations on protection of the general population from the effects of electromagnetic fields generated by radio-transmitting equipment. (In Russian.) No. 2963–84. Moscow, The Ministry.

Other Standards

The Australian standard (Australia, 1985) is essentially the same as the IRPA (1988) guideline except that a 1 mW/cm^2 value was recommended over the microwave range (300 MHz to 300 GHz), as well as the human resonance region (30 to 300 MHz). Details of Western European (Sweden, Finland, Belgium, Norway, France) standards can be found in Mild (1987). The Finnish standard became effective on January 1, 1988, and is available in English translation from the Office of Standards Codes and Information, National Bureau of Standards, Gaithersburg, MD 20899.

Eastern European standards (Czechoslovakia and Poland) have been reviewed by the World Health Organization (WHO, 1981) and Czerski (1985). According to Czerski (1985), the Council of Mutual Economic Co-operation (COMECON) is developing a single set of guidelines on exposure limits that will be adopted by the Eastern European countries belonging to COMECON. He suggests that the COMECON guide will recommend exposure limits similar to those published by the International Non-Ionizing Radiation Committee of IRPA (IRPA, 1988).

REFERENCES

ACGIH (1987). American Conference of Government Industrial Hygienists. Threshold limit values and biological exposure indices for 1987–1988. Cincinnatti, ACGIH.

ANSI (1982). American National Standards Institute. American national standard C95.1, safety levels with respect to human exposure to radio-frequency electromagnetic fields, 300 kHz to 100 GHz. New York, Institute of Electrical and Electronic Engineers, Inc.

ANSI (1988). American National Standards Institute. American national standard safety levels with respect to human exposure to radiofrequency electromagnetic fields, 3kHz to 300GHz. Draft No. 3, 1988 Revision, June 1988. New York, Institute of Electrical and Electronic Engineers, Inc.

AUSTRALIA (1985). Maximum exposure levels—radiofrequency radiation 300kHz-300GHz, Australian Standard 2772–1985. North Sydney, New South Wales, Standards Association of Australia.

BERNHARDT, J.H. (1979). The direct influence of electromagnetic fields on nerve and muscle cells in man within the frequency range of 1Hz and 30MHz. *Radiat. Environ. Biophys. 16*:309–329.

BERNHARDT, J.H. (1985). Evaluation of human exposure to low frequency fields. *In*: AGARD Lecture Series No. 138. The impact of proposed radio-frequency radiation standards on military operations. Nevilly Sur Seine, France, NATO Advisory Group for Aerospace Research and Development (AGARD), pp 8–1 to 8–18.

CZERSKI, P. (1985). Radiofrequency radiation exposure limits in Eastern Europe. *J. Microwave Power 20*:233–239.

DAVYDOV, B.I., TIKHONTCHUK, V.S., AND ANTIPOV, V.V. (1984). Biological effects: standardization and protection against electromagnetic radiation. (In Russian.) Moscow, Meditsina.

DAVYDOV, B.I. (1985). Electromagnetic radiofrequency (microwave) radiation: guidelines, criteria for setting standards and "threshold" dose levels. (In Russian.) *Kosm. Biol. Aviakosm. Med. 19*:8–21.

ELDER, J.A., AND CAHILL, D.F. (eds.) (1984). Biological effects of radiofrequency radiation. U.S. EPA Pub. No. EPA-600/8–83–026f. Research Triangle, N.C., Environmental Protection Agency.

EPA (1986). Environmental Protection Agency. Federal radiation protection guidance: proposed alternatives for controlling public exposure to radiofrequency radiation; notice of proposed recommendations. Federal Register Part II, Vol. 51, No. 146, July 30, 1986, pp. 27318–27339.

FRG (1984). Federal Republic of Germany, Deutsches Institut fur Normen (DIN). Hazards for electromagnetic fields: protection of persons in the frequency range from 10kHz to 300GHz. DIN 578.848, Teil 2, Berlin, DIN (German Standards Institute).

FRG (1986). Federal Republic of Germany. Hazards by electromagnetic fields: protection of persons in the frequency range from 0Hz to 3000 GHz. DIN VDE 0848, Teil 2. Berlin, DIN (German Standards Institute).

GANDHI, O.P. (1985). The ANSI RF safety guideline: its rationale and some of its problems. *In*: Dutta, S.K., and Millis, R.M. (eds.). Biological effects of electropollution. Philadelphia, Information Ventures, pp. 9–19.

GANDHI, O.P. (1988). Advances in dosimetry of radiofrequency radiation and their past and projected impact on the safety standards. Presented to the IEEE Instrumentation and Technology Conference, San Diego, Apr. 19–22, 1988.

GANDHI, O.P., CHATTERJEE, I., WU, D., AND GU, Y.G. (1985). Likelihood of high rates of energy deposition in the human legs at the ANSI recommended 3–30MHz RF safety levels. *Proc. IEEE 73*:1145–47.

GANDHI, O.P., CHEN, J.T., AND RIAZI, A. (1986). Currents induced in a human being for plane-wave exposure conditions 0–50MHz and for RF sealers. *IEEE Trans. Biomed. Eng. 33*:757–767.

GUY, A.W., AND CHOU, C.K. (1985). Very low frequency hazard study. Final report prepared for the USAF School of Aerospace Medicine, Brooks Air Force Base, Tex. Contract No. F33615–83–C–0625.

HEALTH AND WELFARE CANADA (1979). Recommended safety procedures for installation and use of radiofrequency and microwave devices in the frequency range 10MHz–300GHz. Safety Code 6, Environmental Health Directorate, Ottawa, Health and Welfare Canada, Pub. No. 79-EHD-30.

IRPA (1984). International Radiational Protection Association. International Non-Ionizing Radiation Committee. Interim guidelines on limits of exposure to radiofrequency electromagnetic fields in the frequency range from 100MHz to 300GHz. *Health Phys. 46*:975–984.

IRPA (1988). International Radiational Protection Association. Guidelines on limits of exposure to radiofrequency electromagnetic fields in the frequency range from 100MHz to 300GHz. *Health Phys. 54*:115–123.

MILD, K.H. (1987). Western European population and occupational RF protection guides. *In*: Lin, J. (ed.). Proceedings of URSI/BEMS/IRPA Congress, Tel Aviv.

MININ, B.A. (1975). Microwaves and human safety. (English translation.) JRPS Report No. 65506–1 and 65506–2, Arlington, Va. National Technical Information Service (NTIS).

NBOSH (1987). National Board of Occupational Safety and Health. High frequency electromagnetic fields. Stockholm, NBOSH.

NCRP (1986). National Council on Radiation Protection and Measurement. Biological effects and exposure criteria for radiofrequency electromagnetic fields. NCRP Report No. 86, Bethesda, Md., NCRP, p. 381.

NRPB (1989). National Radiological Protection Board. Advice on the protection of workers and members of the general public from the possible hazards of electric and magnetic fields with frequencies below 300 GHz: a consultative document. Didcot, Oxfordshire, U.K., Harwell.

New Soviet population standard: 10 μW/cm^2 at MW frequencies (1985). *Microwave News* V(5):1–5 (June issue).

POLK, C., AND POSTOW, E. (1986). CRC Handbook of biological effects of electromagnetic fields. Boca Raton, Fla., CRC Press, Inc.

REPACHOLI, M.H. (1978). Proposed exposure limits for microwave and radiofrequency radiations in Canada. *J. Microwave Power 13*:199–121.

REPACHOLI, M.H. (1987). Radiofrequency electromagnetic fields exposure standards. *IEEE Eng. Med. Biol.* Magazine 6, March, p. 18–21.

REPACHOLI, M.H. (1988). Introduction to non-ionizing electromagnetic fields. *In*: Repacholi, M.H. (ed.). Non-ionizing radiations: physical characteristics, biological effects and health hazard assessment. Yallambie, Victoria, Aust., International Radiation Protection Association, International Non-Ionizing Radiation Committee, pp. 1–15.

SAVIN, B.N., ET AL. (1983). New trends in the standardization of microwave electromagnetic radiation. *Gig. Tr. Prof. Zabol. 3*:1–4.

SLINEY, D.H. (1988). Current RF safety standards. *In*: Repacholi, M.H. (ed.). Non-ionizing radiations: physical characteristics, biological effects and health hazard assessment. Yallambie, Victoria, Aust., International Radiation Protection Association, International Non-Ionizing Radiation Committee, pp. 219–231.

STUCHLY, M.A. (1987). Proposed revision of the Canadian recommendations on radiofrequency-exposure protection. *Health Phys. 53*:649–665.

STUCHLY, M.A., KRASZEWSKI, A., AND STUCHLY, S.S. (1985). Exposure of human models in the near and far field—a comparison. *IEEE Trans. Biomed. Eng. 32*:609–616.

STUCHLY, M.A., SPIEGEL, R.J., STUCHLY, S.S., AND KRASZEWSKI, A. (1986). Exposure of man in the near-field of a resonant dipole: comparison between theory and measurements. *IEEE Trans. Microwave Theory Tech. 34*:26–31.

STUCHLY, S.S., STUCHLY, M.A., KRASZEWSKI, A., AND HARTSGROVE, G. (1986). Energy deposition in a model of man: frequency effects. *IEEE Trans. Biomed. Eng. 33*:702–711.

SUESS, M.J. (ED.) (1982). Non-ionizing radiation protection. WHO Regional Publication, European Series No. 10. Copenhagen, World Health Organization.

SUESS, M.J., AND BENWELL, D.A. (eds.) (1987). Non-ionizing radiation protection, 2nd ed. Copenhagen, World Health Organization Regional Office for Europe.

U.S.S.R. State Committee on Standards (GOST) (1984a). Occupational safety standards system: electromagnetic fields of radio frequencies; permissible levels on work-places and requirements for control. (In Russian.) GOST 12, 1,006–84. Moscow, Standards Publishers.

U.S.S.R. Ministry of Health Protection (1984b). Temporary health standards and regulations on protection of the general population from the effects of electromagnetic fields generated by radio-transmitting equipment. (In Russian.) No. 2963–84. Moscow, The Ministry.

WHO (1981). World Health Organization. Environmental health criteria 16. Radiofrequency and microwaves. Geneva, WHO.

WHO (1984). World Health Organization. Extremely low frequency (ELF) fields. Environmental Health Criteria No. 35. Geneva, WHO.

WHO (1987). World Health Organization. Magnetic fields. Environmental Health Criteria 69. Geneva, WHO.

3

ANSI Radiofrequency Safety Guide: Its Rationale, Some Problems, and Suggested Improvements

OM P. GANDHI

The American National Standards Institute (ANSI) guide (1982) for safe levels of human exposure to radiofrequency (RF) electromagnetic fields, 300 kHz to 100 GHz, is given in Table 3-1. This radiofrequency protection guide (RFPG) is plotted in Figure 3-1. In the absence of verified reports of injury to or adverse effects on the health of humans who have been exposed to RF electromagnetic (EM) fields, the RFPG was based on the most sensitive measure of biological effects: the behavioral effects on laboratory animals. Because of lack of replicable data on chronic exposure, the assumption was made that reversible disruption during an acute exposure would mean irreversible injury during the chronic exposure. Since the thresholds of reversible behavioral disruption had been found for whole-body-averaged rates of EM energy absorption (specific absorption rates, or SARs) on the order of 4 to 8 W/kg (Justesen, 1979) despite the considerable difference in carrier frequency (600 to 2450 MHz), species (rodents versus primates), and mode of irradiation (cavity, waveguide, and plane wave), the RFPG was prescribed to ensure that the whole-body-average SAR would not exceed 0.4 W/kg for any of the human sizes and age groups. Dosimetric information on EM energy absorption in human beings (Gandhi, 1975, 1979; Durney, 1978, 1980) was used to obtain the power density as a function of frequency so that under the worst-case circumstances (E vector parallel to the length of the body; grounded and ungrounded conditions) the whole-body-averaged SAR would be less than 0.4 W/kg. Recognizing the highly nonuniform nature of SAR distribution, including some regions where there may be fairly high local SARs, the RFPG further prescribes that the local SAR in any 1 g of tissue must not exceed 8 W/kg.

Recent studies have pointed to several problems with this RFPG. These are itemized in the following and discussed at length in this chapter.

1. The high electric fields sanctioned in the RFPG for MF to HF* frequencies may result in significant RF currents flowing through the human body, producing high current densities and SARs for the wet

---

* See Table 1-1 for the definition of frequency bands given by the Institute of Electrical and Electronics Engineers.

TABLE 3-1   Radiofrequency Protection Guide

Frequency range (MHz)	Electric field (V/m)	Magnetic field (A/m)	Power density (mW/cm^2)
0.3–3	632	1.6	100
3–30	1897/f	4.74/f	900/f^2
30–300	63.2	0.16	1.0
300–1500	3.65 f$^{0.5}$	0.009 f$^{0.5}$	f/300
1500–100,000	141	0.35	5.0

Data from American National Standards Institute. (1982). American National Standard C95.1, Safety levels with electromagnetic fields (300kHz-100GHz). New York, Institute of Electrical and Electronic Engineers, Inc. © 1982 IEEE.

f, Frequency in megahertz.

tissues in smaller cross-sectional areas of the body such as the leg and the ankle region (Gandhi, et al., 1985, 1986). Based on measurements with standing human subjects for vertically polarized plane-wave fields, ankle-section SARs as high as 182 to 243 W/kg (current densities of 33 to 41 mA/cm^2) are projected for 1.75 m tall individuals for the RFPG for the frequency band 3 to 40 MHz. The SAR values are considerably larger than the 8 W/kg for any 1 g of tissue assumed in the RFPG.

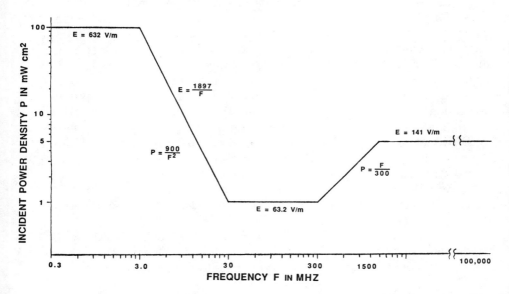

Figure 3-1   ANSI C95.1—1982 safety guide for human exposure to radiofrequency electromagnetic fields.

2. Commonly encountered ungrounded objects such as a car, van, or bus develop open circuit voltages of several hundred volts when exposed to an ANSI-recommended electric field of 632 V/m for the frequency band 0.3 to 3 MHz. When a person touches such a vehicle, large currents may flow through the body that are considerably in excess of those that would cause perception, pain, and even burns in some cases (Gandhi and Chatterjee, 1982; Chatterjee et al., 1986). For example, the current flowing through the hand of a person holding the door handle of an ungrounded automotive van is estimated to be 880 mA, resulting in a local SAR in the wrist of about 1045 W/kg.

3. The depth of penetration of millimeter waves (≥ 30 GHz) in the human skin is less than 1 mm. Since most of the RF absorption at these frequencies is in the region of cutaneous thermal receptors, 0.1 to 1 mm, the sensations of absorbed millimeter-wave energy are likely to be similar to those for far-infrared. For the latter the threshold of perception is near 0.67 mW/cm^2. Millimeter-wave power densities on the order of 8.7 mW/cm^2 are likely to cause sensations of "very warm to hot" with a latency of 1.0 ± 0.6 seconds (Gandhi and Riazi, 1986). If this is validated by psychophysical experiments, the RFPG of 5 mW/cm^2 for this region may be too close to the threshold for sensations of "very warm to hot."

CURRENTS INDUCED IN A STANDING HUMAN BEING FOR VERTICALLY POLARIZED PLANE-WAVE EXPOSURE CONDITIONS

We have previously shown (Gandhi et al., 1985a) that the current I_h flowing through the feet of a standing, grounded human being is given by

$$\frac{I_h}{E} = 0.108 \, h_m^2 \, f_{MHz} \, \frac{mA}{V/m} \tag{1}$$

where E is the plane-wave incident electric field (assumed vertical) in volts per meter, h_m is the height of the individual in meters, and f_{MHz} is the frequency in megahertz. Interestingly, the current in Eq. 1 can be considered as though all the fields falling on an area $1.936 \, h_m^2$ or approximately 5.93 m^2 for a human of height 1.75 m were effectively passed through the human body. Similar results have also been reported by a number of authors, most notably by Hill and Walsh (1985, to 10 MHz), Tell et al. (in press, to 1.47 MHz), Guy and Chou (1982, 0.146 MHz), and Gronhaug and Busmundrud (1982, to 27 MHz). We have found Eq. 1 to be valid to a frequency of 40 MHz for a 1.75 m tall person. Because of the f^2 dependence, currents as high as 13 mA/(V/m) have been measured at 40 MHz for adult humans (Gandhi et al., 1986). This implies a current I_h in excess of 800 mA for the ANSI-recommended E field of 63.2 V/m at this frequency. Anatomical data (Morton et al., 1941) have been used to estimate the effective areas for the flow of currents for the various cross sections of the leg (Gandhi et al., 1985a). The effective area A_e is estimated by the equation

$$A_e = \frac{A_c\sigma_c + A_\ell\sigma_\ell + A_m\sigma_m}{\sigma_c} \quad (2)$$

where A_c, A_ℓ, and A_m are the physical areas of the high-water-content and low-water-content tissues and of the region containing red marrow, having conductivities of σ_c, σ_ℓ, and σ_m, respectively. Since most of the ankle cross section consists of low-conductivity bone or tendon, an effective area of 9.5 cm^2 is calculated for this cross section for an adult human even though the physical cross section is on the order of 40 cm^2 (Gandhi et al., 1985a, 1986). The SARs have been calculated from the equation

$$J^2/\sigma_c\rho = (I_h/2)^2/A_e^2\sigma_c\rho \quad (3)$$

where ρ is the mass density of the tissue, taken to be 10^3 kg/m^3. The current taken for each of the legs is $I_h/2$. For the E fields recommended in the RFPG (Table 3-1), the ankle-section SARs are calculated by using the current I_h from Eq. 1, and the values of the conductivities for high-water-content tissues from Johnson and Guy (1972). The SARs thus calculated are shown in Figure 3-2. A fairly large ankle-section SAR of 243 W/kg is projected for a standing adult of height 1.75 m at a frequency

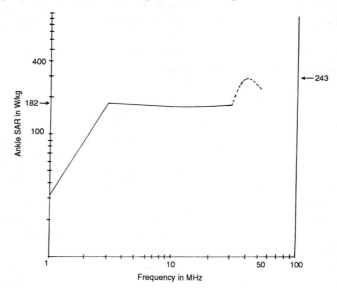

Figure 3-2 Ankle specific absorption rate for an adult man (height 1.75 m) for electromagnetic fields recommended in ANSI–1982 radiofrequency safety guide.

of 40 MHz. This value is of course considerably higher than the ANSI guide of 8 W/kg for any 1 g of tissue.

We have also quantified the currents that would flow through the feet when rubber- or leather-soled shoes are used (Gandhi et al., 1985a,b 1986). We find that the currents for subjects wearing leather-soled shoes and rubber-soled shoes are, respectively, about 90% to 95% and 60% to 80% (the larger values have been measured for higher frequencies) of those for bare feet. The SARs in Figure 3-2 must therefore be multiplied by the square of the appropriate current reduction factors.

SCALING TO OTHER HEIGHTS: 5- AND 10-YEAR-OLD CHILDREN

From Eq. 1, it can be seen that the induced current is proportional to h^2 and is consequently smaller for shorter individuals. Since the cross-sectional dimensions of the body are to a first order of approximation also proportional to (weight)$^{2/3}$ or h^2, the current density J and hence the ankle-section SAR ($= J^2/\sigma_c\rho$) may not be very different at a specific frequency from one height to another. The frequency corresponding to maximum ankle-section current or SAR would, however, increase as $1/h$, to approximately 50.7 MHz for a 10-year-old child ($h = 1.38$ m) and 62.5 MHz for a 5-year-old child ($h = 1.12$ m), in contrast to 40 MHz for an adult. Since the current increases as f, the maximum SARs projected at the new peak SAR frequencies would be considerably higher. Linearly interpolating between the values given at 40.68 and 100 MHz (Johnson and Guy, 1972), we have taken larger conductivities σ_c of the wet tissues at the higher frequencies and have used the values 0.73 and 0.77 S/m at 50.7 and 62.5 MHz, respectively. The highest ankle-section SARs projected for 10- and 5-year-old children for 1 mW/cm^2 incident plane waves ($E = 63.2$ V/m) are estimated to be 371 and 534 W/kg, respectively. Rates of surface temperature elevation have been measured for the ankle section of a healthy human subject for a variety of RF currents and SARs in the frequency band 1 to 50 MHz (Chen and Gandhi, 1988). The observed highest rates of temperature increase in degrees Celsius per minute are given by the best-fit relationship: 0.0045 × SAR in watts per kilogram for the ankle section. Since SARs as high as 182 to 534 W/kg are projected for the ankle section, substantial rates of surface temperature elevation are anticipated.

CONTACT HAZARDS IN THE VLF TO HF FREQUENCY BAND

The problem of RF shock and burns for human contact with commonly encountered metallic bodies has been discussed in the literature (Rogers, 1981; Gandhi and Chatterjee, 1982; Guy and Chou, 1982). Ungrounded objects, such as a car, van, bus, fence, or metallic roof, develop open-circuit voltages on the order of several hundred volts when exposed to the ANSI-recommended electric fields of 632 V/m for the frequency band 0.3 to 3 MHz. Chatterjee et al. (1986) did a study in which the body impedance and threshold currents needed to produce sensations of perception and pain were measured for 367 human subjects (197 male and 170 female) for the frequency range 10 kHz to 3 MHz. The study included various types of contact such as finger contact and grasping a rod electrode to simulate the holding of the door handle of a vehicle. Based on the principles given in an earlier paper (Gandhi and Chatterjee, 1982), we have used the new data to estimate the incident electric fields that will cause perception when a person holds the door handle of various vehicles such as a compact car, van, and school bus. These values are shown in Figure 3-3 for an adult man and scaled therefrom for a 10-year-old child. The sensation is one of tingling or pricking for frequencies less than about 100 kHz and of warming for higher frequencies. Currents of about 250 mA are needed to cause perception for a grasping contact. Although currents needed for threshold of pain could not be obtained from the RF generators available to us, we estimate them to be about 20% higher, based on our experience with finger contact measurements. The threshold

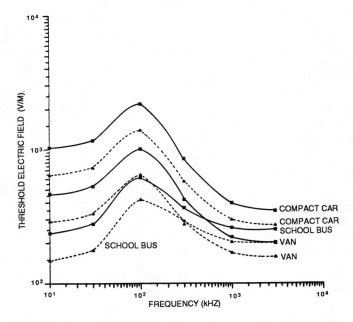

Figure 3-3 Average threshold E field for perception for grounded adult men (*solid curves*) and 10-year-old children (*dashed curves*) in grasping contact with various metallic objects.

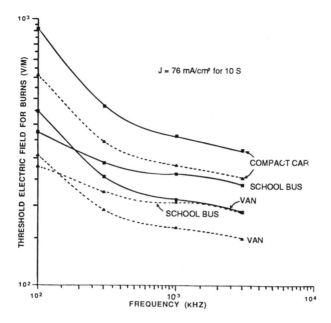

Figure 3-4 Threshold E field for producing burns in adult men (*solid curves*) and 10-year-old children (*dashed curves*) in finger contact with various vehicles (contact area 144 mm^2).

electric fields given in Figure 3-3 may therefore be multiplied by a factor of 1.2 to obtain an estimate of incident E fields that will cause pain when the handle is held. In the literature a current density of 76 mA/cm^2 for 10 seconds is reported to be the threshold for producing RF burns (Dobbie, 1969; Becker et al., 1973). We have used our data to estimate the incident E fields that will cause a current density of 76 mA/cm^2 to flow through the finger upon touching a vehicle (Gandhi et al., 1985b). These fields are shown in Figure 3-4 for adult men and 10-year-old children. From Figures 3-3 and 3-4 it may be seen that the ANSI-recommended E-field level of 632 V/m is considerably higher than the fields that will cause RF perception, pain, and burns in many situations.

COUPLING OF THE HUMAN BODY TO RADIOFREQUENCY MAGNETIC FIELDS

As pointed out earlier, the vertically polarized RF electric field associated with plane waves is capable of inducing fairly significant RF currents in the human body, particularly for conditions of contact with the ground.

Since these conditions result in fairly high SARs in the ankle region, this observation may lead to a future restriction of the RF electric fields in the safety standards for the HF region of frequencies. For example, maximum electric field magnitudes as low as 27.5 V/m have been proposed for the public exposure limit to the frequency band 10 to 400 MHz (IRPA, 1988). In the past, the safety standards generally allowed a magnetic field that was ⅟377 of the electric field, in MKS units. It is therefore of interest to examine the coupling of the RF magnetic field with the human body to see whether a commensurate restriction of the magnetic field component is warranted. Toward this objective we have used the three-dimensional impedance method to calculate the induced currents and the corresponding SARs in the human body where the magnetic field is polarized from front to back (Orcutt and Gandhi, 1988). This orientation was selected because of its strongest coupling to the human body.

We used the inhomogeneous, anatomically based model of the human body described by Sullivan et al. (1988). This model specifies the conductivity and dielectric constant for each of about 144,000, 1.31 cm³ cells in a 59 × 31 × 175 cm prism. About 64,000 of these cells are entirely in air. Figure 3-5 shows the calculated layer-averaged SARs for the model of the human body exposed to a magnetic field of 1 A/m at 30 MHz,

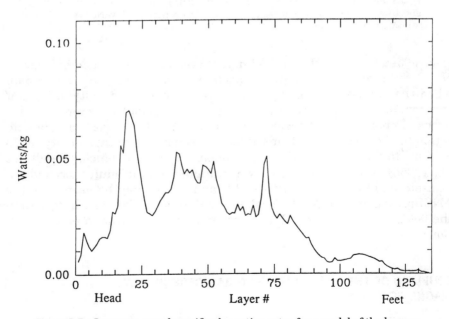

Figure 3-5 Layer-averaged specific absorption rates for a model of the human body, when body is exposed to linearly polarized radiofrequency magnetic field of 1 A/m at 30 MHz, polarized from front to back. Each layer is 1.31 cm thick.

polarized from the front to back of the model. The whole-body-averaged
SAR is 0.03 W/kg. The peak SAR for this case, 0.64 W/kg, occurred in
the cross section through the perineum.

ABSORPTION OF MILLIMETER WAVES BY HUMANS AND BIOLOGICAL IMPLICATIONS

Because of the high loss tangent of water (even deionized water) in the
millimeter-wave band (30 to 300 GHz), which is associated with Debye
relaxation of the water molecule, the millimeter-wave penetration into
the human body is less than 1 to 2 mm, or predominantly in the skin
(Schwan and Piersol, 1954). The data are fairly sparse for the complex
permittivity of the skin, as well as for the other biological tissues in
the millimeter-wave region of the EM spectrum. At 23 GHz, measurements have been made with rabbit skin in vitro (England, 1950), which
has led to a formulation (Cook, 1951) of the complex dielectric constant
of the skin given by the Debye equation

$$\epsilon^*(\omega) = \epsilon_\infty + \frac{\epsilon_s - \epsilon_\infty}{1 + j\omega\tau} + \frac{\sigma}{j\omega\epsilon_0} \tag{3}$$

where $\epsilon_\infty = 4.0$, $\epsilon_s = 42.0$, $\tau = 6.9 \times 10^{-12}$s, $\epsilon_0 = 8.85 \times 10^{-12}$ F/m, and
$\sigma = 1.4$ S/m. We have used Eq. 3 to calculate the power-reflection coefficient
$|\rho|^2$ and the depth δ of penetration (corresponding to the power density
of $1/e^2$ or 13.5% of that at the surface) assuming normally incident plane
waves (Gandhi and Riazi, 1986). The calculated values of power reflection
and absorption coefficients, the depths δ, and the SARs at the surface,
expressed as SAR(0), are given in Table 3-2. Note that the SAR(0) in-

TABLE 3-2   Reflection and Absorption Coefficients, Depths of Penetration, and Surface Specific Absorption Rates for the Human Skin*

Frequency (GHz)	Reflection coefficient ($|\rho|^2$)	Power absorption coefficient ($1 - |\rho|^2$)	Skin depth δ (mm)	P_{inc}[†] 5 mW/cm^2 (SAR[0] W/kg)
30	0.488	0.512	0.782	65.5
60	0.411	0.589	0.426	138.3
100	0.333	0.667	0.318	209.7
150	0.266	0.734	0.271	270.8
200	0.223	0.777	0.249	312.0
250	0.195	0.805	0.238	338.2
300	0.175	0.825	0.231	357.1

* A planar model is assumed for these calculations.
† P_{inc}, Incident power density.

creases rapidly with frequency because of the decreasing δ and the increasing power-coupling coefficient $1 - |\rho|^2$. SARs that are considerably in excess of the ANSI guidelines of 8 W/kg for the peak value are therefore calculated for the millimeter-wave band.

THERMAL SENSATIONS OF MILLIMETER-WAVE IRRADIATION

Owing to the highly superficial nature of its absorption ($\delta \sim 0.23$ to 0.78 mm) and because temperature-sensing nerve endings are distributed in the skin at depths from 0.1 to 1 mm, perception of millimeter-wave absorption is likely to be similar to that of far-infrared (far-IR; $\lambda > 3\ \mu$) irradiation. For the latter the threshold of perception for whole-body irradiation is near 0.67 mW/cm^2 (Hardy and Oppel, 1937).

Experiments have been performed by Lele et al. (1954) to determine the threshold power densities of far-IR irradiation for various sensations (faint warm, warm, and very warm or hot) as a function of the area exposed on the dorsum of the right hand. A sensation of "very warm or hot" was experienced at an average power density of 21.7 ± 4.0 mW/cm^2 for an exposure area of 40.6 cm^2, and a similar sensation occurred for a lower exposure area of 9.6 cm^2 for a larger power density of 55.9 ± 4.9 mW/cm^2. The ratio $21.7/55.9 \simeq 0.4$ in the power densities is similar to that for thresholds of perception for similar surface areas in the earlier article by Hardy and Oppel (1937). Reaction time for the sensation of "very warm or hot" was typically on the order of 1.0 ± 0.6 second. Since there is a reduction by a factor of 2.5 in the threshold of perception for irradiation of the whole body versus that of an area 40.6 cm^2 (Hardy and Oppel, 1937), it is possible that the sensation of "very warm to hot" for larger areas such as the whole body exposed to millimeter-wave irradiation may occur at 21.7/2.5 or 8.7 mW/cm^2. Because of the proximity of this value to the ANSI-recommended safety level of 5 mW/cm^2, there is a need for psychophysical experiments to establish thresholds of perception of millimeter waves with and without clothing. We have previously shown (Gandhi and Riazi, 1986) that, unlike IR energy, millimeter waves may couple through the clothing with the coupling efficiency greater than 90% for clothing of proper thicknesses acting as an impedance-matching transformer.

SUGGESTED RADIOFREQUENCY PROTECTION GUIDE FOR OCCUPATIONAL EXPOSURES

To overcome the problems described above, IRPA and Dr. Maria Stuchly of Health and Welfare, Canada (IRPA, 1988; Stuchly, 1987) have recently proposed new limits for the RFPG. Using the aforementioned data, I

TABLE 3-3   Proposed Radiofrequency Protection Guide for Occupational Exposures

Frequency range (MHz)	Electric field (V/m)	Magnetic field (A/m)	Plane-wave equivalent power density (mW/cm²)
0.003–0.1	614*	163	—
0.1–3.0	614*	16.3/f	—
3–30	1842/f*	16.3/f	—
30–100	61.4*	16.3/f	—
100–300	61.4	0.163	1.0
300–3000	61.4 × (f/300)^{1/2}	0.163 × (f/300)^{1/2}	f/300
3000–300,000	194	0.5	10.0

f, Frequency in megahertz.

* Personnel access areas should be restricted to limit-induced RF body currents and potential for RF shock and burns, as defined in the text.

propose the following modifications of the RFPGs to limit the RF currents that can be induced in the human body (Table 3-3 and Figure 3-6).

Since higher E fields proposed in Table 3-3 for the band 0.003 to 100 MHz, if vertical, would result in high RF-induced body currents

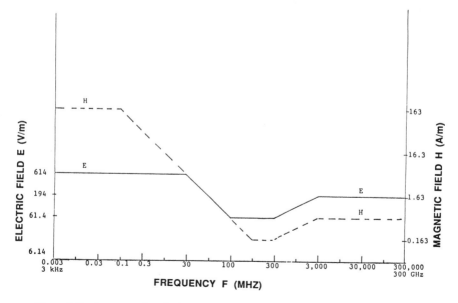

Figure 3-6   A proposed radiofrequency protection guide for occupational exposures.

and a potential for shock and burns from contact with ungrounded metallic bodies, personnel access areas should be limited in the following manner:

1. For freestanding individuals (no contact with metallic bodies) RF current induced in the human body should be less than or equal to 100 mA as measured through both feet or 50 mA through each foot. For a frequency of less than 100 kHz, the allowable induced current should be reduced as follows:

$$I = 1 f_{kHz} \quad mA \tag{4}$$

The above limitations on RF-induced currents are suggested to ensure that the ankle-section SARs for frequencies higher than 0.1 MHz will be no more than 5.8 to 10.7 W/kg for adults of heights 1.75 to 1.5 m. For frequencies lower than 100 kHz the current densities in the ankle section will be slightly lower than those needed for stimulating thresholds for the nerve-muscle system (Bernhardt, 1985; Gandhi et al., 1985a,b; Guy and Chou, 1985; Chatterjee et al., 1986).

For vertically polarized electric fields, the above limitation on current would imply (Gandhi et al., 1986) that the permissible E field is less than (300/f) V/m for frequencies greater than 0.1 MHz.

2. For conditions of contact with metallic bodies, maximum RF current through an impedance equivalent to that of the human body for conditions of grasping contact (Chatterjee et al., 1986), as measured with a contact current meter, should not exceed the following values:

$$I = 0.5 \ f_{kHz} \quad mA \quad \text{for } 3 \le f \le 100 \text{ kHz} \tag{5}$$

$$I = 50 \text{ mA} \qquad \text{for } f > 0.1 \text{ MHz} \tag{6}$$

The current limits given by Eqs. 5 and 6 would help ensure that the current experienced by a human in contact with these metallic bodies is less than that needed for perception or pain at each of the frequencies.

Steps such as grounding and use of safety equipment that result in reduced currents would obviously allow existence of higher fields without exceeding the above limits for conditions of contact with metallic bodies.

Significantly higher RF magnetic fields are recommended in the proposed RFPG of Table 3-3. For the frequency band 0.1 to 100 MHz, the RF magnetic field guideline is

$$H = \frac{16.3}{f} \text{ A/m} \tag{7}$$

For magnetic fields given by Eq. 7, the peak and whole-body-averaged SARs have been estimated through the use of data in the section "Coupling

TABLE 3-4   **Whole-Body-Averaged and Peak Specific Absorption Rates for an Anatomically Realistic Model of an Adult Human for Radiofrequency Magnetic Fields Given by Eq. 7***

Frequency (MHz)	Magnetic field† (A/m)	Whole-body-averaged SAR (W/kg)	Peak current density (mA/cm²)	Peak SAR (W/kg)
0.1	163	0.014	1.17	0.31
0.3	54.3	0.013	1.17	0.29
1.0	16.3	0.012	1.17	0.27
3.0	5.43	0.011	1.17	0.24
10.0	1.63	0.010	1.17	0.22
30.0	0.54	0.009	1.17	0.20
100.0	0.16	0.006	1.17	0.13

* A magnetic field orientation from front to back of the body is assumed to obtain highest possible SARs.

† A magnetic field of 163 A/m corresponds to a magnetic flux of 2.05 G in the gaussian system of units.

to Radiofrequency Magnetic Fields" and Figure 3-5. These are given in Table 3-4 along with the peak internal current densities. A magnetic field orientation from front to back of the body is assumed for these calculations. This orientation was selected because of its strongest coupling to the human body.

For frequencies less than 0.1 MHz, an RF magnetic field of 163 A/m implies a peak current density $\leq 0.0117\, f_{kHz}$ mA/cm², which is considerably lower than the threshold of perception of currents at these frequencies (Bernhardt, 1985; Gandhi et al., 1985a,b; Guy and Chou, 1985; Chatterjee et al., 1986).

SUGGESTED RADIOFREQUENCY PROTECTION GUIDE FOR THE GENERAL PUBLIC

The proposed RFPG for the general public is given in Table 3-5. This RFPG is plotted in Figure 3-7. The explanations for entries a to d in Table 3-5 follow:

a. The electric field E suggested for these frequency bands is lower than the threshold of perception of commonly encountered metallic bodies such as a car or van. It is, however, close to the threshold of perception for finger contact of a school bus by a child (Chatterjee et al., 1986).

TABLE 3-5   Proposed Radiofrequency Protection Guide for the General Population

Frequency range (MHz)	Electric field (V/m)	Magnetic field (A/m)	Plane-wave equivalent power density (mW/cm²)
0.003–0.1	(a) 61.4*†	163	—
0.1–1.0	(a) 61.4*†	16.3/f	—
1.0–3.9	(b) 61.4*‡	16.3/f	—
3.9–100	(c) 240/f*‡	16.3/f	—
30–100	8‡	16.3/f	—
100–5900	0.8 $f^{1/2}$‡	0.163	—
5900–300,000	61.4	0.163	(d) 1*

f, Frequency in megahertz.
* Explanation for (a) to (d) is given in the text.
† Spatially averaged over a volume corresponding to that of an automobile.
‡ Spatially averaged over a volume corresponding to that of a human.

b. For the E field suggested here, the current induced in a freestanding (no contact with metallic bodies) human is less than or equal to 100 mA (one leg current = 50 mA), which is consistent with the access area limitation for occupational exposures.

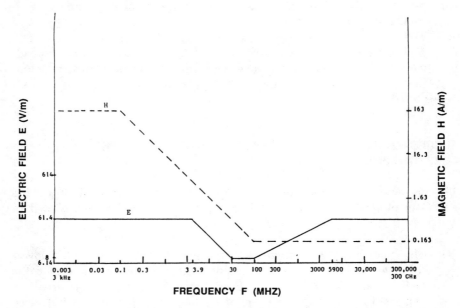

Figure 3-7   A proposed radiofrequency protection guide for general population.

TABLE 3-6   Induced Currents and Ankle-Section Specific Absorption Rates for
an Average Incident E Field of 8 V/m

	Height (m)	Frequency (MHz)	Induced current (mA)	Ankle SAR* (W/kg)
Average adult	1.75	40.0	101.6	3.8
Adult	1.5	46.7	87.2	5.0
10-Year-old child	1.38	50.7	80.1	8.7
5-Year-old child	1.12	62.5	65.0	7.8

* Assuming a conductivity of 0.693 S/m for the high-water-content tissues at 40 and
46.7 MHz (Johnson and Guy, 1972). Somewhat larger conductivities of 0.73 and 0.77
S/m are taken at 50.7 and 62.5 MHz, respectively. The corresponding dielectric constants
taken are 97.3 for 40 and 46.7 MHz and 92.9 and 87.4 for 50.7 and 62.5 MHz, respectively.

c. An average incident electric field of 8 V/m implies the numbers given in Table 3-6 for maximum induced currents and ankle-section SARs.

d. We have previously projected that whole-body-exposure millimeter-wave power densities on the order of 8.7 mW/cm^2 are likely to cause sensations of very warm to hot (Gandhi and Riazi, 1986). At higher frequencies a power density of 1 mW/cm^2 is suggested to prevent threshold of perception of warmth. Also, the suggested power density of 1 mW/cm^2 is consistent with the guideline for the general population recently proposed by the National Council on Radiation Protection and Measurements (NCRP, 1986).

COMPARISON OF THE RECOMMENDED RADIOFREQUENCY PROTECTION GUIDES WITH STANDARDS AT OTHER FREQUENCIES

From Eq. 5 the suggested limit on the contact current is 1.5 mA at 3 kHz. This may be compared with the National Electrical Safety Code (1977), which specifies a maximum leakage current of 0.5 mA from portable electrical tools and household appliances and 0.75 mA for permanently fixed appliances. The threshold current for perception at 3 kHz is approximately 3 times higher than that at 60 Hz (Dalziel and Mansfield, 1950), so a suggested contact current of 1.5 mA is not out of line with the leakage current of 0.5 to 0.75 mA specified in the National Electrical Safety Code.

For higher RF frequencies, the suggested guideline of 10 mW/cm^2 for occupational exposures is in agreement with the occupational standard for IR radiation, and a reduced guideline of 1 mW/cm^2 (Table 3-5) is consistent with the recently proposed NCRP guideline (1986) for the general population.

CONCLUSION

The proposed RFPGs depart from the previous guidelines such as those by ANSI (1982) in two respects:

1. An increase in the safety levels of RF magnetic fields for frequencies less than 100 MHz. This is proposed in recognition of the fact that these fields do not couple as tightly as do the E fields and do not cause substantial SARs.
2. Limitation on the induced currents in the human body to no more than 100 mA for frequencies greater than 100 kHz and a linearly reducing current for lower frequencies. The current under contact situations is limited to 50 mA for frequencies greater than 100 kHz and a proportionally reducing current at lower frequencies.

Identical current limitations are proposed for both occupational and public exposures. Since safety measures can be adapted in the work place, higher field limits are suggested provided steps are taken to limit the currents for contact and noncontact situations. Procedures are available to measure the foot currents through the human body by means of shoe-mounted RF current sensors (Gandhi, 1987). Methods similar to those shown in Figure 3-1 and used by Chatterjee et al. (1986) can be employed to estimate RF currents through the human body for conditions of contact with metallic bodies. For these measurements an impedance equivalent to that of the human body for conditions of grasping contact (Gandhi et al., 1985b; Chatterjee, et al., 1986) may be used.

REFERENCES

ANSI (1982). American National Standards Institute. American national standard C95.1, safety levels with respect to human exposure to radio-frequency electromagnetic fields, 300 kHz to 100 GHz. New York, Institute of Electrical and Electronics Engineers, Inc.

BECKER, C.M., MALHOTRA, I.V., AND HEDLEY-WHYTE, J. (1973). The distribution of radio-frequency current and burns. *Anesthesiology 38*:106–122.

BERNHARDT, J.H. (1985). Evaluation of human exposures to low frequency fields. *In*: AGARD Lecture Series No. 138. The impact of proposed radio-frequency radiation standards on military operations. Neuilly Sur Seine, France, NATO

Advisory Group for Aerospace Research and Development (AGARD), pp. 8.1 to 8.18.

CHATTERJEE, I., WU, D., AND GANDHI, O.P. (1986). Human body impedance and threshold currents for perception and pain for contact hazard analysis in the VLF-MF band. *IEEE Trans. Biomed. Eng.* 33:486–494.

CHEN, J.-Y., AND GANDHI, O.P. (1988). Thermal implications of high SARs in the body extremities at the ANSI-recommended MF-VHF safety levels. *IEEE Trans. Biomed. Eng.* 35:435–441.

COOK, H.F. (1951). The dielectric behavior of some types of human tissues at microwave frequencies. *Br. J. Appl. Phys.* 2:295–300.

DALZIEL, C.F., AND MANSFIELD, T.H. (1950). Effect of frequency on perception current. *AIEE Trans.* G9, Part II, pp. 1162–1168.

DOBBIE, A.K. (1969). The electrical aspects of surgical diathermy. *Biomed. Eng.* 4:206–216.

DURNEY, C.H. (1980). Electromagnetic dosimetry for models of humans and animals: a review of theoretical and numerical techniques. *Proc. IEEE 68:33–40.*

DURNEY, C.H., JOHNSON, C.C., BARBER, P.W., et al. (1978). Radiofrequency radiation dosimetry handbook, 2nd ed. USAF School of Aerospace Medicine, Brooks Air Force Base, Tex., Contract No. SAM-TR-78–22.

ENGLAND, T.S. (1950). Dielectric properties of the human body for wavelengths in the 1–10 cm range. *Nature 166:*480–481.

GANDHI, O.P. (1975). Conditions of strongest electromagnetic power deposition in man and animals. *IEEE Trans. Microwave Theory Tech.* 23:1021–1029.

GANDHI, O.P. (1979). Dosimetry—the absorption properties of man and experimental animals. *Bull. N.Y. Acad. Med.* 55:999–1020.

GANDHI, O.P. (1987). RF personnel dosimeter and dosimetry method for use therewith. U.S. Patent No. 4,672,309, June 9.

GANDHI, O.P., AND CHATTERJEE, I. (1982). Radio-frequency hazards in the VLF to MF band. *Proc. IEEE* 70:1462–1464.

GANDHI, O.P., CHATTERJEE, I., WU, D., AND GU, Y.-G. (1985a). Likelihood of high rates of energy deposition in the human legs at the ANSI recommended 3–30 MHz RF safety levels. *Proc. IEEE* 73:1145–1147.

GANDHI, O.P., CHEN, J.-Y., AND RIAZI, A. (1986). Currents induced in a human being for plane-wave exposure conditions 0–50 MHz and for RF sealers. *IEEE Trans. Biomed. Eng.* 33:757–767.

GANDHI, O.P., AND RIAZI, A. (1986). Absorption of millimeter waves by human beings and its biological implications. *IEEE Trans. Microwave Theory Tech.* 34:228–235.

GANDHI, O.P., et al. (1985b). Very low frequency hazard study. Final report prepared for USAF School of Aerospace Medicine, Brooks Air Force Base, Tex. Contract F 33615–83–R-0613.

GRONHAUG, K.L., AND BUSMUNDRUD, O. (1982). Antenna effect of the human body of EMP. (In Norwegian.) Report No. FFI-NOTAT-82/3013. Kjeller, Norway, Norwegian Defense Research Establishment.

GUY, A.W., AND CHOU, C.K. (1982). Hazard analysis: very low frequency through medium frequency range. Final report, USAF SAM Contract No. F 33615–78-D-0617, Task 0065.

GUY, A.W., AND CHOU, C.K. (1985). Very low frequency hazard study. Final report prepared for the USAF School of Aerospace Medicine, Brooks Air Force Base, Tex., Contract No. F33615–83-C-0625.

HARDY, J.D., AND OPPEL, T.W. (1937). Studies in temperature sensation. III. The sensitivity of the body to heat and the spatial summation of the end organ responses. *J. Clin. Invest.* 16:533–540.

HILL, D.A., AND WALSH, J.A. (1985). Radio-frequency current through the feet of a grounded human. *IEEE Trans. Electromagnet. Comp.* 27:18–23.

IRPA (1988). International Radiation Protection Association. Guidelines on limits of exposure to radio-frequency electromagnetic fields in the frequency range from 100 kHz to 300 GHz. *Health Phys.* 54:115–123.

JOHNSON, C.C., AND GUY, A.W. (1972). Nonionizing electromagnetic wave effects on biological materials and systems. *Proc. IEEE* 60:692–718.

JUSTESEN, D.R. (1979). Behavioral and psychological effects of microwave radiation. *Bull. N.Y. Acad. Med.* 55:1058–1078.

LELE, P.P., WEDDELL, G., AND WILLIAMS, C.M. (1954). The relationship between heat transfer, skin temperature, and cutaneous stability. *J. Psysiol.* 126:206–234.

MORTON, D.J., TRUEX, R.C., AND KELLNER, C.E. (1941). Manual of human cross-section anatomy. Baltimore, Williams & Wilkins Co.

National electrical safety code (1977). ANSI C2, New York, Institute of Electrical and Electronics Engineers, Inc.

NCRP (1986). National Council on Radiation Protection and Measurements. Biological effects and exposure criteria for radio-frequency electromagnetic fields. Report No. 86, Bethesda, Md., NCRP.

ORCUTT, N., AND GANDHI, O.P. (1988). A 3-D impedance method to calculate power deposition in biological bodies subjected to time-varying magnetic fields. *IEEE Trans. Biomed. Eng.* 35:577–583.

ROGERS, R.J. (1981). Radio-frequency burn hazards in the MF/HF band. *In*: Mitchell, J.C. (ed.). Aeromedical review. Proceedings of a Workshop on the Protection of Personnel Against RF Electromagnetic Radiation, Review 3–81, USAF School of Aerospace Medicine, Brooks Air Force Base, Tex., pp. 76–89.

SCHWAN, H.P., AND PIERSOL, G.M. (1954). The absorption of electromagnetic energy in body tissues. *Am. J. Phys. Med.* 33:370–404.

STUCHLY, M.A. (1987). Proposed revision of the Canadian recommendations on radio-frequency exposure protection. *Health Phys.* 53:649–665.

SULLIVAN, D., GANDHI, O.P., AND TAFLOVE, A. (1988). Use of the finite-difference time-domain method in calculating EM absorption in man models. *IEEE Trans. Biomed. Eng.* 35:179–186.

TELL, R., MANTIPLY, E.D., DURNEY, C.H., AND MASSOUDI, H. (In press). Electric and magnetic field intensities and associated induced body currents in close proximity to a 50 kW AM standard broadcast station. *IEEE Trans. Broadcasting.*

Part 2

EM BIOENGINEERING

4

Environmental and Professionally Encountered Electromagnetic Fields

K. Hansson Mild

K. G. Lövstrand

In our modern society we are constantly being exposed to man-made electromagnetic (EM) fields of various frequencies and intensities. EM fields can be of various origins, such as the electric and magnetic fields emanating from high-voltage transmission lines, the radiofrequency (RF) fields from hand-held walkie-talkies, and the microwaves from burglar alarms or automatic door openers. In our environment we also have low-level fields from broadcast radio (AM, FM, shortwave) and television and from radar used for surveillance, navigation, remote sensing, etc. Occupational exposure to EM fields occurs in various industrial processes where electrical energy is used for heating purposes. For example, at lower frequencies, induction heaters are used for melting, forging, annealing, surface hardening, and soldering operations. Dielectric heating equipment usually operates in the shortwave region. This type of heating is used most commonly to speed up gluing of wood, facilitate molding of plastic, remove moisture from materials, or join or seal thin plastic materials. High-frequency heating is also employed in medicine for shortwave therapy (diathermy) and may find increasing applications for EM hyperthermia as an adjunct to cancer therapy. In all of these processes involving high-frequency EM fields, the risk of undesirable or harmful radiation in the work place cannot be overlooked. Occupational exposure to RF fields is not limited to the personnel operating the equipment but includes service and maintenance personnel, who often work close to the radiating parts with the equipment operating at full power.

In this chapter we present an overview of measurements of the electric and magnetic field strengths in the immediate vicinity of some of the most common sources of EM emitting devices.

EXTREMELY LOW-FREQUENCY ELECTROMAGNETIC FIELDS

Power Frequency Environment

Electric power is almost exclusively generated, transmitted, and distributed in alternating current (AC) systems with a frequency of 50 or 60 Hz. For railroad power 16⅔ Hz systems are also used. The electric

and magnetic fields acompanying the power lines have been the subject
of several studies and discussions during the last decade. The focus has
been primarily on high-voltage transmission lines and switchyards and
their EM environment.

Electric Fields

The power frequency electric fields are readily shielded by vehicles,
buildings, and metal or humid wooden towers of transmission lines. Only
under the middle part of a line span between the towers are high field
strengths generally found. Typical fields encountered underneath the
various transmission lines are about 10 kV/m for a 735 kV line, 6 kV/m
for a 420 kV line, and 1 kV/m for a 130 kV line.

Calculations of the electric and magnetic field strengths for numerous transmission line geometries and voltage (Lyskov and Emma, 1975;
Utmischi, 1976; Tell et al., 1977) have been verified by measurements
over flat ground with low vegetation (Sarma Maruvada et al., 1978) (Table
4-1).

Waskaas (1982) has reported local 50% to 100% increases in field
strengths at 1.8 m height in hilly terrain and a complete shielding effect
of trees and bushes. The latter effect has been suggested as a method
to reduce the electric field strength in parks and playgrounds near extra-
high-voltage transmission lines.

The exposure of personnel working near transmission lines is often
unexpectedly low (Table 4-2), although high field strengths are found
in many places (Lövstrand et al., 1978). In exposure measurements near
a 420 kV transmission line in Sweden, very low values were found during
the working periods whereas during the coffee and lunch breaks exposure
values were high. A van with plastic body parked at a high location
below the line was occupied during these breaks. Whereas metallic and
humid wooden structures are effective shields for electric fields, plastics
are relatively transparent.

Some switchyard and transmission line tasks result in high electric
field exposure levels for the operators. This is true especially for the so-
called hot line operations in which work is done on operating high-voltage
lines. Special shielding precautions are often necessary for such operations.

High electric field strengths of power frequency involve some dramatic effects. By capacitive coupling 17 μA of current is fed to a person
of normal height who is standing in a 60 Hz field of 1 kV/m. If insulated
the person will acquire a voltage of about 200 V for each kV/m of field
strength. Large vehicles, fences, and metallic roofs can thus acquire a
voltage of more than 1 kV, which can lead to painful spark discharge,
or a short-circuit current of more than 1 mA (Reilly, 1979). The so-called

TABLE 4-1 Peak Field Strength, E; Width of 50% of Peak Field Strength, and Width of 1 kV/m Field Strength under Transmission Lines of Height h.

Voltage (kV)	h (m)	Peak field strength (kV/m)	Width		Reference
			At 50% peak field strength (m)	At 1 kV/m (m)	
120	6.4	2	20	20	Sarma Maruvada et al. (1978)
130	11.5	1.1	40	25	Waskaas (1982)
300	10.5	4	40	45	Waskaas (1982)
315	7.3	6	25	32	Sarma Maruvada et al. (1978)
420	11.5	6	43	60	Waskaas (1982)
735	11.0	10.5	45	80	Sarma Maruvada et al. (1978)
765	12.0	12	50	90	Tell et al. (1977)
1150	14.5	20	75	180	Lyskov and Emma (1975)

TABLE 4-2 Cumulative Exposure to Several Field Strengths (Expressed as Percentage of Total Exposure Time) for Various Work Operations

Work operation	Voltage (kV)	Measured time (min)	Exposure (% of total time)			
			0–5 kV/m	5–10 kV/m	10–15 kV/m	>15 kV/m
Routine inspection of switch-gear	70	10	100	0	0	0
	200	35	95	5	0	0
	400	40	63	35	2	0.1
	400	42	55	38	6	2
Circuit-breaker work						
Testing	400	60	94	6	0	0
Assembly	400	60	97	3	0	0
Overhaul on top of circuit breaker	400	180	69		21	10
Repair	200	60	100	0	0	0
Insulator testing tower	200	10	72	26	1	1
	400	19	92	6	2	0
General maintenance	130	8	90	10	0	0
	200	19	75	25	0	0
	400	59	48	51	1	0.5
	400	29	41	57	1	0.6
	400	48	44	48	8	0.1

Data from Lövstrand, K.G., et al. (1978). Exposure of personnel to electric fields in Swedish extra high-voltage substations: field strength and dose measurements. *In*: Phillips, R.D., Gillis, M.F., Kaune, W.T., and Mahlum, D.D. (eds.). Biological effects of extremely low frequency electromagnetic fields. Proceedings of the 18th Annual Hanford Life Symposium, pp. 85–92.

let-go current threshold of 7 mA for sensitive persons must be considered in certain cases. Grounding of long fences and similar structures is an efficient precaution in such cases. Some annoying effects can still be found, however. The sparking from a wet umbrella used below a 400 kV high-voltage line, which we have experienced several times, can be very annoying.

Electric fields of power frequency are an environmental factor found exclusively near transmission lines. The fields near power cables in industries or homes are confined to a distance of the order of the cable radius for a one- or three-phase cable, and except for these local fields only weak field strengths of a few volts per meter are measured indoors.

Electrostatic Fields in Industry

In many cases we have measured field strengths of 100 kV/m or more within 1 m of newspaper presses. When the machines are running at high speed of several meters per second, fluctuations of the field strengths of 30% to 40% are often measured with a repetition rate of 10 Hz or more. Therefore AC components of 50 kV/m of "near" power frequency are normally occurring in the working environment of the machine operators. The electric fields in some industries are thus comparable to or stronger than those in the transmission line environment.

Magnetic Fields

Three-phase systems are used for AC high-voltage power transmission and distribution. Such systems consist of three-phase conductors carrying currents with a phase shift of roughly one third of a period between the phases. A system with balanced load carrying equal currents in all phase conductors at any moment thus carries a zero net current. The individual phase currents compensate one another. The electric and magnetic fields from the phase conductors also more or less compensate one another. Only an asymmetry in the distance and direction to the individual conductors results in a net field.

The electric fields near transmission lines are easily predictable because the voltage of the phase conductors is constant within a few percentage points. The magnetic fields are much more variable because the transmitted power, and thus the current of the lines, shows great variations. In transmission networks with the power fed from many power stations, not only the consumption but also the balance between the sources of the power determine the current flow. Diurnal, weekly, and seasonal variations occur, and for generation balance situations, some main high-voltage transmission lines may carry very low currents. For symmetrical loading, the ground current and thus also stray currents in conducting objects in the ground are zero. Any unbalance of the load immediately leads to a net current in the return conductors. Stray currents may then occur in ground return conductors and even enter houses via plumbing systems. Since the loads show large variations, a determination of typical magnetic fields near a power line normally should be based on many measurements over a long time. Especially at places where the stray currents determine the magnetic fields, careful planning of measurements and analysis of measured magnetic field values are necessary.

It is not possible to give exact values for the magnetic fields from a line, but the typical magnetic fields for a certain line can be calculated from maximum loads and average loads, which are determined by the power companies. For a high-voltage transmission line that typically carries 0.5 to 2 kA, magnetic fields of 10 to 40 μT (1 tesla [T] = 10,000 G) are calculated for the region within a 40 m wide strip along the line. The flux densities fall off quickly; at 100 m from the line the flux density is below 1 μT. This value for near-maximum loads for a line should be compared with the fields produced by electrical appliances in homes. Values of 1 mT are typical close to small motors. Magnetic voltage stabilizers sometimes used to feed power to computers were examined in Sweden. Leakage fields of about 1 mT were found within 1 m of the stabilizers with saturated magnetic cores. Some aquarium air pumps used in an experiment to determine bioeffects of weak magnetic fields on small animals generated 10 to 50 μT in the animal cages, which was above the flux densities generated by the intended exposure apparatus. Flux densities on the order of 10 μT have also been measured inside cell incubators.

Whereas the high electric field strengths occur exclusively near high-voltage power lines and are typical for them, the magnetic fields near power lines are comparable to those found in homes. Industrial environments often contain magnetic fields of power frequency 10 to 100 times those near high-voltage power lines. Low-voltage distribution lines may generate fields exceeding those from high-voltage transmission lines.

Typical Electric Field and Magnetic Field Environments

The typical power station and transmission line environment has electric fields of up to 5 kV/m and rarely more than 15 kV/m (which occurs very locally in power stations). For most working situations the electric fields are only a few kilovolts per meter. The magnetic fields are less than 20 μT along lines and may reach 2 mT locally in power stations. In most working situations the flux density is less than 10 μT.

Some industrial processes involving high currents generate magnetic fields that expose the personnel to levels exceeding 10 mT; this is discussed later in the chapter. Machinery typically generates flux densities of 10 to 100 µT. Small motors in office machines and computer terminals may also produce such magnetic fields. The electric fields in industry are low (less than 100 V/m) except in processes involving electrostatic charging in fast-running machines, where 50 kV/m of "near" power frequency may occur.

Electric and Magnetic Fields

In the last decade, interest in 50 to 60 Hz residential magnetic fields has increased because of epidemiological studies indicating a correlation between child and adult cancer and the magnetic field (for instance, Wertheimer and Leeper, 1979, 1982; and Savitz et al., 1988). Several recent reports (such as Czerski, 1988) have also suggested an excess of morbidity or mortality from leukemia among workers exposed to electric and magnetic fields.

As discussed earlier, the overall magnetic field in a house is subject to large hourly, seasonal, and long-term variations depending on the current use. However, an indication of the field strength is of interest. Wertheimer and Leeper (1982) have measured a number of houses and report a median value for the B field of 0.25 µT for houses near what they call "very high current configuration." Houses at so-called end-pole positions had a median value of less than 0.05 µT.

A recent Swedish study (Eriksson et al., 1987) found that the flux density in most residences is lower than 0.1 µT. In houses near high-voltage lines the flux densities could reach a few microtesla. The studies of Kaune et al. (1987) and Male et al. (1987) gave similar results.

In homes the electric fields are low, normally less than 10 V/m except within about 0.1 m of electrical cables and appliances, where a few hundred volts per meter may occur (Kaune et al., 1987; Silva and Kavet, 1987).

The fields emitted from various household appliances and electrical gadgets have been studied by Miller (1974) and Gauger (1984). The B field close to appliances such as hair dryers, electric drills, electric shavers, and color television sets was found to be in the range 0.1 to 2.5 mT. At a distance of 30 cm the electric field was highest (250 V/m) near an electric blanket. Otherwise the E-field values were from a few to a hundred volts per meter. The household appliances usually act essentially as dipoles, with the fields falling off rapidly, approximately as the cube of the distance. This is seen also in the measurements given by Wertheimer and Leeper (1982) from some indoor sources. For example, the B field of an electric drill was 2.5 mT close to the casing, 0.2 µT at 1 m, and not measurable (less than 0.05 µT) at 1.5 m.

Occupational Exposure

Strong electrical currents are used in a variety of industrial processes, and these currents set up related magnetic fields. Lövsund et al. (1982) have reported on measurements of the magnetic fields in electrosteel and welding industries. Field flux densities of 10 mT or less at mostly 50 Hz were found in both types of industries. Examples from these different industrial magnetic field sources and data are summarized in Table 4-3. The measurements give only the magnetic component of the EM field because the various processes studied use very high current with a rather low voltage. Therefore the E field is relatively small as a rule.

Conductive materials can be heated by eddy currents, which are induced by applying alternating magnetic fields to the sample. Induction heating is used mainly for forging, annealing, tempering, brazing, and soldering operations. The operating frequency can reach a few megahertz, but usually this type of equipment works from 50 Hz to about 10 kHz. The frequency is determined mainly by the required penetration depth of the current in the material. The current in the coil producing the magnetic field can be very large; 5000 A is not unusual. Lövsund and Hansson Mild (1978) reported on the magnetic fields around some portable induction heaters. The dimensions of the coils producing the magnetic field were about 10 to 20 cm. Thus there was no high whole-body exposure but rather local exposure of, for instance, the hands. The maximum mag-

TABLE 4-3   Magnetic Flux Densities Accompanying Some Typical Magnetic Sources

Field source	Frequency (Hz)	Magnetic flux density (mT)	Reference
Household appliances and gadgets	60	<3	Lövsund (1980)
Electrosteel furnaces	1–600	<10	Lövsund (1980)
Demagnetizers	50	<50	Lövsund (1980)
Electrolytic processes	0	<50	Lövsund (1980)
Electrical locomotives	16⅔	<50	Lövsund (1980)
Induction heaters	<10,000	<70	Lövsund (1980)
Laboratory work with magnetic materials	0.1–50	<100	Lövsund (1980)
Welding machines	0 or 50	<130	Lövsund (1980)
High-voltage power line (1 kA)	50	0.01	Mantell (1975)
Power station	50	0.3–2	

netic flux density to which the hands of the operator could be exposed was 25 mT. However, in most cases the flux density was less than 1 mT at the hands. In a number of new industrial processes involving the use of superconducting magnets, fusion reactors, and different accelerators, flux densities up to 1 T may be expected (Alpen, 1978).

DIELECTRIC HEATING

Dielectric heating was introduced about 1940 with a 125 kW output generator operating at about 1650 kHz for heating plywood. Since then the frequency has moved upward and now ranges from a few to 120 MHz or more. However, this equipment usually operates on one of the ISM bands at 13.56, 27.12, or 40.68 MHz where the power output of the RF source is unrestricted. Today the total power used for dielectric heating probably exceeds that installed for broadcasting throughout the world (Wilson, 1975).

RF sealers and heaters are used to heat, melt, or cure such materials as plastic, rubber, or glue. These apparatuses are commonly used in manufacture of plastic products such as toys, rain apparel, and plastic tarpaulins; wood lamination; for glue setting; and drying operations in the textile, paper, plastic, and leather industries. For further examples of occupations using RF sealers and heaters see West et al. (1980). They estimate that in the United States alone approximatively 20,000 RF sealers and heaters are in use and about 30,000 to 40,000 workers operate these units. In Sweden we estimate the number of RF sealers to be about 1500, operated by about 1500 operators.

By far the most common equipment used for dielectric heating is the plastic welding machine, employed in sealing or joining sheets of plastic materials. A typical RF sealer consists of a cabinet housing the RF generator and electronic circuitry, a pneumatic press, an applicator or die where the processed material is subjected to the RF energy, and a bed plate to support the material. The RF potential difference over the plastic materials to be joined together varies from about 800 V for thin sheets to 1500 V for thick materials (Eriksson and Hansson Mild, 1985).

In designs where the applicator is enclosed in a tightly fitting or overlapping metal enclosure, the exposure of the personnel to RF stray fields is low. However, these enclosures are present mostly on relatively new machines and not on the old ones, where the applicator is unshielded. This leads to high levels of undesirable radiation in the vicinity of the older machines. Conover et al. (1980) have reported on measurements of E and H fields from 82 different RF sealers in 12 different plants. They found that the majority of the sealers worked at the ISM band located at 27.12 MHz. The duty cycles of the various processes varied from about 0.05 to more than 0.5, but most duty cycles (68%) were found to be in the range 0.05 to 0.2. Tables 4-4 and 4-5 from Conover et al. (1980) show the percentage of the RF measurements exceeding specific field strengths at various anatomical locations. In Table 4-6 the percentage is given for the maximum values of E and H found at each sealer regardless of the anatomical location. These data show that more than 90% of the RF sealers operating at 27.12 MHz exceed the C95.1—1982 guidelines for RF and microwave human exposure of a time-averaged value of no more than 1.22 mW/cm^2 with the corresponding E- and H-field values of 68 V/m and 0.18 A/m, respectively.

Conover et al. (1980) noted that the E field often was higher than the H field when compared on the basis of far-field equivalent power densities. Furthermore, no correlation was observed between RF sealer output power and the field strength exposure levels.

These data can also be considered in view of the tentative National Institute of Occupational Safety and Health (NIOSH) exposure levels of 1 mW/cm^2 with corresponding limits to E and H, but also with a ceiling value of 5 mW/cm^2. The field strength values *not* corrected for duty cycles from Tables 4-4 and 4-5 show that about 95% of the sealers exceed the ceiling value for E field, 140 V/m, and about 70% the value for H field, 0.4 A/m.

In a survey by Cox and Conover (1981) similar results are given. Of 30 operators, 24 (80%) were exposed to fields in excess of the proposed NIOSH time-averaged standard, and for an even higher percentage of operators the exposure exceeded even the proposed ceiling values. Again the E-field values were comparatively higher than those of the H fields.

The same trend is confirmed by our own measurements of more than 100 plastic welding machines, although the percentages might be somewhat different. In Table 4-7 the electric and magnetic field strengths from some of our measurements are given. All these measurements were taken on unshielded welding machines (Figure 4-1). See also Kolmodin-Hedman et al. (1988).

Stuchly et al. (1980) found that the RF fields at the operator locations from sewing machine–type RF sealers exceeded 140 V/m in 58% of the cases and exceeded 0.4 A/m in 42% of the cases. These values correspond to a far-field power density of 5 mW/cm^2. Of the 33 sealers measured, 33% were in excess of 300 V/m (25 mW/cm^2). A Norwegian study by Hannevik and Saxebøl (1983) shows that, of 77 plastic sealers surveyed, 39% exceeded the equivalent power density of 25 mW/cm^2 for either the electric or the magnetic field strength at some anatomical location of the operator.

When survey of a work place is performed, the tester must be aware that fairly strong fields can be found several meters from the RF sources.

TABLE 4-4 Percentage of Radiofrequency Measurements Exceeding Specific Electric Field Strength Values by Anatomical Locations

Anatomical location	Percent RF measurements not corrected for duty cycle			Percent RF measurements corrected for duty cycle		
	>25 V/m	>50 V/m	>200 V/m	>25 V/m	>50 V/m	>200 V/m
Eyes	98.9	96.6	65.5	90.6	74.1	28.2
Neck	98.4	89.1	67.4	89.8	79.5	31.5
Chest	97.5	90.1	59.3	84.8	68.4	20.3
Waist	97.7	95.3	57.4	90.0	70.0	28.3
Gonads	96.3	79.3	31.7	74.1	48.1	3.7
Knees	93.7	80.3	31.5	75.4	51.6	10.3
Ankles	88.3	75.3	11.7	67.1	32.9	1.3

From Conover, D., et al. (1980). Measurement of electric—and magnetic—field strengths from industrial radiofrequency (6–38 MHz) plastic sealers. *Proc. IEEE* 68:17–20. © 1980 IEEE.

TABLE 4-5 Percentage of Radiofrequency Measurements Exceeding Specific Magnetic Field Strength Values by Anatomical Location

Anatomical location	Percent of measurements not corrected for duty cycle			Percent of measurements corrected for duty cycle		
	≥0.05 A/m	>0.15 A/m	>0.5 A/m	≥0.05 A/m	>0.15 A/m	>0.5 A/m
Eyes	86.8	60.5	44.7	73.0	45.9	21.6
Neck	90.0	77.5	55.0	83.5	64.6	16.5
Chest	83.9	67.7	48.4	73.3	53.3	30.0
Waist	89.3	80.0	50.7	82.4	64.9	12.2
Gonads	90.6	71.9	37.5	80.6	48.4	9.7
Knees	89.7	82.1	32.1	84.4	46.8	6.5
Ankles	82.8	69.0	48.3	71.4	46.4	7.1

From Conover, D., et al. (1980). Measurement of electric—and magnetic—field strengths from industrial radiofrequency (6–38 MHz) plastic sealers. *Proc. IEEE* 68:17–20. ©1980 IEEE.

TABLE 4-6 Numbers and Percentage of Radiofrequency Sealers Having at Least One Measurement Exceeding Specific Electric and Magnetic Field Strength Values

	Electric field strength				Magnetic field strength			
	Total	≥25 V/m	>50 V/m	>200 V/m	Total	≥0.05 A/m	>0.15 A/m	>0.50 A/m
Not corrected for duty cycle								
Number	82	81	81	75	66	63	57	45
Percent	100.0	98.8	98.8	91.5	100.0	95.5	86.4	68.2
Corrected for duty cycle								
Number	80	79	77	53	65	58	52	19
Percent	100.0	98.8	96.3	66.3	100.0	89.2	80.0	29.2

From Conover, D., et al. (1980). Measurement of electric—and magnetic—field strengths from industrial radiofrequency (6–38 MHz) plastic sealers. *Proc. IEEE 68*:17–20. © 1980 IEEE.

TABLE 4-7 Electromagnetic Fields near Plastic Welding Machines*

Power (kW)	Eyes Electric (V/m)	Eyes Magnetic (A/m)	Genitalia Electric (V/m)	Genitalia Magnetic (A/m)	Hands on control panel Electric (V/m)	Hands on control panel Magnetic (A/m)	Hands near electrode Electric (V/m)	Hands near electrode Magnetic (A/m)
4	900	0.4	>900	0.7	900	1.2		
4	260	1.1	340	1.3	820	1.5		
	>900†	>1.6†						
3	200		275	1.0	—‡	—‡	>900§	>2.8§
6	250	0.3	170	0.2	>900	0.9		

From Hansson Mild, K. (1980). Occupational exposure to radiofrequency electromagnetic fields. *Proc. IEEE* 68:12–17. © 1980 IEEE.

* Representative results of measurements of electric and magnetic field strength from four different plastic welding machines operating at 27 MHz. The measurements were done at locations corresponding to different anatomical positions on the operator. All measurements were done without the operator's presence.

† In some operations the operator had to bend down close to the electrode to get a better view of the welding process.

‡ Controlled by foot lever.

§ Hands about 15 cm from the electrode.

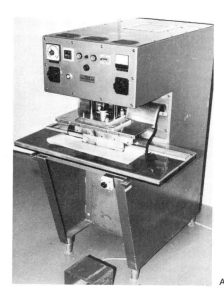

Figure 4-1 Electric and magnetic fields near a plastic sealer. **A,** Sealer that operates at 27.12 MHz with power output of 3 kW. Sealer is equipped with 29 cm long electrode. No shielding is applied to sealer while measurements are made. **B** and **C,** Equivalent isopower density lines for 25 mW/cm^2 for electric field E = 300 V/m and magnetic field H = 0.8 A/m. Measurements were done in a laboratory for work-typical conditions (see also Eriksson and Hansson Mild, 1985).

A

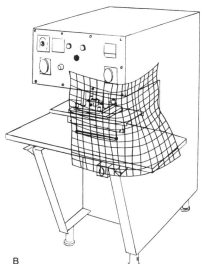

B

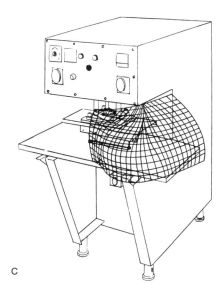

C

In several cases we have noticed that the cables for the power supply are an effective antenna for these frequencies and that the reradiated fields can reach more than 500 V/m in the vicinity of these cables. Large, extended, metallic structures, such as stands and racks, can also act as secondary RF sources. The most effective way to minimize the RF stray field is to shield the electrode by a metallic enclosure, but if this is not possible, other, less efficient methods are available. Some of these are discussed by Stuchly and Repacholi (1980), Ruggera and Schaubert (1982), and Eriksson and Hansson Mild (1985).

In most of the other applications of dielectric heating in industry, the leakage radiation and hence the occupational exposure to RF radiation are much less than in the cases discussed here. The operators may not be required to spend so much time close to the electrodes, since several of these applications are semiautomatic. For much of this heating equipment the power frequency amplitude modulation of the RF fields can be high. In view of the reported biological effects of AM-modulated RF signals on nervous tissue, this might be important in assessing the possible hazard of the RF exposure.

BROADCAST RADIATION

Occupational Exposure

Maintenance work on FM radio and television broadcast towers is often performed while the station is operating at full power. Tower maintenance personnel commonly report a sensation of warmth when climbing energized broadcast towers. The field levels have been measured by Tell (1976) and Hansson Mild (1981), who reported high field strengths.

Tell (1976) measured fields at an FM radio tower at Mount Wilson, Calif., with a total transmitter power of 40 kW distributed on six circularly polarized antennas. The E field inside the tower structure was about 800 V/m at many places. Even higher local fields were found in some areas, especially on the ladder where the hands and feet are exposed during climbing.

Hansson Mild (1981) surveyed 11 large radio stations and FM radio/television broadcasting towers in Sweden. All large stations are built in similar ways. The transmitter equipment is also similar in the different stations. Each of the three Swedish radio programs is transmitted by two transmitters, each with a power of about 3 kW, operating in parallel. Thus the total input power to the antenna for FM broadcasting is about 18 kW ($2 \times 3 \times 3$). The Swedish FM radio band extends from 90 to 100 MHz, in contrast to the 88 to 108 MHz in the United States. The VHF television transmitters are usually in the same room as the FM transmitters, with two transmitters operating simultaneously. The video signal is transmitted with a mean power of about 2 kW from each of the transmitters. Furthermore, for television broadcast there are also two sound transmitters, each with a power of about 0.2 kW. The UHF transmitters are in a separate room. The peak power is 40 kW, and the average power is about 30 kW. The output of the sound transmitter is 4 kW. Only one pair (video and sound) of UHF transmitters is used at the same time. The backup system is turned on only when needed. When a large station is operating with full power, all the transmitters are normally used and 56 kW is being fed to the antenna systems on the tower.

Usually an antenna tower is 330 m high and carries three antenna systems: UHF and VHF television broadcast and FM radio broadcast. The effective radiated power (transmitter power mutliplied by the antenna gain) is 1000 kW for UHF, 60 kW for VHF, and 60 kW for each of the three radio programs. Under normal conditions the level of RF fields in the transmitter room is too low to be measured with ordinary radiation hazard meters. Only very close to the transmitters and feeders (within 0.2 m) can leakage radiation be detected.

One serious problem encountered in the stations is the high RF field strengths found in the transmitter enclosure with the transmitter in question switched off and the cabinet doors open. The transmitter then acts as a tuned receiver for the transmitter operating in parallel and broadcasting at the same frequency. The field strength in the transmitter cabinet often exceeds 200 mW/cm^2 at about 5 cm from the feeder input.

In some circumstances it is necessary to bypass the safety interlock system and have the transmitter switched on while the cabinet door is open. In this case the leakage radiation is substantial; and equivalent power density of 25 mW/cm^2 has been found for the electric field at distances up to 1 m from the transmitter.

When workers are adjusting the UHF transmitter, their hands are exposed to the static magnetic field that comes from the focusing coils of the transmitter tube. This field is about 30 mT on the inside of the coils and about 10 mT outside the coils.

When climbing through the FM antenna, workers cannot avoid direct contact with the coaxial cables feeding the different antenna elements. Around these cables, field strengths are high, up to 600 V/m for the E field and 3 A/m for the H field. The body-to-ground currents have been measured and found to be on the order of 100 to 200 mA.

The VHF television antennas are above the FM antennas. The values of leakage radiation as measured from the ladder in the tower are in most cases below the equivalent of 5 mW/cm^2 for both S_E and S_H. However, high values are found outside the tower near the dipoles. The E field has a maximum at the edge of the dipole and a direction parallel with the long axis of the dipole. The strength is usually around 400 V/m, but values up to 900 V/m are seen in some cases. The magnetic field is circular around the dipole and strongest near the center, where it is about 2 A/m.

The UHF television antennas are at the top of the tower. Since UHF television operates at frequencies of about 600 MHz, measuring only the E field is sufficient. Immediately in front of the dipoles we found a maximum equivalent power density of 100 mW/cm^2. At about 1 m from the dipoles, S_E was about 1 to 3 mW/cm^2. Inside the spire at the lower part, S_E was about 3 mW/cm^2.

The results from these measurements on radio stations and on tall FM radio and television towers show that the personnel may be exposed to high levels of RF radiation when performing certain tasks. Safe passage of maintenance personnel near energized antennas of some types is impossible without a drastic reduction of the transmitted power. When a worker is climbing the ladder through antenna systems, normally only the hands and feet are overexposed. However, if maintenance work is being done, other body parts may also be exposed. Thus it is impossible to work in the tower near an energized antenna without violating the present safety threshold values for RF radiation. In the stations we assessed, the RF leakage radiation was generally low, but when work was done with the cabinet doors of the transmitter open, high field strengths were found in the vicinity of the transmitter even though it was switched off.

Still another aspect has to be taken into account when assessing the health hazard from RF radiation on a tower. Climbing the ladder requires intense physical effort. The RF energy absorbed when a worker passes by an antenna system is added to the already high metabolic level of the body. Under these conditons, body temperature may rise to undesirably high levels more easily than when RF absorption occurs without physical exertion. These problems are discussed in detail by Tell and Harlen (1979).

Population Exposure from Broadcast Radiation

The UHF and VHF braodcast signal field intensities have been measured by Tell and associates (see Tell and Mantiply, 1980, for a review) in 15 metropolitan areas of the United States. The data were obtained at 486 locations and represent approximately 14,000 measurements of VHF (television and FM radio) and UHF (television) signal field strengths. From these data a computer algorithm was developed to allow prediction of the broadcast exposure of the population. The estimated median level (that to which 50% of the population is exposed in 15 surveyed cities) was about 0.005 μW/cm^2. The data also suggest that about 1% of the U.S. population is exposed to levels greater than 1 μW/cm^2. The FM radio broadcast is responsible for most of these field strengths. We are not aware of any similar studies from other countries.

Telecommunications

EM radiation from various telecommunications systems has been measured by Petersen (1980). The maximum power densities in normally accessible areas associated with the operation of tropospheric scatter systems, satellite communication, and point-to point microwave radio systems (power of less than 10 W) were less than 1 μW/cm^2.

If operated improperly, certain satellite communication systems can cause hazardous exposure because of the large on-axis power densities produced at even great distances from the antenna (Hankin, 1974; Stuchly, 1977). Methods for determining the boundaries for these hazardous regions are given by Shinn (1976), who also discusses measures to avoid such hazards.

The problem of determining and eliminating microwave fields aboard naval ships has been treated by Glaser and Heimer (1971).

On merchant vessels the occupational exposure to microwave fields from radar is low. Our measurements indicate that only when working with the transmitter energized and the cabinet safety lock bypassed is it possible to reach locally hazardous field levels. In normal operations the leakage is not measurable with ordinary radiation hazard meters.

Low-power radar is used as weather radar in aircraft, in navigational aids on small boats, and to determine the speed of vehicles. Normally the weather radar is not used while the aircraft is on the ground, but if it is inadvertently turned on, the power density may reach about 3 mW/cm^2 at a distance of 1 m. For marine radar the power density is less than 50 μW/cm^2 at the antenna turntable radius. Immediately in front of the traffic radar antenna (with an output of about 0.1 W), the power density can reach 0.4 mW/cm^2 (see, for example, Janes, 1979).

MICROWAVE OVENS

Microwave ovens have been in use for about 30 years. Most operate at 2450 MHz, and the microwave power levels vary from several hundred watts (typically 500 to 600) in consumer models to 2 kW in some commercial models. Inside the oven the expected power densities are on the order of 1 to 4 W/cm^2 for a 275 ml load.

Microwave leakage from the ovens has been extensively surveyed over the years (see, for example, Osepchuk, 1978). The vast majority of ovens have leakage clearly below 5 mW/cm^2, which is the limit for emission from ovens at a distance of 5 cm, as given by the U.S. Bureau of Radiological Health. Immediately after manufacture the allowed leakage is 1 mW/cm^2. In Sweden the corresponding values are 2 mW/cm^2 when manufactured and this is allowed to degrade to 5 mW/cm^2 over the life of the oven. For ovens in commercial use, control measurements of the leakage are required every third year.

Microwave ovens used in restaurants and cafeterias were surveyed by Skotte (1981), who found that most of the large ovens had leakage

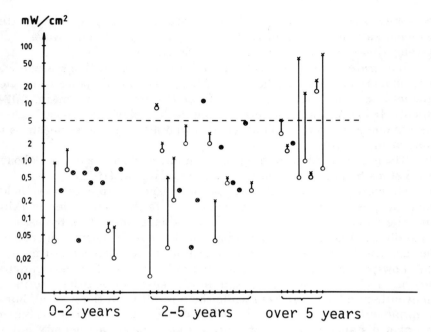

Figure 4-2   Normal (*open circles*) and forced (*x*) leakage from a representative random sample of commercial ovens measured after years in use. (After Skotte, J. [1981] with permission.)

in the range 0.2 to 2 mW/cm^2, with a few over 5 mW/cm^2. The latter typically were older ovens showing obvious signs of insufficient maintenance, such as loose or worn hinges, and warping, and dents in the oven door (see Figure 4-2).

All of Skotte's measurements were taken at a distance of 5 cm from the oven to check compliance with the emission standard for ovens. The exposure of the people working in the vicinity of the oven is much smaller than this. At 1 m the power density is reduced to about 0.02 mW/cm^2, for a maximum leakage of 5 mW/cm^2 at 5 cm.

ELECTROMAGNETIC FIELDS IN MEDICINE

EM fields of high frequency have been used in medicine for more than 50 years. The EM power, in the form of either shortwaves (27 MHz) or microwaves (2450 MHz), is used to heat deep tissues or to stimulate physiological responses in the treatment of certain pathological conditions. Since the introduction of this form of therapy, attention has been paid to the risk of health hazard. As early as 1935 the neurasthenic syndrome was described in connection with occupational exposure to shortwaves. Van Went (1954) even introduced a safety distance of 2 m to the shortwave apparatus during irradiation to minimize the health problems of the attending personnel.

The field strengths in the vicinity of medical equipment have been measured extensively in the last few years (Hansson Mild, 1980; Kalliomäki et al., 1982; Stuchly et al., 1982). The stray fields depend on the type of electrodes that are used. The worst case, from an occupational exposure point of view, occurs when glass capsule electrodes are employed. At 80 cm from such electrodes the E field is still about 430 V/m, corresponding to a far-field-equivalent power density of 50 mW/cm^2. A magnetic field of 1.2 A/m, equivalent to 50 mW/cm^2, is encountered 60 cm from the electrodes. The leakage radiation from the machines used today in physical therapy does not differ much from the earlier ones. For a safety distance of 2 m as introduced by van Went (1954), the fields are not likely to be stronger than those corresponding to an equivalent far field of 0.5 mW/cm^2.

If the physiotherapist adjusts the electrode position while the equipment is working on normal power used for treatment, the exposure can be quite high, certainly more than 2000 V/m and 5 A/m at the hands.

The personnel performing service and maintenance tasks are also exposed to high levels of leakage radiation. When the cover of the shortwave apparatus is removed, the H field at the back of the machine is about 3 A/m and the E field is about 1000 V/m. Furthermore, technicians commonly find out about the status of the diathermy apparatus by placing a hand in the fields between the electrodes and making a subjective judgment of the time taken to feel the sensation of warmth. The fields between the electrodes may reach 40,000 V/m and 100 A/m.

Microwave diathermy apparatus at 2450 MHz also has high levels of leakage radiation. The worst case occurs when the exposure occurs directly in the main beam. At a 2 m distance from the antenna 10 mW/cm^2 is found. In our experience the chassis and cable do not generate as much radiation as for the shortwave apparatus. Usually for occupational safety it is sufficient to stay away from the main beam direction (Ruggera, 1977, 1980).

Safety guidelines for microwave diathermy equipment have been established in Canada (Stuchly et al., 1982), and a proposal for performance standards was issued by the U.S. Food and Drug Administration in 1980. A set of microwave radiation safety considerations has also been developed by the U.S. Bureau of Radiological Health for microwave devices used in cancer therapy by hyperthermia (Bassen and Coakley, 1981).

In surgical diathermy high-frequency currents are used for cutting and for stopping blood flow by coagulation. Surgical diathermy devices operate in the frequency range from 0.5 to 2.4 MHz. The current can be either continuous wave (CW) or amplitude modulated, depending on the mode of operation. The surgeon is handling currents of several amperes, developing up to 1000 W.

Because of the design of diathermy equipment, high levels of undesirable leakage radiation are found near the electrode and the cable (Ruggera, 1977). At 16 cm from the probe lead, an E field of about 1000 V/m, and an H field of about 0.7 A/m were found when the electrosurgical unit was operating at 100% power. The field strengths rapidly decreased with increasing distance from the lead. Our own measurements on a unit with an RF power of 200 W operating at 0.7 MHz indicated E fields well over 1000 V/m at 5 cm from the lead and the probe.

CONCLUSION

Although possible biological effects of 50 or 60 Hz electric fields have been frequently discussed, exposure to high-level field strengths is not a common phenomenon. Only directly below high-voltage lines and in some areas of substations can substantial field strengths be encountered. Also, linemen working near or on energized lines, with either the conventional hot stick method or the barehand method, might be exposed to high field strengths.

Recently interest in the power frequency magnetic field has increased, mainly because of reports indicating a connection between weak extremely low-frequency fields and cancer. In this case the exposure is not confined to the close environment of power and transmission lines. Equipment that generates low-level (50 to 60 Hz) magnetic fields is common in households and industry, and therefore large groups of the population are being exposed. It is important to determine as accurately as possible the small extra risk of cancer resulting from this exposure and consider how best to reduce or eliminate it.

A seldom-mentioned problem is that the electrostatic fields near certain paper-machines and newspaper presses can have large cyclical variations in magnitude, producing an exposure to electric fields comparable to that near high-voltage lines.

RF exposure of the general public is mainly to low-level radio and television transmission. Microwave radio relays, low-power radar, and mobile communication systems make an almost negligible contribution to such exposure (Janes, 1979). In occupational exposure, dielectric heaters, especially RF sealers and heaters, have been found to have RF leakage fields well in excess of the safety standards of most countries. E fields in the range 200 to 1000 V/m and H fields of 0.4 to 2 A/m are fairly common at operator positions. Shortwave and microwave diathermy equipment used in physical therapy can also give rise to substantial exposure of the therapist if a safe distance of about 1 m from the electrodes is not maintained.

The use of RF and microwave energy for new and novel modes of communication and for industrial applications is burgeoning (Gandhi, 1982). The communication applications involve fairly low radiated powers and hence low power densities. Other uses involve high power—for instance, for potential applications in fusion and in satellite power stations—and must therefore be carefully controlled to keep the exposure of occupied regions sufficiently low. Some of the new medical applications, such as hyperthermia in cancer therapy, also involve relatively high powers, but with the use of direct-contact applicators this need not cause any problem.

REFERENCES

ALPEN, E.L. (1978). Magnetic field exposure guidelines. In: Tenforde, T. (ed.). Proceedings of the Biomagnetic Workshop. Lawrence Berkeley Laboratory Report No. LBL-7452, Berkeley, University of California, pp. 19–26.

BASSEN, H.I., AND COAKLEY, R.F., JR. (1981). United States radiation safety and regulatory considerations for radiofrequency hyperthermia systems. J. Microwave Power 16:215–226.

CONOVER, D., MURRAY, W., FOLEY, E., LARY, J., AND PARR, W. (1980). Measurement of electric—and magnetic—field strengths from industrial radiofrequency (6–38 MHz) plastic sealers. Proc. IEEE 68:17–20.

COX, C., AND CONOVER, D. (1981). Industrial hygiene survey report in support of epidemiologic study of RF heat sealer operators at National Blank Book Company, Inc., Holyoke, Massachusetts. Cincinnati, Ohio. National Institute of Occupational Safety and Health. Pub. No. PB 83–151630.

CZERSKI, P. (1988). Extremely low frequency magnetic fields: biological effects and health risk assessment. In: Repacholi, M.H. (ed.). Non-ionizing radiations: physical characteristics, biological effects and health hazard assessment. Proceedings of the International Non-Ionizing Radiation Workshop, Melbourne, Aust., Apr. 5–9, 1988, pp. 291–301. Available from: Australian Radiation Laboratory, Lower Plenty Road, Yallambie, Victoria, Australia.

ERIKSSON, A., AND HANSSON MILD, K. (1985). Radiofrequency electromagnetic leakage fields from plastic welding machines: measurements and reducing measures. J. Microwave Power 20:95–107.

ERIKSSON, A., HANSSON MILD, K., LIND, TH., PAULSSON, L.-E., WALTRÉ, M., AND ÖSTMAN, U. (1987). 50 Hz magnetic fields in residences. Stockholm, Swedish National Board of Occupational Safety and Health Investigation Report No. 6.

GANDHI, O.P. (1982). Present and future benefits: applications of radiofrequency and microwave energy. In: Steneck, N.H. (ed.). Risk/benefit analysis: the microwave case. San Francisco, San Francisco Press, Inc.

GAUGER, J.R. (1984). Household appliance magnetic field survey. Tech Report No. EO6549–3, Chicago, II T Research Institute.

GLASER, Z.R., AND HEIMER, G.M. (1971). Determination and elimination of hazardous microwave fields aboard naval ships. *IEEE Trans. Microwave Theory Tech.* MTT-19:232–238.

HANKIN, N.N. (1974). An evaluation of selected satellite communication systems as sources of environmental microwave radiation. Washington, D.C. Report No. EPA-520 2–74–008, Environmental Protection Agency, Office of Radiation Programs.

HANNEVIK, M., AND SAXEBØL, G. (1983). A survey on radiofrequency radiation in plastic and furniture industry. (In Norwegian.) Österås, Norway, SIS Report No. 1983:2, State Institute of Radiation Hygiene.

HANSSON MILD, K. (1980). Occupational exposure to radiofrequency electromagnetic fields. *Proc. IEEE* 68:12–17.

HANSSON MILD, K. (1981). Radiofrequency electromagnetic fields in Swedish radio stations and tall FM/TV towers. *Bioelectromagnetics* 2:61–69.

JANES, D.E., JR. (1979). Radiation surveys—measurement of leakage emissions and potential exposure fields. *Bull. N.Y. Acad. Med.* 55:1021–1041.

KALLIOMÄKI, P.L., HIETANEN, M., KALLIOMÄKI, K., KOISTINEN, O., AND VALTONEN, E. (1982). Measurements of electric and magnetic stray fields produced by various electrodes of 27 MHz diathermy equipment. *Radio Sci.* 17:29S–34S.

KAUNE, W.T., STEVENS, R.G., CALLAHAN, N.J., SEVERSON, R.K., AND THOMAS, D.B. (1987). Residential magnetic and electric fields. *Bioelectromagnetics* 8:315–335.

KOLMODIN-HEDMAN, B., HANSSON MILD, K., HAGBERG, M., JÖNSSON, E., ANDERSSON, M.-C., AND ERIKSSON, A. (1988). Health problems among operators of plastic welding machines and exposure to radiofrequency electromagnetic fields. *Int. Arch. Occup. Environ. Health* 60:243–247.

LÖVSTRAND, K.G., LUNDQUIST, S., BERGSTRÖM, S., AND BIRKE, E. (1978). Exposure of personnel to electric fields in Swedish extra high-voltage substations: field strength and dose measurements. *In*: Phillips, R.D., Gillis, M.F., Kaune, W.T., and Mahlum, D.D. (eds.). Biological effects of extremely low frequency electromagnetic fields. Proceedings of the 18th Annual Hanford Life Symposium, Richland, Wa. pp. 85–92.

LÖVSUND, R. (1980). Biological effects of alternating magnetic fields with special reference to the visual system. Linköpings studies in science and technology. Dissertation No. 47, Linköpings University, Sweden.

LÖVSUND, P., AND HANSSON MILD, K. (1978). Low frequency electromagnetic field near some induction heaters. Stockholm, Investigation Rep. No. 1978:38, National Board of Occupational Health and Safety, Sweden.

LÖVSUND, P., ÖBERG, P.Å., AND NILSSON, S.E.G. (1982). ELF magnetic fields in electrosteel and welding industries. *Radio Sci.* 17:35S–38S.

LYSKOV, Y.I., AND EMMA, Y.S. (1975). Electrical field as a parameter considered in designing electric power transmission of 750 kV; the measuring methods, the design practices and direction of further research. *In*: Symposium on EHV-

AC Power Transmission, Joint American/Soviet Committee on Cooperation in the Field of Energy, Washington, D.C., Feb. 17–27, 1975.

MALE, J.C., NORRIS, W.T., AND WATTS, W. (1987). Exposure of people to power-frequency electric and magnetic fields. *In*: Anderson, L.E., Kelman, B.J., and Weigel, R.J. (eds.). Interaction of biological systems with static and ELF electric and magnetic fields. Proceedings of the 23rd Hanford Life Sciences Symposium, Oct. 2–4, 1984, Richland, Wash. Richland, Wash., Pacific Northwest Laboratory, pp. 407–418.

MANTELL, B. (1975). Untersuchungen über die Wirkung eines magnetischen Wechselfeldes 50 Hz auf den Menschen. Dissertation, der Albert-Ludwigs-Universität, Freiburg, Federal Republic of Germany.

MILLER, D.A. (1974). Electric and magnetic fields produced by commercial power systems. *In*: Llaurado, J.G., Sances, A., Jr., and Battocletti, J.H. (eds.). Biologic and clinical effects of low-frequency magnetic and electric fields. Springfield, Ill., Charles C Thomas, Publishers, pp. 62–69.

OSEPCHUK, J.M. (1978). A review of microwave oven safety. *J. Microwave Power* 13:13–26.

PETERSEN, R.C. (1980). Electromagnetic radiation from selected telecommunications system. *Proc. IEEE* 68:21–24.

REILLY, J.P. (1979). An approach to the realistic-case analysis of electric field induction from AC transmission lines. Presented at the 3rd International Symposium on High Voltage Engineering, Milan, Aug. 28–31, 1979.

RUGGERA, P.S. (1977). Near-field measurements of RF-fields. *In*: Hazzard, D.G. (ed.). Symposium on Biological Effects and Measurements of Radio Frequency Microwaves, Rockville, MD., Feb. 16–18, 1977, HEW Pub. No. (FDA) 77–8026, pp. 104–114, available from NTIS, Springfield, VA 22161.

RUGGERA, P.S. (1980). Measurements of emission levels during microwave and shortwave diathermy treatments. HHS Pub. No. (FDA) 80–8119, available from NTIS, Springfield, VA 22161.

RUGGERA, P.S., AND SCHAUBERT, D.H. (1982). Concepts and approaches for minimizing exposure to electromagnetic radiation from RF sealers. HHS Pub. No. (FDA) 82–8192, available from NTIS, Springfield, VA 22161.

SARMA MARUVADA, P., HYLTEN-CAVALLIUS, N., AND GIAO TRIAH, N. (1978). Electrostatic field effects from high voltage power lines and in substations. Presented at the International Conference on Large High Voltage Electric Systems, Aug. 25–Sept. 2, 1976, no. 36–04.

SAVITZ, D.A., WACHTEL, H., BARNES, F.A., JOHN, E.M., AND TVRDIK, J.G. (1988). Case-control study of childhood cancer and exposure to 60-hertz magnetic fields. *Am. J. Epidemiol.* 128:21–38.

SHINN, D.H. (1976). Avoidance of radiation hazards from microwave antennas. *Marconi Rev.* 39:61–80.

SILVA, J.M., AND KAVET, R. (1987). Estimating public exposure to power-frequency electric fields. *In*: Anderson, L.E., Kelman, B.J., and Weigel, R.J. (eds.). Interaction of biological systems with static and ELF electric and magnetic fields.

Proceedings of the 23rd Annual Hanford Life Sciences Symposium, Oct. 2–4, 1984, Richland, Wash. Richland, Wash., Pacific Northwest Laboratory, pp. 419–435.

SKOTTE, J. (1981). Undersøgelse af mikrobølgeovne i storkøkkener. (In Danish.) Arbejdstilsynet, Denmark, Report No. 6.

STUCHLY, M.A. (1977). Potentially hazardous microwave radiation sources: a review. *J. Microwave Power 12*:369–381.

STUCHLY, M.A., AND REPACHOLI, M.H. (1980). Dielectric (rf) heaters: guidelines for limiting radiofrequency radiation. Ottawa, Health and Welfare Canada, Environmental Health Directorate Pub. No. 80-EHD-58.

STUCHLY, M.A., REPACHOLI, M.H., LECUYER, D., AND MANN, R. (1980). Report on the survey of radiofrequency heaters. Ottawa, Health and Welfare Canada, Environmental Health Directorate Pub. No. 80-EHD-47.

STUCHLY, M.A., REPACHOLI, M.H., LECUYER, D.W., AND MANN, R.D. (1982). Exposure to the operator and patient during short wave diathermy treatments. *Health Phys. 42*:341–366.

TELL R.A. (1976). A measurement of RF field intensities in the immediate vicinity of an FM broadcast station antenna. Las Vegas, Nev., Tech. Note ORP/EDA-76–2, Environmental Protection Agency.

TELL, R.A., AND HARLEN, F. (1979). A review of selected biological effects and dosimetry data useful for development of radiofrequency safety standards for human exposures. *J. Microwave Power 14*:405–424.

TELL, R.A., AND MANTIPLY, E.D. (1980). Population exposure to VHF and UHF broadcast radiation in the United States. *Proc. IEEE 68*:6–12.

TELL, R.A., NELSON, J.C., LAMBDIN, D.L., WHIT ATHEY, T., HANKIN, N.N., AND JANES, D.E., JR. (1977). An examination of electric fields under EHV overhead power transmission lines. Las Vegas, Nev., Pub. No. EPA-520/2–76–008. Environmental Protection Agency.

UTMISCHI, D. (1976). Das elektrische feld unter hochspannungsfreileitungen. Dissertation, Technischen Universität, München, Federal Republic of Germany.

VAN WENT, J.M. (1954). Ultrasonic and ultrashort waves in medicine. Amsterdam, Elsevier.

WASKAAS, M. (1982). Elektriske felt i høgspenningsanlegg. (In Norwegian.) State Institute of Radiation Hygiene, Norway, SIS Rapport 1982:5.

WERTHEIMER, N., AND LEEPER, E. (1979). Electrical wiring configurations and childhood cancer. *Am. J. Epidemiol. 109*:273–284.

WERTHEIMER, N., AND LEEPER, E. (1982). Adult cancer related to electrical wires near the home. *Int. J. Epidemiol. 11*:345–355.

WEST, D., GLASER, Z., THOMAS, A., et al. (1980). Radiofrequency (RF) sealers and heaters: potential health hazards and their prevention. *Am. Ind. Hyg. Assoc. J. 41*:A22-A38.

WILSON, T.L. (1975). Dielectric heating—a useful industrial tool. Electromagnetic Compatibility Symposium Record, San Antonio, Tex., IEEE 68LG EMC, pp. 333–336.

5

Electrical Properties of Biological Substances

MARIA A. STUCHLY
STANISLAW S. STUCHLY

Interest in the electrical properties of biological substances results from many considerations, on both the fundamental biophysical level and the applied one, as for example in elucidating interaction mechanisms of electromagnetic (EM) fields with biological systems and in medical diagnosis and therapy.

The electrical properties of biological substances have been studied extensively since the beginning of the century, initially at low radiofrequencies (below 100 MHz) and after World War II at microwave frequencies up to 10 GHz. In the 1970s and 1980s the studies also included in vivo measurements of biological tissues.

In this chapter macroscopic properties of biological substances are defined and related to molecular properties followed by descriptions of mathematical models and graphical representations. The data base on electrical properties is reviewed starting with molecules and cells in solutions and continuing with tissues at low frequencies and radio and microwave frequencies. A few specific topics are highlighted, such as in vivo versus in vitro properties, comparison between species, and properties of the tumor tissues.

Because most of the investigations of the electrical properties of biological substances are experimental, a brief review of various experimental techniques is given. Various sample holders for in vivo and in vitro studies are also discussed.

Finally, various physical interaction mechanisms are discussed. These include relaxation phenomena, field-induced forces, and recently postulated nonequilibrium phenomena.

Electrical properties of biological substances and systems have been of great interest since the discovery of the bioelectric effect in early 1800s. Very generally, the properties can be divided into two groups: the active properties, which describe the ability to generate electrical potentials and fields, and the passive properties, which characterize the responses to externally applied electrical stimuli. Only the latter properties are considered in this chapter.

The reasons for interest in the passive electrical properties of biological materials, subsystems, and systems are many and varied. On the fundamental research level, the electrical properties provide an insight into the structure and function of molecules, cells, and subcellular systems and of organized systems, such as tissues. Knowledge of electrical properties is essential to elucidation of interaction mechanisms of EM fields with biological systems. On the applied level, knowledge of electrical properties is needed to assess the rate of the energy absorption (the specific absorption rate, SAR) and its spatial distribution in biological bodies exposed to EM fields. The specific absorption rate is used to quantify the effects of EM fields on various species, including humans. The SAR is considered sufficient in most cases to quantify the effects of the deposition of thermal energy in the biological system, resulting from exposure to EM fields. In cases where the effect depends on the rate of temperature change, the temporal changes of SAR have to be determined.

The SAR and other essential exposure parameters can also be used in defining exposure conditions for nonthermal biological effects, such as calcium efflux (Adey, 1981) or stimulation of bone growth (Watson, 1981). EM dosimetry dealing with theoretical and experimental determination of SAR together with scientific data base on experimentally induced biological effects and epidemiological studies forms a sound basis for an assessment of health hazards from exposure and development of rational protection standards. The situation is more complicated in case of nonthermal interactions, particularly when their mechanisms are not understood.

Knowledge of electrical properties of biological media is also important in medical diagnosis and therapy. Diagnostic applications are cardiography, plethysmography, and cancer detection by microwave radiometry. Therapeutic applications include diathermy, hyperthermia treatment of cancer, and stimulation of bone growth and wound healing.

Investigations of electrical properties of biological substances and systems have been carried out in two cooperative streams. Mathematical models for biological structures and functions have been proposed and experiments to confirm them carried out, and conversely, the experimental data have led to the development of mathematical or physical (equivalent circuit) models. A hypothesis of Bernstein of 1902, that the cell consists of the electrolyte surrounded by a poorly permeable membrane, was confirmed in 1910 by measurements performed by Hoeber and led to development of a complete model by Fricke in 1925 (Cole, 1962; Schwan, 1981a). During the next 10 years many cellular systems were measured and analyzed by Fricke, Cole, and Curtis. Furthermore, Cole (1962) elegantly showed at that time that the electrical properties of cell suspensions and cell membranes can be modeled on the basis of Maxwell's and Rayleigh's mixture theories. In the late 1930s Osswald and Rajewsky measured electrical properties of tissues (Stoy et al., 1982). All the measurements before World War II were performed at frequencies between a few kilohertz and 100 MHz. After the war the frequency range of measurements was extended to lower frequencies and higher frequencies up to about 10 GHz. In that period the monumental contribution by Schwan stands out. Relaxation mechanisms responsible for the electrical behavior were analyzed (Schwan, 1957; Pauly and Schwan, 1966; Foster and Schwan, 1986; Stoy et al., 1982).

By the late 1970s an increased interest in the electrical properties of tissues became evident. In addition to the ever-present interest in these properties for understanding of the basic biophysical interaction mechanisms, this revival of interest can be attributed to the concern about health hazards of exposure to EM fields and to the new applications of these fields in medicine, particularly in cancer therapy and stimulation of bone growth. While most of the previous measurements were done on tissues in vitro, recent advances in measurement techniques have made in vivo measurements feasible (Athey et al., 1982; Burdette et al., 1980; Kraszewski et al., 1982; Stuchly et al., 1982a,b,c). A more detailed history of developments in dielectric spectroscopy are given by Foster and Schwan (1986).

The average electrical properties, as determined by dielectric spectroscopy, account basically for the events taking place under steady-state conditions in equilibrium systems. While these conditions are representative for many molecular biological systems, some of the biological entities may be in nonequilibrium state (Fröhlich, 1980; Illinger, 1982). Only very recently the analytical tools of nonequilibrium thermodynamics have become available (Illinger, 1982), and some hypotheses regarding biological systems have been postulated (Fröhlich, 1980; Adey, 1981). Experimental verification of these and future hypotheses appears to be particularly difficult. Nevertheless, since some of the experimentally observed interactions of EM fields cannot be explained on the basis of available knowledge, the field of electrical properties of biological systems and interaction mechanisms remains open to new theories and experimentation.

In this chapter basic electrical properties of biological substances in equilibrium systems are defined, their microscopic origin is explained, and macroscopic representation is outlined. The data base of electrical properties is summarized, and measurement techniques are briefly described. Well-established interaction mechanisms (for equilibrium systems) and some new proposed theories (nonequilibrium systems) are reviewed.

MACROSCOPIC AND MICROSCOPIC ELECTRICAL PROPERTIES

Macroscopic Properties

The interactions of the electric field with matter is described in terms of the complex permittivity, $\hat{\epsilon}$:

$$\hat{\epsilon} = \epsilon' - j\epsilon'' = D/E \tag{1}$$

where D is the electric flux density, E is the electric field intensity, ϵ' is the dielectric constant, and ϵ'' is the loss factor ($j = \sqrt{-1}$). The dielectric constant ϵ' is a measure of the ability to store electric field energy. The loss factor ϵ'' describes a fraction of energy dissipated in the material per hertz.

The permittivity represents a combined macroscopic effect of various molecular phenomena causing electrical polarization.

Frequently the relative permittivity is used, that is, the permittivity normalized to that of free space (vacuum)

$$\hat{\epsilon}_r = \epsilon'_r - j\epsilon''_r = \frac{\hat{\epsilon}}{\epsilon_0} = \frac{\epsilon'}{\epsilon_0} - j\frac{\epsilon''}{\epsilon_0} \tag{2}$$

where ϵ_0 is the permittivity of the free space, $\epsilon_0 \simeq 8.85 \times 10^{-12}$ f/m.

The loss factor ϵ'' is related to the conductivity of the material σ in the following way:

$$\epsilon''_r = \frac{\sigma}{\omega\epsilon_0} \tag{3}$$

where $\omega = 2\pi f$, and f is the frequency. The unit of conductivity is siemens per meter (S/m). The conductivity σ consists of two terms: the static conductivity resulting from ionic conduction and the conductivity resulting from various polarizabilities.

Frequently a parameter called the loss tangent, tan δ, is used. It is defined as

$$\tan \delta = \frac{\epsilon''}{\epsilon'} = \frac{\sigma}{\omega\epsilon'_r\epsilon_0} \tag{4}$$

A parameter called resistivity ρ is also used (particularly in plethysmography):

$$\rho = 1/\sigma \tag{5}$$

The units of resistivity are ohm-meter (Ω-m) or, more frequently, ohm-centimeter (Ω-cm).

The interaction of materials with the magnetic field is described on the macroscopic level by the permeability. However, most biological substances are nonmagnetic or very weakly diamagnetic and their permeability can be assumed equal to that of vacuum (1.26×10^{-6} H/m). Some bacteria, insects, and some tissues of birds exhibit weak magnetic properties (Adey, 1981).

Molecular Properties

Atoms and molecules respond to an external electric field because they contain charged carriers that are permanently displaced or can be displaced by the field. Matter in general is characterized by four types of polarizability as illustrated in Figure 5-1 (von Hippel, 1954). Application of an external electric field results in a slight displacement of electrons with respect to the nuclei producing electronic polarization. Atoms in molecules normally do not share their electrons symmetrically, since the electrons are displaced toward stronger binding atoms. Thus atoms acquire charges of opposite polarity, and an external field acting on these net charges tends to change the equilibrium positions of the atoms. This displacement of charged atoms or groups of atoms with respect to one another results in the atomic polarization of the dielectric. The asymmetrical charge distribution between the unlike components of a molecule gives rise to permanent dipole moments that exist also in the absence of the external field. Such molecules tend to orient themselves in the direction of the field. Consequently, an orientation (or dipole) polarization arises.

These three mechanisms of polarization, characterized by the electronic polarizability, the atomic polarizability, and the orientation or dipole polarizability, result from charges that are locally bound in atoms, molecules, or structures of solids and liquids. In addition, free-charge

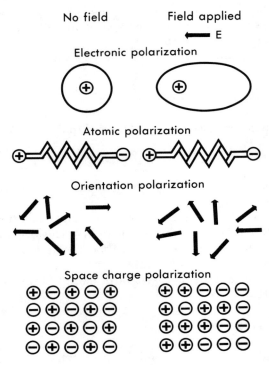

Figure 5-1 Polarization mechanisms. (From von Hippel, 1954.)

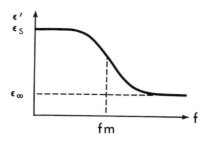

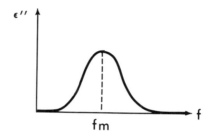

Figure 5-2 Dielectric properties of a material exhibiting a Relaxation frequency f_m.

carriers (ions) that can migrate in the dielectric usually exist. When such carriers are impeded in their motion, either because they become trapped in the material or on interfaces or because they cannot be freely discharged or replaced at the electrodes, space charges and a macroscopic field distortion result. This nonuniform space charge distribution in the dielectric is responsible for a space charge (interfacial) polarization.

Any of the preceding outlined polarization phenomena result in a relaxation-type behavior and in corresponding changes in the permittivity illustrated in Figure 5-2.

For biological materials two polarization mechanisms are of particular importance: the space charge polarization from existence of membranes and ions and dipolar polarization. The relaxation frequencies for electronic and atomic polarization are higher than 300 GHz.

Mathematical and Graphical Representation

The electrical properties of biological materials are frequently represented by electrical equivalent circuits, mathematical formulas, and special graphs. Only the most frequently used representations are briefly discussed here; additional information can be found in Foster and Schwan (1986). A single relaxation process resulting from permanent dipoles can be represented by an electrical circuit consisting of a resistor and two capacitors (von Hippel, 1954), or a membrane behavior described by the

Maxwell-Wagner relaxation can be represented by two resistors and a capacitor (Takashima and Schwan, 1974).

A single relaxation process can be described by the Debye equation

$$\hat{\epsilon} = \epsilon_\infty + \frac{\epsilon_s - \epsilon_\infty}{1 + j\omega\tau} \tag{6}$$

where ϵ_∞ and ϵ_s are the permittivities at frequencies much higher and much lower than the relaxation frequency, respectively, and τ is the relaxation time constant, $\omega = 2\pi f$, in which f is the frequency. The relaxation frequency is equal to

$$f_m = \frac{1}{2\pi\tau} \tag{7}$$

Eq. 6 yields:

$$\epsilon' = \epsilon_\infty + \frac{\epsilon_s - \epsilon_\infty}{1 + (\omega\tau)^2} \tag{8}$$

and

$$\sigma = \sigma_0 + (\sigma_\infty - \sigma_0)\frac{(\omega\tau)^2}{1 + (\omega\tau)^2} \tag{9}$$

where σ_0 and σ_∞ represent contributions not resulting from the relaxation process or to relaxation processes at frequencies far removed from the relaxation frequency (Foster and Schwan, 1986).

The electrical properties that can be described by the Debye equation are represented as a semicircle (the Cole-Cole plot) in the complex plane of ϵ (*dashed circle*, Figure 5-3). Also, the existence of linear relationships between $\hat{\epsilon}'$, and ϵ'' and f/f_m can be demonstrated. These linear relationships and the Cole-Cole plot are useful in analyzing measurements data (Foster and Schwan, 1986).

Many materials, for example, long-chain molecules, or polymers, show a broad distribution of relaxation times. Their behavior is described by the Cole-Cole equation rather than the Debye equation and is represented by a shifted arc in the complex plane as shown in Figure 5-3 (*solid circle*) (Foster and Schwan, 1986).

$$\hat{\epsilon} = \epsilon_\infty + \frac{\epsilon_s - \epsilon_\infty}{1 + (j\omega\tau)^{1-\alpha}} \tag{10}$$

For heterogeneous materials, such as solutions of biological molecules and tissues, mixture theories provide a useful tool for analyzing various component contributions to the dielectric polarization.

For a suspension of spherical particles of complex permittivity $\hat{\epsilon}_p$,

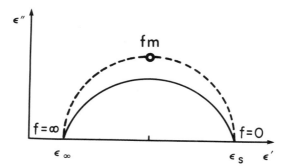

Figure 5-3 Cole-Cole plot for a material having a single relaxation time (*dashed line*) and for material having distribution of relaxation time (*solid line*). f = 0, frequency equal to zero; f = ∞, infinitely high frequency; f_m = relaxation frequency.

in a solvent of complex permittivity $\hat{\epsilon}_w$, the mixture permittivity is (Schwan, 1957):

$$\hat{\epsilon} = \hat{\epsilon}_w \frac{2\hat{\epsilon}_w (1 - p) + \hat{\epsilon}_p (2p + 1)}{\hat{\epsilon}_w (2 + p) + \hat{\epsilon}_p (1 - p)} \tag{11}$$

where p is the volume fraction of the suspension. For nonspherical particles each factor 2 should be replaced by a function of the particle shape (Foster and Schwan, 1986).

ELECTRICAL PROPERTIES OF BIOLOGICAL SUBSTANCES: DATA BASE

Molecules and Cells in Solution

Suspension of biological molecules and cells in solutions have been extensively investigated to infer their structure and electrical properties. The measurement techniques, methods of analysis, and some results are described in detail by Grant et al. (1978), and an analysis of behavior is reviewed by Takashima and Minakata (1975) and Foster et al. (1982).

In studies of aqueous solutions, knowledge of the electrical properties of water is essential. These properties are rather well characterized up to about 12 GHz (Schwan et al., 1976), with some recent data also available at higher frequencies (Grant et al., 1981). The average electrical properties of water in solutions of biological molecules and cells are frequently different from those of free or bulk water. This is because of the water in the immediate vicinity of the molecules, the so-called bound water. Bound water exhibits dielectric relaxation at frequencies between 100 and 1000 MHz at 37° C, depending on the molecule to which water is attached and its viscosity. The static permittivity, ϵ_s, of bound water is close to the static permittivity of free water (Schwan, 1965).

Studies of protein suspensions (Oncley, 1942; Schwan, 1957, 1965; Essex et al., 1977) indicated rotational relaxation of proteins at frequencies between 100 kHz and 50 MHz. Owing to nonspherical shape of the molecules, more than one relaxation time is typical. Protein molecules are highly charged with a nearly equal number of positive and negative charges nearly uniformly distributed on the surface. However, because of large dimensions of the molecules, a relatively small asymmetry in the charge distribution results in a large dipole moment. Typical values of dipole moments are μ = 200 to 1000 Debye units (1 D = 3.33 × 10^{-30} C/m). Dielectric saturation for proteins occurs at the electric field intensities of 10 to 100 kV/cm (Schwan, 1981b).

One thoroughly investigated macromolecule is hemoglobin (Grant and Sheppard, 1974; Schwan, 1965, 1983). Hemoglobin exhibits a distributed-relaxation-time dispersion owing to the polar nature of the molecule at about 2 MHz. The distribution of the relaxation times probably results from molecule-molecule interactions at high concentrations of hemoglobin. A small dispersion between 10 and 100 MHz is a result of the relaxation of polar side chains extending from the molecule surface. Bound water attached to hemoglobin, with an approximate hydration value of 0.2 ± 0.05 g/g of hemoglobin, is responsible for a dispersion at frequencies of about 500 to 1000 MHz.

Investigations of erythrocytes (Bianco et al., 1979; Jenin and Schwan, 1980; Schwan, 1983) indicated β-dispersion at a few megahertz owing to polarization of red blood cell membranes (Maxwell-Wagner relaxation). Erythrocyte water appears to have electrical properties similar if not identical to those of free water (Schwan, 1983).

Peptides and amino acids, being much smaller than proteins, exhibit relaxation at higher frequencies, between 0.5 and 3 GHz. Their dipole moment is a few tens of Debye units.

Investigations of yeast, blood, bacteria, vesicles, synaptosomes, and cellular organelles have contributed to an understanding of the role of cell membranes in the polarization processes (Schwan, 1981b). The essential electrical parameters of the membrane are capacitance and conductance per unit area. For a large number of membranes the unit capacitance is 1 μF/cm^2, remains constant in relation to frequency, and is unaffected by physiological processes. Conductance is 1 to 100 mS/cm^2 and is frequency dependent at low frequencies; for example, for a squid axon membrane, capacitance decreases from 1 to 0.6 μF/cm^2 and conductance increases from 1.2 to 40 mS/cm^2 for frequencies between 1 and 50 kHz (Takashima and Schwan, 1974).

The membranes separate regions of different dielectric properties, so that charged interfaces are formed and Maxwell-Wagner relaxation takes place. This is called β-dispersion and typically occurs at a few tens of kilohertz to a few hundred megahertz (Foster and Schwan, 1986).

Tissues: Low-Frequency Data

Data on the specific resistance of various tissues were summarized by Geddes and Baker (1967), and data on dielectric constant and specific resistivity were recently reviewed by Foster and Schwan (1986).

At low (audio) frequencies a strong dispersion phenomenon called α-dispersion is observed. Many tissues, for example, muscle, have anisotropic properties at low frequencies because of directional arrangement of fibers, and the resistivities may differ by a factor of a few depending on the fiber orientation (Foster and Schwan, 1986). Recently the dielectric constant and conductivity of skeletal muscle were measured at frequencies from 20 Hz to 1 MHz for the fiber orientation perpendicular and parallel to the electric field (Epstein and Foster, 1983). The properties were found to be anisotropic. The conductivity and the dielectric constant are greater for the parallel fibers than for the perpendicular fibers.

Nonlinear properties of tissues, that is, the dependence of their electrical properties on the density of the current passed through them, have also been investigated. Sekeletal muscle has linear properties at frequencies from 10 Hz to 10 kHz for a current density below 2 mA/cm^2 (Schwan and Kay, 1956). The specific resistivity of skin depends on the current density of about 10 to 100 μA/cm^2 depending on frequency and species (Yamamoto and Yamamoto, 1981). The current density limit is lower and the variations are greater at lower frequencies (below 10 Hz). Ionic conduction in the keratin layer is suggested to be responsible for the nonlinearity. Sweat pores, in species that have them, can also contribute significantly to the nonlinearity.

Tissues: Radiofrequency and Microwave Data

Tables 5-1 and 5-2 give references where the most recent detailed data on the electrical properties of tissues in vitro and in vivo at radio and microwave frequencies can be found. Numerous other data can be found in other publications (Stuchly and Stuchly, 1980a; Stoy et al. 1982; Foster and Schwan, 1986). Very few data are available on the electrical properties of tissues at frequencies above 10 GHz. Representative ranges of values of the dielectric constant and conductivity are given in Tables 5-3 and 5-4, respectively. These data indicate two major relaxation phenomena, β and γ, with a small δ relaxation. The β-dispersion with a broad distribution of relaxation times takes place at a few tens of kilohertz to a few megahertz. The γ-dispersion occurs at about 20 GHz, the same as the relaxation frequency of free water. The δ-dispersion results from

TABLE 5-1   Tissue Permittivity In Vitro

Species	Tissue	Frequency range	Reference
Giant barnacle	Muscle	0.01–17 GHz	Foster et al. (1980)
Dog	Brain	0.1–100 MHz	Stoy et al. (1982)
	Brain	0.01–10 GHz	Foster et al. (1979)
	Brain	0.14–4 GHz	Nightingale et al. (1980)
	Kidney	0.1–10 GHz	Burdette et al (1980)
	Skeletal muscle	0.1–100 MHz	
	Spleen	0.1–100 MHz	Stoy et al. (1982)
	Pancreas	0.1–100 MHz	
	Liver	0.1–100 MHz)	
Cat	Skeletal muscle	10 kHz–8 GHz	
	Spleen	10 kHz–8 GHz	Kraszewski et al. (1982)
	Kidney	10 kHz–8 GHz	Surowiec et al. (1986a)
	Liver	10 kHz–8 GHz	
	Brain	10 kHz–8 GHz	
Rat	Bone	10 Hz–100 MHz	Kosterich et al. (1983, 1984)
	Skeletal muscle	0.1–100 MHz	Stoy et al. (1982)
	Skeletal muscle	40–90 GHz	Edrich and Hardee (1976)
Mouse	Brain	0.07–5 GHz	Thurai et al. (1984)
Rabbit	Brain	1–18 GHz	Steel and Sheppard (1985)
	Liver	0.1–100 MHz	Stoy et al. (1982)
	Lens	0.1–6 GHz	Dawkins et al. (1981a)
		0.01–10 GHz	Gabriel et al. (1983) and Gabriel and Grant (1985)
		2–18 GHz	Steel and Sheppard (1986)
	Bone marrow	1 kHz–1 GHz	Smith and Foster (1985)
	Bone	1 kHz–1 MHz	Reddy and Saha (1984)
Cow	Fat	40–90 GHz	Edrich and Hardee (1976)
	Fat	1 kHz–1 GHz	Smith and Foster (1985)
	Liver	0.02–100 MHz	
	Kidney	0.02–100 MHz	Surowiec et al. (1985)
	Spleen	0.02–100 MHz	
	Brain	0.02–100 MHz	Surowiec et al. (1986b)
Human	Lens	0.1–16 GHz	Dawkins et al. (1981a)
	Skin	0.01–10 GHz	Gabriel et al. (1987)
	Breast	0.02–100 MHz	Surowiec et al. (1988)

TABLE 5-2   Tissue Permittivity In Vivo

Species	Tissue	Frequency range	Reference
Dog	Skeletal muscle	0.1–10 GHz	Burdette et al. (1980)
	Fat	0.1–10 GHz	
	Kidney	0.1–10 GHz	
Cat	Muscle	10 kHz–8 GHz	Kraszewski et al. (1982)
	Brain	10 kHz–8 GHz	Stuchley et al. (1982a,b)
	Liver	10 kHz–8 GHz	
	Kidney	10 kHz–8 GHz	Surowiec et al. (1986a,b)
	Spleen	10 kHz–8 GHz	
	Lung	0.01–100 MHz	Surowiec et al. (1987)
Rat	Skeletal muscle	0.1–10 GHz	Stuchly et al. (1982c)
	Brain	0.1–10 GHz	
	Spleen	0.1–10 GHz	
	Liver	0.1–10 GHz	
Human	Skin	8–18 GHz	Hey-Shipton et al. (1982)

bound water. In some tissues, for example, skeletal muscle (Schwan and Foster, 1977; Foster et al, 1980), water appears to be mostly in the free state. Other tissues contain a significant amount of water (10% to 20%) in bound state (Stuchly et al., 1982c).

In Vivo Versus In Vitro Tissue Properties

The electrical properties of tissues in situ, freshly excised and some time after death, are expected to be different. The most profound differences result from breakdown of cellular structure and cell membrane function (Foster and Schwan, 1986). These occurrences result in the redistribution of intracellular and extracellular ions. Additionally, tissue excision or death can result in loss of blood and water. The greatest differences between in vivo and in vitro properties and the fastest change after excision are at low frequencies in the range of the α-dispersion. These changes in tissue properties are due to change in metabolic activity and ionic milieu of the cells. Pronounced changes can be observed within hours (Schwan, 1957). The changes in the electrical properties in the β-dispersion region are slower, since the rate of change depends on the rate of disintegration of cell membranes (Schwan, 1957; Surowiec et al., 1985, 1986b). At high frequencies (microwave range) the differences between the in vivo and in vitro properties result mostly from blood and water content variations (Schwan, 1957).

More recently, measurements of bone properties indicated that the

TABLE 5-3 Dielectric Constant at 37° C of Various Tissues at Radio and Microwave Frequencies

Tissue	Frequency						
	100 kHz	1 MHz	10 MHz	100 MHz	1 GHz	10 GHz
Skeletal muscle	$(14.4-24.8) \times 10^3$	$(1.9-2.5) \times 10^3$	162–204	64–90	57–59	43–45
Liver	$(9.8-13.7) \times 10^3$	1.97×10^3	251–338	65–82	47–49	35
Spleen	3.3×10^3	1.45×10^3	321–410	69–101	50–55	41
Kidney	$(10.9-12.5) \times 10^3$	$(2.39-2.69) \times 10^3$	190–204	66–95	42–50	40
Brain	$(1.96-3.8) \times 10^3$	$(0.54-1.25) \times 10^3$	163–352	57–90	37–55	38–44
Bone	280	87	37	23		

TABLE 5-4 Conductivity at 37° C of Various Tissues at Radio and Microwave Frequencies in Siemens per Meter

Tissue	Frequency					
	100 kHz	1 MHz	10 MHz	100 MHz	1 GHz	10 GHz
Skeletal muscle	0.38–0.59	0.58–0.85	0.69–0.96	0.75–1.05	1.38–1.45	11.5
Liver	0.15–0.16	0.27–0.3	0.42–0.47	0.6–0.72	0.95–1.1	8.9
Spleen	0.62	0.63	0.5–0.84	0.73–1.05	1.09–11.3	10.1
Kidney	0.24–0.25	0.36–0.37	0.50–0.68	0.66–1.05	0.95–1.0	9.7
Brain	0.12–0.17	0.14–0.21	0.21–0.63	0.48–0.95	0.81–1.2	8–10.8
Bone	0.014	0.017	0.024	0.057		

low-frequency conductivity of freshly excised bone increases by 5% to 15% over a 50-hour period (Kosterich et al., 1983).

Dielectric properties in vivo and in vitro at radiofrequencies (10 kHz to 100 MHz) and microwave frequencies (100 MHz to 8 GHz) were recently measured and compared (Kraszewski et al., 1982; Surowiec et al., 1986a). Differences between in vivo and in vitro properties were observed at frequencies below 100 MHz (Surowiec et al., 1986a). Furthermore, the differences increase as a function of time after animal death or tissue excision (Surowiec et al., 1985, 1986b). At frequencies greater than 100 MHz the dielectric constant and the conductivity of all the tissues in vitro, when measured a few hours after the animal's death, were found to be the same as those in vivo, within the measurement uncertainty limits (less than 3%) (Kraszewski et al., 1982). In view of the previous discussion, the lack of significant difference between the dielectric properties in vitro and in vivo at frequencies greater than 100 MHz is not surprising.

Comparison between Species

The general behavior of the electrical properties as a function of frequency is the same in various tissues for different species. Illustration is given in Figures 5-4 and 5-5 (Stuchly et al., 1982c). The differences in the electrical properties are rather small (not more than 15%) and in this frequency range can be attributed to different water content. This conclusion applies only to mammalian tissues of nonaquatic species.

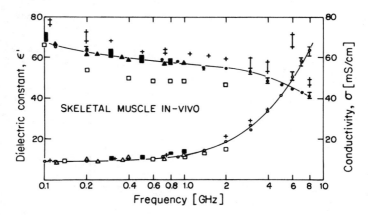

Figure 5-4 Dielectric constant and conductivity of skeletal muscle tissue. ●○, Cat, $T = 34 \pm 0.5°$ C (Stuchly et al., 1982c); ▲△, rat, $T = 34 \pm 0.5°$ C (Stuchly et al., 1982c); ■, cat, $T = 31 \pm 0.5°$ C (Stuchly et al, 1981); +, rat, $T = 31°$ C (Burdette et al., 1980); □, dog, $T = 34°$ C (Burdette et al., 1980). Bars indicate estimated uncertainty of measurements.

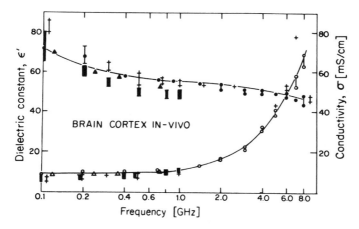

Figure 5-5 Dielectric constant and conductivity of brain cortex tissue. ●○, Cat, $T = 35 \pm 1°$ C (Stuchly et al., 1982c); ▲△, rat, $T = 35 \pm 1°$ C (Stuchly et al., 1982c); ■, cat, $T = 33 \pm 0.5°$ C (Stuchly et al., 1981); +, rat, $T = 32°$ C (Burdette et al., 1980). Bars indicate estimated uncertainty of measurements.

For the same species, dielectric properties of some tissues, such as brain, change as the animal grows into maturity (Thurai et al., 1984).

Tumor Tissues

Knowledge of the differences in the permittivity of cancerous and healthy tissues of the same type is essential if EM techniques are to be applied to the detection and treatment of tumors. Studies of the properties of tumor tissues (Schepps and Foster, 1980; Foster and Schepps, 1981; Rogers et al., 1983; Surowiec et al., 1988) indicate that the dielectric constant and conductivity of many tumors are greater than those of the surrounding healthy tissue. The differences vary with frequency. Similarly, many lung tumors have dielectric properties close to those of high-water-content tissues, such as muscle, rather than the low values representative for healthy lung tissue. However, properties of some other tumors are not significantly different from the properties of the healthy tissue, for example, adenocarcinoma. For human breast tissue the dielectric properties of the apparently healthy tissue adjacent to the tumor are considerably different from those of healthy breast tissue at frequencies from 20 kHz to 100 MHz (Surowiec et al., 1988).

Analysis of the permittivity data for normal and tumor tissues at frequencies between 10 MHz and 17 GHz (Schepps and Foster, 1980; Foster and Schepps, 1981) indicate that many tumors contain, on the average, 83% water (ranging between 80% and 92%), while normal high-water-content tissues contain, on the average, 75% water (for example, skeletal muscle 79.5%, brain white matter 74%, gray matter 84%). For this reason the dielectric constant is usually higher (by about 25%) than that of the normal tissue. More important, the difference in the conductivities is even greater.

EXPERIMENTAL TECHNIQUES

General Considerations

Experimental methods for measuring electrical properties of biological tissues have several common features, as outlined here. At lower frequencies (f ≤100 MHz) a quasistatic approach to the design of a sample holder is generally justified. At these frequencies the sample holder usually consists of a parallel-plate or coaxial capacitor whose impedance is measured with and without the sample by means of appropriate bridges, vector voltmeters, Q-meters, or network analyzers. Both time and frequency domain techniques are used. At frequencies above 1 GHz the wave character of the studied phenomena has to be taken into account. The sample is normally placed in a coaxial line or waveguide rather than in a capacitor, and properties of reflected or transmitted waves are measured as they are related to the dielectric properties of the test material. At frequencies above approximately 40 GHz, free space quasioptical techniques are also used. As at low frequencies, both time and frequency domain techniques are used.

Great progress has recently been made in frequency-domain measurements because of the introduction of ultrastable synthesized signal sources and very sensitive, low-noise, field-effect transistor (FET) based receivers and the proliferation of low-cost microcomputers and minicomputers, which are used for on-line experiment control, calibration, and data processing. Owing to these developments the uncertainty of measurements of the dielectric constant and the conductivity decreased to less than 1% at most frequencies, and further improvements are likely.

Well-known impedance measurement techniques must be modified to suit biological substances for accurate results. The investigation of dielectric dispersion phenomena can be carried out in both time and frequency domain by means of transient and steady-state methods, respectively. The two approaches are equivalent, and for linear systems the transformation of observed data from either of these domains into the other is rather straightforward.

Low Radiofrequency Measurement Techniques

Electrode polarization makes low-frequency (less than 100 kHz) dielectric measurements of biological samples difficult. Two opposing requirements must be balanced. A large electrode separation is desirable to minimize the effect of electrode polarization, but such a large separation leads to uncontrolled stray fields affecting the accuracy of the dielectric constant measurements (capacitance of the sample holder) and to a lesser degree the conductivity (conductance) (Schwan and Li, 1953; Schwan, 1964).

Electrode polarization is one of the major sources of error in measurements of biological substances, and this is particularly pronounced at frequencies less than 100 kHz. When a metal electrode comes in contact with an ionic solution, a DC-boundary potential arises between them. When an alternating current passes through the boundary, this DC potential is modulated and the resulting effect of electrode polarization can be represented as a series combination of resistance and capacitance, which are functions of frequency (Schwan, 1964; Geddes, 1972). The capacitance changes with $f^{-0.3}$ to $f^{-0.5}$, and the resistance varies with $f^{-0.5}$ in the frequency range from 10 Hz to 1 MHz. Details regarding selection of the metal and preparation of the electrode can be found in Geddes (1972). Sandblasted platinum black electrodes have been found to have the highest capacitance and therefore the lowest series impedance. In practice the effects of electrode polarization can be minimized by using properly prepared platinum black electrodes, whose polarization impedance can be determined experimentally by using a known ionic solution and applying appropriate correction factors (Schwan, 1964).

A typical low-frequency sample holder for biological work consists of a parallel-plate capacitor with variable electrode separation surrounded by a temperature-control chamber (van der Touw et al., 1975a). At frequencies less than 100 MHz, commercially available measuring bridges, vector voltmeters, and network analyzers are used to determine the input impedance of the sample holder. Significant improvements have recently been introduced in the design of both the sample holders and the associated bridge circuitry (van der Touw et al., 1975b). At frequencies greater than 1 MHz a coaxial cell with variable height has been used (van Beek et al., 1985), and with changes in the sample length, some measurement errors, particularly electrode polarization effects, can be eliminated.

A large body of work exists on use of transient techniques to measure dielectrics at low and extremely low frequencies. Kent (1980) reviewed time-domain techniques at low frequencies and applied these techniques in a frequency range of 20 Hz to 10 kHz. An attempt to use time-domain techniques for in vivo studies of biological tissues in a frequency range 0.1 to 100 kHz has also been reported (Singh et al., 1979).

Radio and Microwave Measurement Techniques

Time-domain techniques.   The term "time-domain spectroscopy" (TDS) is used to describe experimental techniques for determining the permittivity $\hat{\epsilon}(\omega)$ from measurements performed in the time domain. Originally employed at low frequencies in the 1950s, it has expanded toward higher frequencies. At present the TDS methods cover the frequency range from a fraction of a hertz to approximately 15 GHz (Nicolson and Ross, 1970; Iskander and Stuchly, 1972; van Gemert and Suggett, 1975; Cole, 1975; Dawkins et al., 1979, 1981b, 1981c; Boned and Peycelasse, 1982).

A block diagram of a typical TDS system is shown in Figure 5-6. In all TDS methods a fast rise time step voltage is propagated in a low-loss coaxial line and the signals reflected by or transmitted through a test sample placed in the coaxial line are monitored by a sampler connected to a sampling oscilloscope.

The propagation of EM waves in a coaxial transmission line is described by two characteristic parameters: the propagation constant $\gamma(\omega)$ and the characteristic impedance $Z(\omega)$. For a coaxial line of negligible conductor loss filled with the test sample of the permittivity $\hat{\epsilon}(\omega)$:

$$Z(\omega) = \frac{Z_0}{\sqrt{\hat{\epsilon}(\omega)}} \tag{13}$$

$$\gamma(\omega) = \gamma_0 \sqrt{\hat{\epsilon}(\omega)} \tag{14}$$

where Z_0 and γ_0 are the characteristic impedance and the propagation constant of the air-filled line, respectively.

The reflection and transmission coefficients of a section filled with the test sample are given by:

$$\Gamma(\omega) = \frac{Z(\omega) - Z_0}{Z(\omega) + Z_0} \tag{15}$$

$$T(\omega) = \frac{2Z(\omega)}{Z(\omega) + Z_0} \tag{16}$$

These coefficients can be obtained from the measured reflected and transmitted signals in the time domain by means of Fourier transforms.

The time window used may be either very short to encompass only the first reflection from the air-dielectric interface or long enough to take in essentially all the successive reflections including those from the section behind the sample.

Frequency-domain techniques.   The term "frequency-domain spectroscopy" (FDS) is associated with experimental techniques for determining the permittivity $\hat{\epsilon}(\omega)$ from measurements performed in the frequency domain by means of a selected monochromatic signal. Since the beginning of the century the FDS has been used in a variety of configurations and with a multitude of sample holders. It has undergone a rapid develop-

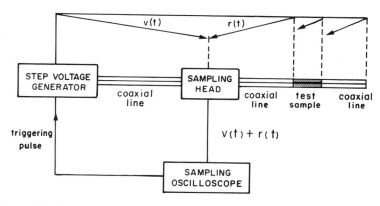

Figure 5-6   Basic diagram of time-domain spectroscopy. v(t), transmitted wave; r(t), reflected wave.

ment with the introduction of the automatic network analyzer, which is capable of accurate measurements of transmission and reflection coefficients in a wide band of frequencies, typically from a few hertz to 100 GHz.

A block diagram of an automatic computer-based network analyzer system is shown in Figure 5-7. Even higher accuracy and convenience of measurements are obtained when most recent network analyzers, such as model no. HP8510B or HP3577, are used. The reflection or transmission

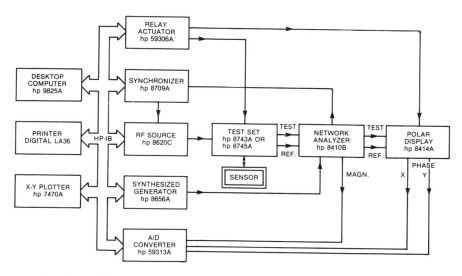

Figure 5-7   Block diagram of automatic computer-controlled network analyzer system for measuring permittivity.

coefficient is measured by comparing the amplitudes and phases of the reflected and transmitted waves with those of the incident wave by means of a calibrated superheterodyne receiver. The permittivity of the sample, usually placed in a coaxial line or waveguide sample holder, is then calculated from Eqs. 13 and 14.

A modern FDS technique we developed for measuring the in vivo permittivity of biological tissues in the frequency range from 10 MHz to 10 GHz illustrates a frequency-domain method.

The measurement system was based on the model no. HP8407 and HP8410 network analyzers and consists of a sensor and a computer-controlled network analyzer. The sensor translates changes in the permittivity of a test sample into changes in the input reflection coefficient of the sensor. These impedances are then measured by the network analyzer. An open coaxial line, placed in contact with the test sample (Figure 5-8), is used as a sensor. The sample must be homogeneous within a sufficiently large volume to approximate a slab that is electrically infinite in size. The equivalent circuit of the sensor consists of two elements (Figure 5-8, B): a lossy capacitor ($C[\hat{\epsilon}] = \hat{\epsilon}C_0$, where C_0 is the capacitance when the line is in air) and a capacitor C_f, which accounts for the fringing field in the Teflon. This equivalent circuit is valid at frequencies where the dimensions of the line are small compared with the wavelength so that the open end of the line is not radiating and all the energy is concentrated in the fringe or reactive near field of the line. At higher frequencies the value of the capacitance C_0 increases with frequency (Kraszewski et al., 1983b), owing to the increase in the evanescent TM modes being excited at the junction discontinuity. When the evanescent modes are taken into account, an expression $C_0 + Af^2$, where A is a constant depen-

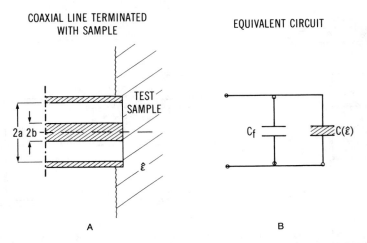

Figure 5-8   Open-ended coaxial line sensor. **A,** Geometry. **B,** Equivalent circuit.

dent on the line dimensions, should be used instead of C_0. Recent calculations (Grant et al., 1986) indicate that radiation of the open-ended sensor becomes significant at frequencies greater than 3 GHz (for the 3 mm line), particularly when the sensor is in contact with a test sample with high dielectric constant, and such contact is almost always the case in studies of biological materials. A more detailed, although incomplete, analysis of the open-ended coaxial line has been presented by Mosig et al. (1981). When the frequencies are sufficiently low that the equivalent circuit of Figure 5-8, B, is applicable, the input reflection coefficient at the plane of the discontinuity can be calculated from:

$$\hat{\Gamma} = \Gamma e^{j\phi} = \frac{1 - j\omega Z_0[C(\hat{\epsilon}) + C_f]}{1 + j\omega Z_0[C(\hat{\epsilon}) + C_f]} \tag{17}$$

Solving for the permittivity we get:

$$\hat{\epsilon} = \frac{(1 - \hat{\Gamma})}{j\omega Z_0 C_0(1 + \hat{\Gamma})} - \frac{C_f}{C_0} \tag{18}$$

It has been shown (Stuchly et al., 1974; Rzepecka and Stuchly, 1975) that the greatest accuracy in determining the permittivity of materials having tan $\delta < 1$ and for a given accuracy of the reflection coefficient measurement is obtained when:

$$C_0 = \frac{1}{\omega Z_0 \sqrt{\epsilon'^2 + \epsilon''^2}} \tag{19}$$

This expression holds strictly only when the uncertainties in the magnitude and phase of the reflection coefficient are approximately the same, that is, $\Delta\phi \simeq \Delta\Gamma/\Gamma$. In other cases this is still a good compromise because the optimum C_0 is different for ϵ' and ϵ'', these values being smaller and larger or vice versa than the value given by Eq. 19.

The total capacitance in air, $C_T = C_0 + C_f$, is a function of the line dimensions, the permittivity of the dielectric filling the line, and the frequency. The capacitance C_T was calculated analytically (Gajda and Stuchly, 1983) and also determined experimentally (Kraszewski and Stuchly, 1983).

The following criteria for the probe selection should be considered: the optimum capacitance condition; size, especially for in vivo measurements; compatibility with liquid, semiliquid, and solid samples; and range of operating frequencies.

Approximate values of the optimum capacitance, calculated from Eq. 19, for several biological substances and reference materials are given in Table 5-5. The total capacitance C_T values for a few commercially available coaxial lines are listed in Table 5-6.

From a comparison of the values presented in Tables 5-5 and 5-6

TABLE 5-5 Optimum Capacitance for an Open-Ended Coaxial Line Probe in pF

Material	Frequency (GHz)						
	0.01	0.05	0.1	0.5	1.0	5.0	10
Muscle, 37° C	0.25	0.25	0.25	0.08	0.035	0.017	0.007
Fat, 37° C	0.8	0.8	0.8	0.45	0.23	0.16	0.08
Water, 25° C	4	0.8	0.2	0.08	0.04	0.01	0.005
0.02N NaCl, 25° C	0.37	0.37	0.37	0.08	0.04	0.01	0.005
0.08N NaCl, 25° C	0.19	0.19	0.19	0.08	0.04	0.01	0.005
0.25N NaCl, 25° C	0.08	0.07	0.07	0.055	0.035	0.01	0.005

TABLE 5-6   Capacitance of Open Coaxial Lines

Line	a(mm)	b(mm)	$C_{T(pF)}$
14 mm, air	7.15	3.10	0.14
7 mm, air	3.50	1.52	0.075
8.3 mm, Teflon	3.62	1.12	0.055
6.4 mm, Teflon	2.66	0.815	0.040
3.6 mm, Teflon	1.50	0.456	0.023
2.2 mm, Teflon	0.836	0.256	0.013

it is evident that smaller Teflon lines, when used as probes, offer nearly optimum measurement conditions for high-water-content tissues, such as muscle, brain, liver, and kidney, at higher frequencies (0.5 to 2 GHz). However, at lower frequencies and for low-moisture-content tissues, special sensors are required. Such sensors have recently been developed (Stuchly et al., 1986; Esselle and Stuchly, 1988).

Selection of sensor dimensions and configuration to satisfy the optimum capacitance condition for a given dielectric material is important if measurement accuracy is required. In measurements of biological tissues, a compromise between the line diameter and configuration and the optimum capacitance has to be achieved.

Other sample holders.   The majority of present-day radiowave and microwave sample holders for studies of biological materials are based on a standard coaxial line equipped with a standard connector, a 7 mm rigid 50-ohm coaxial line and an APC-7 precision connector being most popular.

Available sample holders can be classified as two port and single port. In the two-port sample holder used in transmission measurements, the sample usually fills the space between inner and outer conductors of a coaxial line, while two dielectric low reflection beads are used to confine the sample to a required length (Cole, 1975; van Gemert and Suggett, 1975). However, most dielectric studies of biological materials are performed in single-port, reflection-type sample holders. A comprehensive review of the available configurations has been published (Stuchly and Stuchly, 1980b). Variations of the sample holder consisting of a section of a coaxial line filled with the test sample have been reported for reflection measurements by several authors (Cole, 1975; Stuchly et al., 1978; Schepps and Foster, 1980). An advanced design of a traveling-wave, single-port sample holder has also been reported (Szwarnowski and Sheppard, 1979; Szwarnowski, 1982). Shielded open-ended coaxial sample holders proposed by Cole (1975) and Giese and Tiemann (1975) have been successfully used for liquids by Bianco et al. (1980) and for granular

materials by Bussey (1980). A detailed error analysis for this method
has also been reported (Scott and Smith, 1986).

Finally, the open-ended coaxial lines described before have been
used for in vivo studies of biological materials (Westhphal, 1954; Tanabe
and Joines, 1976; Burdette et al., 1980; Stuchly et al., 1982a, 1982c).

Approximate mathematical analysis of the coaxial sample holders
is available for the majority of configurations currently used (Stuchly
and Stuchly, 1980a). Analytical expressions linking the permittivity of
the test sample and the measured parameters of the sample holder (transmission or reflection coefficients) exist in most cases. This, in principle,
permits evaluation of the relative uncertainty of permittivity measurements for a given uncertainty in the transmission or reflection measurements, whether performed in the frequency or time domain.

INTERACTION MECHANISMS

General Considerations

Passive electrical properties of biological entities, as described previously, have been extensively investigated and have proved essential in
elucidating mechanisms of interaction of EM fields with biological systems. Various relaxation phenomena resulting from nonuniform spatial
distribution of electrical charges within components or subsystems of
biological bodies have been identified. These properties provide reliable
and efficient tools in explaining and quantifying numerous interactions
of EM fields with living matter.

Until fairly recently, debate concentrated on divisions of biological
effects of EM fields into thermal and nonthermal on the basis of measurable whole-body or partial-body temperature increases. This division is
not a reliable criterion for at least two reasons. Living biological systems
are equipped with abilities to compensate for thermal loading. This property of course may result in biological effects, but no temperature increases. The other factor is a limited ability to measure the spatial temperature changes in living systems. A more appropriate division into
thermal and nonthermal effects can be based on whether the effect is
resulting from heating because of exposure to EM energy or because of
direct interactions. It is essential to realize that biological effects of heating
by EM energy can be profoundly different from effects caused by other
means of thermal loading. Exposure to EM fields results in a highly
nonuniform energy deposition within biological bodies. Furthermore, the
rate of the energy deposition can be very high, resulting in rapid temperature increases, particularly in the case of pulse-modulated fields. However,
some effects have been shown to be directly related to the field interactions,

for example, field-induced forces, and the accurate interaction mechanism for other effects remains an open subject of investigation.

Very weak fields at specific frequencies (in the extremely low-frequency [ELF] range, or other frequencies modulated at ELF) have been shown to interact with biological systems (for a review see Adey, 1981, or Chapters 9 and 10 of this book). The character of the interactions, namely the very low rate of energy deposition, specific sensitivity to the modulation frequency, and intensity of the field, practically preclude explanation by classical biophysics as related to thermal equilibrium processes. Since biological systems or at least some processes are known to be in nonequilibrium, explanation of these effects has been sought on the basis of nonequilibrium thermodynamics. The initial stimulus provided by the impressed EM field is amplified in the biological system to elicit specific responses. Various theories of interactions have been proposed in recent years. Amplification of stimuli in biological systems is well established in biochemical events, for example, enzymic reactions (Goldbeter and Koshland, 1982).

The following brief review describes the well-established interaction mechanisms resulting from relaxation processes and field-induced forces and of interaction mechanisms currently under investigation, such as piezoelectricity and nonequilibrium phenomena.

Relaxation Phenomena

Biological tissues as described earlier exhibit three strong relaxation phenomena (the α-, β-, and γ-dispersions) and one weak (the δ-dispersion). The molecular phenomena responsible for the α-dispersion are the least understood (Schwan, 1981a,b). Intracellular structures, for example, the tubular apparatus in muscle cells, relaxational behavior of membranes themselves and relaxation of counterions about the charged cellular structure, all may contribute to this dispersion to varying degrees. The β-dispersion results mostly from a nonhomogeneous structure, the resulting interfacial polarization causing the Maxwell-Wagner type of relaxation. Smaller contributions result from relaxation of proteins. The γ-dispersion results from free water relaxation, and the δ-dispersion results from relaxation of bound water, amino acids, and charged side groups of proteins (Foster and Schwan, 1986).

All relaxation phenomena lead to conversion of EM energy of the interaction field into thermal energy. The thermal energy is then responsible for various biological responses. The amount of energy dissipated at any location of a biological body depends on the intensity of the electric field at that location and the tissue conductivity. Biological responses to electromagnetically induced thermal stimuli can be significantly different from responses to other thermal stimuli.

Field-Induced Forces

High-intensity electric fields can interact with nonpolar biological molecules and cells through ponderomotoric forces. Effects that can be observed in alternating fields include pearl chain formation, directional orientation, dielectrophoresis (movement of particles in nonhomogeneous fields), cell deformation, cell destruction, cell fusion, and cell rotation (Schwan, 1982).

Pearl chain formation is the alignment of particles into chainlike structures in a direct or alternating current (DC or AC) electric field. The alignment results from field-induced dipole moments. Pearl chains are formed only above a certain threshold intensity of the electric field. This threshold intensity depends on the particle size and ranges from 8 V/m in situ for a particle radius of 100 μm to 8 kV/m for a radius of 1 μm (Schwan, 1982).

Nonspherical particles are oriented in an electric field of a sufficient intensity according to their induced moments and the general tendency to minimize their potential energy. The threshold field intensity is estimated to be 2 or 3 times lower than that for pearl chain formation (Schwan, 1982).

Cell destruction occurs when the induced membrane potential reaches the dielectric breakdown level. This level is about 0.1 to 1 V across the membrane, that is, the required in situ field intensities are about 10^4 to 10^6 V/m in situ depending on the membrane thickness.

Nonequilibrium Phenomena

Numerous interactions of EM waves with biological systems can be interpreted on the basis of the complex permittivity and permeability of the systems. Some recent experimental results have stimulated interest in other avenues toward their explanation. A few theories have been postulated that assume nonlinear interactions in systems in thermal nonequilibrium. None of the theories has, however, been cohesively supported by experimental evidence.

Experimental evidence (discussed in Adey, 1981, and other chapters of this book indicates that weak EM fields can interact with biological systems in ways that can be explained only in terms of nonlinear, nonequilibrium phenomena. Several general theories of nonlinear interactions of EM waves with biological systems in nonequilibrium states have been proposed. Although experiments indicate that such interactions indeed occur, the exact mechanisms involved have yet to be elucidated. Any of the theories or a combination of some of them may prove applicable. They may, after further development, be capable of explaining the interactions not only in very general qualitative terms, but also in more precise quantitative terms. A brief review of interaction mechanisms currently considered possible follows. More comprehensive information can be found in Adey (1981), Fröhlich, (1980), and Illinger (1982). Not only can externally imposed EM fields interact with biological functions, but weak intrinsic EM fields also appear to control numerous phenomena in living organisms.

Fröhlich (1980) has developed a theory of long-range coherent vibrations in biological systems. Oscillations of biological membranes or their sections with displacement perpendicular to the surface correspond to vibrating electric dipoles. Oscillations of individual proteins within the membrane may also be treated as oscillating dipoles. Furthermore, electric vibrations may arise from the plasma modes of unattached electrons. The interactions of the oscillating systems can be considered as bands of modes as in solid-state physics. Some of these modes extend spatially over relatively large regions; others are restricted to the surroundings of certain molecules. Energy may be supplied to the modes of a band of electric polarization waves by metabolic processes. A small but critical additional amount for triggering strong excitations is supplied by EM energy. The frequencies expected for the coherent vibrations can be calculated on the basis of the size and elastic properties of the system. The frequencies have been estimated as 10^{10} to 10^{11} Hz for membranes, 10^{12} to 10^{14} Hz for proteins, and 10^9 Hz for DNA or RNA. Owing to large sizes of the individual systems and interactions between the systems, mode softening may shift the bands into much lower frequencies.

Another interaction mechanism postulated by Fröhlich (1980) involves metastable highly polar states. The electrical energy state of a weakly polarized material depends on the polarizability and shape. Deformation leads to a change in the electrical energy, and, conversely, polarization of the material causes its deformation. From considerations of the total energy of such material, consisting of elastic and electrical energy, it can be shown that under certain conditions the minimum energy state corresponds to a highly polarized state that is stable only against small displacements (a metastable state). If a large molecule, such as a protein, possesses a metastable state, and if that molecule is embedded in a membrane, the molecule becomes exposed to the membrane field and its metastable state becomes stable. A different situation arises when the molecule in the metastable state is in an ionic solution. The small ions of the solution surround and screen the molecule within a very short range, stabilizing the metastable state. This system is then not involved in long-range interactions, but the forces exerted by the molecule on ions may be important in reducing activation energies in enzymatic reactions.

The Fröhlich model of coherent excitations is hypothesized also to account for the documented interactions at extremely low frequencies

(1 to 100 Hz) (Fröhlich, 1980). Coherent vibrations in enzymes and sub-strates may lead to long-range interaction and oscillation of collective enzymatic processes at a frequency determined by the rate of spontaneous recombination of an activated enzyme and the rate of long-range attraction of substrates. None of these rates is known at present, but theoretically they could lead to the frequencies of interaction observed experimentally. Similarly, as previously formulated, the main energy supply to the oscilla-tions is provided by the relevant collective chemical processes, with EM energy playing only the role of a trigger. This is not inconsistent with sensitivity amplification in enzymatic processes (Goldbeter and Koshland, 1982).

Experimental studies of the effects of weak ELF fields (0.1 to 300 Hz) and ELF-modulated radio waves and microwaves point at membranes as primary interaction sites. Although a typical transmembrane electrical gradient is about 10^7 V/m and a typical shift resulting from release of the neural transmitter is about 10^5 V/m, fields as low as EEG gradients, that is, about 5 V/m or even less, are capable of interaction under specific conditions. Two nonequilibrium types of reactions can account for interac-tions of such small stimuli resulting in profound effects: cooperative pro-cesses and dispersive processes with reaction-diffusion effects and soliton formation (Adey, 1981; Lawrence and Adey, 1982).

Cooperative processes involve many sites within a system with all the sites having identical energy levels, so they can be considered coherent. A very weak stimulus at one site of this coherent domain causes an alteration of its energy state. The altered energy state spreads to adjacent sites of the coherent domain. Only a small initial amount of energy is provided by the trigger (for example, the EM field), with the vast majority of the energy supplied by the affected system (Adey, 1981). The membrane structure and function, as described by the greater membrane concept and the fluid mosaic model of Singer and Nicolson (1972), appears to offer a possibility for cooperative interactions of EM fields. In these models the lipid bilayer of the plasma membrane displays a fluidlike behavior. In particular, longitudinal movements of intramembranous molecules are possible. Many of these molecules have protrusions that extend inside and outside the membrane itself. Some of the external protrusions are glycoproteins with fixed-charge anionic binding sites. Long-range interac-tions between charged sites along the membrane surface may be possible when electrochemical gradients near one site are perturbed by an EM field (Adey, 1981). The interactions are likely to be through transductive coupling of weak stimuli to membrane glycoproteins, but interaction with the membrane's lipid bilayer cannot be excluded (Adey, 1981).

A model of membrane function, based on the classical theory of ionic reaction-diffusion processes and the Davydov soliton, has been devel-oped (Lawrence and Adey, 1982). This model can account for initiation and propagation of the action potential. It can also explain interactions of EM waves, including field effects, on transmembrane fluxes, on the propagation of extracellular disturbances, and on the dynamic properties of molecules bound to the membrane. The model is based on the premise that interactions of phonons and excitons along linear molecules produce nonlinear molecular vibrations in the form of soliton waves. Solitons exist in a minimal energy state and are extremely long lived in comparison with linear oscillations. At one end of a long-chain molecule a chemical event may produce energy that can be transferred, in the form of a soliton, along that molecule toward the cell's interior, where it initiates a second-ary chemical event. Alternatively, a few photons from the EM field may be absorbed by a long-chain molecule, and a soliton wave induced; the consequences of the soliton may be the same as in the case of the chemical trigger. Another possibility is that soliton waves can transfer energy along the gel-lipid domain in the membrane from one protein site to another (Lawrence and Adey, 1982).

CONCLUSION

Experimental and theoretical investigations of passive electrical proper-ties of biological systems have helped to develop understanding of the structure and of properties of various biological entities and to elucidate mechanisms of interaction of EM fields. The experimental and theoretical works have complemented each other, experimental data leading to devel-opment of models and new advanced models in turn being verified experi-mentally. This by now classical area of biophysics describes the systems behavior in terms of linear thermodynamics of systems in thermal equilib-rium. A significant amount of data and reliable qualitative models are available. However, a few areas deserve further investigation. Among others, they include in vivo electrical properties of tissues at low frequen-cies (below 10 kHz), the molecular mechanisms responsible for dielectric dispersion at very low frequencies (the α-dispersion), and, to some extent, tissue electrical properties at millimeter waves.

Experimental data obtained during the last decade have indicated that at least some interactions of EM fields with biological systems cannot be explained on the basis of well-established biophysical theories as appli-cable to equilibrium systems. Since some phenomena in living organisms can definitely be classified as being due to thermal nonequilibrium, possi-ble explanations of these interactions have been contemplated in terms of dynamics of nonequilibrium systems. Several theories of interaction mechanisms have been postulated. One common feature of all these hy-potheses is that a weak stimulus provided by an imposed EM field is amplified in the biological system to elicit a significant response. Furthermore, a high degree of cooperativity in the system is expected to be involved, and membranes have been postulated to be the primary sites of the interactions. A major weakness of the present theories is their lack of quantitative experimental verification. Although they may plausibly explain the observed biological effects in very general terms, they have not been sufficiently developed, and specific experiments have not been carried out to confirm or reject them. Experiments that could verify the theories appear difficult to design and perform.

REFERENCES

ADEY, W.R. (1981). Tissue interactions with nonionizing electromagnetic fields. *Physiol. Rev. 61*:435–514.

ATHEY, T.W., STUCHLY, M.A., AND STUCHLY, S.S. (1982). Measurement of radiofrequency permittivity of biological tissues with an open-ended coaxial line. Part I. *IEEE Trans. Microwave Theory Tech. 30*:82–87.

BIANCO, B., DRAGO, G.P., MARCHESI, M, MARTINI, C., MELO, G.S., AND RIDELLA, S. (1979). Measurements of complex dielectric constant of human sera and erythrocytes. *IEEE Trans. Instrum. Measure. 28*:290–295.

BIANCO, B., DRAGO, G., MARCHESI, M., et al. (1980). Physical measurements of dielectric properties of biological substances. *Alta Frequenza 49*:95–100.

BONED, C., AND PEYCELASSE, J. (1982). Automatic measurements of complex permittivity (from 2 MHz to 8 GHz) using time domain spectroscopy. *J. Phys. E. Sci. Instrum. 15*:535–538.

BURDETTE, E.C., CAIN, F.L., AND SEALS, J. (1980). in vivo probe measurement technique for determining dielectric properties at VHF through microwave frequencies. *IEEE Trans. Microwave Theory Tech. 28*:414–427.

BUSSEY, H.E. (1980). Dielectric measurements in a shielded open circuit coaxial line. *IEEE Trans. Instrum. Measure. 29*:120–124.

COLE, K.S. (1962). The advance of electrical models for cells and axon. *Biophys. J. 2*:101–119.

COLE, R.H. (1975). Evolution of dielectric behavior by time domain spectroscopy. I. Dielectric response by real time analysis. *J. Phys. Chem. 79*:1459–1474.

DAWKINS, A.W.J., GABRIEL, C., SHEPPARD, R.J., AND GRANT, E.H. (1981a). Electrical properties of lens material at microwave frequencies. *Phys. Med. Biol. 26*:1–9.

DAWKINS, A.W.J., GRANT, E.H., AND SHEPPARD, R.J. (1981b). An on-line computer-based system for performing tissue domain spectroscopy. II. Analysis of the errors in total reflection TDS. *J. Phys. E. Sci. Instrum. 14*:1260–1265.

DAWKINS, A.W.J., GRANT, E.H., AND SHEPPARD, R.J. (1981c). An on-line computer-based system for performing time domain spectroscopy. III. Presentation of results for total reflection TDS. *J Phys. E. Sci. Instrum. 14*:1429–1434.

DAWKINS, A.W.J., SHEPPARD, R.J., AND GRANT, E.H. (1979). An on-line computer-based system for performing time domain spectroscopy. I. Main features of the basic system. *J. Phys. E. Sci. Instrum. 12*:1091–1099.

EDRICH, J., AND HARDEE, P.C. (1976). Complex permittivity and penetration depth of muscle and fat tissues between 40 and 90 GHz. *IEEE Trans. Microwave Theory Tech. 24*:273–275.

EPSTEIN, B.R., AND FOSTER, K.R. (1983). Anisotropy in the dielectric properties of skeletal muscle. *Med. Biol. Eng. Comput. 21*:51–55.

ESSELLE, K., AND STUCHLY, S.S. (1988). Capacitive sensors for in-vivo measurements of the dielectric properties of biological materials. *IEEE Trans. Instrum. Measure. 37*:101–105.

ESSEX, C.G., SYMONDS, M.S., SHEPPARD, R.J., et al. (1977). Five-component dielectric dispersion in bovine serum albumin solution. *Phys. Med. Biol. 22*:1160–1167.

FOSTER, K.R., AND SCHEPPS, J.L. (1981). Dielectric properties of tumor and normal tissues at radio through microwave frequencies. *J. Microwave Power 16*:107–119.

FOSTER, K.R., SCHEPPS, J.L., AND EPSTEIN, B.J. (1982). Microwave dielectric studies on proteins, tissues, and heterogeneous suspensions. *Bioelectromagnetics 3*:29–43.

FOSTER, K.R., SCHEPPS, J.L., AND SCHWAN, H. P. (1980). Microwave dielectric relaxation in muscle, a second look. *Biophys. J. 29*:271–282.

FOSTER, K.R., SCHEPPS, J.L., STOY, R.D., AND SCHWAN, H.P. (1979). Dielectric properties of brain tissue between 0.01 and 10 GHz. *Phys. Med. Biol. 24*:1177–1187.

FOSTER, K.R., AND SCHWAN, H.P. (1986). Dielectric properties of tissues. *In*: Polk, C., and Postow, E. (eds.). Handbook of biological effects of electromagnetic fields. Boca Raton, Fla., CRC Press, pp. 27–96.

FRÖHLICH, H. (1980). The biological effects of microwaves and related questions. *Adv. Electronics Electron Physics 53*:85–152.

GABRIEL, C., BENTALL, R.H., AND GRANT, E.H. (1987). Comparison of the dielectric properties of normal and wounded human skin material. *Bioelectromagnetics 8*:23–27.

GABRIEL, C., AND GRANT, E.H. (1985). Dielectric properties of ocular tissue in the supercooled and frozen state. *Phys. Med. Biol. 30*:975–983.

GABRIEL, C., SHEPPARD, R.J., AND GRANT, E.H. (1983). Dielectric properties of ocular tissue. *Phys. Med. Biol. 28*:43–49.

GAJDA, G., AND STUCHLY, S.S. (1983). Numerical analysis of open-ended coaxial lines. *IEEE Trans. Microwave Theory Tech. 31*:380–384.

GEDDES, L.A. (1972). Electrodes and measurements of bioelectric events. New York, John Wiley & Sons.

GEDDES, L.A., AND BAKER, L.E. (1967). The specific resistance of biological material—a compedium of data for the biomedical engineer and physiologist. *Med. Biol. Eng. 5*:271–293.

GIESE, K., AND TIEMANN, R. (1975). Determination of the complex permittivity from thin-sample time-domain reflectometry improved analysis of the step response waveform. *Adv. Molec. Relaxation Processes* 7:45–59.

GOLDBETER, A., AND KOSHLAND, E.E. (1982). Sensitivity amplification in biochemical systems. *Q. Rev. Biophys.* 15:555–591.

GRANT, E.H., AND SHEPPARD, R.J. (1974). Relationship between the electrical permittivity of whole blood and the haemoglobin content. *Phys. Med. Biol.* 19:153–160.

GRANT, E.H., SHEPPARD, R.J., AND SOUTH, G.P. (1978). Dielectric behaviour of biological molecules in solution. Oxford, Eng., Clarendon Press.

GRANT, E.H., SZWARNOWSKI, S., AND SHEPPARD, R.J. (1981). Dielectric properties of water in the microwave and far-infrared regions. *In:* Illinger, K.H. (ed.). Biological effects of nonionizing radiation, American Chemical Society Symposium Series No. 157, Washington, D.C., pp. 47–56.

GRANT, J.P., CLARKE, R.N., SYMM, G.T., AND TPYROU, N.M. (1986). A critical study of the open-ended coaxial line sensor for medical and industrial dielectric measurements. Presented at the IEE Colloquium, May 9, 1986, London, Digest 1986/73.

HEY-SHIPTON, G.L., MATTHEWS, P.A., AND McSTAY, J. (1982). The complex permittivity of human tissue at microwave frequencies. *Phys. Med. Biol.* 27:1067–1071.

ILLINGER, K.H. (1982). Spectroscopic properties of in vivo biological systems: boson radiative equilibrium with steady-state nonequilibrium molecular systems. *Bioelectromagnetics* 3:9–16.

ISKANDER, M.F., AND STUCHLY, S.S. (1972). A time-domain technique for measurement of the dielectric properties of biological substances. *IEEE Trans. Instrum. Measure.* 21:425–429.

JENIN, P.C., AND SCHWAN, H.P. (1980). Some observations on the dielectric properties of hemoglobin's suspending medium inside human erythrocytes. *Biophys. J.* 30:285–294.

KAATZE, V., AND GIEZE, K. (1980). Dielectric relaxation spectroscopy of liquids: frequency domain and time domain experimental methods. *J. Phys. E. Sci. Instrum.* 13:133.

KENT, M. (1980). Time domain technique for low frequency dielectric measurements. *J. Phys. E. Sci. Instrum.* 13:457–460.

KOSTERICH, J.D., FOSTER, K.R., AND POLLACK, S.R. (1983). Dielectric permittivity and electrical conductivity of fluid saturated bone. *IEEE Trans. Biomed. Eng.* 30:81–86.

KOSTERICH, J.D., FOSTER, K.R., AND POLLACK, S.R. (1984). Dielectric properties of fluid-saturated bone—the effect of variation in conductivity of immersion fluid. *IEEE Trans. Biomed. Eng.* 831:369–374.

KRASZEWSKI, A., STUCHLY, M.A., AND STUCHLY, S.S. (1983a). Calibration method for measurements of dielectric properties. *IEEE Trans. Instrum. Measure.* 32:385–387.

KRASZEWSKI, A., STUCHLY, M.A., STUCHLY, S.S., AND SMITH, A.M. (1982). In vivo and in vitro dielectric properties of animal tissues at radio frequencies. *Bioelectromagnetics 3*:421–433.

KRASZEWSKI, A., AND STUCHLY, S.S. (1983). Capacitance of open-ended dielectric-filled coaxial lines—experimental results. *IEEE Trans. 32*:517–519.

KRASZEWSKI, A., STUCHLY, S.S., STUCHLY, M.A., AND SYMONS, S. (1983b). On the measurement accuracy of the tissue permittivity in vivo. *IEEE Trans. Instrum. Measure. 32*:37–42.

LAWRENCE, A.F., AND ADEY, W.R. (1982). Nonlinear wave mechanisms in interactions between excitable tissue and electromagnetic fields. *Neurol. Res. 4*:115–153.

MOSIG, J.R., BESSON J.-C., GEX-FABY, M., AND GARDIOL, F.E. (1981). Reflection of an open-ended coaxial line and application to nondestructive measurement of materials. *IEEE Trans. Instrum. Measure. 30*:46–51.

NICOLSON, A.M., AND ROSS, G.F. (1970). Measurement of the intrinsic properties of materials by time-domain techniques. *IEEE Trans. Instrum. Measure. 19*:377–382.

NIGHTINGALE, N.R.V., DAWKINS, A.W.J., SHEPPARD, R.J., GRANT, E.H., GOODRIDGE, V.D., AND CHRISTIE, J.L. (1980). The use of time domain spectroscopy to measure the dielectric properties of mouse brain at radiowave and microwave frequencies. *Phys. Med.. Biol. 25*:1161–1165.

ONCLEY, J.L. (1942). The investigation of proteins by dielectric measurements. *Chem. Rev. 30*:433–450.

PAULY, H., AND SCHWAN, H.P. (1966). Dielectric properties and ion mobility in erythrocytes. *Biophys. J. 6*:621–639.

REDDY, G.N., AND SAHA, S. (1984). Electrical and dielectric properties of wet bone as a function of frequency. *IEEE Trans. Biomed. Eng. 31*:296–302.

ROGERS, J.A., SHEPPARD, R.J., GRANT, E.H., BLEEHEN, N.M., AND HONESS, D.J. (1983). The dielectric properties of normal and tumour mouse tissue between 50 MHz and 10 GHz. *Br. J. Radiol. 56*:335–338.

RZEPECKA, M.A., AND STUCHLY, S.S. (1975). A lumped capacitance method for the measurement of the permittivity and conductivity in the frequency and time domain—a further analysis. *IEEE Trans. Instrum. Measure. 24*:27–32.

SCHEPPS, J.R., AND FOSTER, K.R. (1980). The UHF and microwave dielectric properties of normal and tumour tissues: variation in dielectric properties with tissue water content. *Phys. Med. Biol. 25*:1149–1159.

SCHWAN, H.P. (1957). Electrical properties of tissues and cell suspensions. *Adv. Biol. Med. Phys. 5*:147–209.

SCHWAN, H.P. (1964). Electrical characteristics of tissues, a survey, *Biophysics 1*:198–208.

SCHWAN, H.P. (1965). Electrical properties of bound water. *Ann. N.Y. Acad. Sci. 125*:344–354.

SCHWAN, H.P. (1981a). Electrical properties of cells: principles, some recent results and some unresolved problems. *In*: The biophysical approach to excitable systems. Honoring K.S. Cole's 80th Birthday. New York, Plenum Publishing Corp.

SCHWAN, H.P. (1981b). Dielectric properties of biological tissue and biophysical mechanisms of electromagnetic-field interaction. *In*: Illinger, K.H. (ed.). Biological effects of nonionizing radiation. American Chemical Society Symposium Series 157, Washington, D.C., pp. 109–131.

SCHWAN, H.P. (1982). Nonthermal cellular effects of electromagnetic fields: AC-field induced ponderomotoric forces. *Br. J. Cancer 45*(supp. V):220–224.

SCHWAN, H.P. (1983). Electrical properties of blood and its constitutents: alternating current spectroscopy. *Blut 46*:1–13.

SCHWAN, H.P., AND FOSTER, K.R. (1977). Microwave dielectric properties of tissue. *Biophys. J. 17*:193–197.

SCHWAN, H.P., AND KAY, C.F. (1956). Specific resistance of body tissues. *Circ. Res. 4*:664–670.

SCHWAN, H.P., AND LI, K. (1953). Capacity and conductivity of body tissues at ultrahigh frequencies. *Proc. IRE 41*:1735–1740.

SCHWAN, H.P., SHEPPARD, R.J., AND GRANT, E.H. (1976). Complex permittivity of water at 25°C. *J. Chem. Phys. 64*:2257–2258.

SCOTT, W.R., AND SMITH, G.S. (1986). Error analysis for dielectric spectroscopy using shielded open-circuited coaxial lines of general length. *IEEE Trans. Instrum. Measure. 35*:130–137.

SINGER, S.J., AND NICOLSON, G.L. (1972). The fluid mosaic model of the structure of cell membranes. *Science 175*:720–731.

SINGH, B., SMITH, C.W., AND HUGHES, R. (1979). In vivo dielectric spectrometer. *Med. Biol. Eng. Comput. 17*:45–60.

SMITH, S.R., AND FOSTER, K.R. (1985). Dielectric properties of low-water-content tissues. *Phys. Med. Biol. 30*:965–973.

STEEL, M.C., AND SHEPPARD, R.J. (1986). Dielectric properties of lens tissue at microwave frequencies. *Bioelectromagnetics 7*:73–81.

STEEL, M.C., AND SHEPPARD, R.J. (1985). Dielectric properties of mammalian brain tissue between 1 and 18 GHz. *Phys. Med. Biol. 7*:621–630.

STOY, R.D., FOSTER, K.R., AND SCHWAN, H.P. (1982). Dielectric properties of mammalian tissues from 0.1 to 100 MHz: a summary of recent data. *Phys. Med. Biol. 27*:501–513.

STUCHLY, M.A. (1979). Interaction of radiofrequency and microwave radiation with living systems. *Radiat. Environ. Biophys. 16*:1–14.

STUCHLY, M.A., AND STUCHLY, S.S. (1980a). Coaxial line reflection methods for measuring dielectric properties of biological substances at radio and microwave frequencies—a review. *IEEE Trans. Instrum. Measure. 29*:176–183.

STUCHLY, M.A., AND STUCHLY, S.S. (1980b). Dielectric properties of biological substances—tabulated. *J. Microwave Power 15*:19–26.

STUCHLY, M.A., ATHEY, T.W., SAMARAS, G.M., AND TAYLOR, G. (1928b). Dielectric properties of biological substances of radio frequencies. II. Experimental results. *IEEE Trans. Microwave Theory Tech. 30*:87–92.

STUCHLY, M.A., ATHEY, T.W., STUCHLY, S.S., SAMARAS, G.M., AND TAYLOR, G. (1982a). Dielectric properties of animal tissues in vivo at frequencies 10 MHz–1 GHz. *Bioelectromagnetics 2*:93–103.

STUCHLY, M.A., KRASZEWSKI, A., STUCHLY, S.S., AND SMITH, A.M. (1982c). Dielectric properties of animal tissues in vivo at radio and microwave frequencies—comparison between species. *Phys. Med. Biol.* 27:927–936.

STUCHLY, S.S., GAJDA, G., ANDERSON, L., AND KRASZEWSKI, A. (1986). A new sensor for dielectric measurements. *IEEE Trans. Instrum. Measure.* 35:138–141.

STUCHLY, S.S., RZEPECKA, M.A., AND ISKANDER, M.F. (1974). Permittivity measurements at microwave frequencies using lumped elements. *IEEE Trans. Instrum. Measure.* 23:56–62.

STUCHLY, S.S., STUCHLY, M.A., AND CARRARO, B. (1978). Permittivity measurements in a resonator terminated by an infinite sample. *IEEE Trans. Instrum. Measure.* 27:436–439.

SUROWIEC, A.J., STUCHLY, S.S., BARR, J.R., AND SWARUP, A. (1988). Dielectric properties of breast carcinoma and the surrounding tissues. *IEEE Trans. Biomed. Eng.* 35:257–262.

SUROWIEC, A., STUCHLY, S.S., KEANEY, N., AND SWARUP, A. (1986a). In vivo and in vitro dielectric properties of feline tissue at low radiofrequencies. *Phys. Med. Biol.* 8:901–909.

SUROWIEC, A.J., STUCHLY, S.S., KEANEY, M., AND SWARUP, A. (1987). Dielectric polarization of animal lung at radio frequencies. *IEEE Trans. Biomed. Eng.* 34:62–67.

SUROWIEC, A., STUCHLY, S.S., AND SWARUP, A. (1985). Radiofrequency dielectric properties of animal tissues as a function of time following death. *Phys. Med. Biol.* 30:1131–1141.

SUROWIEC, A., STUCHLY, S.S., AND SWARUP, A. (1986b). Postmortem changes of the dielectric properties of bovine brain tissue at low radiofrequencies. *Bioelectromagnetics* 7:31–43.

SZWARNOWSKI, S. (1982). A transmission line cell for measuring the permittivity of liquids over the frequency range 90 MHz to 2 GHz. *J. Phys. E. Sci. Instrum.* 15:1068–1072.

SZWARNOWSKI, S., AND SHEPPARD, R.J. (1979). A coaxial line system for measuring the permittivity of conductive liquids. *J. Phys. E. Sci. Instrum.* 12:937–940.

TAKASHIMA, S., AND MINAKATA, A. (1975). Dielectric behavior of biological macromolecules. *Dig. Dielectric Literature* 37:602–653.

TAKASHIMA, S., AND SCHWAN, H.P. (1974). Passive electrical properties of squid axon membrane. *J. Membrane Biol.* 17:51–68.

TANABE, E., AND JOINES, W.T. (1976). A nondestructive method for measuring permittivity of dielectric materials at microwave frequencies using an open transmission line resonator. *IEEE Trans. Instrum. Measure.* 25:222–226.

THURAI, M., GOODRIDGE, V.D., SHEPPARD, R.J., AND GRANT, E.H. (1984). Variation with age of the dielectric properties of mouse brain cerebrum. *Phys. Biol. Med.* 9:1133–1136.

VAN BEEK, W.M., VAN DER TOUW, F., AND MANDEL, M. (1985). A measuring device for the determination of the electric permittivity of conducting liquids in the frequency range 1–100 MHz. *J. Phys. E. Sci. Instrum.* 9:385–391.

VAN DER TOUW, F., DE GOEDE, J., VAN BEEK, W.M., AND MANDEL, M. (1975a). A measuring device for the determination of the electric permittivity of conducting liquids in the frequency range 2–500 kHz. I. The bridge. *J. Phys. E. Sci. Instrum.* *8*:840–844.

VAN DER TOUW, F., SELIER, G., AND MANDEL, M. (1975b). A measuring device for the determination of the electric permittivity of conducting liquids in the frequency range 2–500 kHz. II. The measuring cell. *J. Phys. E. Sci. Instrum.* *8*:844–846.

VAN GEMERT, M.J.C., AND SUGGETT, A. (1975). Multiple reflection time domain spectroscopy. II. A lumped element approach leading to an analytical solution for the complex permittivity. *J. Chem. Phys. 62*:2720.

VON HIPPEL, A.R. (1954). Dielectric materials and applications. Cambridge, Mass., MIT Press.

WATSON, J. (1981). Electricity and bone healing. *Proc. IEE (U.K.) 128*:329–335.

WESTHPHAL, W.B. (1954). Dielectric measuring techniques. *In*: von Hippel, A.R. (ed.). Dielectric materials and applications. New York. John Wiley & Sons, pp. 63–122.

YAMAMOTO, T., AND YAMAMOTO, Y. (1981). Non-linear electrical properties of skin in the low frequency range. *Med. Biol. Eng. Comput. 19*:302–310.

6

Numerical Methods for Specific Absorption Rate Calculations

OM P. GANDHI

Knowledge of the specific absorption rate (SAR) and temperature distributions in the human body in response to electromagnetic (EM) exposures is of basic interest in the assessment of biological effects and medical applications of EM energy. Several methods have been described in the literature for numerical calculations of SAR distributions (Taflove and Brodwin, 1975a; Chen and Guru, 1977; Hagmann et al., 1979). Although experiments must be done to verify the accuracy of any theoretical procedure, the numerical methods allow a detailed modeling of the anatomically relevant human inhomogeneities that are not easy to model experimentally. Two excellent review articles summarize the status of the field (Durney, 1980; Spiegel, 1984), although these are somewhat outdated at the present time. Maxwell's equations have been solved in both the integral and differential equation form for the distribution of electric and magnetic fields and mass-normalized rates of energy deposition (SARs). For temperature calculations the bioheat equation is solved for a cylindrical thermal model in which the human body is represented by six cylindrical segments for the head, torso, arms, hands, legs, and feet (Stolwijk, 1970; Stolwijk and Hardy, 1977; Stolwijk, 1980). Each segment consists of four concentric cylinders representing layers of skin, fat, muscle, and core tissue. Recognizing that such formulations are incapable of properly accounting for the painstakingly obtained SAR distributions, we have developed an inhomogeneous thermal block model of a human using heterogeneous thermal properties obtained from the anatomical data for 476 cells (Chatterjee and Gandhi, 1983). Since SARs are now available with a higher degree of resolution than ever in the past, a 5432-cell inhomogeneous thermal model of the human body has also been developed recently (Gandhi and Hoque, to be published).

This chapter focuses on the numerical methods for SAR calculations and does not discuss the thermal models for temperature calculations. To simplify computational requirements, several authors have also used two-dimensional formulations for individual cross sections of the body. Since this is not an accurate description of the three-dimensional (3-D) nature of the human body problem, this chapter does not discuss these techniques. The focus instead is on techniques that lend themselves to high-resolution 3-D modeling of the body for either far-field or near-field

EM exposures. For SAR calculations the most promising techniques at present are the finite-difference time-domain (FDTD) method (Spiegel, 1984; Spiegel et al., 1985; Sullivan et al., 1987, 1988) and the sinc-basis fast Fourier transform (FFT)–conjugate gradient (CG) method (Borup et al., to be published), which is a modified version of the traditional method of moments (Chen and Guru, 1977; Hagmann et al., 1979). For lower frequencies at which quasistatic approximations may be made (≤ 40 MHz for the human body), the impedance method has been found to be highly efficient numerically and has been used for a number of applications (Armitage et al., 1983; Gandhi et al., 1984; Gandhi and DeFord, 1988; Orcutt and Gandhi, 1988).

METHOD OF MOMENTS

The method of moments (MOM) (Harrington, 1968) has been extensively used to calculate SAR distributions in block model representations of the human body (Livesay and Chen, 1974; Chen and Guru, 1977; Gandhi et al., 1979; Hagmann and Gandhi, 1979; Hagmann et al., 1979). In this procedure the fields $\mathbf{E(r)}$ within the body are solved from the solution of the electric field integral equation (EFIE) obtained from Maxwell's equations. The EFIE for an isotropic, nonmagnetic, arbitrarily inhomogeneous body is as follows:

$$\mathbf{E}^i(\mathbf{r}) = \mathbf{E(r)} - (k_0^2 + \nabla\nabla \cdot) \int_{v'} (\epsilon_r^*(\mathbf{r}) - 1)\, \mathbf{E(r')}\, g\,(\mathbf{r} - \mathbf{r'})\, dv' \qquad (1)$$

where $\mathbf{E}^i(\mathbf{r})$ are the incident fields at the individual locations within the body, if the body were absent, $\mathbf{E(r')}$ are the unknown total fields at the various locations, k_o is the wave number in free space, ϵ_r^* are the complex dielectric constants at the various locations, the equation

$$g(\mathbf{r} - \mathbf{r'}) = \frac{e^{-jk_0|\mathbf{r}-\mathbf{r'}|}}{4\pi|\mathbf{r} - \mathbf{r'}|}$$

is the 3-D free-space Green's function, and the integral v' is taken over the entire volume of the body.

The unknown fields $\mathbf{E(r)}$ are involved both outside and inside the integral sign of Eq. 1. With pulse-basis function, which implies that the electric field is assumed constant over the volume of the individual cells, the EFIE can be expressed in the form of a matrix equation

$$\overset{\leftrightarrow}{A} \cdot \mathbf{E} = \mathbf{E}^i \qquad (2)$$

where $\overset{\leftrightarrow}{A}$ is a $3N \times 3N$ matrix that describes coupling between the various cells, $\mathbf{E}$ is a vector of $3N$ unknown field components, 3 for each of the N

cells into which the body is divided, and $\mathbf{E}^i$ is a vector of $3N$ known field components that would be incident at the same N cells if the body did not exist. Solution of this matrix equation by conventional methods such as Gauss elimination or the conjugate gradient method with matrix multiplication requires order $(3N)^2$ storage and order $(3N)^2$ to $(3N)^3$ computation steps. Both of these computational requirements expand rapidly as the number of cells N is increased. Consequently, it has not been possible to apply the traditional MOM to block model representation of the human body with N larger than 1132 (DeFord et al., 1983). Despite the difficulty of handling a larger number of cells, image theory has been used to modify the Green's function in lieu of the free-space Green's function, thereby allowing SAR calculations in human models with grounding and reflector effects (Hagmann and Gandhi, 1979).

FAST FOURIER TRANSFORM–CONJUGATE GRADIENT METHOD OF MOMENTS

Because of the convolutional nature of the EFIE (Eq. 1), iterative algorithms based on the highly efficient FFT have been developed recently to allow the heterogeneous modeling of the human body by up to 5607-cell models (Borup et al., to be published). In this method, as in all moment methods, the numerical solution of Eq. 1 begins with approximation of the source polarization current $J_p = (\epsilon_r^* - 1)\,\mathbf{E}$ with a finite basis expansion. In the present approach the tensor product sinc basis is used

$$\mathbf{J}(x,y,z) = \frac{\delta^3}{\pi^3}\sum_n\sum_m\sum_l \mathbf{J}\,(n\delta, m\delta, l\delta)$$
$$\frac{\sin\frac{\pi}{\delta}(x - n\delta)\,\sin\frac{\pi}{\delta}(y - m\delta)\,\sin\frac{\pi}{\delta}(z - l\delta)}{(x - n\delta)\,(y - m\delta)\,(z - l\delta)} \quad (3)$$

where δ is the grid increment. Inserting Eq. 3 into Eq. 1 and enforcing the equality of Eq. 1 at the grid points results in a linear system of equations.

$$\mathbf{E}^i\,(i,j,k) = \mathbf{E}\,(i,j,k) +$$
$$\sum_n\sum_m\sum_l \overline{\overline{G}}\,(i - n, j - m, k - l)\cdot[(\epsilon_{nml}^* - 1)\,\mathbf{E}\,(n,m,l)]$$

where

$$\overline{\overline{G}}(n,m,l) = (k_0^2 + \nabla\nabla\,\cdot)$$

$$\left\{ \frac{e^{-jk_0 r}}{4\pi r} * \frac{\delta^3}{\pi^3} \frac{\sin\left(\frac{\pi x}{\delta}\right)}{x} \frac{\sin\left(\frac{\pi y}{\delta}\right)}{y} \frac{\sin\left(\frac{\pi z}{\delta}\right)}{z} \right\} \Bigg|_{\substack{x = n\delta \\ y = m\delta \\ z = l\delta}} \tag{4}$$

and * denotes a 3-D convolution.

Because an equally spaced grid has been used, Eq. 4 has inherited the convolutional form of Eq. 1. This form can be exploited to provide a means of computing the sum in Eq. 4 in order $N \log_2 N$ arithmetic operations. In addition, no matrix need be stored because only the 3-D FFTs of the components of $\overline{\overline{G}}$ are needed. This provides an efficient method to compute the matrix products $A\bar{x}$ and $A^H\bar{x}$ where A is the matrix operator implicit in Eq. 4 (the superscript H denotes the complex conjugate transpose matrix). To solve the system (Eq. 4), the efficient calculation of the matrix-vector products is used in the implementation of a conjugate gradient–type iteration method (CGM). The CGM has recently become popular as a means of solving linear systems obtained with the MOM. Hestenes and Stiefel (1952) originated the most-used version of this algorithm, and Sarkar et al. (1981) introduced it for EM problems. Unfortunately, this method often requires a large number of iterations to obtain a converged solution because the CGM applies only to positive definite, hermition matrices. This method is applied to nonhermition systems by first "squaring" the original system, $A\bar{x} = \bar{y}$, with the conjugate transpose matrix to give the normal equations, $A^H A\bar{x} = A^H\bar{y}$. The conjugate gradient method is then applied to the hermition system $A^H A$. The problem with this is that the formation of the normal equations squares the spectral condition number of the linear system. Because the number of iterations needed for convergence is asymptotically equal to the square root of the condition number, this procedure can lead to slow convergence.

To alleviate this difficulty we have replaced the CGM with a biconjugate gradient method (BCGM) developed by Fletcher (1975). The BCGM applies directly to nonhermition matrices without the formation of the normal equations and has been found to converge nearly as rapidly as the CGM applied to similarly sized and conditioned hermition systems. Our experience is that the use of the BCGM requires far fewer iterations than the CGM applied to the normal equations for systems obtained from Eq. 4.

After testing the accuracy of the new formulation with homogeneous and layered lossy dielectric sphere test problems, we have used it with

5607-cell human models (2.62 cm cubical cells) exposed to 30 and 100 MHz plane waves with and without a ground plane. Typical run times are about 10 minutes when a Cray II is used.

FINITE-DIFFERENCE TIME-DOMAIN METHOD

Perhaps the most successful and the most promising of the numerical methods for SAR calculations is the FDTD method. This method was first proposed by Yee (1966) and later developed by Taflove and colleagues (Taflove and Brodwin, 1975a,b; Taflove, 1980; Umashankar and Taflove, 1982), Holland (1977), and Kunz and Lee (1978). Recently it has been extended for calculations of the distribution of EM fields in a human model for incident plane waves (Spiegel, 1984; Spiegel et al., 1985; Sullivan et al., 1987, 1988; Chen and Gandhi, 1989b) and for exposures in the near fields (Chen and Gandhi, 1989a; Wang and Gandhi, 1989). In this method the time-dependent Maxwell's curl equations

$$\nabla \times \mathbf{E} = -\mu \frac{\partial \mathbf{H}}{\partial t}, \quad \nabla \times \mathbf{H} = \sigma \mathbf{E} + \epsilon \frac{\partial \mathbf{E}}{\partial t} \tag{5}$$

are implemented for a lattice of cubic cells. The components of $\mathbf{E}$ and $\mathbf{H}$ are positioned about a unit cell of the lattice (Figure 6-1) and evaluated alternately with half-time steps. The goal of the method is to model the propagation of an EM wave into a volume of space containing dielectric and/or conducting structures by time stepping, that is, repeatedly implementing a finite-difference analogue of the curl equations at each cell of the corresponding space lattice. The incident wave is tracked as it first propagates to the dielectric structure and interacts with it via surface current excitation, spreading, penetration, and diffraction. Wave tracking is completed when a sinusoidal steady-state behavior for $\mathbf{E}$ and $\mathbf{H}$ fields

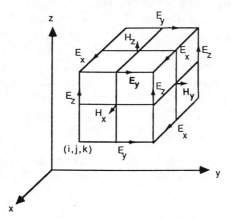

Figure 6-1 Unit cell of Yee lattice indicating positions for various field components.

is observed for each lattice cell. A second approach is to illuminate the body with a pulse of radiation in the time domain. If the medium is nondispersive (that is, its dielectric properties do not change with frequency), this method has the advantage of giving the performance of the medium at various frequencies from the inverse Fourier transform of the calculated fields. Although Spiegel and his collaborators (Spiegel, 1984; Spiegel et al., 1985) have followed this approach, we have used the sinusoidal variation of the illuminating fields, since the dielectric properties of the tissues are highly dependent on frequency.

The Maxwell's equations (Eq. 5) can be rewritten as difference equations. We assume the media to be nonmagnetic, that is, $\mu = \mu_o$ and a grid point of the space defined as (i, j, k) with coordinates $(i\delta, j\delta, k\delta)$ where δ is the cell size.

Upon substituting

$$\tilde{\mathbf{E}} = \sqrt{\frac{\epsilon_o}{\mu_o}}\, \frac{\mathbf{E}}{2} \qquad (6)$$

the equations in difference form for E_z and H_z, for example, can be written as:

$$\tilde{E}_z^{n+1}(i,j,k+1/2) = CA_z(i,j,k+1/2)\,\tilde{E}_z^n(i,j,k+1/2) + CB_z(i,j,k+1/2) \cdot$$
$$\left[\begin{array}{l} H_y^{n+1/2}(i+1/2,j,k+1/2) - H_y^{n+1/2}(i-1/2,j,k+1/2) \\ + H_x^{n+1/2}(i,j-1/2,k+1/2) - H_x^{n+1/2}(i,j+1/2,k+1/2) \end{array}\right] \qquad (7)$$

$$H_z^{n+1/2}(i+1/2,j+1/2,k) = H_z^{n+1/2}(i+1/2,j+1/2,k)$$
$$+ \left[\begin{array}{l} \tilde{E}_x^n(i+1/2,j+1,k) - \tilde{E}_x^n(i+1/2,j,k) \\ + \tilde{E}_y^n(i,j+1/2,k) - \tilde{E}_y^n(i+1,j+1/2,k) \end{array}\right] \qquad (8)$$

where

$$CA_z(i,j,k+1/2) = \left[1 - \frac{\sigma_z(i,j,k+1/2)\,\delta t}{2\epsilon_z(i,j,k+1/2)}\right]\left[1 + \frac{\sigma_z(i,j,k+1/2)\,\delta t}{2\epsilon_z(i,j,k+1/2)}\right]^{-1} \qquad (9)$$

$$CB_z(i,j,k+1/2) = \frac{\epsilon_0}{4}\left[\epsilon_z(i,j,k+1/2) + \frac{\sigma_z(i,j,k+1/2)\,\delta t}{2}\right]^{-1} \qquad (10)$$

where the superscript n denotes the time $n\,\delta t$ in terms of the incremental time or time step δt. The time step δt is determined by the cell size and must satisfy the stability condition (Taflove and Brodwin, 1975b)

$$v_{\max}\,\delta t < \left[\frac{1}{\delta x^2} + \frac{1}{\delta y^2} + \frac{1}{\delta z^2}\right]^{-1/2} \qquad (11)$$

where $v_{\max}$ is the maximum wave phase velocity within the model. For the cubic cell model $\delta x = \delta y = \delta z = \delta$, the following relationship is usually taken

$$\delta t = \frac{\delta}{2c_{\max}} \tag{12}$$

where $c_{\max}$ is the maximum velocity of EM waves in the interaction space. We have taken $c_{\max}$ corresponding to velocity of EM waves in air. The ϵ and σ may be different for E_x, E_y, and E_z in the inhomogeneous media, because as shown in Figure 6-1 the components of **E** are not positioned at the same point for the same cell in Yee's algorithm. Thus we have ϵ_x, ϵ_y, ϵ_z, σ_x, σ_y, and σ_z for each of the cells.

A basic problem with any finite-difference solution of Maxwell's equations is the treatment of the field components at the lattice truncation. Because of the limited computer storage, the lattice must be restricted in size. Proper truncation of the lattice requires that any outgoing wave disappear at the lattice boundary without reflection during the continuous time stepping of the algorithm. An absorption boundary condition for each field component is therefore needed at the edge of the lattice. In our formulation the absorption boundary conditions in second approximation derived by Mur (1981) are used. The condition for E_z at $i = 1$, for example, can be written as

$$\tilde{E}_z^{n+1}(1, j, k + 1/2) = -\tilde{E}_z^{n-1}(2, j, k + 1/2)$$

$$+ \frac{c_\ell\,\delta t - \delta}{c_\ell\,\delta t + \delta} [\tilde{E}_z^{n+1}(2, j, k + 1/2) + \tilde{E}_z^{n-1}(1, j, k + 1/2)]$$

$$+ 2\left(\frac{\delta}{c_\ell\,\delta t + \delta} - \frac{(c_\ell\,\delta t)^2}{\delta(c_\ell\,\delta t + \delta)}\right) [\tilde{E}_z^n(1, j, k + 1/2) + \tilde{E}_z^n(2, j, k + 1/2)]$$

$$+ \frac{(c_\ell\delta t)^2}{2\delta(c_\ell\delta t + \delta)} \begin{bmatrix} \tilde{E}_z^n(1, j + 1, k + 1/2) + \tilde{E}_z^n(1, j - 1, k + 1/2) \\ + \tilde{E}_z^n(2, j + 1, k + 1/2) + \tilde{E}_z^n(2, j - 1, k + 1/2) \\ + \tilde{E}_z^n(1, j, k + 3/2) + \tilde{E}_z^n(1, j, k - 1/2) \\ + \tilde{E}_z^n(2, j, k + 3/2) + \tilde{E}_z^n(2, j, k - 1/2) \end{bmatrix} \tag{13}$$

where c_ℓ is the phase velocity of the medium at the lattice truncation.

ANATOMICALLY BASED INHOMOGENEOUS HUMAN MODEL

As previously described in Sullivan et al. (1987, 1988), the model for the human body is developed from information in the book *A Cross-Section Anatomy*, by Eycleshymer and Schoemaker (1911). This book contains cross-sectional diagrams of the human body that were obtained by making cross-sectional cuts about 1 inch apart in human cadavers. The process for creating the data base of the human model was the following: First, a quarter-inch grid was taken for each single cross-sectional diagram, and each cell on the grid was assigned a number corresponding to one of the 14 tissue types given in Table 6-1, or air. Thus the data associated with a particular layer consisted of three numbers for each square cell: x and y positions relative to some anatomical reference point in this layer, usually the center of the spinal cord, and an integer indicating which tissue that cell contained. Since the cross-sectional diagrams available in Eycleshymer and Schoemaker (1911) are for somewhat variable separations, typically 2.3 to 2.7 cm, a new set of equispaced layers was defined at ¼-inch intervals by interpolating the data onto these layers. Because the cell size of quarter-inch is too small for the memory space of present-day computers, the proportion of each tissue type was calculated next for somewhat larger cells of ½ inch or 1 inch combining the data for $2 \times 2 \times 2 = 8$ or $4 \times 4 \times 4 = 64$ cells of the smaller dimension. Without changes in the anatomy, this process allows some variability in the height and weight of the body. We have taken the final cell size of 1.31 or 2.62 cm (rather than ½ inch or 1 inch) to obtain the whole-body weight of 69.6 kg for the model. The numbers of cells either totally or partially within the human body for the two models are 41,256 and 5628, respectively.

TABLE 6-1   Tissue Properties Used at Various Frequencies

Tissue type	Mass density (1000 kg/m³)	27.12 MHz		100 MHz		350 MHz	
		$\sigma_{S/m}$	ϵ_r	$\sigma_{S/m}$	ϵ_r	$\sigma_{S/m}$	ϵ_r
Air	0.0012	0.00	1	0.0	1	0.0	1
Muscle	1.05	0.74	106	1.0	74	1.33	53.0
Fat, bones	1.20	0.04	29	0.07	7.5	0.072	5.7
Blood	1.00	0.28	102	1.1	74	1.2	65.0
Intestines	1.00	0.29	60	0.55	36	0.66	26.5
Cartilage	1.00	0.04	29	0.07	7.5	0.072	5.7
Liver	1.03	0.51	132	0.62	77	0.82	50.0
Kidney	1.02	0.79	209	1.0	90	1.16	53.0
Pancreas	1.03	0.69	206	1.0	90	1.16	53.0
Spleen	1.03	0.69	206	0.82	100	0.9	90.0
Lung	0.33	0.17	34	0.34	75	1.1	35.0
Heart	1.03	0.64	210	0.75	76	1.0	56.0
Nerve, brain	1.05	0.45	155	0.53	52	0.65	60.0
Skin	1.00	0.74	106	0.55	25	0.44	17.6
Eye	1.00	0.45	155	1.9	85	1.9	80.0

IMPEDANCE METHOD

For low-frequency dosimetry ($\leq$ 40 MHz for the human body) problems in which quasistatic approximations may be made, the impedance method has been found to be highly efficient numerically (Armitage et al., 1983; Gandhi et al., 1984; Gandhi and DeFord, 1988; Orcutt and Gandhi, 1988). In this method the biological body or the exposed part thereof is represented by a 3-D network of impedances whose individual values are obtained from the complex conductivities $\sigma + j\omega\epsilon$ of the various body regions. Using homogeneous and layered cylindrical bodies (DeFord, 1985) or spherical bodies (Orcutt and Gandhi, 1988) as test cases, where the analytical solutions are available (Harrington, 1961), we have established the maximum frequency limit for the impedance method to be approximately 30 to 40 MHz for a tissue-equivalent cylinder or sphere of diameter of 30 cm, similar to the dimensions of the human torso. The frequency limit was established by obtaining solutions for cases of transverse electric (TE) plane-wave irradiation of the cylindrical or the spherical body using the impedance method and comparing them with the analytical solutions at various frequencies. The effect of the incident electric field is to introduce currents into the model given by $j\omega\epsilon_0 E_{ext}$, where E_{ext} is the external electric field (incident + scattered) at the surface of the body. The contribution from the H field is to set up emfs in the circuit loops of the model given from Faraday's law of induction by $j\omega\mu_0 H_n \delta^2$ where H_n is the magnetic field normal to the plane of the loop of area δ^2. With the anatomically based human models (nominal ½- or 1-inch resolution), the impedance method has been used for the following applications:

1. Calculation of SAR distributions for operator exposure to a radiofrequency (RF) induction heater. In the article by Gandhi and DeFord (1988), SARs are obtained for an anatomically based model of the human torso for spatially varying vector magnetic fields because of a 450 kHz RF induction heater.

2. SAR distributions in the anatomically based model of the human body for linear or circularly polarized spatially variable magnetic fields representative of magnetic resonance imagers. In a paper by Orcutt and Gandhi (1988), a 1.31 cm resolution model of the human body is used to calculate SAR distributions for RF magnetic fields employed for magnetic resonance imaging of the torso and the head regions of the body. The layer-averaged SAR distribution calculated for a circularly polarized RF magnetic field (in the cross-sectional plane of the body) is shown in Figure 6-2. The layer-numbering system used for the model of the human body is shown in Figure 6-3. Each layer is 1.31 cm from its neighbors. Layer 1 is 0.655 cm below the top of the head.

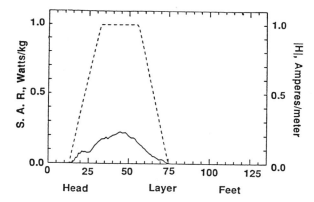

Figure 6-2   Layer-averaged specific absorption rates (SARs) for model of human body exposed to magnetic field at 63 MHz, circularly polarized in x-y plane. Spatial variation of field strength is shown by dashed line. Peak SAR for this case, 0.98 W/kg, occurred in layer 48. Whole-body-averaged SAR was 0.03 W/kg.

3. SAR distributions in the human body because of the magnetic field component of incident plane waves. The calculated layer-averaged SAR distribution for an incident RF magnetic field of 1 A/m at 30 MHz is given in Figure 3-5. It is concluded that the body-averaged SAR because

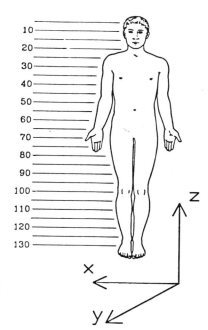

Figure 6-3 Layer-numbering system used in model of human body. Each layer is 1.31 cm from its neighbors. Layer 1 is 0.655 cm below top of head.

of the magnetic field (0.03 W/kg) is considerably smaller than that for the electric field component of the plane waves at 30 MHz.

4. SAR distributions because of the spatially variable vector magnetic fields of Magnetrode applicators for hyperthermia. Cylindrical current-carrying conductor or Magnetrode-type applicators have been used for hyperthermia that is caused by induced currents in the body because of time-varying magnetic fields (Elliott et al., 1982). Using the impedance method, we have obtained internal current and SAR distributions accounting for the spatially variable vector magnetic fields of such an applicator. Whereas a 2-D sectional model of the human body was used earlier (Gandhi et al., 1984), a 3-D model of the human torso has been used by DeFord (1985).

5. SAR distributions because of capacitor-type electrodes used for hyperthermia. Whereas a 3-D, 2.54 cm resolution model of the human torso has been used by DeFord (1985), a 1.31 cm resolution model of the whole human body has recently been used for these applicators (Orcutt and Gandhi, 1990), which are fairly popular in Japan.

6. SAR distributions for interstitial RF needle applicators in irregularly shaped tumors. In the article by Zhu and Gandhi (1988) a model based on computerized tomographic (CT) scans of the human head is used to find the optimum locations of the 0.5 MHz RF needles for minimum standard deviations of the SAR distributions in the volume of the identified brain tumor. The procedure described in this article could be used in planning thermotherapy for a number of tumors, such as those of the vaginal cuff, colon-rectum, and head and neck, for which local hyperthermia by RF needle applicators has been found useful (Manning and Gerner, 1981).

Even though isotropic electrical properties have been used for the applications of the impedance method to date, directional averaging of the electrical properties done at the stage of going from smaller to larger cells would have yielded anisotropic properties for the cells. Furthermore, at lower frequencies the tissue properties are known to be anisotropic, which would also result in directionally dependent impedances that must be used for each of the cells. A natural application of the impedance method would be for dosimetry for 50/60 Hz EM fields because of power transmission lines.

APPLICATIONS OF THE FINITE-DIFFERENCE TIME-DOMAIN AND THE SINC-FUNCTION FAST FOURIER TRANSFORM METHOD OF MOMENTS

I have alluded to several problems in which these newly developed approaches may be used for SAR calculations. Following are some of these applications:

1. SAR and induced current distributions for exposures to plane-wave fields for grounded and ungrounded conditions. Both the FDTD and the sinc-function FFT MOM have been used for calculations of SAR distributions in human models for grounded and ungrounded conditions. For example, the layer-averaged SAR distributions calculated at 100 MHz are shown in Figures 6-4 and 6-5 for ungrounded and grounded model conditions, respectively. The dielectric properties for the various

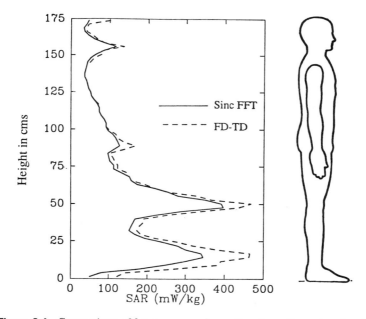

Figure 6-4 Comparison of layer-averaged specific absorption rates for sinc-function fast Fourier transform method of moments (FFT MOM) and finite-difference time-domain (FDTD) method for ungrounded man exposed to vertically polarized, frontally incident plane wave with intensity 1 mW/cm². Calculations were made with 2.62 cm resolution, 5628-cell model of man. FFT MOM average specific absorption rate is 101 mW/kg. FDTD method gives 116 mW/kg.

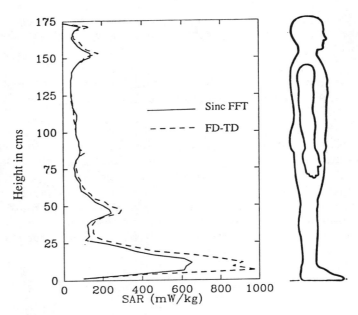

Figure 6-5 Comparison of layer-averaged specific absorption rates for sinc-function fast Fourier transform method of moments (FFT MOM) and finite-difference time-domain (FDTD) method for grounded man exposed to vertically polarized, frontally incident plane wave with intensity 1 mW/cm². Calculations were made with 2.62 cm resolution, 5628-cell model of man. FFT MOM average specific absorption rate is 93 mW/kg. FDTD method gives 106 mW/kg.

tissues are taken from Table 6-1. Even though radically different procedures are used for the FFT MOM and FDTD methods (integral versus differential equation formulation of the Maxwell's equations), fairly similar layer-averaged SAR distributions are obtained (Figures 6-4 and 6-5). The slight discrepancies between the SARs for the knee and ankle sections may occur because only few cells have been used for these two sections and the SARs calculated by both methods are somewhat lower than those estimated from measurements of currents induced in human subjects (Gandhi et al., 1986). Higher-resolution models are needed for calculations at higher frequencies. Therefore the 1.31 cm cell size, 41,256-cell human model has been used for calculations of SAR distributions at 350 MHz (Sullivan et al., 1988). The contour diagram of the SAR distribution for the cross section through the eyes is shown in Figure 6-6 to illustrate the kind of detail that can be obtained. As expected, the highest SARs are obtained for the frontal region of the cross section. The calculated whole-body-averaged SARs for grounded and isolated human models are shown in Figure 6-7 for the frequency band 20 to 100 MHz (Chen and Gandhi, 1989b). Also shown for comparison are the experi-

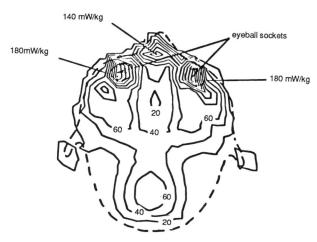

Figure 6-6 Contour diagram of specific absorption rate distribution through head of inhomogeneous man model. Incident plane wave was 1 mW/cm^2 at 350 MHz. Each contour is 20 mW/kg.

mental data by Hill (1984) with human subjects and by Guy et al. (1984) with a homogeneous model. Whereas excellent agreement is seen with Hill's data (1984) for human subjects, higher SARs are obtained for the inhomogeneous model used for the present calculations than those for the homogeneous model (Guy et al., 1984). As shown in Figures 6-8 and 6-9, substantial RF currents are induced in the legs. Because of the large bone content of the legs, an inhomogeneous model properly accounts for the lower effective conductivities in the region, which results in higher SARs.

The calculated E fields can be used to determine the local current densities from the relationship $\mathbf{J} = (\sigma + j\omega\epsilon)\,\mathbf{E}$. The z-directed currents for any of the layers in Figure 6-3 can be obtained by summing up the terms from the individual cells in a given layer as follows:

$$I = \delta^2 \sum_i (\sigma_i + j\omega\epsilon_i)\,E_{zi} \qquad (14)$$

where δ^2 is the cross-sectional area for each of the cells. The layer-averaged induced current distributions are given in Chen and Gandhi (1989b) for isolated and grounded conditions at frequencies of 27 to 90 MHz. The induced current distributions are shown in Figures 6-8 and 6-9 for frequencies of 50 and 60 MHz, which were chosen for illustration because they are close to the resonant frequencies for grounded and ungrounded conditions, respectively (Figure 6-7). Since E fields of 61.4 V/m have been recommended as safe in the ANSI C95.1–1982 RF safety guideline

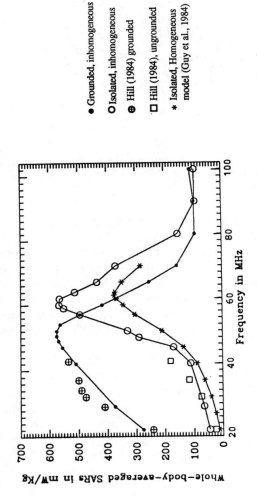

Figure 6-7 Whole-body averaged specific absorption rates for grounded and isolated man model. Also shown for comparison are human subject data of Hill (1984) and homogeneous, isolated model data of Guy et al. (1984).

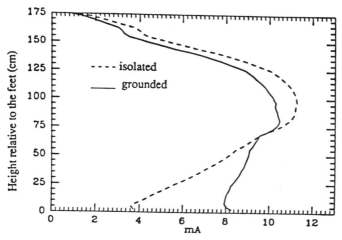

Figure 6-8 Induced radiofrequency current distributions for grounded and isolated human model at 50 MHz under 1 V/m plane-wave exposure condition.

(1982) for the frequency band 30 to 300 MHz, substantial RF currents are obviously implied from the data given in Figures 6-8 and 6-9.

2. SARs and induced current distributions for leakage fields of a parallel-plate dielectric heater. In a recent article by Chen and Gandhi (1989a), the FDTD method has been used to calculate the local, layer-averaged, and whole-body-averaged SARs and induced RF currents in

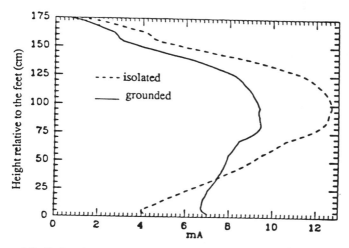

Figure 6-9 Induced radiofrequency current distributions for grounded and isolated human model at 60 MHz under 1 V/m plane-wave exposure condition.

a 5628-cell (cell size 2.62 cm) human model for spatially variable EM fields of a parallel-plate applicator representative of RF dielectric heaters used in industry. Included in the calculations are the shape and dimensions of the applicator plates (57.6 × 15.7 cm parallel plates with a separation of 2.62 cm), as well as a typical separation of 21 cm to the human operator (geometry shown in Figure 6-10). The calculated leakage field components without the human model are in agreement with the experimentally measured values. The human model is considered under the following conditions of exposure: isolated from ground, feet in contact with ground, and with an additional grounded top plate 13.1 cm above the head to simulate screen rooms that are occasionally used for RF sealers. Also considered is the model with a separation layer of rubber (ϵ_r = 4.2) of thickness 2.62 cm between feet and ground to simulate shoes. The layer-averaged SAR and current distributions calculated for the various conditions are shown in Figures 6-11 and 6-12, respectively, for an irradiation frequency of 27.12 MHz. Since foot currents can be measured for a human subject by means of a bilayer sensor detailed in Gandhi et al. (1986), we have made these measurements for a human subject in front of a parallel-plate applicator of dimensions identical to those used for the calculations. The ground plane underneath the current sensor was provided by a $\frac{1}{16}$-inch thick aluminum plate of dimensions 1.2 × 2.4 m. The foot currents have been measured for grounded conditions and for a subject wearing electrical "safety shoes" (size 11, Vibram Manu-

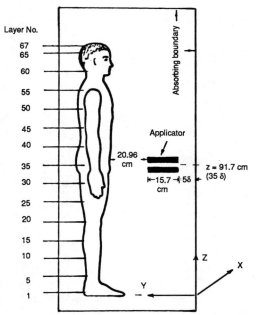

Figure 6-10 Geometry of applicator and human model.

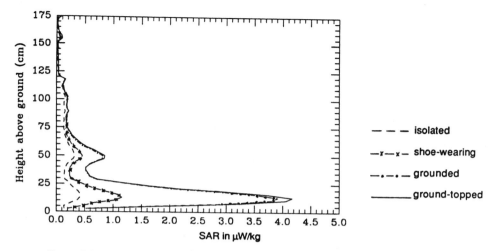

Figure 6-11 Layer-averaged specific absorption rate distributions for isolated, shoe-wearing, grounded, and ground-topped human model at 27.12 MHz under near-field exposure conditions. Maximum Erms = 1 V/m at 21 cm in front of parallel-plate applicator.

facturing Company, rubber sole thickness 1.75 cm). For the so-called isolated condition, the foot current was measured by using a sufficient styrofoam thickness (typically larger than 12.7 cm) under the feet to "isolate" the subject from ground. For such thicknesses the currents were

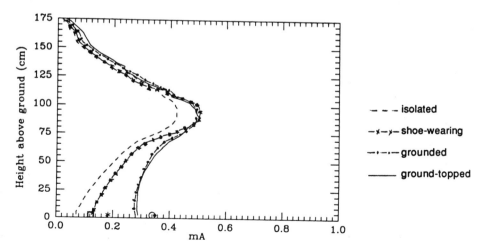

Figure 6-12 Induced vertical current distributions for isolated, shoe-wearing, grounded, and ground-topped human model at 27.12 MHz under near-field exposure conditions. Maximum Erms = 1 V/m at 21 cm in front of parallel-plate applicator.

found to be independent of the thickness of styrofoam. The measured currents are shown for comparison in Figure 6-12. The results are in reasonable agreement with the calculated values of the currents through the feet for the various irradiation conditions. A spatially maximum E field of 1 V/m RMS has been used for the plots shown in Figures 6-11 and 6-12. Because peak E fields as high as 1000 to 2700 V/m have been measured at industrial locations typically occupied by the operator, significant internal RF currents on the order of 0.5 to 2.3 A are projected, scaling the calculated values given in Figure 6-12.

3. SAR distributions for annular-phased arrays (APAs) of aperture and dipole antennas for hyperthermia. One of the challenging tasks in EM hyperthermia is to develop applicators for selectively heating a deep-seated tumor in the human body. Because of the difficulty of experimentation with inhomogeneous, let alone anatomically realistic, models, all of the electromagnetic applicators at the present time are characterized with homogeneous phantoms. This characterization is relatively worthless and not pertinent to the EM deposition patterns for the human body. The knowledge of the SAR distribution in anatomically based models is likely to aid in the design of the applicators in regard to the frequency, size, and magnitude and phase of the various elements (if a multielement applicator is used) to obtain the highest SAR in the tumor vis-à-vis the surrounding tissues.

One of the most popular means of heating internal tissues is the APAs (Turner, 1984a,b). We have used the FDTD method to calculate the SAR distributions in a 17,363-cell, 1.31 cm resolution model of the human torso (Figure 6-13) that was surrounded by deionized water to simulate the water bolus typically used (Wang and Gandhi, 1989). Eight element arrays of aperture and dipole antennas located around a cylinder of radius 23.6 cm concentric with the central axis of the model are assumed for the calculations to simulate the APAs commonly used. Test runs on the calculation of fields in the water-filled interaction space and with homogeneous circular- and elliptical-cylinder phantoms correlate well with the experimental data (Turner, 1984a,b). The anatomically based model of the torso shown in Figure 6-13 is then used for SAR calculations. Shown on the left are the layer numbers used for the model and for displaying the calculated SARs. Three cases have been considered for the parallel-plate applicators. In all cases the frequency is 100 MHz and the total incident power is 100 W.

In Figure 6-14 the layer-averaged SARs are shown for the model of the torso for three cases: (1) eight radiating elements each with a separation of 33δ or 43.23 cm, (2) eight elements, each with a separation of 15δ or 19.65 cm, and (3) five elements on the side close to the liver

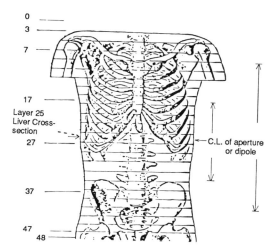

Figure 6-13 Diagram of human torso showing levels at which data were calculated with finite-difference time-domain method. Also shown are relative sizes of apertures or dipoles.

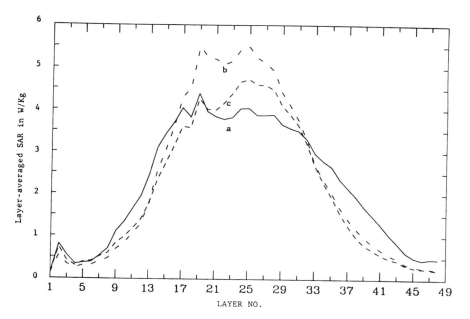

Figure 6-14 Layer-averaged specific absorption rate distributions for model of torso. a, Eight parallel-plate applicators, each with separation of 43.23 cm (33δ). b, Eight parallel-plate applicators, each with separation of 19.65 cm (15δ). c, Five elements surrounding liver are energized, each with separation of 19.65 cm (15δ). Frequency is 100 MHz. Input power is 100 W.

to focus the energy preferentially into this organ. The mass densities for the various tissues given in Table 6-1 are used to calculate the weights of the individual cells, which are then used to convert the volume densities $\frac{1}{2}\sigma E^2$ of absorbed power to the SARs for the respective cells. As expected, the energy absorption is somewhat more focused in the central layers for the narrower apertures of separation, 15δ, than for the wider-aperture APA. Figure 6-15 gives the contours of the calculated SARs for layer No. 25 (Figure 6-13), corresponding to the centerline of the apertures for the three cases identified above. Similar diagrams on the SAR distributions are of course available for each of the other layers as well.

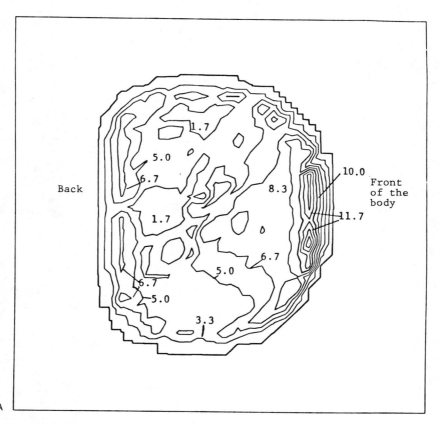

A

Figure 6-15 Specific absorption rate distributions for layer 25 corresponding to central line of applicators. **A,** Eight parallel-plate applicators, each with separation of 43.23 cm (33δ).

Figure 6-16 shows the comparison of normalized layer-averaged SARs for the torso model for an eight-aperture APA (*b* of Figure 6-14) and an eight-dipole APA at a frequency of 100 MHz. Identical dipole length and aperture separations each of 15δ or 19.65 cm have been used for the calculations. Consistent with experimental observations (P. F. Turner, personal communication), fairly similar layer-averaged SAR distributions are calculated for aperture- and dipole-type APAs.

As mentioned before, we have recently developed an anatomically based, thermal block human model (Gandhi and Hoque, to be published) and have used it to calculate the temperature distributions for exposure to plane-wave irradiation conditions. Because the cell sizes of this thermal model are compatible with those used here, SARs obtained here could be used to calculate the temperature distributions for the various APAs.

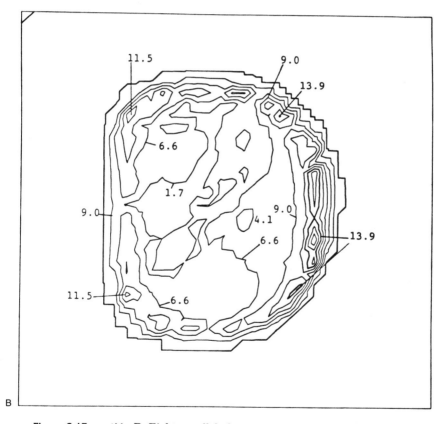

Figure 6-15, cont'd   B, Eight parallel-plate applicators, each with separation of 19.65 cm (15δ).

Continued.

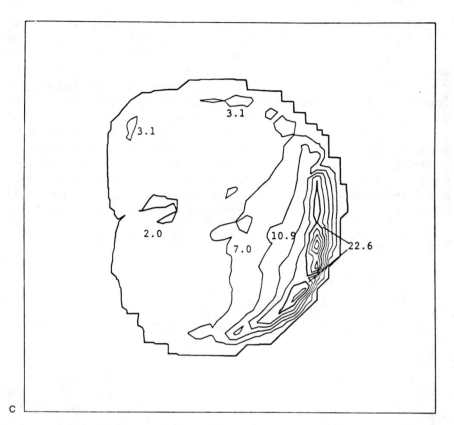

C

Figure 6-15, cont'd C, Five elements surrounding liver are energized, each with separation of 19.65 cm (15δ). Frequency is 100 MHz. Input power is 100 W.

An attempt will be made to use inhomogeneous models obtained from the CT scans of an individual patient so that the size and the location of the tumor can be properly modeled.

CONCLUSION

The numerical models for SAR calculations have reached a level of sophistication that would have been unthinkable a few years ago. These models are consequently being applied to some very realistic situations both in assessing RF safety and for medical applications. The 3-D thermal models are not so sophisticated as the models for SAR calculations. In addition to improvements in the thermal models, efforts are needed in using individualized models based on the CT scans of a patient so that size and location of the tumor can be properly modeled.

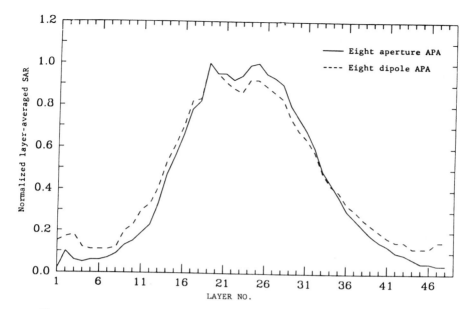

Figure 6-16 Comparison of normalized layer-averaged specific absorption rates for eight aperture and eight dipole annular-phased arrays. Frequency is 100 MHz.

REFERENCES

ANSI (1982). American National Standards Institute. American national standard C95.1, safety levels with respect to human exposure to radio-frequency electromagnetic fields, 300 kHz to 100 GHz. New York, Institute of Electrical and Electronic Engineers, Inc.

ARMITAGE, D.W., LEVEEN, H.H., AND PETHIG, R. (1983). Radio-frequency induced hyperthermia: computer simulation of specific absorption rate distributions using realistic anatomical models. *Phys. Med. Biol.* 28:31–42.

BORUP, D.T., GANDHI, O.P., AND JOHNSON, S.A. A novel sinc basis FFT-CG method for calculating EM power deposition in anatomically-based man models. *IEEE Trans. Microwave Theory Tech.* Submitted for publication.

CHATTERJEE, I., AND GANDHI, O.P. (1983). An inhomogeneous thermal block model of man for the electromagnetic environment. *IEEE Trans. Biomed. Eng.* 30:707–715.

CHEN, J.Y., AND GANDHI, O.P. (1989a). Electromagnetic deposition in anatomically-based model of man for leakage fields of a parallel-plate dielectric heater. *IEEE Trans. Microwave Theory Tech.* 37:174–180.

CHEN, J.Y., AND GANDHI, O.P. (1989b). RF currents induced in an anatomically-based model of a human for plane-wave exposures 20–100 MHz, *Health Phys.* 57:89–98.

CHEN, K.M., AND GURU, B.S. (1977). Internal EM field and absorbed power density in human torsos induced by 1–500 MHz EM waves. *IEEE Trans. Microwave Theory Tech. 25*:746–755.

DEFORD, J.F. (1985). Impedance method for solving low-frequency dosimetry problems. M.S. Thesis, University of Utah, Salt Lake City.

DEFORD, J.F., GANDHI, O.P., AND HAGMANN, M.J. (1983). Moment-method solutions and SAR calculations for inhomogeneous models of man with large number of cells. *IEEE Trans. Microwave Theory Tech. 31*:848–851.

DURNEY, C.H. (1980). Electromagnetic dosimetry for models of humans and animals: a review of theoretical and numerical techniques. *Proc. IEEE 68*:33–40.

ELLIOTT, R.S., HARRISON, W.H., AND STORM, F.K. (1982). Hyperthermia: electromagnetic heating of deep-seated tumors. *IEEE Trans. Biomed. Eng. 29*:61–64.

EYCLESHYMER, A.C., AND SCHOEMAKER, D.M. (1911). A cross-section anatomy. New York, D. Appleton & Co.

FLETCHER, R. (1975). Conjugate gradient methods for indefinite systems. *In*: Watson, G.A. (ed.). Numerical analysis, Dundee Lecture Note 506, Berlin, Springer-Verlag, pp. 73–89.

GANDHI, O.P., CHEN, J.Y., AND RIAZI, A. (1986). Currents induced in a human being for plane-wave exposure conditions 0–50 MHz and for RF sealers. *IEEE Trans. Biomed. Eng. 33*:757–767.

GANDHI, O.P., AND DEFORD, J.F. (1988). Calculation of EM power deposition for operator exposure to RF induction heaters. *IEEE Trans. Electromagnet. Comp. 30*:63–68.

GANDHI, O.P., DEFORD, J.F., AND KANAI, H. (1984). Impedance method for calculation of power deposition patterns in magnetically-induced hyperthermia. *IEEE Trans. Biomed. Eng. 31*:644–651.

GANDHI, O.P., HAGMANN, M.J., AND D'ANDREA, J.A. (1979). Part-body and multibody effects on absorption of radio-frequency electromagnetic energy by animals and by models of man. *Radio Sci. 14*:6(suppl.) 15–21.

GANDHI, O.P., AND HOQUE, M. An inhomogeneous thermal block model of man for electromagnetic exposure conditions. *IEEE Trans. Biomed. Eng.* Submitted for publication.

GUY, A.W., CHOU, C.K., AND NEUHAUS, B. (1984). Average SAR and SAR distributions in man exposed to 450-MHz radio-frequency radiation. *IEEE Trans. Microwave Theory Tech. 32*:752–763.

HAGMANN, M.J., AND GANDHI, O.P. (1979). Numerical calculation of electromagnetic energy deposition in models of man with grounding and reflector effects. *Radio Sci. 14*:6(suppl.) 23–29.

HAGMANN, M.J., GANDHI, O.P., AND DURNEY, C.H. (1979). Numerical calculation of electromagnetic energy deposition for a realistic model of man. *IEEE Trans. Microwave Theory Tech. 27*:804–809.

HARRINGTON, R.F. (1961). Time harmonic electromagnetic fields. New York, McGraw-Hill Book Co., pp. 232–238.

HARRINGTON, R.F. (1968). Field computations by moment methods. New York, Macmillan, Inc.

HESTENES, M., AND STIEFEL, E. (1952). Method of conjugate gradients for solving linear systems. *J. Res. Nat. Bur. Standards* 49:409–436.

HILL, D.A. (1984). The effect of frequency and grounding on whole-body absorption of humans in E-polarized radio-frequency fields. *Bioelectromagnetics* 5:131–146.

HOLLAND, R. (1977). THREDE: a free-field EMP coupling and scattering code. *IEEE Trans. Nucl. Sci.* 24:2416–2421.

KUNZ, K.S., AND LEE K.-M. (1978). A three-dimensional finite-difference solution of the external response of an aircraft to a complex transient EM environment. The method and its implementation. *IEEE Trans. Electromagnet. Comp.* 20:328–332.

LIVESAY, D.E., AND CHEN, K.M. (1974). Electromagnetic fields induced inside arbitrary-shaped bodies. *IEEE Trans. Microwave Theory Tech.* 22:1273–1280.

MANNING, M.R., AND GERNER, E.W. (1981). Interstitial thermoradiotherapy. *In*: Storm, F.K. (ed.). Hyperthermia in cancer therapy.

MUR, G. (1981). Absorbing boundary conditions for the finite-difference approximation of the time-domain electromagnetic field equations. *IEEE Trans. Electromagnet. Comp.* 23:377–382.

ORCUTT, N.E., AND GANDHI, O.P. (1988). A 3-D impedance method to calculate power deposition in biological bodies subjected to time-varying magnetic fields. *IEEE Trans. Biomed. Eng.* 35:577–583.

ORCUTT, N.E., AND GANDHI, O.P. (1990). Use of the impedance method to calculate 3-D power deposition patterns for hyperthermia with capacitive plate electrodes. *IEEE Trans. Biomed. Eng.* 37.

SARKAR, T.K., SIARKIEWICZ, K.R., AND STRATTON, R.F. (1981). Survey of numerical methods for solution of large systems of linear equations for electromagnetic field problems. *IEEE Trans. Antennas Prop.* 29:847–856.

SPIEGEL, R.J. (1984). A review of numerical models for predicting the energy deposition and resultant thermal response of humans exposed to electromagnetic fields. *IEEE Trans. Microwave Theory Tech.* 32:730–746.

SPIEGEL, R.J., FATMI, M.B.E., AND KUNZ, K.S. (1985). Application of a finite-difference technique to the human radio-frequency dosimetry problem. *J. Microwave Power* 20:241–254.

STOLWIJK, J.A.J. (1970). Mathematical model of thermoregulation. *In*: Hardy, J.D., Gagge, A.P., and Stolwijk, J.A.J. (eds.). Physiological and behavioral temperature regulation. Springfield, Ill., Charles C Thomas, Publisher, pp. 703–721.

STOLWIJK, J.A.J. (1980). Mathematical models of thermal regulation. *Ann. N.Y. Acad. Sci.* 335:98–106.

STOLWIJK, J.A.J., AND HARDY, J.D. (1977). Control of body temperature. *In*: Lee, D.H.K. (ed.). Handbook of physiology. Bethesda, Md., American Physiological Society, pp. 44–68.

SULLIVAN, D.M., BORUP, D.T., AND GANDHI, O.P. (1987). Use of the finite-difference time-domain method in calculating EM absorption in human tissues. *IEEE Trans. Biomed. Eng. 34*:148–157.

SULLIVAN, D.M., GANDHI, O.P., AND TAFLOVE, A. (1988). Use of the finite-difference time-domain method for calculating EM absorption in man models. *IEEE Trans. Biomed. Eng. 35*:179–186.

TAFLOVE, A. (1980). Application of the finite-difference time-domain method to sinusoidal steady-state electromagnetic-penetration problems. *IEEE Trans. Electromagnet. Comp. 22*:191–202.

TAFLOVE, A., AND BRODWIN, M.E. (1975a). Computation of the electromagnetic fields and induced temperatures within a model of the microwave irradiated human eye. *IEEE Trans. Microwave Theory Tech. 23*:888–896.

TAFLOVE, A., AND BRODWIN, M.E. (1975b). Numerical solution of steady-state electromagnetic scattering problems using the time-dependent Maxwell's equations. *IEEE Trans. Microwave Theory Tech. 23*:623–630.

TURNER, P.F. (1984a). Hyperthermia and inhomogeneous tissue effects using an annular phased array. *IEEE Trans. Microwave Theory Tech.* 32:874–882.

TURNER, P.F. (1984b). Regional hyperthermia with an annular phased array. *IEEE Trans. Biomed. Eng. 31*:106–114.

UMASHANKAR, K., AND TAFLOVE, A. (1982). A novel method to analyze electromagnetic scattering of complex objects. *IEEE Trans. Electromagnet. Comp. 24*:397–405.

WANG, C.Q., AND GANDHI, O.P. (1989). Numerical simulation of annular phased arrays for anatomically-based models using the FDTD method. *IEEE Trans. Microwave Theory Tech. 37*:118–126.

YEE, K.S. (1966). Numerical solution of initial boundary value problems involving Maxwell's equations in isotropic media. *IEEE Trans. Antennas Prop. 14*:302–307.

ZHU, X.L., AND GANDHI, O.P. (1988). Design of RF needle applicators for optimum SAR distributions in irregularly-shaped tumors. *IEEE Trans. Biomed. Eng. 35*:382–388.

7

Experimental Techniques and Instrumentation

HOWARD I. BASSEN

TADEUSZ M. BABIJ

ROLE OF EXPERIMENTAL TECHNIQUES AND INSTRUMENTATION IN BIOELECTROMAGNETICS

Strong electromagnetic (EM) fields can produce both detrimental as well as therapeutic effects in exposed personnel and other biological subjects. They can also render critical medical electronic systems unsafe (Bassen, 1986). Determination of the intensity of radiofrequency (RF) EM fields (with frequencies ranging from several kilohertz to several hundred giga-hertz) is mandatory when studying the biological effects of EM fields on laboratory animals. Quantification of human exposure, in both the work place and nonoccupational settings, is also required to determine compliance with applicable safety standards (Wacker and Bowman, 1971; Aslan, 1983). The nature of actual external exposure fields and the result-ing absorption in biological systems is complex. Therefore the measure-ment of exposure fields and the performance of dosimetry (quantification of RF absorption in biological tissues) is often best accomplished through experimental methods rather than, or in addition to the use of mathemati-cal techniques. The estimation of exposure field strengths that could induce a biological effect in humans can be extrapolated from the results of experiments performed on irradiated laboratory animals. This is accom-plished by using information on the rate of energy absorption inside the animal, the specific absorption rate (SAR). The SAR is expressed in terms of whole-body average or spatially localized values in units of watts per kilogram. A large body of knowledge on experimental measure-ment techniques for RF exposure fields exists and is summarized in several books (ANSI, 1981; Elder and Cahill, 1984; Durney et al., 1986; Polk and Postow, 1986; Michaelson and Lin, 1987; ANSI, in press; Tell et al., in press). This chapter attempts to supplement the information in these publications by presenting important new or unreported informa-tion.

The views of Howard I. Bassen do not reflect the views of the Department of the U.S. Army or the Department of Defense.

IRRADIATION SYSTEMS FOR BIOEFFECTS EXPERIMENTS

Techniques for Implementing Exposures In Vivo and In Vitro

General goals for in vivo exposure systems.   Various exposure systems have been developed for biological effects research. Exposure systems designed to irradiate the whole body of a live animal should produce a relatively uniform spatial distribution of internal SARs. A stationary subject should not have localized SARs induced in it that differ by more than an order of magnitude. However, when an animal assumes various positions with respect to the **E** and **H** vectors of the exposure field, a highly varied SAR distribution results. Variations in the local SAR can be minimized in most exposure systems by maintaining the animal in a fixed orientation with respect to the external E- and H-field vectors. "RF-transparent" restrainers can be used during the irradiation of un-anesthetized laboratory animals. These restrainers are usually planar sheets of plastic, which must have a thickness of less than 0.1 wavelength (including the foreshortening effects of the dielectric constant of the material). This type of restrainer does not excessively perturb exposure fields (Lin et al., 1977).

For behavioral and certain other types of research, animals should be irradiated in an environment where the ventilation, temperature, lighting, and sound levels are similar to those in the animals' normal housing. A solid metal cavity or waveguide exposure system does not meet these requirements. The use of nonmetallic restrainers during animal exposures can introduce stress and other factors that affect the validity of certain biological effects experiments. For long-term exposures, water and food must be provided without altering the fields or shocking the animal when it is feeding or drinking (Guy and Chou, 1976).

General goals for in vitro exposure systems.   The exposure of in vitro samples requires that a uniform SAR be induced throughout the sample volume and that the temperature, exchange of gases, and other environmental factors be maintained within certain limits. The special considerations required in development of sample holders and exposure systems are described later in the chapter.

Free-Field Exposure Techniques

The principal goal of free-field exposure techniques is to irradiate one or more biological subjects with uniform electric and magnetic fields of known magnitude and polarization. It is difficult to deposit significant RF power in a subject that is small compared with the irradiating wavelength using free-field exposure systems or systems such as a transverse electromagnetic (TEM) cell that produce exposures similar to those encountered under free-field conditions. The following are the most common implementations of free-field exposure systems.

Far-field, plane-wave exposure systems.   One of the most widely used techniques for microwave irradiation of biological subjects has been the plane-wave "free-space" exposure chamber for frequencies above about 900 MHz. Typically an anechoic chamber is illuminated by a horn antenna with RF power supplied to the antenna by a microwave generator. The test object is placed in the far field of the antenna. The "far field" exists at distances greater than 2 times R, where R is defined in Eq. 1.

$$R = (2\,D^2)/\lambda \tag{1}$$

where R is the distance in meters from the electrical center of the antenna to the point in space where the irradiated subject is placed, D is the maximum linear dimension in meters of the transmitting antenna's radiating aperture, and λ is the wavelength in meters of the RF that is radiated from the transmitting antenna.

For the case of simple antennas the maximum linear dimension is equal to the length of a dipole antenna, the diameter of a loop antenna, or the longest side of the rectangular aperture of a horn antenna. In the far field $\mathbf{E}$ is perpendicular to $\mathbf{H}$, and both vectors are perpendicular to the direction of propagation (a TEM mode exists). Also, in the far field the ratio of the E to H field has a constant value (termed the intrinsic impedance of free space) of 377 ohms. Since the power density is the vector cross-product of $\mathbf{E}$ and $\mathbf{H}$, the following far-field relationships can be derived with the most commonly used units (mW/cm^2) for these parameters:

$$\mathbf{S} = \mathbf{E}^2/3770 = \mathbf{H}^2 \times 37.7 \tag{2}$$

where $\mathbf{S}$ is the power density (mW/cm^2), $\mathbf{E}$ is the electric field strength (V/m), and $\mathbf{H}$ is the magnetic field strength (A/m). In the near field these equations are not valid (since E/H is not 377 ohms). However, the preceding equations have been frequently applied by instrument manufacturers and their users to specify "equivalent far-field power density" in the near field, when either the E or the H field is measured.

One significant advantage of the use of true plane-wave exposures over other exposure systems is the degree of standardization afforded. Two laboratories can use different plane-wave exposure facilities, yet produce nominally identical whole-body SARs in animals with identical size, weight, and orientation to the E- and H-field vectors. Also, approximately the same regional distribution of SAR is produced in all exposed animals. Furthermore, most quantitative data published on SAR versus exposure for a wide variety of animals and humans involve plane-wave irradiation conditions (Durney et al., 1986; S. Stuchly, 1987).

One disadvantage of plane-wave exposures performed in an anechoic chamber is that high-power generators (hundreds or thousands of watts) must be used to produce several milliwatts per square centimeter. Also, anechoic chambers become extremely large and costly for use at frequencies less than about 500 MHz. Finally, a plane-wave exposure system provides unilateral irradiation (the surface receiving illumination has a much higher local SAR than the opposite surface).

Corner reflector exposure devices for creating increased power density. Devices have been developed for use in anechoic chambers to increase the power density in a small area within a metallic reflector (Gandhi et al., 1977) (Figure 7-1). This type of exposure system reduces the transmitter power needed to produce a given power density and illuminates both the front and back body surfaces of the subject in the reflector. Careful E-field mapping within the reflector must be performed to locate the enhancement region where a biological subject should be placed. Misplacement of the subject by approximately one eighth of a wavelength can reduce the SAR in the subject drastically. If the subject is not anesthetized, it must be restrained as mentioned previously. Finally, the SAR delivered to the subject in a corner reflector must be verified by in situ measurements of a physical replica (phantom) or a cadaver whose size and position are identical to those of the actual experimental subject.

Multiple animal exposure systems.   Several means for simultaneous exposure of several animals in free-space fields have been developed.

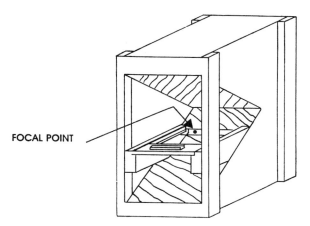

FOCAL POINT

Figure 7-1 Corner reflector exposure system. Shaded area is metal, and all other parts are made of plastic foam.

Judicious arrangement of a group of animals in a plane-wave exposure system can provide equal exposures to all animals (Oliva and Catravas, 1977). Adequate spacing of the animals minimizes the effect of reflections from the neighboring animals. Alternatively, a monopole antenna, placed over a large groundplane, can be used to expose many animals at once (Figure 7-2). Animals are placed along the circumference of a circular locus in the far field of the radiator (D'Andrea et al., 1986).

Enclosed Exposure Systems

Enclosed exposure systems provide users with an economical means for exposing biological subjects under well-controlled conditions. Under normal circumstances a relatively small amount of power (1 to 20 W) and less expensive RF sources can be used to deliver reasonably high SARs to small animals or samples. If the input, reflected, and output powers for these systems are measured, the total power absorbed by the subject can be determined. This is possible because no RF energy is radiated from enclosed exposure systems. However, since the test subject intercepts virtually all the power delivered to the exposure system, the input impedance and reflected power depend largely on the size and orientation of the specimen within the enclosed system. Impedance matching devices or isolators, or both, are usually placed between the RF generator and the input port of these exposure systems to minimize the reflected power from the biological subject.

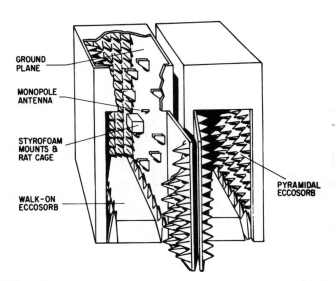

GROUND PLANE

MONOPOLE ANTENNA

STYROFOAM MOUNTS & RAT CAGE

WALK-ON ECCOSORB

PYRAMIDAL ECCOSORB

Figure 7-2 Exposure system using a monopole above a groundplane.

Transverse electromagnetic (TEM) cells.   The TEM cell may be used to generate precisely known values of E and H fields (Crawford, 1974). With this type of enclosed exposure system, small biological subjects can be exposed to a pseudo–plane wave over a frequency range of 10 to about 500 MHz. The TEM cell is an expanded coaxial transmission line in which the center conductor is a flat metal strip and the outer (ground) conductor has a rectangular cross section (Figure 7-3). The usable volume that may be occupied by a subject in the TEM cell is limited. The height of this usable volume is approximately one third of the separation distance between the center conductor and the outer wall of the cell. Larger objects destroy the pure TEM mode existing in the cell so that uniform pseudo–plane wave conditions no longer exist. Also, for preservation of the TEM mode and "plane-wave" conditions, an upper frequency limit must not be exceeded. This limit is inversely proportional to the cell's cross-sectional dimensions and is specified by the cell's manufacturer.

Waveguide exposure systems.   Hollow, rectangular waveguides are readily available for use at frequencies higher than about 750 MHz. The internal dimensions are proportional to the wavelength of the lowest frequency that can be propagated in the waveguide. These waveguides may be used to fabricate a variety of exposure systems for partial- and whole-body irradiation of laboratory animals and for in vitro samples. These systems are inherently capable of carrying extremely high levels of peak power (megawatts). The effects of exposure to high-peak-power pulsed RF (such as radar) may be studied by means of waveguide exposure systems.

Waveguide exposure systems for whole-body irradiation.   Standard rectangular microwave waveguides have been used extensively to expose laboratory rats and other small animals in vivo (Ho et al., 1973). Ideally a single animal should be placed with its long axis aligned with the electric field vector (that is, parallel to the shortest side of the cross section of a rectangular waveguide). At frequencies greater than approxi-

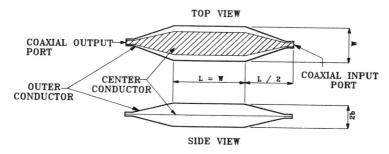

TOP VIEW

COAXIAL OUTPUT
PORT

OUTER
CONDUCTOR

CENTER
CONDUCTOR

L = W   L / 2

COAXIAL INPUT
PORT

2b

SIDE VIEW

Figure 7-3   Basic configuration of a transverse electromagnetic cell.

mately 1200 MHz, only subjects as small as a mouse can be exposed in this manner because of the relatively small dimensions of the waveguide (for example, the WR650 waveguide with dimensions of 6.50 by 3.25 inches). One disadvantage of waveguide exposure systems is that a highly nonuniform SAR is induced in an animal if the long axis of its body is aligned with the direction of propagation of the waveguide. Under these conditions the end of the animal facing the incident microwaves (the head or tail end) absorbs most of the microwave energy. However, without restraint or anesthesia, larger animals reorient themselves and even turn around during the course of an experiment. This produces a more uniform but unpredictable regional SAR distribution.

Waveguide systems for partial-body and in vitro exposures. The waveguide affords a convenient means for irradiating selected regions of a laboratory animal's body or an entire in vitro sample. Microwave power can be deposited in one region such as the animal's head if this part of the subject is inserted through the narrow sidewall or end of a standard waveguide (Lenox et al., 1976). In vitro samples, such as a test tube filled with a buffer solution plus a tissue sample, may be inserted through the broad sidewall of a rectangular waveguide. The long axis of the sample holder is aligned with the E-field vector, maximizing the coupling of energy to the sample. Gas- or water-carrying lines may be placed outside the waveguide, so that only the in vitro sample is irradiated while aeration is provided without disrupting the exposure procedure (Creighton et al., 1987).

Cavity exposure systems. Metallic cavities that are large compared with the wavelength of microwave irradiation are well suited for whole-animal exposure systems. They are capable of inducing relatively uniform SAR distributions in laboratory animals, especially when a mechanical mode stirrer, similar to the device used in microwave ovens, is incorporated (Justesen et al., 1971). These cavities can be fabricated with cylindrical and rectangular geometries. A specially designed cylindrical waveguide-cavity exposure system that produces a circularly polarized TE_{11} mode has been designed (Guy and Chou, 1976). It induces a relatively uniform distribution of SAR throughout a test animal's body. Little microwave power is reflected at the input port of this cavity, regardless of the animal's position. In addition, this system is formed with wire mesh to provide visibility and ventilation through the walls of the waveguide.

Resonant cavity systems can be designed to allow good coupling to very small biological samples. With this type of system the effects of pulsed, high-peak, low-average-power microwave radiation have been studied. An instantaneous peak SAR of 20 MW/kg can be induced in the brain of a mouse with a 200 kW peak input power when the cavity exposure system shown in Figure 7-4 is used (Bassen et al., 1988).

Other Exposure Systems

Microwave aperture "applicators."   Microwave "applicators" have been designed with open-ended waveguides as antennas to selectively expose portions of a laboratory animal. Miniaturized applicators are often produced by filling their interior waveguide structure completely with a high dielectric constant material (a ceramic or deionized water). This makes the applicator capable of operating at frequencies whose free-space wavelength is much larger than the applicator's output (aperture) size (Magin, 1979). However, the dielectric loading of a miniaturized applicator produces a significant reduction in the depth of penetration in biological tissue, compared with full-sized, air-filled applicators operating at the same frequency (Cheever, 1987).

Helical coil exposure system.   A unique apparatus has been developed for the uniform deposition of RF energy in biological materials and for therapeutic heating at a selected frequency in the 10 to 100 MHz range (Ruggera and Kantor, 1984). This device is a multiturn, resonant helical coil with an air core. It is capable of delivering a relatively uniform SAR throughout the cross section of a cylindrical, lossy dielectric object, such as a human leg or a small animal. No contact between the subject and the coil occurs. A single helical coil exposure device has been used to irradiate several laboratory rodents simultaneously, producing relatively uniform SAR in each animal. The coil provides ambient air and visibility through the spaces between windings of the coil.

In the 10 to 100 MHz range both the helical coil and the TEM cell can be used as RF exposure systems. However, the coil couples energy into biological objects that are small compared with the RF wavelength

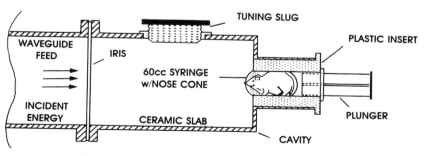

Figure 7-4   Waveguide resonant-cavity exposure system.

whereas the TEM cell does not. Other differences include the fact that
the helical coil is a resonant, narrow-band device, designed for use at a
specific frequency, whereas the TEM cell is broad band and can be used
easily at any frequency in its specified operating frequency band.

INSTRUMENTATION

Instruments for Radiofrequency Exposure-Field Measurements

General physical configurations of field strength measurement systems. Instruments intended to quantify RF field strengths (from about
1 MHz to greater than 18 GHz) under near- and far-field conditions
must be designed to accommodate a variety of parameters of the fields.
Many RF "hazard" or survey monitors are constructed with a sensor
enclosed in a plastic sphere or cylinder that has a diameter of 10 to 20
cm. The sensor is usually an array of three small antennas with integral
RF detectors (Figure 7-5, *A*). Many RF probes have a tubular handle
30 to 60 cm long. The handle is attached to the sensor at one end and
contains signal readout leads that emerge at the other end of the tube
(Figure 7-5, *B*). The signal leads range from about 1 to more than 5 m
and are connected to a readout box containing electronic components
and a visual field-strength data display. The sensor is kept away from
the user's body when the user grips the opposite end of the handle.
This reduces RF coupling and interaction between the user's body and
the sensors.

Other field measurement instruments are constructed as integrated,
enclosed systems with the antennas emerging from the sides of a small,
metallic cube (Figure 7-5, *C*). The cubical box contains RF detection and
processing circuitry and a data display. Some field measurement instruments
have a remote data display attached to the field-sensing device
with long resistive or fiber-optic signal leads. This eliminates the need
to have a person in the close proximity of the system's antennas. This
minimizes errors introduced by reflections from the operator's body.

Important performance parameters for E- and H-field instruments. The following characteristics are either essential or highly desirable
for surveying or monitoring EM exposure fields (Wacker and Bowman, 1971; ANSI, in press):

1. The probe's response should be independent of the angular orientation or polarization of the E- or H-field vectors and the direction

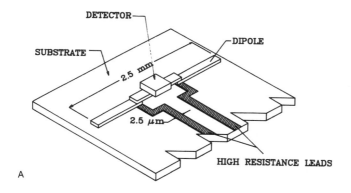

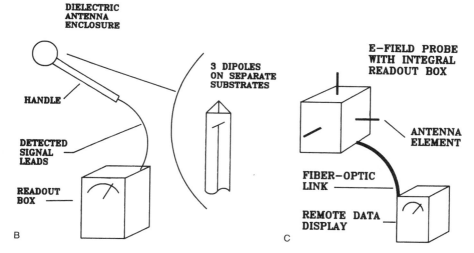

Figure 7-5   **A,** E-field-probe antenna/detector design. **B,** Conventional E-field-probe system. **C,** Integrated E-field-probe system with fiber-optic data link.

of the incident radiation. (That is, an isotropic receiving pattern is required.)

2. An exposure field instrument's accuracy should not be adversely affected by strong E fields. Such problems sometimes occur at low frequencies (below several megahertz) because of E-field "pickup" on the electrical leads attached to the probe's sensor array and in its handle.

3. The probe, its readout device, and interconnecting cables should not cause a large amount of scattering of the incident field or alteration of the emission characteristics of the RF source being measured. Such a probe is described as "nonperturbing."

4. The probe should be able to resolve the gradients and standing waves of the fields being measured. Resolution should be a fraction of a wavelength or, in the near field, several centimeters, regardless of frequency.
5. The instrument should measure the true RMS field strength, regardless of the magnitude of the E or H field and the amount of amplitude modulation imposed on the RF field.
6. The probe should provide a constant sensitivity, independent of the frequency of any signals being measured. It should not respond excessively to fields whose frequencies lie outside the probe's intended range of use.
7. The instrument's RF sensors, electronics, and display device should be insensitive to changes in ambient temperatures, orientation of the readout device, and other physical conditions.

E-field probe.   The type of RF electric field measurements associated with biological effects and personnel safety require data only on the magnitude of the E or H field, but not its phase (Wacker and Bowman, 1971; Bassen and Smith, 1983). Isotropic E-field probes use three orthogonal dipoles, each with its own detector (Figure 7-5, A). Each dipole antenna has two arms of equal length and a detector (diode or thermocouple) between the arms. To be nonperturbing and have good spatial resolution, the antenna must have a small total length in comparison with the wavelength being measured. The use of three orthogonal, electrically small antennas with individual square-law detectors enables isotropic, polarization-independent performance. Resistive dipole elements that are not small compared with the wavelength of the field being measured are often incorporated in E-field probes. These antennas provide very wide operating bandwidths that include centimeter or millimeter wavelength fields, while maintaining isotropic response (Hopfer and Adler, 1980). If each antenna has its own square-law detector (whose output voltage is proportional to the field strength squared), the sum of the squares of the three E-field vector components may be obtained easily with a simple "summing" operational amplifier. High-resistance leads that do not interact with the RF field or act as parasitic antennas are often used to convey the detected RF signal from the sensor to the base of the probe handle and even to the readout electronic components box. This ensures isotropic, nonperturbing probe performance.

To alleviate the problem of inadequate isolation of the resistive leads from the probe's antennas at low RF frequencies (less than several megahertz), a miniature electrical to optical data converter and fiber-optic leads may be employed (Bassen and Hoss, 1978). This approach has been incorporated in several commercially available broad-band EM measurement systems. A completely passive, nonelectronic technique for measuring E fields is emerging as a practical alternative to the previously described designs. Photonic or electrically sensitive optical crystals can be used as an antenna and sensor with fiber optics and broad-band (0 to 5 GHz) optical detectors (Bassen and Smith, 1983; Wyss and Sheeran, 1985).

H-field probe. Probes for measuring RF magnetic fields are constructed in a manner similar to RF electric field probes. The principal difference is that in an H-field probe an array of three small, orthogonal loops is used as an isotropic receiving antenna. Each loop delivers an RF voltage to a square-law detector whose output is then summed to produce a signal proportional to the total H field. Magnetic field probes that are available commercially have an upper frequency limit of about 300 MHz and a lower limit of several megahertz (Nesmith and Ruggera, 1982).

E-H field probe. Complete near-field RF measurements require determination of both E- and H-field strengths. This necessitates the use of two different isotropic probes. A problem arises under certain measurement conditions. Both the ratio of E to H and the generation of RF emissions by industrial or medical devices change rapidly with time or location. It is often impossible to measure the brief emission of both fields at a single location, simultaneously. When isotropic E and H sensors are incorporated in the same small volume, this problem can be avoided with the following approach. An array of three orthogonal dipoles, each with its own square-law detector, can be employed to provide a single DC voltage that is proportional to the total E-field strength, via a summing amplifier. A second detected voltage proportional to the total H-field strength can be provided simultaneously by an array of three orthogonal loops with individual square-law detectors. This approach yields data on the magnitudes of the total electric and the total magnetic field at a single location at any instant in time (Babij and Bassen, 1980, 1986). The E-H measurement system design concept is illustrated in Figure 7-6. Proper physical arrangements of the three orthogonal dipoles and loops minimize coupling between the six antennas. If these antennas are thin and electrically small and the loops use a common-center configuration, a highly isotropic pattern is achieved (Aslan, 1987). Several E-H probe designs are available from commercial sources for use at frequencies below 50 MHz.

Personal radiofrequency dosimeters. Personal dosimeters are commonly used for protective monitoring of personnel exposed to x-rays and other forms of ionizing radiation. These body-mounted devices measure

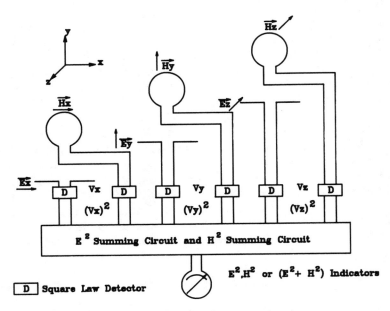

Figure 7-6   E-H probe measurement system.

a person's cumulative exposure. An RF dosimeter (which measures cumulative exposures to field strengths that exceed a certain level) has been sought by the radiation protection community for many years. To conform with contemporary RF safety standards, an RF dosimeter must be accurate over a wide frequency range, be lightweight and have a small physical configuration, have an omnidirectional pattern, and be capable of recording time-integrated exposure or SAR data.

Commercially available personal dosimeters have not provided these performance parameters (Bassen, 1979). The inaccuracies of these dosimeters are produced because of the shielding effect of the wearer's body. Also, if a dosimeter of this type is located on or very near the body surface, its antennas are subject to loading from RF reflections. This causes variations in measured field strengths, depending on the frequency and the distance from the body (Beischer and Reno, 1975). In contrast to this inadequate design approach, a different method for personal dosimetry has been demonstrated successfully. At frequencies below the resonance of the wearer (about 40 MHz), total current flow through the body may be measured noninvasively with a thin insolelike measurement device incorporated in a pair of shoes. This approach provides a reasonably accurate basis for personal dosimetry in certain frequency regions (Gandhi, 1987).

Measurement of Internal Fields and Radiofrequency Absorption in Biological Systems

Measurement of whole-body versus local specific absorption rates. SAR is commonly measured as a spatially localized quantity (that is, at one point in a large, heterogeneous biological object). However, whole-body-averaged SAR has been the dosimetric quantity most commonly cited as the basis for contemporary RF personnel safety standards. "Whole-body-averaged" refers to the volume averaged SAR for the body. Even when the whole body of a biological subject is exposed to plane-wave (far-field) RF irradiation, local internal hot spots are induced. In hot spots the local SAR in a few grams of tissue often exceeds the average whole-body SAR by factors of 20 to 100 (Stuchly et al., 1986). Therefore most contemporary experimental dosimetry is performed by taking many SAR data points within a biological subject or model. These data can be integrated later to obtain a coarse approximation of whole-body-averaged SAR. Only calorimetry provides an experimentalist with a means for measuring the whole-body SAR accurately (Phillips et al., 1975).

Defining specific absorption rate in terms of internal E fields or rate of temperature rise. Use of the absorbed dose rate (power delivered to a local volume) within the subject is the key to determining the precise level where a biological response occurs in an exposed animal, regardless of the external exposure circumstances. Microwave power deposition in biological tissue is termed specific absorption rate (SAR). The SAR is expressed in units of watts per kilogram.

The SAR is directly proportional to the electric field strength squared in biological tissue (Eq. 3) and is also proportional to the initial rate of temperature rise in exposed tissue (Eq. 4).

$$\text{SAR} = (\sigma \mathbf{E}^2) / \rho \tag{3}$$

where σ is conductivity of the tissue at the location of interest (siemens/meter), ρ is mass density of the tissue (kilograms/cubic meter), and $\mathbf{E}$ is magnitude of the electric field strength (volts/meter).

$$\text{SAR} = c(dT/dt) \tag{4}$$

where dT/dt is rate of temperature rise in tissue (degrees Celsius/s) and c is specific heat capacity of the tissue (joules/[kilogram − degree Celsius]).

Important performance parameters for internal radiofrequency absorption measurement instruments. Certain general characteristics are desirable for SAR-measuring (or dosimetric) instruments. They should not be affected by strong EM fields other than those at the intended sensor location. The presence of any part of the instrument's sensor or signal leads should not alter the internal SARs or temperatures being measured. The instrument should be able to resolve the steep gradients in the SAR that occur in the biological subject being studied.

Instruments for Measuring Specific Absorption Rates

Implantable temperature probes.   Specially designed temperature probes provide a practical means for determining local SARs. Measurements can be made in tissue-equivalent phantoms, in the cadavers of laboratory animals, or in humans undergoing therapeutic heating via selective RF irradiation. A typical probe contains a temperature sensor and signal leads, both having a diameter of 1 mm or less. In addition to being electrically nonperturbing, the signal leads must not conduct heat into or out of the region where the RF-induced temperature rise is being measured. Electrical signal leads are usually made of high-resistance materials such as carbon-filled Teflon (Bowman, 1976), and the sensor is a miniature thermistor chip. Optical temperature probes with sensors made of temperature-sensitive phosphors are used with fiber-optic signal leads (Wickersheim and Sun, 1987). The smallest detectable SARs with these probes are a few watts per kilogram because of the resolution of commercially available temperature probes (typically 0.01° to 0.1° C). Modern temperature measurement systems contain four to 16 sensors, either as separate probes with their own individual signal leads or as a single probe with a linear array of temperature sensors (Figure 7-7). These multisensor thermometry systems allow the simultaneous determination of SARs at a number of locations in an irradiated subject.

Researchers with limited budgets have often performed RF dosimetry with inexpensive thermocouple or thermistor temperature probes that have metallic readout wires. This approach leads to a variety of significant measurement errors and should therefore be avoided. Sources of error include internal field perturbations and thermodynamic problems, which are discussed later in this chapter.

Thermographic camera.   Guy (1971) described a method for the evaluation of the distribution of SAR throughout an entire inner surface of a bisected cadaver, or of a biological model composed of tissue-simulating materials. The test object is encapsulated in a low-loss dielectric mold or shell, which is split open briefly for thermographic viewing immediately before and after high-power irradiation. The temperature distribution is observed on the midplane of the bisected model (Figure 7-8). The thermographic camera detects and displays an image of the infrared (IR) emissions from the surface of an object. The intensity of these IR emissions

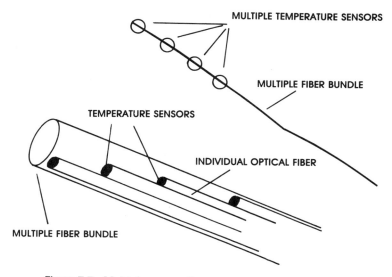

Figure 7-7 Multiple-sensor, linear array temperature probe.

is proportional to the temperature of the surface of the bisected object. Each half of the bisected object must be covered by an IR-transparent membrane (plastic or silk screen) across the entire plane of bisection. This very thin membrane prevents physical deformation and leakage of

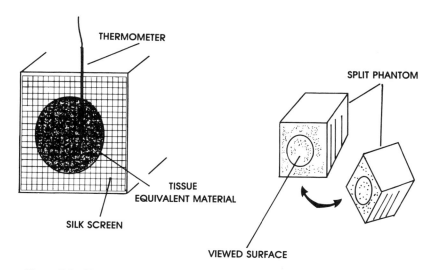

Figure 7-8 Use of a split test object for dosimetric measurements made with a thermographic camera.

the moist tissue or tissue-equivalent material when the bisected phantom is separated for viewing by the thermographic camera.

Implantable E-field probes for specific absorption rate measurements. Internal E-field probes provide the ability to measure the RF electric field strength at a single point continuously or to scan and map the E field along a selected path within a test object. A typical probe consists of a thin-film dipole, 0.5 to 3 mm long, with a microelectronic diode detector chip placed across the gap, between the two arms of the dipole antenna (Figure 7-5). A pair of very narrow, high-resistance leads on a ceramic, plastic, or glass substrate carries the detected (DC) signal from the diode to a remote readout device. The dipole is encapsulated with a few millimeters of a low-dielectric-constant insulating material. This eliminates large changes in the probe's calibration factor, which is proportional to the particular dielectric constant of the material immediately surrounding the probe (Smith, 1979). E-field probes are more sensitive for SAR measurements than temperature probes and can detect SARs as low as 0.2 W/kg (Stuchly et al., 1986). The size of the dipole of an E-field probe determines its spatial resolution (typically several millimeters). A low-frequency limit of several hundred megahertz exists for this type of probe, since the high-resistance leads cannot reject spurious RF pickup adequately at lower frequencies.

Calorimeters. A variety of calorimeters have been used to measure the total energy delivered to a whole-animal cadaver by brief, intense exposure to RF irradiation. Gradient layer (Gandhi et al., 1979), Dewar (Blackman and Black, 1977), and twin-well (Phillips et al., 1975) calorimeters have been used by investigators to determine whole-body-averaged SAR in animals. The twin-well technique uses two nominally identical cadavers or biological models, one irradiated and one as a thermal reference object. This approach eliminates the need to know the average specific heat of the subject. Although calorimetry provides a means for very accurate determinations of whole-body-averaged SAR, it cannot provide information about SAR distribution within the irradiated subject.

Instruments for noninvasive measurements of whole-body or regional current flow in exposed personnel. A few methods have been developed to enable noninvasive measurements of regional SAR or RF currents flowing through the body. For exposure situations involving RF fields below the resonant frequency of a subject (about 40 MHz for a human standing on a conducting ground plane), the total RF current flowing through the body to ground can be measured as described in the section of this chapter on personal dosimeters. It is more difficult to estimate regional SAR (for example, SAR in the arm) when only the magnitude of the total current flowing through the body to ground is known. A technique for the noninvasive measurement of RF currents flowing in human extremities has been used at frequencies both below and above the resonant frequency of the human body. A current probe, fabricated with high-resistance, carbon-loaded, fluorocarbon "wire," is used to obtain current flow data on the same principle as an electrician's clamp-on amme- ter (Hagmann and Babij, 1988).

Measurement of Exposure Fields: Sources of Errors and Techniques to Minimize Them

The accurate measurement of external RF exposure fields is difficult even for experienced personnel. Several documents provide a detailed discussion of the theoretical basis and practical techniques for performing RF exposure field surveys (ANSI, 1981; ANSI, in press; Tell et al., in press). The following discussion presents the fundamental concepts needed to perform accurate measurements. Many factors affect the accu- racy of the measurement of complex RF fields, and each must be addressed through the selection of appropriately designed instruments and the use of special techniques.

Standing waves. Standing waves occur when a radiated EM wave strikes a reflecting surface (the ground or other large conducting object such as a wall, or the field measurement instrument plus the body of the person holding it). Multipath effects occur when these reflections interact with the incident wave, creating an interference pattern (standing wave) with periodic maxima and minima. Under worst-case conditions the peaks of this standing wave may be twice the field strength of the incident field and the periodic minima may have an amplitude of zero. To locate and measure fields at these maxima, the experimentalist should perform scans at several heights above the ground, with an isotropic RF survey meter along two, orthogonal, linear paths parallel to the ground. Sampling measurements can also be made in this grid, at intervals of about one eighth of the wavelength of the field under study.

Polarization and omnidirectional radiofrequency sources. RF fields may have either linear or elliptical polarizations. Often the polarization of an exposure field is unknown or may change significantly over a small area, depending on the RF source and nearby reflecting objects. Isotropic survey probes minimize errors caused by polarization uncertainty. In addition, in the far field of one or more RF sources, the direction of propagation may be unknown and a probe with an omnidirectional an- tenna receiving pattern is needed to measure true field strength.

Multiple frequencies.   During measurements of unknown exposure environments, different fields from several RF sources or a single source with strong harmonic content may produce a complex EM environment containing several RF frequencies (Hopfer and Adler, 1980; Kanda, 1987). Therefore exposure measurement probes must have a frequency-independent, broad-band response. Also, the probes should not have excessively high sensitivity to fields whose frequency is outside the instrument's intended range of use.

Complex modulation.   RF fields often have some form of modulation imposed on them, depending on the nature of the source. For example, radar transmitters impose 100% amplitude modulation and have a unique pulse repetition rate. Most microwave ovens have a "mode stirrer" that significantly changes the amplitude of RF leakage every few seconds.

Spurious responses of E and H probes.   Strong E and H fields with an unknown ratio exist in the near field of an RF emitter. Therefore an H-field probe must not be sensitive to electric fields. Pickup of E fields by the metallic leads and readout box of a survey instrument can produce highly erroneous data (Nesmith and Ruggera, 1982). This problem can be identified by a user if the probe tip with RF sensors is kept in a fixed location while the handle and readout cable are placed first perpendicular and then parallel to a known, uniform E field. A significant change in readings obtained for these probe orientations can indicate the presence of spurious E-field pickup by an isotropic E- or H-field probe.

Interaction of radiofrequency hazard probes with nearby scattering or radiating objects.   Users of RF survey probes often express concern about the effects on measurement accuracy of a reflecting object or a person near the probe. Also, the accuracy of a measurement is unclear when it is made close to an RF radiator (for example, a leaking RF heater or a hand-held transmitter).

Errors from E and H probes near reflecting objects.   Measurement errors can result when a probe is near an RF-reflecting object that can alter the impedance of the probe's antenna. For an electrically small dipole with a diode detector, placed close to an infinite, conducting plane that is illuminated by a plane wave, the worst-case errors are as follows (Smith, 1979). A 0.2-wavelength-long dipole (tip to tip) separated by 0.2 wavelength from the reflector produces a 10% error in the measurement of the E field (about 20% for $\mathbf{E}^2$ or power density). For example, at 300 MHz these error values result when the probe-to-reflector separation and the probe's dipole dimensions are both 20 cm. Similar, relatively insignificant errors can be expected from H-field loops near a reflector if the loop diameter is small compared with a wavelength.

Measurement errors from E and H probes near an active radiator.   If a probe is very close to an active radiator, several factors degrade measurement accuracy. Coupling may occur between the probe's antennas and the radiator. Also, backscatter from the hazard probe can alter the radiator's emission characteristics (Rudge and Knox, 1970). In addition, spatial averaging of the radiator's fields (with their steep spatial gradients) occurs over the volume of the probe's sensors. A separation of 5 probe antenna lengths ensures a worst-case spatial averaging error of less than approximately 3 dB. An antenna length is the tip-to-tip length of an E probe's dipoles or the diameter of an H probe's loops (ANSI, in press). A conservative estimate of the largest antenna length of a probe can be made by assuming that this length is equal to the largest physical dimension of the probe tip's protective housing (usually a foam plastic sphere or cylinder).

Measurement of Internal Fields and Specific Absorption Rates: Sources of Errors and Techniques to Minimize Associated Inaccuracies

Techniques for specific absorption rate determination via temperature measurements and errors caused by thermodynamic factors.   The use of temperature measurements (via thermometry or thermography) can provide accurate SAR data if several thermodynamic phenomena are accounted for. The SAR distribution is highly variable in virtually all biological subjects in any RF irradiation environment. This causes large thermal gradients to be induced in the subject. Thermal conduction, diffusion, and convection cause heat to flow from the hottest spots in the irradiated object to cooler spots. Also, in living systems, active thermoregulation alters the RF-induced temperature distribution. These sources of SAR measurement errors can be minimized by limiting the maximum temperature rise in any portion of the irradiated object to the smallest practical value while ensuring a sufficient temperature rise for precise measurements. Also, temperature measurements should be made only during the first few seconds from the start of irradiation.

Measurement techniques and sources of error for determination of specific absorption rates via temperature probes.   Although many researchers perform SAR measurements with temperature probes, few are fully aware of the factors that affect the accuracy of their SAR measurements. These factors include the probe's resolution and response time. For example, with a probe having a resolution of $\pm 0.1°$ C and a response time of 1 second, SAR data will have uncertainties of at least 20% when RF irradiation induces a rise of $2°$ C in 10 seconds. Longer periods of irradiation will invoke errors owing to thermodynamic effects, and shorter irradiation periods will exceed the probe's response time capabilities. The temperature should be recorded continuously, along with the RF radiation source's output power. Recording should begin at least 10 seconds before and continue 10 seconds after irradiation. Determination of the initial rate of temperature rise (slope) yields true SAR data. In tissue-equivalent models the rate of rise is affected by heat flow from hot spots to cooler areas after the first 10 to 20 seconds of irradiation (Figure 7-9). Also, SAR data can be erroneous if too few spatial samples are taken throughout the volume of the irradiated subject. Intervals of less than 1 to 2 cm along three orthogonal axes should be used to locate and record the maximum SAR, regardless of RF frequency.

Measurement techniques and sources of error for determination of specific absorption rate via thermography. Use of a thermographic camera to evaluate SAR distribution in a bisected phantom (model) or cadaver is described previously in this chapter. A delay between the cessation of irradiation and opening of the phantom or cadaver to view the RF-induced heating can introduce significant errors because of thermodynamic factors. A nonperturbing temperature probe inserted in the subject at the location of highest SAR (Figure 7-8) helps the user determine and correct this source of error (Hochuli, 1981). The silk screen or thin plastic sheet covering each half of the bisected surfaces must be in tight contact during irradiation. This eliminates air gaps that alter RF current flow and the resulting SAR induced in the phantom. In general, silk screen is preferred for low-frequency, near-field irradiation (Moon, 1988). Plastic membranes offer advantages for SAR evaluation under far-field microwave irradiation or for evaluation of SAR induced by waveguide aperture applicators, when the E-field vector and the direction of RF current flow are not perpendicular to the membrane's surface (Cetas, 1978).

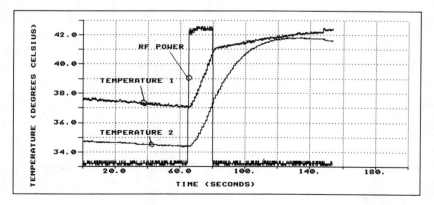

Figure 7-9 Experimental data plot of temperature rise versus time.

Techniques and sources of error for measuring specific absorption rate via implantable E-field probes.   The use of implantable E-field probes is most advantageous when the spatial distribution of low values of SAR must be measured. Continuous mechanical scans with E probes in tissue-equivalent phantoms enable quick mapping of SAR. Since commercial sources for these devices are scarce, the developer or user usually calibrates and evaluates performance of custom-designed probes. Therefore sources of measurement error must be understood and avoided. Detailed discussions on the use of implantable probes have been published (Bassen et al., 1977; Stuchly et al., 1984).

INSTRUMENT CALIBRATION TECHNIQUES

Exposure-Field Instrument Calibrations

Many users and researchers evaluate and calibrate E- or H-field probes by means of a calculable standard E or H field. Several approaches can be used, each with its own technical and economic advantages and limitations.

Plane-wave calibration of radiofrequency probes.   Calibration of electric field probes at frequencies above about 500 MHz is often performed in the far field of a horn antenna in an anechoic chamber. The approach used is discussed earlier in this chapter. To generate a power density with an uncertainty of less than ±1 dB, a series of meticulous calibrations and measurements with specialized methods must be performed for all antennas, waveguide or transmission line components, and power meters (Bassen and Herman, 1977; ANSI, 1981).

Probe calibration procedures using transverse electromagnetic cells. The TEM cell is well suited for the calibration of E- and H-field probes at frequencies below about 500 MHz (Babij and Trzaska, 1976; ANSI, 1981). A typical TEM cell setup for the calibration of E- and H-field probes is shown in Figure 7-10. The probe sensor is placed inside the cell, centered midway between the cell's outer wall and the flat center conductor. The maximum dimensions of the sensor under test must be less than one third of the space between the flat center conductor and the outer conductor. This keeps field perturbations within acceptable limits and minimizes capacitive coupling errors that degrade the calibration (Crawford, 1974). An uncertainty of about ±10% in field strength is the best that can be achieved for a probe calibrated carefully in a TEM cell system.

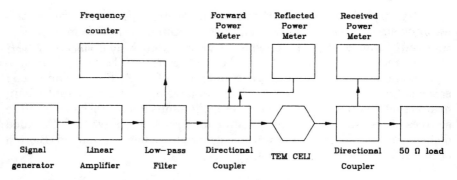

Figure 7-10 Instrumentation configuration for the generation of known electromagnetic field strengths in a transverse electromagnetic cell.

Probe calibration procedures using waveguide systems. Standard rectangular waveguides may be used to calibrate E-field probes fabricated with electrically small dipoles (Aslan, 1975; ANSI, 1981). A section of rectangular waveguide with a slot in its narrow wall can be used in a system that has a configuration similar to the one in Figure 7-10, except that the slotted waveguide section is substituted for the TEM cell.

Calibration system errors. Several sources of error are common among the various calibration systems. These include power measurement uncertainties, the presence of standing waves in the exposure fields, and the perturbation of fields by the probe under test and its readout cable. These can be minimized with special measurement techniques (Bassen and Herman, 1977; ANSI, 1981).

Calibration of Internal Field and Specific Absorption Rate Instruments

Calibration of implantable E-field probes. Implantable E-field probes may be calibrated in a sphere composed of high-water-content, tissue-equivalent materials. Calibration is done with the probe moved radially through the sphere while the sphere is irradiated by a plane wave (Bassen et al., 1979; Stuchly et al., 1984). Calibrations may also be performed in waveguides filled with lossy dielectric liquids (Hill, 1982). Finally, the SAR in an irradiated dielectric object may be determined at one point with a nonperturbing temperature probe. Then the E-field probe can be placed at precisely the same location and its output voltage can be equated with a known SAR. For any of these methods the probe's calibration uncertainty is typically several decibels when the probe is implanted in biological tissue containing a large percentage of water, such as muscle, brain, and internal organs but not bone or fat (Bassen et al., 1977; Bassen and Smith, 1983). Care must be taken when calibrating E-field probes with any of the methods just described. The SAR varies significantly over distances of 1 cm or more in any lossy dielectric object.

Calibration of temperature probes used to measure specific absorption rates.   Nonperturbing temperature probes must be calibrated with their method of use in mind. Precision (resolution and linearity) are more important than absolute accuracy, since SAR is determined by measurement of temperature change rather than the absolute value of the temperature. Modern optical and thermistor-based temperature probes require calibration at intervals ranging from once a day to once a year, depending on the stability of the probe's electronic and optical components and its temperature sensor. Two approaches may be used for temperature probe calibrations. Calibrations can be performed at several fixed temperatures over the range of intended use. This is accomplished with a standard reference thermometer in a stable water bath. A second, dynamic temperature calibration technique uses a standard reference thermometer and the probe under calibration in a water bath whose temperature is slowly increased at a steady rate. A computer data acquisition system performs instantaneous and simultaneous readings from both the reference thermometer and the nonperturbing temperature probe. Details of the problems and solutions associated with these calibration techniques may be found in several papers (Cetas, 1977; Hochuli, 1981; ANSI, in press).

Calibration of thermographic specific absorption rate measurement systems.   A thermographic camera may be calibrated with a commercially available black-body IR source. When a calibrated thermographic camera is used, several error sources must be taken into account, including IR radiometric parameters. Detailed means for recognizing and minimizing these errors are described by Cetas (1977).

SIMULATED BIOLOGICAL TISSUES FOR EXPERIMENTAL DOSIMETRY

Estimates of the SAR distribution induced by RF radiation in real biological subjects may be obtained more conveniently when physical replicas (phantoms) of biological subjects are used instead of cadavers. SARs may be measured in these phantoms with temperature or E-field probes or a thermographic camera. Phantoms are fabricated with materials that simulate the dielectric properties of various biological tissues (such as fat, muscle, brain, and bone). The physical characteristics of phantom materials range from liquids to solids.

Simulated Soft-Tissue Materials: Semisolid Gels

Many formulations of high-water-content tissues (muscle, brain, viscera) have been developed. The primary component of most of these tissue-equivalent materials is salt water (saline solution). Gels or liquids of varying viscosity are made by adding other soluble and insoluble materials to the gel. A gel is formed into the desired geometrical shape by means of a mold made of plastic foam or thin-walled plastic or epoxy-fiberglass whose inner shape is a replica of the outer surface of a biological subject. An epoxy-fiberglass shell can simulate a layer of skin and subcutaneous fat. The most commonly used formulations of soft-tissue simulants are composed of saline solution, polyethylene powder, and a gelling agent (Johnson and Guy, 1972). This form of phantom material is very viscous, pliable, and puttylike. It is well suited for constructing bisected phantoms for thermographic evaluation. Mixing techniques and the exact grain size of polyethylene powder affect the homogeneity and dielectric properties significantly. Once poured into a mold, this gel has a tendency to entrap air pockets. A less viscous gel can be made with saline solution and hydroxethyl cellulose (HEC). Polyethylene powder or sugar must be added for use above 100 MHz (Hartsgrove et al., 1987). Inserting and repositioning of probes does not leave permanent voids in low-viscosity HEC gel. Air bubbles can migrate upward naturally and escape through filling holes in the shell of a model filled with HEC gel (Allen et al., 1988). Visual inspection for air bubbles and the position of implanted probes can be performed simply in the optically transparent HEC gel. Preservation with a bactericide and refrigeration are necessary with either formulation of these simulated soft-tissue gels. Also, evaporation of the water in these gels must be prevented by proper sealing of their containers (the molds or shells containing the gel).

Bone-Equivalent Simulants

Solid material has been developed to simulate live, moist bone. The dielectric properties of live bone are significantly different from those of dry, dead bone. Since dielectric properties of bone and fat are almost identical over a wide range of RF frequencies, a bone simulant is commonly used to simulate fat as well. Hollow shells of this rigid material have been cast in the shape of the human skull (Cleveland and Athey, 1989) and in the approximate shape of the human torso (Allen et al., 1988) to simulate the outer layer of subcutaneous fat of a human. These rigid bone– and fat-equivalent materials are composed of polyester resins filled with materials such as carbon, acetylene black, and either aluminum powder or barium titanate powder (Johnson and Guy, 1972; Durney et al., 1986). Care must be taken to ensure that the powders do not settle during the fabrication process. The settling problem has been alleviated by using formulations without powders (Hartsgrove et al., 1987).

Liquid Tissue-Simulating Formulations

Low-viscosity liquids have been used to simulate internal body tissues. They are poured to fill rigid, outer shells of simulated subcutaneous fat. The result is an RF phantom in the shape of a full-size human containing simulated skeletal bones (Stuchly et al., 1987). Implantable E-field probes can be easily moved in a continuous path through these liquid-filled phantoms with mechanical scanners. This provides an efficient means for mapping local SAR distributions throughout models with complex shapes such as the human extremities.

Thermal and Physical Properties of Tissue-Equivalent Materials and Biological Tissues

Knowledge of the precise thermal properties of tissue-equivalent materials is important whenever thermal dosimetry is performed in models composed of tissue simulants. Although tissue simulants and their corresponding biological tissues have similar dielectric properties, their thermal properties are not identical. Examination of Eq. 4 indicates that both the specific heat and the rate of temperature rise must be known precisely for the determination of SAR from experimental data. The thermal properties of biological tissues and their corresponding tissue simulants are presented in Table 7-1. The muscle and brain simulants in this table are composed of saline solution, polyethylene powder, gelling agent, and (for 27 MHz) aluminum powder. Adipose (fat) simulant is composed of aluminum powder, carbon powder, polyester resin, and acetylene black (Johnson and Guy, 1972).

Electrical Properties of Tissue-Equivalent (Phantom) Materials

To calculate SAR from measured, internal E-field data, the investigator must know the dielectric properties and mass density of the irradiated material (see Eq. 3). Data on the dielectric properties of these materials versus frequency are presented in Chapter 5. The mass density of phantom materials is presented in Table 7-1.

CONCLUSION

We agree with other specialists in dosimetry that the uncertainties associated with external and internal EM field measurements have frequently

TABLE 7-1 Thermal Properties and Mass Density of Tissue-Equivalent Materials and Actual Biological Tissues

Material	Thermal conductivity ([W/(m − °C)] × 10³)	Specific heat ([J/(kg − °C)] × 10³)	Thermal diffusivity ([m²/s] × 10⁻⁶)	Mass density ([kg/m³] × 10³)
Muscle simulant*	0.535	3.70	0.145	1.00
Muscle simulant†	0.657	3.58	0.167	1.10
Brain simulant*	0.478	3.41	0.143	0.98
Fat tissue simulant†‡	0.352	1.07	0.230	1.43
Muscle in vitro	0.197–0.545	3.51	0.183	1.07
Brain in vitro	0.497–0.566	3.47	0.134–0.143	1.07
Fat tissue in vitro	0.132–0.371	1.21–1.55	0.230	1.06
Bone	—	1.26–2.97	—	1.25–1.79

* Data for tissue formulated for use at 2450 MHz.
† Data for tissue formulated for use at 27 MHz.
‡ Simulated fat material has dielectric properties that are almost identical to living bone.
From Leonard, J., Foster, K., and Athey, T.W. (1984). Thermal properties of tissue equivalent phantom materials. *IEEE Trans. Biomed. Eng.* 31:533–536. © 1984 IEEE.

been underestimated by biological effects researchers and radiation protection specialists (ANSI, in press). Specific problems that limit the accuracy of these measurements are described below.

Limitations on the Accuracy of Measurements of Radiofrequency Exposure Fields

The measurement of EM exposure fields is a difficult task. Even under ideal, plane-wave, far-field conditions, fields cannot be measured experimentally with an absolute accuracy of greater than approximately ± 0.5 to ± 1 dB ($\pm 10\%$ to $\pm 20\%$ for power density, or field strength squared) (Bassen and Herman, 1977; ANSI, in press). In addition, complex EM environments, which are the most commonly encountered, cannot be measured as accurately or precisely as plane-wave fields. Therefore field strength measurement data should be expressed only to two significant figures (for example, 1.1 V/m or 2.2 mW/cm^2). Uncertainty limits should accompany any published exposure field data.

Limitations on the Accuracy of Measurements of Absorption of Radiofrequency Energy (Specific Absorption Rate)

Internal field strengths and the resulting dose rates or SARs in biological subjects usually have large measurement uncertainties. Under plane-wave exposure conditions, the maximum local (point) SAR can be 20 to 100 times higher than the whole-body-averaged SAR (S. Stuchly et al., 1986). Steep gradients in the internal E fields and thermodynamic factors increase the magnitude of measurement errors of the SAR when determined by E-field or thermal measurements. Therefore an absolute accuracy of about ± 3 dB (a factor of 2:1) is the best-case measurement uncertainty that can be achieved when attempting to determine the maximum and minimum internal EM fields or SARs within an irradiated biological body. Calorimetric measurements of the whole-body-averaged SAR are accurate within several percentage points (Gandhi et al., 1979). However, whole-body-averaged SAR, as well as local SAR distributions, vary significantly as a biological subject changes position while being irradiated. Therefore measured SAR data should be expressed with realistic precision (no more than two significant figures), and the limits of the uncertainty of the SAR measurements should be stated explicitly.

REFERENCES

ALLEN, S., KANTOR, G., BASSEN, H.I., AND RUGGERA, P.F. (1988). CDRH RF phantom for hyperthermia systems evaluations. *Int. J. Hyperthermia* 4:17–23.

ANSI (1981). American National Standards Institute. American national standard C95.5–1981, recommended practice for the measurement of hazardous electromagnetic fields—RF and microwave, New York, Institute of Electrical and Electronics Engineers, Inc.

ANSI (In press). ANSI C95. American National Standard—recommended practice for the measurement of potentially hazardous electromagnetic fields—RF and microwave, New York, Institute of Electrical and Electronics Engineers, Inc.

ASLAN, E. (1987). A combined electric and magnetic field radiation monitor. *J. Microwave Power 22*:79–83.

ASLAN, E. (1983). An ANSI radiation protection guide conformal probe. *Microwave J. 26*:87–92.

ASLAN, E. (1975). Simplify leakage probe calibration. *Microwaves 14*:52–57.

BABIJ, T.M., AND BASSEN, H.I. (1980). Isotropic instruments for measurements of electric and magnetic fields in the 10–100 MHz range. *Bioelectromagnetics 1*:248 (abstract).

BABIJ, T.M., AND BASSEN, H.I. (1986). Broadband isotropic probe system for simultaneous measurement of complex E and H fields, U.S. Patent No. 4,558,993.

BABIJ, T.M., AND TRZASKA, H. (1976). Accuracy limitations of the Crawford cell. *In*: Proceedings of the IEEE Conference on Precision Electromagnetic Measurements, Boulder, Colo., pp. 145–149.

BASSEN, H.I. (1986). From problem reporting to technological solutions, *Med. Instrum. 20*:17–26.

BASSEN, H.I. (1979). A limited evaluation of the Cicoil "personal RF radiation detector," *Health Phys. 3*:171–174.

BASSEN, H.I., HERCHENROEDER, P., CHEUNG, A., AND NEUDER, S.M. (1977). Evaluation of an implantable electric field probe within finite, simulated tissues. *Radio Sci. 12*:15–25.

BASSEN, H.I., AND HERMAN, W. (1977). Precise calibration of plane wave microwave power density using power equation techniques. *IEEE Trans. Microwave Theory Tech. 25*:701–706.

BASSEN, H.I., AND HOSS, R. (1978). An optically-linked telemetry system for use with electromagnetic field hazard probes. *IEEE Trans. Electromagnet. Comp. 20*:483–488.

BASSEN, H.I., MOON, C., AND BROWN D. (1988). 20 megawatt/kg exposure system for in vivo pulsed biological effects research. *In*: Abstracts of the 10th Annual Meeting of the Bioelectromagnetics Society, Portland, Ore., June 1988, p. 93.

BASSEN, H.I., AND SMITH, G.S. (1983). The electric field probe—a review. *IEEE Trans. Antennas Prop. 31*:710–718.

BEISCHER, D., AND RENO, V. (1975). Microwave energy distribution measurements and their practical application. *Ann. N.Y. Acad. Sci. 247*:473–480.

BLACKMAN, C., AND BLACK, J. (1977). Measurement of microwave radiation absorbed by biological systems. II. Analysis by Dewar flask calorimetry. *Radio Sci. 12*:9–14.

CETAS, T. (1978). Practical thermometry with thermographic camera-calibration, transmittance, and emittance measurements. *Rev. Sci. Inst. 49*:245–254.

CHEEVER, E., LEONARD, J., AND FOSTER, K. (1987). Depth of penetration of fields from rectangular apertures into lossy media. *IEEE Trans. Microwave Theory Tech.* 35:865–867.

CLEVELAND, R., AND ATHEY, T. (1989). Specific Absorption Rate (SAR) in models of the human head exposed to hand-held UHF portable radios. *Bioelectromagnetics* 10(2):173–186.

CRAWFORD, M. (1974). Generation of standard EM fields using TEM transmission cells. *IEEE Trans. Electromagnet. Comp.* 16:185–195.

CREIGHTON, M.L., LARSEN, P., STEWART-DeHAAN, J., et al. (1987). In vitro studies of microwave induced cataract. *Exp. Eye Res.* 45:357–373.

D'ANDREA, J., DeWITT, J., GANDHI, O., STENSASS, S., LORDS, J., AND NIELSON, H. (1986). Behavioral and physiological effects of microwave irradiation of the rat at 0.5 mW/cm², *Bioelectromagnetics* 7:45–56.

DURNEY, C., MASSOUDI, H., AND ISKANDER, M. (1986). Radiofrequency radiation dosimetry handbook, 4th ed. Report No. USAFSAM-TR-85–73, USAF School of Aerospace Medicine, Brooks Air Force Base, Tex.

ELDER, J., AND CAHILL, D., (eds.). (1984). Biological effects of radiofrequency radiation, Report No. EPA-600/8–83–026F, Environmental Protection Agency, Research Triangle Park, N.C.

GANDHI, O.P. (1987). RF personnel dosimeter and dosimetry method for use therewith, U.S. Patent No. 4,672,309.

GANDHI, O.P., HAGMANN, M.J., AND D'ANDREA, J.A. (1979). Part-body and multi-body effects on absorption of radio-frequency electromagnetic energy by animals and by models of man. *Radio Sci.* 14:15–21.

GANDHI, O.P., HUNT, E.L., AND D'ANDREA, J.A. (1977). Deposition of electromagnetic energy in animals and in models of man with and without grounding and reflector effects. *Radio Sci.* 12:39–47.

GUY, A.W. (1971). Analyses of electromagnetic fields in biological tissues by thermographic studies on equivalent phantom models, *IEEE Trans. Microwave Theory Tech.* 19:205–214.

GUY, A.W., AND CHOU, C.K. (1976). System for chronic exposure of a population of rodents to UHF fields. *In*: Johnson, C.C., and Shore, M.L. (eds.). Biological effects of electromagnetic waves, Vol. II. HEW Pub. No. (FDA) 77–8011, Rockville, Md., Food and Drug Administration, pp. 389–410.

HAGMANN, M.J., AND BABIJ, T.M. (1988). Device for non-perturbing measurement of current as a dosimeter for hyperthermia. *In*: Abstracts of the 9th Annual Meeting of the North American Hyperthermia Group, Philadelphia, April 1988, p. 51.

HARTSGROVE, G., KRASZEWSKI, A., AND SUROWIEC, A. (1987). Simulated biological materials for electromagnetic radiation absorption studies. *Bioelectromagnetics* 8:29–36.

HILL, D. (1982). Waveguide techniques for the calibration of miniature electric field probes for use in microwave-bioeffects studies. *IEEE Trans. Microwave Theory Tech.* 30:92–94.

HO, H.S., GINN, E.I., AND CHRISTMAN, C.L. (1973). Environmentally controlled waveguide irradiation facility. *IEEE Trans. Microwave Theory Tech. 21*:837–840.

HOCHULI, C. (1981). Procedure for evaluating non-perturbing thermometers in microwave fields. Report No. (FDA) 81–8143, Rockville, Md., Food and Drug Administration.

HOPFER, S., AND ADLER, Z. (1980). An ultra broad-band (200 kHz–26 GHz) high sensitivity probe. *IEEE Trans. Instrum. Measure. 23*:445–451.

JOHNSON, C., AND GUY, A.W. (1972). Nonionizing electromagnetic wave effects in biological materials and systems. *Proc. IEEE 60*:692–718.

JUSTESEN, D., LEVINSON, D., CLARK, R., AND KING, N. (1971). A microwave oven for behavioral and biological research: electrical and structural modifications, calorimetric dosimetry, and functional evaluation. *J. Microwave Power 6*:237–258.

KANDA, M., AND DRIVER, L. (1987). An isotropic electric-field probe with tapered resistive dipoles for broad-band use, *IEEE Trans. Microwave Theory Tech. 35*:124–133.

LENOX, R.H., GANDHI, O.P., MEYERHOFF, J.L., AND GROVE, H.M. (1976). A microwave applicator for in vivo rapid inactivation of enzymes in the central nervous system. *IEEE Trans. Microwave Theory Tech. 24*:58–61.

LIN, J.C., BASSEN, H.I., AND WU, C. (1977). Perturbation effect of animal restraining materials on microwave exposure, *IEEE Trans. Biomed. Eng. 24*:80–83.

MAGIN, R. (1979). A microwave system for the controlled production of local tumor hyperthermia in animals, *IEEE Trans. Microwave Theory Tech. 27*:78–83.

MICHAELSON, S.M., AND LIN, J.C. (eds.). (1987). Biological effects and health implications of radiofrequency radiation. New York, Plenum Publishing Corp.

MOON, C. (1988). Comparative study of shortwave heating patterns in phantoms with polyethylene and silk partitions. *Bioelectromagnetics 9*:79–86.

NESMITH, B., AND RUGGERA, P. (1982). Performance evaluation of RF electric and magnetic field measuring instruments, Report. No. FDA 1–81–8185, Rockville, Md., Food and Drug Administration.

OLIVA, S.A., AND CATRAVAS, G.N. (1977). A multiple-animal array for equal power density microwave irradiation, *IEEE Trans. Microwave Theory Tech. 25*:433–436.

PHILLIPS, R., HUNT, E., AND KING, N. (1975). Field measurement, absorbed dose, and biologic dosimetry of microwaves. *Ann. N.Y. Acad. Sci. 247*:499–509.

POLK, C., AND POSTOW, E. (eds.) (1986). Handbook of biological effects of electromagnetic fields. Boca Raton, Fla.; CRC Press.

RUDGE, A., AND KNOX, R. (1970). Near field instrumentation. Pub. No. BRH/DEP 70–16, Rockville, Md., Food and Drug Administration.

RUGGERA, P.S., AND KANTOR, G. (1984). Development of a family of RF helical coil applicators which produce transversely uniform axially distributed heating in cylindrical fat-muscle phantoms. *IEEE Trans. Biomed. Eng. 31*:98–106.

SMITH, G.S. (1979). The electric-field probe near a material interface with application to probing of fields in biological bodies. *IEEE Trans. Microwave Theory Tech. 27*:270–278.

STUCHLY, M.A., STUCHLY, S.S., AND KRASZEWSKI, A. (1984). Implantable electric field probes—some performance characteristics. *IEEE Trans. Biomed. Eng.* *31*:526–531.

STUCHLY, S. (1987). Specific absorption rate distributions in a heterogeneous model of the human body at radiofrequencies. Report No. PB87–201356, Ottawa University, Ottawa, Ontario, Canada.

STUCHLY, S.S., STUCHLY, M.A., KRASZEWSKI, A., AND HARTSGROVE, G. (1986). Energy deposition in a model of man: frequency effects. *IEEE Trans. Biomed. Eng.* *33*:702–711.

TELL, R. (ed.). (In press). A practical guide to determination of human exposures to radiofrequency radiation. Scientific Subcommittee 78, Bethesda, Md., National Council on Radiation Protection and Measurements.

WACKER, P.F., AND BOWMAN, R.R. (1971). Quantifying hazardous electromagnetic fields, scientific basis and practical considerations. *IEEE Trans. Microwave Theory Tech.* *19*:178–187.

WICKERSHEIM, K., AND SUN, M. (1987). Fiberoptic thermometry and its applications. *J. Microwave Power 22*:85–94.

WYSS, G., AND SHEERAN, S. (1985). A practical optical modulator and link for antennas, *J. Lightwave Tech. 3*:316–321.

8

Electromagnetic Energy Absorption in Humans and Animals

OM P. GANDHI

Biological studies of the effects of electromagnetic (EM) radiation have used experiments with laboratory animals such as rats, monkeys, and rabbits, to determine behavioral and/or biochemical changes. For these studies to have any projected meanings for humans, quantification of the whole-body power absorption and its distribution for the irradiation conditions is necessary. Furthermore, dosimetric information must be known for humans subjected to irradiation at different frequencies and for realistic exposure conditions. This knowledge is vital to evaluate and establish radiation safety standards and to design EM applicators for medical applications such as hyperthermia.

Unlike the field of ionizing radiation, where the absorption cross section of a biological target is directly related to its geometrical cross section, the whole-body EM energy has been shown (Gandhi, 1974; Durney et al., 1975) to be strongly dependent on frequency, polarization (orientation of electric, or E, field of incident waves), and physical environment, such as conducting ground and other reflecting surfaces. This chapter summarizes the state of knowledge in this area. The knowledge about whole-body absorbed dose is well established, particularly for far-field irradiation conditions that are typically used for animal experiments (Durney et al., 1978, 1980, 1986). Unfortunately, the same cannot be said about the distribution of absorbed energy (distributive dosimetry), where the knowledge is in a fairly elementary stage.

The whole-body absorbed dose under different exposure conditions is known for the following:

1. Far-field irradition conditions ($E \perp H \perp k$).
2. Different frequencies and polarizations of irradiation.
3. Isolated animals and, to a lesser extent, regularly spaced multiple animals (Gandhi, 1980)
4. Near-field exposure conditions for aperture-type sources (Chatterjee et al., 1980b, 1982).
5. Near-field irradiation from simple loop and dipole and monopole antennas (Durney et al., 1980; Karimullah et al., 1980; Chatterjee

et al., 1985; M. Stuchly et al., 1986, 1987) and from parallel-plate radiators representative of RF sealers (Chen and Gandhi, 1989a).

An area of less knowledge is the distribution of absorbed dose or distributive dosimetry, although the picture here is improving dramatically with the development of new high-resolution numerical procedures (see Chapter 6) and a computer-controlled scanning system that can be used to determine internal E-field distributions in a full-scale human model (M. Stuchly et al., 1986, 1987; S. Stuchly et al., 1986, 1987). A major reason for less progress in this area is that the dose distributions are highly variable (to a much larger extent than even the whole-body dose) depending on irradiation conditions, body size, and posture, and tools are not yet available for proper modeling at higher frequencies either numerically or experimentally.

MEASUREMENT TECHNIQUES

Whereas proportioned, reduced-scale models of the human body were used to obtain specific absorption rates (SARs) in the past (Gandhi et al., 1977b), full-scale human models, either homogeneously or heterogeneously filled, have been used recently (Guy et al., 1984; M. Stuchly et al., 1986, 1987; S. Stuchly et al., 1986, 1987). A large transverse electromagnetic (TEM) cell has been used to obtain a simulated plane-wave irradiation, and human volunteers have been used to obtain the effect of frequency and grounding on whole-body absorption of RF fields (Hill, 1984). The highlights of the results with models have also been checked by experimentation with small laboratory animals (Gandhi et al., 1977a, 1979) from 25 g mice to 2245 g rabbits. The SARs are determined by measuring the colonic temperature elevation of anesthetized animals or by calorimetric determination of the absorbed dose by freshly euthanized animals.

Prolate spheroidal (Durney et al., 1975; Barber, 1977; Iskander et al., 1983) and ellipsoidal (Massoudi et al., 1977) models have been used for theoretical calculations of whole-body absorption for humans and animals. For very high frequencies a geometric optics method has been developed to estimate the power absorption in prolate spheroidal (Rowlandson and Barber, 1979) and cylindrical (Massoudi et al., 1979) human models. It has been shown that the dependence of whole-body-averaged SAR on both frequency and polarization of the incident fields may be estimated with such models. Because of their inappropriate shape and dielectric properties, these models are of course not meant for distributive dosimetry.

For distributive dosimetry it is necessary to use inhomogeneous models, for which dielectric properties are obtained from anatomical diagrams of the body. The numerical procedures for SAR calculations are discussed in detail in Chapter 6. Models with 5000- to 41,000-cell representations of the human body have been developed and used for plane-wave exposures, as well as for spatially nonuniform fields representative of some industrially relevant exposure conditions (Gandhi and DeFord, 1988; Chen and Gandhi, 1989a,b). Experimental procedures have used either homogeneously filled models (Guy et al., 1984; Chatterjee et al., 1985; M. Stuchly et al., 1986; S. Stuchly et al., 1986). or the four-tissue (skeleton, lungs, brain, and muscle) heterogeneous model (M. Stuchly et al., 1987; S. Stuchly et al., 1987).

The effects of the layered nature of the tissues on energy absorption have been studied in human models (Barber et al., 1979; Massoudi et al., 1979). The layering information required for the multilayered models was obtained from cross sections of the human anatomy. Specific tissue thicknesses were used for horizontal cross sections, and a layering resonance (interpreted as being due to impedance matching provided by the thicknesses of the outer layers) was calculated for each of the cross sections. These calculations show a broad, layering-caused enhancement in absorption for the frequency region 1 to 2 GHz, with an average SAR somewhat less than twice that for homogeneous models.

FREE-SPACE PLANE-WAVE IRRADIATION CONDITIONS

The whole-body absorption of EM waves by biological bodies is strongly dependent (Gandhi, 1974; Durney et al., 1975) on frequency and the orientation of the electric field $\mathbf{E}$ relative to the longest dimension $\mathbf{L}$ of the body. The highest rate of energy deposition occurs for $\mathbf{E}\|\mathbf{L}$ ($\mathbf{E}$-orientation) for frequencies such that the major length is approximately 0.36 to 0.4 times the free-space wavelength (λ) of radiation (Gandhi, 1975). Peaks of whole-body absorption for the other two configurations (major length oriented along the direction $\mathbf{k}$ of propagation, $\mathbf{k}\|\mathbf{L}$ or $\mathbf{k}$-orientation, or along the vector $\mathbf{H}$ of the magnetic field $\mathbf{H}\|\mathbf{L}$ or $\mathbf{H}$ orientation) have also been reported (Gandhi, 1974; Gandhi et al., 1977a) for $\lambda/2$ on the order of weighted average circumference of the animals.

Curves for whole-body absorption (fitted to the experimental data; Gandhi et al., 1977a,b) for human models exposed to radiation in free space are given in Figure 8-1. Figure 8-2 shows a comparison between the experimental data (Guy et al., 1984; Hill, 1984) and the various theoretical models (Hagmann et al., 1979; Chen and Gandhi, 1989b) for the most absorbing $\mathbf{E}$ orientation. For this orientation the whole-body absorption curves (Figure 8-2) may be discussed in terms of five regions:

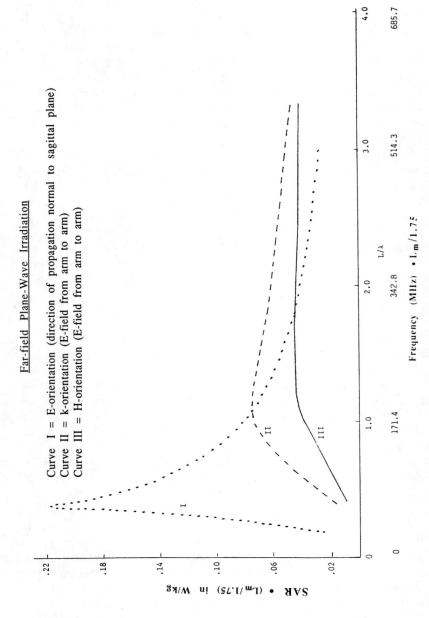

Figure 8-1 Whole-body-averaged specific absorption rate for human models for incident fields at 1 mW/cm². (From Gandhi, O. P. [1980]. *Proc. IEEE 68*:24–32.)

Far-field Plane-Wave Irradiation

Curve I = E-orientation (direction of propagation normal to sagittal plane)
Curve II = k-orientation (E-field from arm to arm)
Curve III = H-orientation (E-field from arm to arm)

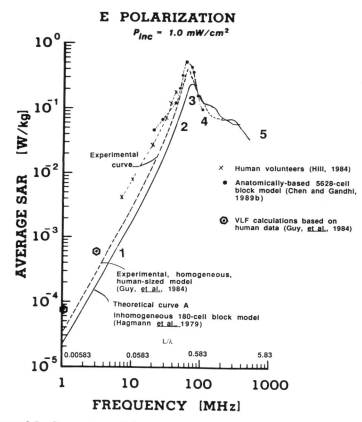

Figure 8-2   Comparison of theoretical and experimentally measured whole-body-averaged specific absorption rates for isolated man exposed at various frequencies.

1. Frequencies well below resonance ($L/\lambda <$ 0.1 to 0.2). An f^2-type dependence has been derived theoretically and checked experimentally by Durney et al. (1978).

2. Subresonant region ($0.2 < L/\lambda < 0.36$). An $f^{2.75}$ to f^3 dependence of total power deposition has been experimentally observed for this region (Gandhi et al., 1977a; Hill, 1984).

3. Resonant region ($L/\lambda \simeq 0.36 - 0.4$). A relative absorption cross section (Gandhi et al., 1977b), defined by EM absorption cross section*/physical cross section, S_{res} on the order of $0.665L/2b$ (derivable also from antenna theory) has been measured for this region, where

---

* Electromagnetic absorption cross section is defined as the power absorbed divided by the incident power density in watts per square meter.

L is the major length of the body and $2\pi b$ is its weighted average circumference. For a 70 kg, 1.75 m tall adult human, $L/2b \simeq 6.3$ and therefore S_{res} is approximately 4.2 at the resonance frequency. The resonance frequency f_r in megahertz is approximately (62 to 68) $\times$ $1.75/L_m$, where L_m is the height of the individual in meters.

4. Above-resonance region to frequencies on the order of $1.6\ S_{res}$ times the resonance frequency (for humans, this covers the region $f_r < f < 7 f_r$). A whole-body absorption reducing as f_r/f from the resonance values has been experimentally observed.

5. $f \gg f_r$ region. The EM absorption cross section should asymptotically approach the "quasioptical" value, which is (1 − power reflection coefficient) or about one half the physical cross section.

A major contribution of the numerical calculations with the block human model (see curve A in Figure 8-2) is that it reveals a fine structure to whole-body absorption in the above-resonance region. Minor peaks in this region at 150 and at 350 MHz are ascribed to maxima of energy deposition in the various body parts (Hagmann et al., 1979) such as the arm and the head, respectively. From Figure 8-2 it should be noted that the SARs measured with a full-scale human-sized phantom by Guy et al. (1984) are larger by a factor of almost 2:1 than the theoretical values obtained with a 180-cell block human model (Hagmann et al., 1979) for below-resonance frequencies. For above-resonance frequencies, on the other hand, the data for the block model are in much better agreement with the experimental results. This may be due to the fewer cells used in a 180-cell inhomogeneous block model representation. However, DeFord et al. (1983) obtained an SAR at 27.12 MHz that was about 2 times larger than the SAR calculated with the 180-cell model (Hagmann et al., 1979) and about the same as the value measured by Guy et al. (1984).

Another point to note from Figure 8-2 is that the SARs measured for the human volunteers by Hill (1984), or more recently calculated by Chen and Gandhi (1989b) using a finely discrete, anatomically based human model, are even larger than those measured with homogeneously filled human-sized phantoms (Guy et al., 1984), as has also been observed by Guy et al. from their very low-frequency analysis of human volunteers. This is because substantial radiofrequency currents are induced in the legs (see Figures 6-8 and 6-9). Higher SARs are therefore induced in the legs owing to their large bone content and this phenomenon is not modeled properly by the measurements with the homogeneously-filled phantom.

Analytically calculated SARs are shown in Figure 8-3 for E polarization for humans and some of the commonly used experimental animals, such as a rhesus monkey (3.5 kg), a medium rat (320 g), and a medium

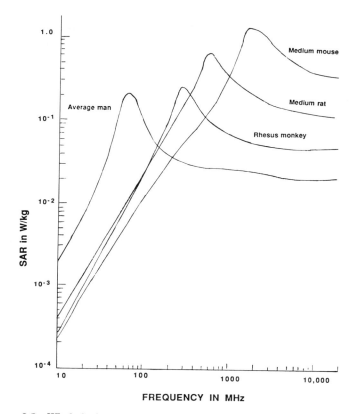

FREQUENCY IN MHz

Figure 8-3   Whole-body-averaged specific absorption rate of prolate spheroidal models of average man, rhesus monkey, medium rat, and medium mouse for E polarization at incident plane-wave power density of 1 mW/cm². (From Durney, C. H., Johnson, C. C., Barber, P. W., et al. [1978]. Radiofrequency radiation dosimetry handbook, 2nd ed. Pub. No. SAM-TR-78-22, USAF School of Aerospace Medicine (RZP), Aerospace Medical Division (AFSC), Brooks Air Force Base, Tex.)

mouse (20 g). The smaller the animal, the higher its resonant frequency and peak SAR.

For the highest-absorption E orientation, empirical equations have been obtained for SAR as a function of frequency (Gandhi et al., 1977a, 1979; Durney et al., 1979). These are given in Table 8-1. The empirical equations have been checked by experiments with six animal species from 25 g mice to 2250 g rabbits. The data are given in Table 8-2 (Gandhi et al., 1979).

For the data in Table 8-2 the animals were anesthetized (with sodium pentobarbital, 45 mg/kg⁻¹, to prevent movement and maintain a fixed orientation and also to limit pharmacologically the animals' normal

TABLE 8-1   Empirical Equations for Whole-Body-Averaged Specific Absorption Rates of Human Models under Conditions of Free-Space Irradiation

E polarization

Resonant frequency $f_r = 11{,}400/L_{cm}$ MHz

For *subresonant* region—$0.5\,f_r < f < f_r$:

$$SAR \text{ in } mW/g \text{ for } 1\ mW/cm^2 \text{ incident plane-wave field} = \frac{0.52\,L_{cm}^{\ 2}}{mass\ in\ g}\left(\frac{f}{f_r}\right)^{2.75}$$

For *above-resonant* region—$f_r < f < 1.6\,S_{res}f_r$:

$$SAR \text{ in } mW/g \text{ for } 1\ mW/cm^2 \text{ incident plane-wave field} = \frac{5950\,L_{cm}}{f_{MHz}\cdot mass\ in\ g}$$

where L_{cm} is the long dimension of the body in centimeters, and

$$S_{res} = 0.48\,\sqrt{\frac{L_{cm}^{\ 3}}{mass\ in\ g}}$$

thermoregulatory functions (Putthoff et al., 1977). The experimental SAR was calculated from the increase in colonic temperature (cloacal temperature in the case of lizards and birds) after 3 minutes of irradiation at 100 mW/cm². For the 500 g rat and 120.3 g dove, freshly killed animals were used and a calorimeter (Thermonetics model No. 2401A) was employed to determine the whole-body dose; the procedure was similar to that employed by Phillips et al., (1975). From Table 8-2 it can be seen that SARs from the empirical equation correlate well with experimental measurements on several species ranging in mass from 18.8 to 2245 g and in length from 8 to 44 cm. For these animals a whole-body SAR varying by a factor of 36:1 is observed for 2450 MHz irradiation.

GROUND EFFECTS

For a standing person with feet in conductive contact with a perfect ground, there is a drastic alteration in the whole-body-averaged SAR and its distribution. For E polarization the new resonant frequency is lower than that given by Eq. 1 for free-space irradiation (see Table 8-1). The whole-body-averaged SARs calculated for different models and the experimental data of Hill (1984) and Gandhi et al. (1979) are shown in Figure 8-4. As expected, higher SARs are obtained for the recent, finely discrete human model (Chen and Gandhi, 1989b) than for the previous, relatively crude 180-cell block human model (Hagmann and Gandhi, 1979). With the advent of larger computers and the use of the

TABLE 8-2   Whole-Body-Averaged Specific Absorption Rates for E Polarization of Several Species of Laboratory Animals Irradiated by 2450 MHz Energy in Free Space*

Weight (g)	Length† (cm)	SAR for 50 mW/cm² fields (mW/g)		Percent error
		From measurements	From empirical equation	
Long-Evans rat (*Rattus norvegicus*)				
355	21	11.72	11.43	+2.5
490	25	8.47	9.86	−14.1
499	26	9.41	10.07	−6.5
506	26	9.41	9.92	−5.1
508	25	8.47	9.51	−10.9
550	26	7.53	9.13	−17.5
500	—	9.48	—	—
Rabbit (New Zealand white)				
2000	44	3.80	4.25	−10.6
2000	44	4.27	4.25	+0.5
2245	43	3.90	3.71	+5.1
Vole (*Microtus montanus*)				
24	9	68.61	72.48	−5.3
22	8.5	72.94	74.67	−2.3
23	8.5	70.40	71.43	−1.4
Deer mouse (*Peromyscus maniculatus*)				
29	8.5	58.90	56.63	+4.0
24	8.0	68.61	64.41	+6.5
Ring dove (*Streptopelia risoria*)				
141.5	14.0	30.13	19.12	—
143.2	15.5	37.66	20.92	—
144	13.0	29.03	17.45	—
144	13.0	28.60	17.45	—
120.3	—	29.76	—	—
Whiptail lizard (*Cnemidophorus tigris*)			Effective length from empirical equation	
24	9.5 + 21 cm tail	124.55	15.46	—
23	9.5 + 9 cm tail	133.95	15.95	—
20.5	8.5 + 22 cm tail	124.77	13.26	—
18.8	9.5 + 10 cm tail	92.15	8.95	—

* Freshly euthanized animals and a Thermonetics model No. 2401-A gradient-layer calorimeter were used to measure the 500 g rat and the 120.3 g dove. Other measurements are based on anesthetized animals.
† The length of the animals was measured from snout to posterior portion of animal body excluding the tail.

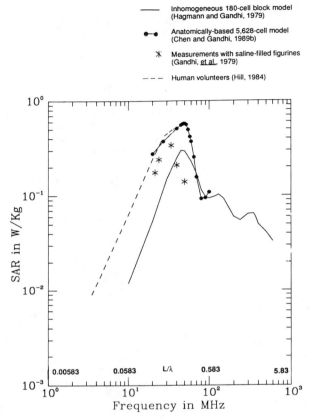

Figure 8-4 Comparison of theoretical and experimental whole-body-averaged specific absorption rates for grounded man exposed at various frequencies.

numerically efficient finite-difference time-domain (FDTD) procedure (see Chapter 6), it has been possible recently to use a superior theoretical representation of the human body (5,000- to 41,000-cell models), which as shown in Figure 8-4 gives a better correlation of the data obtained with human volunteers (Hill, 1984). An advantage of the numerical procedure is that it is possible to obtain SAR distributions for the anatomically based human model. Shown in Figures 8-5 and 8-6 are the calculated section-averaged SAR distributions for 50 and 60 MHz for a grounded and a free-space human model (Chen and Gandhi, 1989b) of height 1.75 m. (See Chapter 6 for the procedure by which the anatomically based model was developed.) The 50 and 60 MHz frequencies are chosen for illustration because they are close to the resonant frequencies for grounded and free-space irradiation conditions, respectively (see Figures

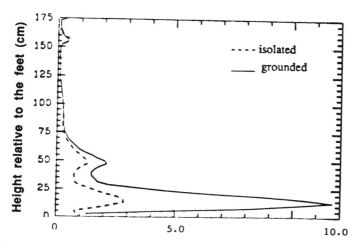

Figure 8-5 Layer-averaged specific absorption rate (SAR) distributions for grounded and isolated man model at 50 MHz with vertical E-field polarization. All SARs are result of 1 mW/cm² incident plane wave.

8-2 and 8-4). From Figures 8-5 and 8-6 it can be seen that the highest SARs are calculated for the sections through the neck, knee, and ankle, the former because of a smaller cross section and the latter two because they also have high bone content. The section-averaged SARs for the ankle, knee, and neck sections calculated for grounded and free-space

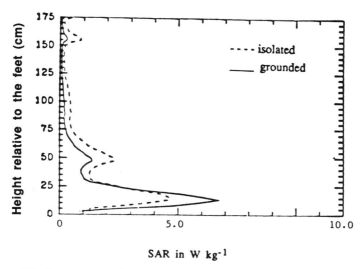

SAR in W kg⁻¹

Figure 8-6 Layer-averaged specific absorption rate (SAR) distributions for grounded and isolated man model at 60 MHz with vertical E-field polarization. All SARs are result of 1 mW/cm² incident plane wave.

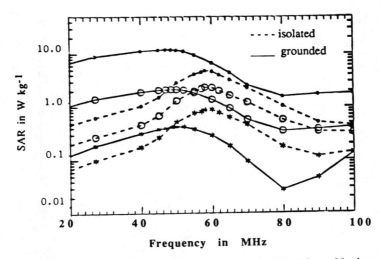

Figure 8-7 Layer-averaged specific absorption rates (SARs) for ankle, knee, and neck sections under grounded and isolated conditions. All SARs are result of 1 mW/cm^2 incident plane wave. ●, Ankle section; ○, knee section; ⋆, neck section.

irradiation conditions are shown in Figure 8-7 (Chen and Gandhi, 1989b) for frequencies of 20 to 100 MHz. This frequency band was selected to include the important whole-body resonance region of frequencies for grounded and free-space irradiation conditions.

NEAR-FIELD EXPOSURE CONDITIONS

Near-field exposure conditions are perhaps of greater interest than far-field irradiation conditions because they are encountered in industrial and occupational situations.

In some near-field environments the sources are tightly coupled to the human operator, in which case the incident field is altered by the presence of the operator. In such cases the field distributions are obtained by using coupled integral equations or iterative methods (Durney et al., 1980; Karimullah et al., 1980; M. Stuchly et al., 1987; S. Stuchly et al., 1987; Chen and Gandhi, 1989a). Since in real life a multitude of near-field conditions exist, these approaches can be cumbersome because they have to be repeated for each individual circumstance. For a majority of situations, particularly those involving leakage fields, coupling back to the source may be neglected. Chatterjee et al., (1980a) have used the plane-wave spectrum approach to study this class of problems. The procedure developed is general and can be used for any incident fields prescribed at a two-dimensional plane. However, to avoid the complexity resulting from rapidly varying fields, particularly for the near-field regions, these authors have standardized most of their calculations to fields that are prescribed by measurements or otherwise over a vertical plane just in front of the operator's feet in the intended location. The prescribed fields are represented as a superposition of plane waves propagating toward the target at different angles. Up to 2^{12}, or 4096, component plane waves, many of them evanescent with decaying amplitudes, have generally been used to find the EM energy absorption and its distribution within the biological target. Since the fields emanating from any localized sources are likely to roll off monotonically to negligible values in the two dimensions of the plane, most of the calculations have been performed for prescribed electric fields having a half-cycle cosine variation along both the vertical and horizontal axes. Several test cases have shown that with such approximated fields, whole-body SAR calculations are within 5% to 10% of the values that would have been obtained with exactly prescribed fields (Chatterjee et al., 1980b), owing perhaps to the spatial integrative nature of the body.

For each set of the prescribed fields (E components in the vertical and horizontal directions, respectively), the remaining body-normal E component and components of H are obtained from Maxwell's equations and used for the calculations. The phase variation of the prescribed fields is important for exact calculations of SAR. However, it has been shown (Chatterjee et al., 1980b) that the worst-case absorption (maximum whole-body SAR) is always obtained for assumed constant phase of the incident fields. Since the upper bound of the absorbed energy is often the desired quantity, constant phase is therefore assumed when rates of energy deposition are calculated for the 180-cell block human model shown in Figure 8-8 (Hagmann et al., 1979). The whole-body-averaged SAR is found to satisfy an empirical equation (Chatterjee et al., 1981, 1982) for frequencies up to 915 MHz.

$$\text{SAR}|_{\text{near fields}} = \frac{\text{SAR}|_{\text{far fields}}}{\left[1 + \left(\dfrac{A_v}{\Delta_v}\right)^2\right]\left[1 + \left(\dfrac{A_h}{\Delta_h}\right)^2\right]} \tag{1}$$

In Eq. 1, Δ_v and Δ_h are the vertical and horizontal widths of the best-fit half-cycle cosine functions to the prescribed leakage fields. The dimensional constants A_v and A_h for the vertical and horizontal directions, respectively, have been obtained from the numerical calculations of the SAR for the inhomogeneous block model and are plotted in Figure 8-9 for various frequencies for P polarization (no component of incident E directed arm to arm) and for N polarization (incident E directed arm to arm). In Eq. 1 the SAR for far fields corresponding to the maximum

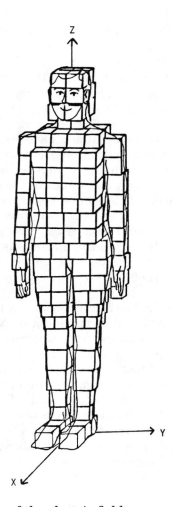

Figure 8-8 A 180-cell block human model of man. (From Hagmann et al. [1979]. *IEEE Trans. Microwave Theory Tech.* 27:804–809. © 1979 IEEE.)

magnitudes of the electric field components E_v and E_h are obtained from curves I and II of Figure 8-1. From Figure 8-9 it can be seen that for both P and N polarizations the dimensional constants A_v and A_h are relatively constant for frequencies below whole-body resonant frequency. For the case of P polarization, the values for these constants A_v and A_h are of the order of 2.5 and 1.1 m, respectively, corresponding to 1.4 times the height and 2.1 times the width of the human model. Consistent with the physical intuition, for field distributions considerably broader than the physical dimensions of the block model ($\Delta_v \gg 1.75$ m, $\Delta_h \gg 0.53$ m), the SAR given by Eq. 1 is the far-field value. With N polarization at low frequencies, the deposition at the vertical extremities (head, neck, and legs) is less pronounced so that A_v need not be so large a fraction of the height of the model to approach plane-wave deposition.

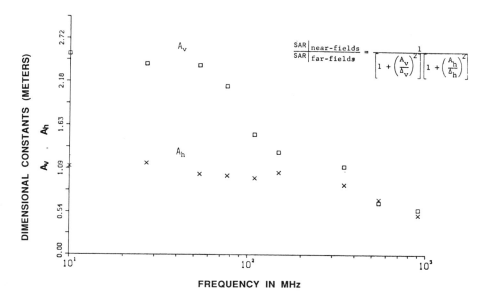

Figure 8-9 Dimensional constants for Eq. 1 for P and N polarizations. (From Chatterjee et al. [1982]. *IEEE Trans. Microwave Theory Tech. 30*:2000–2005. © 1982 IEEE.)

The validity of the near-field empirical Eq. 1 has been confirmed with reduced-scale saline solution–filled figurines (Chatterjee et al., 1982). A point to note from Eq. 1 is that, for near-field exposures, SARs considerably lower than those for far-field exposure conditions are observed when the physical extents of fields Δ_v and Δ_h are much less than A_v and A_h, respectively. This is often the case with leakage-type fields such as those from RF sealers. Measurements of leakage E fields in front of RF dielectric heat sealers have indicated that the P-polarized components of the E field are the dominant ones and Δ_v and Δ_h are typically about 1 m each (Conover et al., 1980). With the recent development of the FDTD procedure for EM dosimetry (Sullivan et al., 1987, 1988), it has become possible to include coupling back to the source, which was neglected by Chatterjee et al., (1980b, 1982). Also, because of the high numerical efficiency of the FDTD procedure, it is now possible to use anatomically based human models with 5000 to 41,000 cells, giving resolutions considerably superior to those possible with the 180-cell model. Chen and Gandhi (1989a) have used the FDTD method in a 5628-cell human model to calculate the SAR distributions resulting from fields of an RF sealer–simulant, parallel-plate applicator of dimensions 57.6 × 15.7 cm (see Chapter 6).

Another important occupationally encountered source of EM radiation is the RF induction heater. Induction heating caused by time-varying magnetic fields is used extensively for metal product heating or melting, heating and drawing optical fibers, and for zone refining, and crystal growth in the semiconductor industry. Gandhi and DeFord (1988) have used the impedance method to calculate SAR distributions in an anatomically based model of the human torso for spatially varying vector magnetic fields produced by a current-carrying coil that represents a 450 kHz RF induction heater. SARs of a few microwatts per kilogram are found for magnetic fields of about 1.8 A/m at the central plane of the model. This implies that fairly low SARs (microwatts or milliwatts per kilogram) would result from the leakage magnetic fields of 1 to 20 A/m that have been reported for RF induction heaters at 450 kHz (Stuchly and Lecuyer, 1985; Conover et al., 1986). The SARs would rise, of course, as H^2 if higher magnetic fields are used, and approximately as f^2 with increasing frequency.

For near-field exposure conditions, maximum SARs are likely for body parts in regions of the highest incident fields. Distribution of SAR is therefore likely to be important in assessing the safety of near-field exposure conditions. With the recent development of the numerically efficient FDTD and impedance methods, technology is now available to estimate the SAR distributions accurately. Some of the applications to date for near-field exposure conditions are discussed in Chapter 6.

AREAS OF LESS KNOWLEDGE

As mentioned previously, the distribution of absorbed dose, or distributive dosimetry, is an area of less knowledge. Two reasons for less progress in this area are that the dose distributions are highly variable (to a much larger extent than even the whole-body dose, depending on irradiation conditions, body size, and posture and that experimental determination is tedious for all the conditions one might encounter.

For experimental dosimetry, Guy (1971) has developed a thermographic technique that can be used with phantom models or sacrificed animals. The method uses a thermographic camera to determine the temperature distribution for a given plane or over a given surface of the body as a result of exposure to far- or near-field EM fields. Although primarily qualitative, the method offers the advantage of rapidly identifying regions of high SARs. In living systems, however, the presence of blood flow is likely to smear the so-called electrical hot spots. Thermal hot spots therefore may not occur at these locations. Olsen et al. (1980; Olsen and Griner, 1982) have measured the SAR distributions for muscle-equivalent models of a sitting rhesus monkey and for a full-size human model. D'Andrea et al. (1985) have also done some work in this area with rats.

CONCLUSION

Even though considerable progress has been made in microwave radiation dosimetry, most of it pertains to the quantification of whole-body-averaged SARs at various frequencies and for different orientations of the body relative to the incident fields. Progress has also been made in analyzing some of the important near-field exposure conditions such as leakage fields from RF sealers, induction heaters, and transceiver antennas. Distribution of absorbed energy is likely to be important for determining biological effects, yet there is still little experimental or theoretical knowledge of irradiation conditions at which the SARs are maximum in the critical organs of exposed animals. It is true that distributive dosimetry varies with every slight movement of the animals, but nevertheless much more work should be done to allow experimenters to focus on conditions of maximum absorption in the critical organs for study of the biological effects. The development of finely discretized, inhomogeneous, experimentally verified models for distributive dosimetry is therefore of great importance. Also needed are inhomogeneous thermal models that can be used to translate the absorption dose distributions into temperature increases for the various parts of the body. The thermal models developed to date (Spiegel et al., 1980; Chatterjee and Gandhi, 1983) are fairly elementary and should be considered only the first steps in the development of thermal models that are needed.

REFERENCES

Barber, P.W. (1977). Electromagnetic power absorption in a prolate spheroidal model of man and animals at resonance. *IEEE Trans. Biomed. Eng.* 24:513–521.

Barber, P.W., Gandhi, O.P., Hagmann, M.J., and Chatterjee, I. (1979). Electromagnetic absorption in a multilayered model of man. *IEEE Trans. Biomed. Eng.* 26:400–405.

Chatterjee, I., and Gandhi, O.P. (1983). An inhomogeneous thermal block model of man for the electromagnetic environment. *IEEE Trans. Biomed. Eng.* 30:707–715.

Chatterjee, I., Gandhi, O.P., and Hagmann, M.J. (1982). Numerical and experimental results for near-field electromagnetic absorption in man. *IEEE Trans. Microwave Theory Tech.* 30:2000–2005.

Chatterjee, I., Gandhi, O.P., Hagmann, M.J., and Riazi, A. (1980a). Plane-wave spectrum approach for the calculation of electromagnetic absorption under near-field exposure conditions. *Bioelectromagnetics* 1:363–377.

Chatterjee, I., Gu, Y.G., and Gandhi, O.P. (1985). Quantification of electromagnetic absorption in humans from body-mounted communication transceivers. *IEEE Trans. Vehicular Tech. 34*:55–62.

CHATTERJEE, I., HAGMANN, M.J., AND GANDHI, O.P. (1980b). Electromagnetic energy deposition in an inhomogeneous block model of man for near-field irradiation conditions. *IEEE Trans. Microwave Theory Tech. 28*:1452–1459.

CHATTERJEE, I., HAGMANN, M.J., AND GANDHI, O.P. (1981). An empirical relationship for electromagnetic energy absorption in man for near-field exposure conditions. *IEEE Trans. Microwave Theory Tech. 29*:1235–1238.

CHEN, J.Y., AND GANDHI, O.P. (1989a). Electromagnetic deposition in an anatomically-based model of man for leakage fields of a parallel-plate dielectric heater. *IEEE Trans. Microwave Theory Tech. 37*:174–180.

CHEN, J.Y., AND GANDHI, O.P. (1989b). RF currents induced in an anatomically-based model of a human for plane-wave exposures (20–100 MHz). *Health Phys. 57*:89–98.

CONOVER, D.L., MURRAY W.E., JR., FOLEY, E.D., LARY, J.M., AND PARR, W.H. (1980). Measurement of electric- and magnetic-field strengths from industrial radio-frequency (6–38 MHz) plastic sealers. *Proc. IEEE 68*:17–20.

CONOVER, D.L., MURRAY W.E., JR., LARY, J.M., AND JOHNSON, P.H. (1986). Magnetic field measurements near RF induction heaters. *Biolectromagnetics 7*:83–90.

D'ANDREA, J.A., EMMERSON, R.Y., BAILEY, C.M., DEWITT, J.R., OLSEN, R.G., AND GANDHI, O.P. (1985). Microwave radiation absorption in the rat: frequency-dependent SAR distribution in body and tail. *Bioelectromagnetics 6*:199–206.

DEFORD, J.F., GANDHI, O.P., AND HAGMANN, M.J. (1983). Moment-method solutions and SAR calculations for inhomogeneous models of man with large number of cells. *IEEE Trans. Microwave Theory Tech. 31*:848–851.

DURNEY, C.H., ISKANDER, M.F., MASSOUDI, H., ALLEN, S.J., AND MITCHELL, J.C. (1980). Radiofrequency radiation dosimetry handbook, 3rd ed., Pub. No. SAM-TR-80-32, USAF School of Aerospace Medicine, Aerospace Medical Division (AFSC), Brooks Air Force Base, Tex.

DURNEY, C.H., ISKANDER, M.F., MASSOUDI, H., AND JOHNSON, C.C. (1979). An empirical formula for broadband SAR calculations of prolate spheroidal models of humans and animals. *IEEE Trans. Microwave Theory Tech. 27*:758–762.

DURNEY, C.H., JOHNSON, C.C. BARBER, P.W., ET AL. (1978). Radiofrequency radiation dosimetry handbook, 2nd ed. USAF School of Aerospace Medicine (RZP), Aerospace Medical Division (AFSC), Brooks Air Force Base, Tex., Contract No. SAM-TR-78-22.

DURNEY, C.H., JOHNSON, C.C., AND MASSOUDI, H. (1975). Long wavelength analysis of plane-wave irradiation of a prolate spheroid model of man. *IEEE Trans. Microwave Theory Tech. 23*:246–253.

DURNEY, C.H., MASSOUDI, H., AND ISKANDER, M.F. (1986). Radiofrequency radiation dosimetry handbook, 4th ed. Pub. No. USAF SAM-TR-85-73, USAF School of Aerospace Medicine, Aerospace Medical Division (AFSC), Brooks Air Force Base, Tex.

GANDHI, O.P. (1974). Polarization and frequency effects on whole-animal absorption of RF energy. *Proc. IEEE 62*:1166–1168.

GANDHI, O.P. (1975). Conditions of strongest electromagnetic power deposition in man and animals. *IEEE Trans. Microwave Theory Tech. 23*:1021–1029.

GANDHI, O.P. (1980). State of the knowledge for electromagnetic absorbed dose in man and animals. *Proc. IEEE 68*:24–32.

GANDHI, O.P., AND DEFORD, J.F. (1988). Calculation of EM power deposition for operator exposure to RF induction heaters. *IEEE Trans. Electromagnet. Comp. 30*:63–68.

GANDHI, O.P., HAGMANN, M.J., AND D'ANDREA, J.A. (1979). Part-body and multibody effects on absorption of radiofrequency electromagnetic energy by animals and by models of man. *Radio Sci. 14*:6(suppl.), 15–22.

GANDHI, O.P., HUNT, E.L., AND D'ANDREA, J.A. (1977a). Electromagnetic power deposition in man and animals with and without ground and reflector effects. *Radio Sci. 12*:6(suppl.), 39–47.

GANDHI, O.P., SEDIGH, K., BECK, G.S., AND HUNT, E.L. (1977b). Distribution of electromagnetic energy deposition in models of man with frequencies near resonance. *In*: Biological effects of electromagnetic waves, vol. II, selected papers of the USNC/URSI annual meeting, Boulder, Colo., Oct. 20–23, 1975, HEW Pub. No. (FDA) 77–8011, pp. 44–67. Available from National Technical Information Service (NTIS), Springfield, Va.

GUY, A.W. (1971). Analysis of electromagnetic fields induced in biological tissues by thermographic studies on equivalent phantom models. *IEEE Trans. Microwave Theory Tech. 19*:205–214.

GUY, A.W., CHOU, C.K., AND NEUHAUS, B. (1984). Average SAR and SAR distribution in man exposed to 450-MHz radiofrequency radiation. *IEEE Trans. Microwave Theory Tech. 32*:752–763.

HAGMANN, M.J., AND GANDHI, O.P. (1979). Numerical calculations of electromagnetic energy deposition in man with ground and reflector effects. *Radio Sci. 14*:6(suppl.), 23–29.

HAGMANN, M.J., GANDHI, O.P., AND DURNEY, C.H. (1979). Numerical calculation of electromagnetic energy deposition for a realistic model of man. *IEEE Trans. Microwave Theory Tech. 27*:804–809.

HILL, D.A. (1984). The effect of frequency and grounding on whole-body absorption of humans in E-polarized radiofrequency fields. *Bioelectromagnetics 5*:131–146.

ISKANDER, M.F., LAKHTAKIA, A., AND DURNEY, C.H. (1983). A new procedure for improving the solution stability and extending the frequency range of the EBCM. *IEEE Trans. Antennas Prop. 31*:317–324.

KARIMULLAH, K., CHEN, K.M., AND NYQUIST, D.P. (1980). Electromagnetic coupling between a thin wire antenna and a neighboring biological body: theory and experiment. *IEEE Trans. Microwave Theory Tech. 28:1218–1225*.

MASSOUDI, H., DURNEY, C.H., BARBER, P.W., AND ISKANDER, M.F. (1979). Electromagnetic absorption in multilayered cylindrical models of man. *IEEE Trans. Microwave Theory Tech. 27*:825–830.

MASSOUDI, H., DURNEY, C.H., AND JOHNSON, C.C. (1977). Long wavelength analysis of plane-wave irradiation of an ellipsoidal model of man. *IEEE Trans. Microwave Theory Tech. 25*:41–46.

OLSEN, R.G., AND GRINER, T.A. (1982). Electromagnetic dosimetry in a sitting rhesus model at 225 MHz. *Bioelectromagnetics* 3:385–389.

OLSEN, R.G., GRINER, T.A., AND PRETTYMAN, G.D. (1980). Far-field microwave dosimetry in a rhesus monkey model. *Bioelectromagnetics* 1:149–160.

PHILLIPS, R.D., HUNT, E.L., AND KING, N.W. (1975). Field measurements, absorbed dose, and biologic dosimetry of microwaves. *Ann. N.Y. Acad. Sci.* 247:499–509.

PUTTHOFF, D.L., JUSTESEN, D.R., WARD, L.B., AND LEVINSON, D.M. (1977). Drug-induced ectothermia in small mammals: the quest for a biological microwave dosimeter. *Radio Sci.* 12:6(suppl.), 73–80.

ROWLANDSON, G.I., AND BARBER, P.W. (1979). Absorption of higher frequency RF energy by biological models: calculations based on geometrical optics. *Radio Sci.* 14:6(suppl.), 43–50.

SPIEGEL, R.J., DEFFENBAUGH, D.M., AND MANN, J.E. (1980). A thermal model of the human body exposed to an electromagnetic field. *Bioelectromagnetics* 1:253–270.

STUCHLY, M.A., KRASZEWSKI, A., STUCHLY, S.S., HARTSGROVE, G.W., AND SPIEGEL, R.J. (1987). RF energy deposition in a heterogeneous model of man: near-field exposures. *IEEE Trans. Biomed. Eng.* 34:944–950.

STUCHLY, M.A., AND LECUYER, D.W. (1985). Induction heating and operator exposure to electromagnetic fields. *Health Phys.* 49:693–700.

STUCHLY, M.A., SPIEGEL, R.J., STUCHLY, S.S., AND KRASZEWSKI, A. (1986). Exposure of man in the near-field of a resonant dipole: comparison between theory and measurements. *IEEE Trans. Microwave Theory Tech.* 34:26–31.

STUCHLY, S.S., KRASZEWSKI, A., STUCHLY, M.A., HARTSGROVE, G.W., AND SPIEGEL, R.J. (1987). RF energy deposition in a heterogeneous model of man: far-field exposures. *IEEE Trans. Biomed. Eng.* 34:951–957.

STUCHLY, S.S., STUCHLY, M.A., KRASZEWSKI, A., AND HARTSGROVE, G. (1986). Energy deposition in a model of man: frequency effects. *IEEE Trans. Biomed. Eng.* 33:702–711.

SULLIVAN, D.M., BORUP, D.T., AND GANDHI, O.P. (1987). Use of the finite-difference time-domain method in calculating EM absorption in human tissues. *IEEE Trans. Biomed. Eng.* 34:148–157.

SULLIVAN, D.M., GANDHI, O.P., AND TAFLOVE, A. (1988). Use of the finite-difference time-domain method for calculating EM absorption in man models. *IEEE Trans. Biomed. Eng.* 35:179–186.

Part 3

BIOLOGICAL EFFECTS AND HEALTH IMPLICATIONS

9

Biological Effects of Extremely Low-Frequency and 60 Hz Fields

L. E. ANDERSON

Until the last few decades, the natural background levels of atmospheric electric and magnetic fields were extremely low; however, they have since dramatically increased. The industrialization and electrification of society have resulted in the exposure of people, animals, and plants to a complex milieu of elevated electromagnetic (EM) fields that span all frequency ranges. One of the most significant contributors to this changing electrical environment has been the technological advances associated with the growth of electrical power generation and transmission systems. In addition, EM field–generating devices have proliferated in industrial plants, office buildings, public transportation systems, homes, and elsewhere. Other chapters in this book address the potential impacts of a broad range of frequencies. This chapter focuses on the effects of extremely low-frequency (ELF) fields, primarily at 50 and 60 Hz, on biological systems.

EM fields, which may extend far beyond their sources, are mostly imperceptible to people. In the past, there was considerable controversy as to whether fields in the ELF portion of the EM spectrum could even cause significant biological effects, let alone pose a hazard to health. However, research and clinical experience have shown that biological effects from such fields are not precluded simply because they are not perceived. Recent data confirm some of the earlier reports that ELF fields do cause changes in certain biological systems. Thus it is both reasonable and timely to evaluate the interactions between the modern EM environment and living organisms, including humans, and to investigate whether such interactions are beneficial or detrimental, transient or permanent.

In the past two decades, research programs throughout the world have greatly expanded in scope and depth to address such issues. Significant progress has been achieved, both in defining the ways living organisms interact with ELF fields and in describing biological effects, real and potential, from such fields. Much of this effort has been directed toward electric fields of power frequencies. However, frequencies other than 50 and 60 Hz have also been examined, research has been expanded to include magnetic as well as electric fields. Although it is now clear that ELF EM fields do cause biological effects, the basis for these effects

Work supported by the U.S. Department of Energy, Office of Energy Storage and Distribution, under Contract No. DE-AC06-76RLO-1830.

and the underlying mechanisms of interaction remain largely unknown, and the health implications for humans and animals have yet to be fully determined.

As in other areas of scientific investigation, the research conducted on ELF bioeffects has been performed at several levels: human studies (primarily epidemiological), animal experiments, and cellular (mechanistic) studies. The relationship among these general elements is depicted in Figure 9-1. Results from each of these areas of investigation have specific strengths but also exhibit inherent weaknesses.

Some of the earliest efforts to examine health-related issues of ELF field exposures were focused on the impacts of such fields in humans. Despite the obvious desirability of obtaining such data, they are the least complete. Often, even the results available suffer from some combination of the following problems:

1. Monitoring of symptoms is subjective and often poorly defined.
2. Quantitative evaluation of effects either is not performed or is not clearly described.
3. Control populations are ill matched with exposure groups or are nonexistent.
4. Electric and magnetic fields have been confounded by secondary factors (such as exposure to microshocks or chemicals).
5. Duration of observations is often limited to short time periods that poorly represent real environmental exposure.
6. Exposure levels vary widely and are not documented, making it

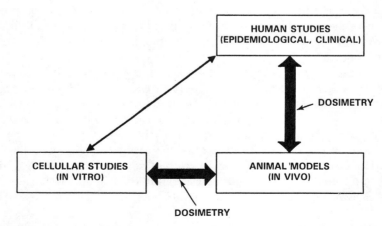

Figure 9-1 Three major levels of investigation in extremely low-frequency electric and magnetic field research.

difficult to estimate accurately the magnitude and duration of exposure.

7. Many of the earlier studies have insufficient numbers of subjects to establish the statistical significance of putative effects.

As addressed in Chapter 17, more recent and ongoing epidemiological studies have addressed many of these concerns and promise to contribute valuable information on ELF health effects.

Although the impact of ELF exposure on humans is of primary importance and concern, many areas of biological investigation are more appropriately and efficiently conducted with cellular systems or animal models. This chapter specifically examines the biological effects of exposure to ELF EM fields observed in in vitro and in vivo studies. An attempt is made to help the reader evalute experimental results and, insofar as possible, interpret them with respect to potential health implications. An overview of current concepts and possible mechanisms is given, and possible future directions of research are discussed.

PHYSICAL CONSIDERATIONS FOR COMPARING EXTREMELY LOW-FREQUENCY EXPOSURE BETWEEN SPECIES

Electric field coupling to living organisms has been investigated from both a theoretical and an experimental perspective. Theoretical treatments, addressed in earlier chapters of this book, have been extensively reviewed elsewhere (Kaune, 1985; Kaune and Phillips, 1985; Polk and Postow, 1986) and therefore are not discussed in this chapter. Experimental modeling is briefly reviewed because it provides important scaling and dosimetric information for extrapolating data from animals to humans. A more detailed treatment of the subject can be found in recent papers by Kaune and Forsythe (1985) and Tenforde and Kaune (1987).

In animals or models exposed to an electric field, an easily determined electrical parameter is the short-circuit current induced in the grounded subject. Although most of the data collected to date were obtained at only one frequency and body weight, currents at other frequencies f and body weights W can be determined with an $fW^{2/3}$ dependence (Kaune, 1981). The total short-circuit currents in humans and various animals have been compared during exposure to a constant vertical ELF electric field (Table 9-1).

Another method of comparison is a simple relationship, described by Deno (1977), in which the external electric fields acting on the surface of a body are measured. Kaune and Phillips (1980) used such measures to compare surface electric fields and induced-current distributions in grounded models of rats and pigs. Current densities were estimated from

---

TABLE 9-1   Short-Circuit Currents Induced in Grounded Humans and Animals by Vertical Extremely Low-Frequency Electric Fields*

Species	Short-circuit current* (μA)
Human	15.0
Horse	8.5
Cow	8.6
Pig	7.7
Guinea pig	4.2
Rat	4.0

Reprinted with permission from Tenforde, T.S., and Kaune, W.T. (1987). Interaction of extremely low frequency electric and magnetic fields with humans. *Health Phys. 53*:585–606.

* $I \times 10^8/f W^{2/3} E_0$, where I = current (A), f = frequency (Hz), W = weight (g), and E_0 = electric field intensity (V/m).

the induced current data. By combining data derived from Deno's human measurements and Kaune's animal data, researchers have determined peak surface electric fields and current densities (Figure 9-2). All three models shown in the figure were exposed to identical 60 Hz electric fields of 10 kV/m. An evaluation of the data shows that, despite comparable exposure, the doses of electric fields received by the three models are quite different. If dose is represented by either the induced axial (along the long axis of the body) current density or the peak surface electric field, the values are considerably larger in the human than in the animal models. Therefore, if one wishes to extrapolate biological data from one species to another, adjustments must be made to scale the exposure parameters. Since exposures are usually given as unperturbed field levels (that is, fields with no bodies present), a multiplier (scaling factor) must be used to equalize differences between species. A complicating element is that the value of the scaling factor depends on the internal or external quantity being scaled. For example, at the top of the body the surface fields (180, 67, and 37 kV/m for human, pig, and rat, respectively) require scaling factors of about 1:2.7:4.9 for these respective species. If, on the other hand, axial current density in the neck is the desired comparison, the scaling factors are about 1:13.8:19.6 for the three species. These values change to 1:12.5:125, respectively, for current densities through the lower abdomen. Although the general principle of scaling is applicable and necessary, precise, quantitative extrapolation of data across species requires additional knowledge about the specific site of action for a particular biological end point.

More precise current-density data have recently been obtained by measuring more than one component of the total internal current-density

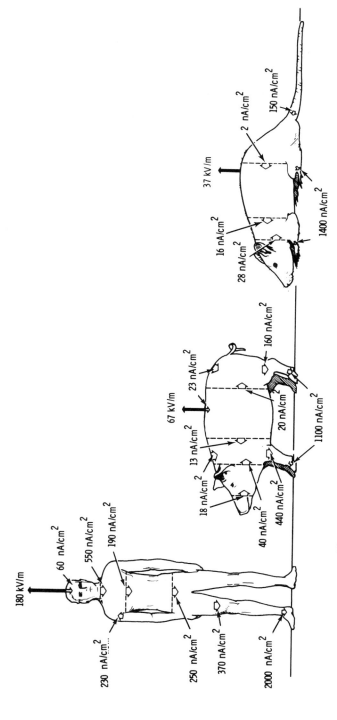

Figure 9-2 Electric field intensity comparisons for highest point on surface of grounded man, pig, and rat exposed to 10 kV/m, 60 Hz electric field. Estimated average axial current densities are also compared for same species through body sections as shown. Also given for man and pig are current densities calculated as perpendicular to body surface. Relative body sizes are not to scale. (From Kaune, W.T., and Phillips, R.D. [1980]. *Bioelectromagnetics 1*:117–129.)

vector. Representative data for a human model exposed to a vertical, 10 kV/m electric field are shown in Figure 9-3 (Kaune and Forsythe, 1985). Similar data have been obtained for animal models as well (Kaune and Forsythe, 1988). Methods have also been developed to extrapolate data obtained with grounded subjects to the ungrounded condition (Kaune et al., 1987).

Coupling of humans or animals to ELF magnetic fields is different from the electric field coupling discussed previously. Although biological organisms do not perturb an incident ELF magnetic field, they serve as a conductive pathway in which eddy currents are induced. These circulating currents lie in planes perpendicular to the direction of the incident magnetic field (Tenforde, 1986). The magnitude of an electric field induced by an external magnetic field depends mainly on the loop size of the induced current. Equivalent doses for subjects exposed to a magnetic field can be obtained by using a scaling factor based roughly on the size of the animal or human in question.

As described in a paper by Tenforde and Kaune (1987), if the relative magnitudes of the electric field induced in a human by electric (10 kV/m) and magnetic (30×10^{-4} T) fields (simulating the fields close to a high-voltage power transmission line) are compared, the internal fields induced by the electric field are roughly an order of magnitude larger than those induced by the magnetic field. That much of ELF bioeffects research has been focused on electric field exposure can be partially explained by this large difference in induced internal electric fields.

REVIEW OF HUMAN STUDIES

Concern about possible deleterious effects of ELF EM fields on human health grew out of observations in the Soviet Union during the late 1960s and early 1970s. These reports claimed a variety of exposure-related symptoms, including headaches, poor digestion, cardiovascular changes, decreased libido, loss of sleep, and increased irritability in switchyard workers subsequent to prolonged exposure to E fields (up to 26 kV/m) (Asanova and Rakov, 1966; Korobkova et al., 1972). Because of the subjective nature of the reports, it was not possible to conclude that the functional changes resulted exclusively from exposure to EM fields, especially in view of the presence of spark discharges at the substations. However, the findings led to increased research in the Soviet Union and throughout the rest of the world. Numerous studies were initiated in a wide range of investigations to assess the potential biological consequences of exposing humans to ELF EM radiation.

In human studies conducted to date, the principal sources of information on effects of ELF fields are surveys of utility workers and of people

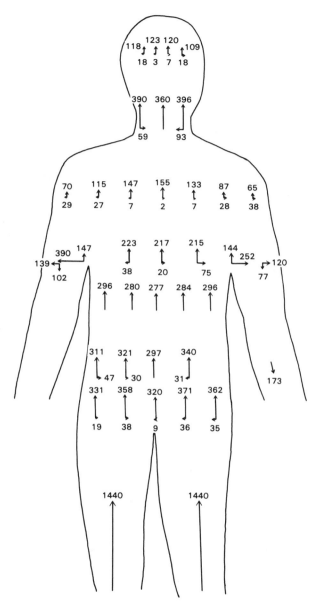

Figure 9-3 Induced current densities (nA/cm^2) measured in saline model of man exposed to 10 kV/m, 60 Hz electric field. Axial and radial components of induced densities are represented by vertical and horizontal arrows, respectively, with length of arrows roughly comparable to intensity value of current. (Reprinted with permission from Tenforde, T.S., and Kaune, W.T. [1987]. Interaction of extremely low frequency electric and magnetic fields with humans. *Health Phys. 53*:585–606. Copyright 1987, Pergamon Press.)

living near high-voltage lines, a few laboratory and clinical studies, and several epidemiological studies. Aspects and results of the epidemiological studies are discussed in Chapter 17. A small number of laboratory studies on human response to ELF fields are briefly described here.

Laboratory Investigations

Relatively few laboratory and clinical studies of ELF exposure effects on humans have been performed. The most extensive laboratory experiments on human physiology and affect were conducted by Hauf. In 1974 he began a comprehensive clinical evaluation of more than 100 volunteer subjects who were exposed for relatively brief periods to fields of 1, 15, or 20 kV/m at 50 Hz (Hauf, 1974, 1976a). Among the many parameters tested, only a few field-related effects were observed, including slight decreases in reaction time and slight increases in white blood cell counts in exposed subjects. A slight elevation in their levels of norepinephrine was also observed. Hauf proposed that this might reflect minor stress. In a further attempt to define the cause of the slight variations observed, Hauf studied the effects of injected currents (200 μA) in humans. These currents, calculated to equal the displacement currents expected from previous electric field exposures, did not alter either reaction time or electroencephalograms (EEGs). Hauf concluded that the slight effects previously observed in subjects exposed to an electric field were probably due to "nonspecific excitation" (Hauf, 1976b). The results of Hauf's studies were confirmed and extended by Kuhne (1978). Data from all these studies are summarized in a World Health Organization document (Hauf, 1982).

In a similar study conducted in Poland, the conscious reaction to sound and light stimuli was measured in 35 volunteers exposed to 50 Hz E fields. At field strengths greater than 10 kV/m, the reaction was prolonged for both types of stimuli (Szuba and Nosol, 1985).

Additional information on human exposure comes from a medical evaluation study involving 32 subjects exposed intermittently for more than 20 years in a 380 kV facility (Bauchinger et al., 1981). No effects of exposure were noted in sister chromatid exchange analyses or in hematological, hormonal, and behavioral tests.

In another study involving laboratory exposure of human subjects, conducted by Cabanes and Gary (1981), the threshold for perception of a 50 Hz electric field was evaluated. Seventy-five subjects were exposed to varying electric fields in three body positions. Threshold levels for responses that showed field perception ranged from 0.35 kV/m (in 4% of the subjects) to greater than 27 kV/m. Approximately 40% could not detect 27 kV/m with their arms against the body. Data supporting these results were obtained by Deno and Zaffanella (1982), who conducted similar experiments with 60 Hz fields. They reported comparable results, with 5% of exposed subjects able to detect a 1 kV/m field and a median value for perception of 7 kV/m. If such a large perceptual threshold variation holds true in other species, it might provide some explanation for the great variability in biological data obtained to date.

In three laboratory studies of ELF magnetic fields, involving short-term exposures of human subjects, hematologic and serum chemistry changes were the biological end points of interest (Beischer et al., 1973; Mantell, 1975; Sander et al., 1982). With the exception of one report of increased serum triglyceride levels in exposed subjects (Beischer et al. 1973), no effects of magnetic field exposure were observed. Additional observations were made in more than 100 subjects exposed to time-varying magnetic fields (5 Hz to 1 kHz, B less than 100 mT). EEGs, electrocardiograms, and blood pressure and body temperature measurements showed no effects of exposure (Silney, 1979).

The most widely studied biological effect of magnetic field exposure in humans is a visual phenomenon known as "phosphenes" (Lovsund et al., 1979). This phenomenon appears to arise from the induction of electrical currents that stimulate the retina. It is highly frequency dependent, with maximum effects at 20 Hz (Lovsund et al., 1980).

Recently reported experimental work with humans has been done at the Midwest Research Institute in Kansas City, Missouri, and at Manchester University in England. In the former study, volunteer male subjects were exposed to both electric and magnetic fields (60 Hz) below the level of perception for 8-hour periods (Fotopoulos et al., 1987; Graham et al., 1987). Although some differences appeared to exist between exposed and sham-exposed subjects, particularly in some endocrine parameters and heart rate, the effects were not consistent across time and lay within the normal biological variations. The Manchester work (Bonnell et al., 1985; Stollery, 1987) involved male volunteers subjected for $5\frac{1}{2}$ hours to 50 Hz currents, injected via electrodes on the skin to simulate exposure to a 36 kV/m electric field. Tests of mood, memory, attention, and verbal reasoning skills revealed no clear effects of the exposure.

In contrast to the slight effects observed in bone fracture repair in animals exposed to sinusoidal electric fields, biological effects of pulsed magnetic field (PMF) exposure appear to be marked. Since the early 1970s, PMFs with repetition frequencies in the ELF range have been used clinically to provide electrical stimulation in noninvasive treatment of bone nonunions and pseudarthroses (Basset, 1978; Bassett et al., 1974, 1982; Sedel et al., 1981). Pulsed field applicators, used for fracture therapy, induce current densities in bone of approximately 20 mA/cm^2. Initial clinical trials with such magnetic stimulation have achieved a high rate of success (up to 85% in fracture healing). The biophysical mechanisms of the interaction between bone tissue and PMF have been investigated in a number of studies. These investigations have suggested that bidirectional PMF may enhance the synthesis of collagen and alter the synthesis of cell surface glycoproteins in cultures of bone-forming cells and fibroblasts (Cain et al., 1987; Fitton-Jackson and Bassett, 1980; Norton, 1982). Two excellent reviews address medical applications of time-varying ELF magnetic fields and present detailed information on the interaction of these fields with living tissue (Tenforde, 1986; Tenforde and Budinger, 1985).

REVIEW OF ANIMAL STUDIES

Although the interaction of humans with electric and magnetic fields is of prime importance and concern, many areas of biological investigation are more efficiently and appropriately conducted with various other animal species. Animals provide an integrated system that can be used in prospective studies, in contrast to the retrospective studies usually done with humans. A major challenge of using data from animal studies is the question of extrapolation to human exposure conditions as discussed previously.

By far the largest body of information on biological effects of ELF fields has been obtained in experimental research on animals exposed to electric fields. Experiments have been performed primarily on rodents (rats and mice), but a wide variety of other subjects have also been used, including insects, birds, cats, dogs, swine, and nonhuman primates. A broad range of exposure levels has been employed, and an equally large number of biological end points have been examined for evidence of possible electric and/or magnetic field effects. These multitudinous studies have been reviewed several times (NAS, 1977; Phillips and Kaune, 1977; Sheppard and Eisenbud, 1977; WHO, 1984; Anderson and Phillips, 1985; Graves, 1985). Summaries of the important findings are presented in this chapter, arranged according to the biological systems that appear to be principally involved: neural and neuroendocrine systems (including behavior), reproductive systems (including fertility, growth, and development), and other functions (including cardiovascular and blood chemistry, bone growth and repair, and cellular and membrane properties).

Biological research conducted at power-frequency electric fields of 50 to 60 Hz has produced the preponderance of experimental data. More limited work, including many in vitro studies (to be discussed in Part 5), has been conducted at lower frequencies (15 to 35 Hz); very few studies have been performed at frequencies between 100 and 300 Hz. Only relatively recently have investigators begun to focus on the effects of ELF magnetic fields or combined electric and magnetic field exposures on biological systems.

Neural and Neuroendocrine Systems

Many of the biological effects observed in animals exposed to ELF fields appear to be directly or indirectly associated with the nervous system. This apparent relationship might be anticipated, since the nervous system is composed of tissues and processes that are unusually responsive to electrical signals. In addition, both the structure and function of this system are fundamentally involved in the interaction of an animal with its environment. The major features of this interaction—transmittal of sensory input from external stimuli, central processing of such information, and subsequent efferent innervation of tissues and organs—may provide the basis for explaining possible links between ELF exposure and observed biological consequences.

In early experimental studies, nervous system parameters were measured only occasionally, although many of the observed effects, primarily behavioral, were related to nervous system function. Before the late 1970s, studies on ELF exposure relating to nervous system function could generally be classified in three categories: assessments of activity or startle-response behavior, evaluations of stress-related hormones (such as corticosteroids), and general measurements of central nervous system responses (such as EEGs and interresponse times). Results were often contradictory, with claims of both effects and no effects from ELF electric field exposure. However, because of the apparent sensitivity of the nervous system to ELF fields, subsequent studies included a broader range of neurological assessments. Concomitant with this increased emphasis, specific nervous system responses, in addition to behavior, began to be sought in experiments. This effort was mounted to determine the extent and nature of ELF-tissue interactions and also to clarify the mechanisms underlying the observed biological effects.

Behavior.   Among the most sensitive measures of perturbations in a biological system are tests that determine modifications in the behavioral patterns of animals. This sensitivity is especially valuable in studying environmental agents of relatively low toxicity.

Behavioral studies in several species provide evidence of electric field perception and of the possibility the field may directly alter behavior. The threshold of detection reported by Stern et al. (1983) is between 4 and 10 kV/m in rats. Human volunteers were able to detect a 9 kV/m, 60 Hz field in certain postures (Graham et al., 1987). Thresholds for perception of the field in other animal species, reportedly in the 25 to 35 kV/m ranges, include mice (Moos 1964; Rosenberg et al. 1983), pigs (Kaune et al., 1978), and pigeons and chickens (Graves et al., 1978a,b). It appears that a change in other environmental factors, such as relative humidity, has the potential to alter perception threshold values (Weigel and Lundstrom, 1987).

Cutaneous sensory receptors that respond to a 60 Hz electric field have been identified in the cat paw (Weigel et al., 1987). Whether such receptors exist in human skin is unknown.

An evaluation of the preference/avoidance behavior of animals for remaining in or out of the E-field has been conducted at several field strengths for 60 Hz electric fields. At 100 V/m, no effect of exposure, either in preference behavior or temporal discrimination, was evident in monkeys (deLorge, 1974). At 25 kV/m, rats preferred to spend their inactive period in the field, whereas at 75 to 100 kV/m they avoided exposure (Hjeresen et al., 1980). Swine (Hjeresen et al., 1982) remained out of the field (30 kV/m) at night but demonstrated few other observable behavioral changes. Alterations in activity have also been reported in animals exposed to ELF fields, including a transitory, increased activity response on initial exposure of rats or mice at 25 to 35 kV/m (Hjeresen et al., 1980; Rosenberg et al., 1983).

Much of the behavioral work with nonhuman primates has been performed at very low field strengths (7 to 100 V/m), where essentially no effects of exposure were reported (summarized in NAS, 1977). Gavalas et al. (1970) and Gavalas-Medici and Day-Magdaleno (1976) observed changes in interresponse time of monkeys during exposure, but no other effects. At much higher field strengths (30 kV/m), Rogers et al. (1987) reported minor behavioral changes in exposed baboons that appear related to the animals' perception of the field. The observed effects do not seem to be permanent or deleterious.

In studies examining the effect of ELF magnetic fields on behavior, many of the investigations carried out at low field intensities have shown behavioral alterations, primarily activity changes (Persinger, 1969; Persinger and Foster, 1970; Smith and Justesen, 1977). In contrast, studies conducted at higher field intensities have shown no evidence of a field-associated effect on animal behavior (Creim et al., 1985; Davis et al., 1984).

In the experimental studies that have been conducted to determine whether ELF fields cause behavioral alterations, remarkably few robust effects have been demonstrated (Lovely, 1988). Effects that have been observed, usually arousal or activity responses, are probably due to the animal's detection and possible perception of the electric field.

Biological rhythms. Far from being static, living organisms exhibit marked dynamics in metabolism and function. Major elements of such dynamics are the endogenous rhythms of varying frequencies (such as ultradian, circadian, and infradian). These biological rhythms, which respond to exogenous environmental cues, are normally a complex mix of phase-locked rhythms and have significant impacts on the physiological and psychological well-being of the organism. Biochemical processes, cellular communications, and functional systems are all intimately associated with endogenous rhythms, as is overall systemic response to the environment. Dysfunctions in these underlying rhythms can profoundly affect the organism and lead to a variety of biological effects.

A number of investigations have been conducted to examine the effects of ELF electromagnetic fields on natural biological rhythms. After Wever's significant findings (1971) on the influence of electromagnetic fields on humans, several studies were reported. Dowse (1982) claimed that a 10 Hz, 150 V/m field affected the locomotor rhythm of individual fruit flies. Researchers in Ehret's laboratory (Duffy and Ehret, 1982; Rosenberg et al., 1983) used metabolic indicators to examine both circadian and ultradian rhythms in rats and mice exposed to 60 Hz electric fields. They observed no effects of exposure in rats, but they reported that the activity and rhythms of oxidative metabolism in male mice could be phase shifted by exposure.

Wilson et al. (1981, 1983) directly examined another aspect of circadian activity in rats by measuring the cyclical pineal production of indolamines and enzymes. A significant reduction in the normal nighttime rise of melatonin and biosynthetic enzymes in the pineal gland was observed in rats exposed to either 1.5 or 40 kV/m. Furthermore, the change in pineal indole response occurred only after at least 3 weeks of chronic exposure (Wilson et al., 1986). In other studies, nocturnal pineal components in mice and rats have been shown to be sensitive to rotated magnetic fields (Semm, 1983; Welker et al., 1983; Kavaliers et al., 1984). Recent evidence suggests that retinal sensors may be involved in the pineal response to EM fields (Olcese et al., 1985; Reuss and Olcese, 1986).

Sulzman and Murrish (1987) investigated the effects of ELF fields on circadian function in squirrel monkeys. In an examination of exposure to a range of electric field intensities (2.6, 26, and 39 kV/m), accompanied by a 100 T magnetic field, they reported apparent intensity-related effects. None of the monkeys exposed to 2.6 kV/m showed any change in activity or feeding after 2 weeks of exposure. However, 33% of the monkeys exposed to 26 kV/m and 75% of those exposed to 39 kV/m had significant changes in their circadian cycles.

Although firm conclusions cannot yet be made regarding potential health impacts from ELF effects on circadian or biological rhythms, it is apparent that EM fields alter the circadian timing mechanisms in mammals. Much work remains to be accomplished before the observed effects and their biological consequences are clearly understood. It seems probable that ELF effects on rhythms, particularly those mediated by neuroendocrine systems, could play an important role in other areas of observed bioeffects, such as behavior and development.

Neurophysiology. The relationship between the neurotransmitters norepinephrine and epinephrine and the physiological responses of stress and arousal is well established. As researchers began to look for potential biological effects of ELF electric fields, measuring these transmitters became one of the assessments used to examine the nervous system for evidence of a stress response in animals. This approach, which benefited from the ease of measuring these chemicals in serum, urine, or brain tissue, addressed reports that ELF fields acted as mild stressors (Dumansky et al., 1977; Marino and Becker, 1977). Unfortunately, potential methodological problems raised serious questions about the validity of the early reports (Michaelson, 1979) and have also been problematic in some of the more recent studies.

Groza et al. (1978) measured catecholamines in both urine and blood after exposure of rats to 100 kV/m, 60 Hz fields. They reported significant increases in epinephrine levels in both blood and urine after acute (6-hour to 3-day) exposures but no changes in norepinephrine or epinephrine with longer-term (12-day) exposures.

A report of increased norepinephrine in serum of rats exposed to 50 Hz (50 V/m and 5.3 kV/m) is found in the work of Mose (1978). A companion paper by Fischer et al. (1978) examined norepinephrine content in brain tissue of rats exposed to 5.3 kV/m for 21 days; after 15 minutes of exposure the levels increased rapidly. However, after 10 days of exposure, levels were significantly lower than in a control group. Portet and Cabanes (1988) reported no changes in adrenal epinephrine or norepinephrine in 2-month-old rats exposed to a 50 kV/m, 50 Hz field for 8 hours a day. In contrast, Wolpaw et al. (1987) reported decreases in cerebrospinal fluid concentrations of the major metabolites of dopamine and serotonin, homovanillic acid, and 5-hydroxyindoleacetic acid in macaques exposed to electric and magnetic fields. In addition to possible species-specific response differences, some of the discrepancies between results of various laboratories may be explained in light of results described by Vasquez et al. (1988). Because of circadian fluctuations in levels of neurotransmitters, the time of sampling may be critical in determining whether an ELF effect is observed. Vasquez et al. reported significant changes in diurnal patterns of several biogenic amines when rats were exposed to 60 Hz electric fields for 4 weeks.

Examining another neurochemical parameter, Kozyarin (1981) measured the acetylcholinesterase (AChE) enzyme levels in rats exposed to 50 Hz electric fields. He reported that serum AChE activity was approximately 25 times baseline levels in both young and old animals exposed to 15 kV/m for 60 days, 30 minutes a day. Brain levels of AChE decreased in exposed animals, although not by such large percentages. Further important measurements were made to estimate the course of recovery from the observed effects. All values had returned to normal 1 month after cessation of exposure. The author concluded that electric fields can cause changes in the functional condition of the central nervous system, although the changes appear to be temporary.

In general, neurochemical data provide relatively weak evidence that exposure to electric fields in the power-frequency range may cause slight changes in nervous system function. The number of experiments is not large, and there are significant questions about the validity of several of the studies. Nevertheless, the findings support the hypothesis that ELF exposure alters internal rhythms, increases arousal in animals, and is transient in its effect.

Measurements of corticosteroids in animals exposed to electric fields have resulted in a somewhat confusing picture, perhaps because of the quick response to stimuli of these adrenal steroids (Michaelson, 1979). Studies at Pennsylvania State University examined the hypothesis that 60 Hz electric fields act as a biological stressor (Hackman and Graves, 1981). In that study an acute, transient increase in plasma corticosterone levels occurred in mice exposed to 25 or 50 kV/m. Serum levels of the steroid returned to normal within 1 day. In some studies conducted in the Soviet Union, Dumansky et al. (1976) showed an increase in corticosteroids in rats exposed for 1, 3, or 4 months at 5 kV/m.

In a study conducted by Marino et al. (1977), serum corticosteroid levels were decreased in animals exposed to 15 kV/m for 30 days. This study, however, used pooled, grouped samples of serum. It also had several other technical problems: cages varied, and in four experiments exposed rats were individually housed, whereas control rats were housed in groups.

Results that appear to contradict Marino's and Dumansky's data have been described by Free et al. (1981) and Portet and Cabanes (1988), who exposed rats or rabbits to 100 and 50 kV/m, respectively, for 30 or 120 days. No differences in corticosterone levels were observed between exposed and control animals. Providing additional support for these data was a study by Gann (1976) in which dogs exposed to 15 kV/m showed no effects of E-field exposure on corticosterone secretion. Quinlan et al. (1985) collected blood samples from rats via carotid artery cannulas during exposure or sham exposure to an 80 kV/m, 60 Hz electric field. No statistically significant differences in corticosterone levels were noted.

Several laboratories have examined the morphology of brain tissue from animals exposed to ELF electric fields. Carter and Graves (1975) and Bankoske et al. (1976) exposed chicks to 40 kV/m E fields and saw no effects on central nervous system morphology. This finding was supported by those of Phillips et al. (1978), who examined rats exposed to 100 kV/m for 30 days. Again, no morphological evidence of an electric field effect was observed. In a study in Sweden (Hansson 1981a,b) dramatic changes in cell structure were reported in the cerebella of rabbits exposed to a 14 kV/m E field. Exposed animals showed disintegration of Nissl bodies and the three-dimensional endoplasmic reticulum structure, as well as the abnormal presence of many lamellar bodies, particularly in the Purkinje cells of the cerebellum. Reduced numbers of mitochondria, reduced arborization of the dendritic branches, and an absence of hypolemmal cisterns were also evident in these cells. However, these reported changes must be interpreted with caution. The animals were exposed outdoors and showed evidence of significant health deficits (whether resulting from the electric field, other environmental conditions, or some combinations of these factors is not clear). Furthermore, results from these studies are in conflict with experiments conducted by Portet and Cabanes (1988), in which no ultrastructural changes occurred in the cerebella of young rabbits exposed to 50 kV/m. These questions concerning neuroanatomical changes have yet to be resolved. However, the lack of obvious, significant functional deficits in the central nervous systems of thousands of animals exposed to date suggests that the dramatic morphological alterations in exposed rabbits may result from conditions unrelated to electric field exposure. The possibility of synergistic effects from the E field and a stressful environment cannot be ruled out.

Because the nervous system is by nature electrically sensitive, it has been assumed to be particularly sensitive to influence by external ELF fields. To some degree this assumption has been borne out by experimental results, although in the area of neurophysiology a confusing array of studies have claimed both effects and no effects of ELF field exposure. A case in point is the commonly used measure of general central nervous system activity, the EEG. When chicks were exposed for 3 weeks to 60 Hz E fields of up to 80 kV/m, Graves et al. (1978b) noted no changes in EEGs recorded via electrodes implanted after exposure. Similarly, no effects were observed in the EEGs of cats exposed to 80 kV/m at 50 Hz (Silney, 1981). Earlier, Blanchi et al. (1973) reported significant changes in EEG activity when guinea pigs were exposed for $\frac{1}{2}$ hour to a 100 kV/m, 50 Hz field. Takashima et al. (1979) examined EEGs from rabbits exposed at 1 to 10 MHz, modulated at 15 Hz. Before exposure, these animals had silver electrodes implanted in their skulls for recording the EEG. After 2 to 3 weeks of exposure, abnormal responses were observed in the EEGs, although it was subsequently determined that the EEG returned to normal when the electrodes were removed during exposure. The investigators thus concluded that the effect on the EEG was due to the local fields created by the presence of the electrodes in the cranial cavity. Gavalas et al. (1970) noted that 7 and 10 Hz E fields of only 7 V/m affected EEGs recorded from monkeys via implanted electrodes. The significance of these results is unclear, since they may be due to an artifact caused by the implanted electrodes as noted previously.

EEGs from cats exposed to 50 Hz magnetic fields (8 hours a day at 20 mT) showed short-term decreases in power density spectra (Silney,

1979). This response was observed only for a short time after the magnetic field was switched on.

In an assessment of a more specific electric "fingerprint" of the brain, the visual evoked response (VER), no effects of exposure were observed in adult or developing rats. Jaffe et al. (1983) assessed the VER in 114 rats exposed in utero through 20 days post partum. The dams, fetuses, and subsequent pups were exposed to a 65 kV/m, 60 Hz electric field. No consistent, statistically significant effects of exposure were observed. Wolpaw and associates (1987) examined evoked potentials in pig-tailed macaques exposed to combined electric and magnetic fields. As in Jaffe's studies, the VER and the auditory evoked potential showed no changes caused by exposure. However, an attenuation of the late components of the somatosensory evoked potentials was demonstrated in exposed animals. The authors suggest that these abnormalities may have been due to a particularly large number of stimuli giving rise to a change in the mechanisms of attention.

Two other excellent neurophysiological studies have had clear, replicable results. Jaffe et al. (1980) examined synaptic junctions from chronically exposed rats (60 Hz and 100 kV/m for 30 days). In these studies, presynaptic fibers were stimulated with a pair of above-threshold pulses. The height ratio of the resultant action potentials, observed as a function of the interspike interval, demonstrated an enhanced neuronal excitability in nerves from exposed animals. However, many other parameters tested in these nerves showed no changes in exposed animals. In a second experiment Jaffe et al. (1981) examined a wide range of physiological parameters of the peripheral nervous system and neuromuscular function. The only effect observed was slightly faster recovery from fatigue after chronic stimulation in one class of muscle, the soleus, slow-twitch muscle.

In summary, numerous studies have been initiated to determine how greatly an electrical environment containing electric or magnetic fields of ELF affects the nervous system. Many of the experiments have not confirmed any neuropathological effects, even after prolonged exposures to high-strength (100 kV/m) electric fields and high-intensity (5 mT) magnetic fields (Tenforde, 1985). As discussed previously, nervous system effects that have been observed include altered neuronal excitability, altered circadian levels of pineal hormones, and behavioral aversion to or preference for the field. In addition, in several instances where unconfirmed or controversial data exist, observed effects may or may not be real. Examples are changes in serum catecholamines or corticosteroids, morphology of brain tissue, and EEG waveforms. Possibly these and other putative effects are due to a direct interaction of the electric field with tissue or to an indirect interaction, such as a physiological response owing to detection or stimulation of sensory receptors by the field. The nature of the physical mechanisms involved in field-induced

effects is obscure, and elucidating them is one of the urgent goals of current research.

The behavioral tests that most frequently showed an effect of exposure were those relating to detection of the field or to activity. Most other behaviors did not change with ELF field exposure. It should also be noted that influences of the nervous system on other biological systems are often mediated indirectly through neuroendocrine or endocrine responses.

Reproduction and Development

Developing organisms, including prenatal and postnatal mammals, are generally considered more sensitive to physical or chemical agents than are adult animals (Mahlum et al., 1978). This greater sensitivity, when it occurs, is thought to originate in subtle effects on the increased number and activity of processes and controls that guide the developing cellular interactions. A number of studies have examined the effects of ELF exposure on reproduction and development of both mammalian and nonmammalian species. These studies have been assessed by other reviewers (Chernoff, 1985; Sikov, 1985) and are only briefly summarized here.

Most of the nonmammalian studies have been performed on chickens or pigeons. Many studies have indicated that electric field exposure of chicks at several field strengths, before and after hatching, did not significantly affect viability, morphology, behavior, or growth (Krueger et al., 1972; Reed and Graves, 1984; Veicsteinas et al., 1987). However, in one series of experiments chicks exposed to 40 or 80 kV/m on days 1 to 22 after hatching showed significantly less motor activity during the week after removal from the field (Graves et al., 1978b).

Few studies have examined the effects of ELF magnetic fields on growth and development of birds. Krueger et al. (1972) exposed chicks from hatching through 28 days of age to a nonuniform, 45 Hz, 1.4×10^{-4} T field. Growth rates were depressed, but no other parameters were affected. Great interest has been shown in the reports of Delgado et al. (1982), who observed a marked increase in malformation rate in chick eggs exposed to low levels of pulsed magnetic fields (0.12 or 12×10^{-6} T). It was subsequently reported that an important determinant of the results was the wave shape of the pulse (Ubeda et al., 1983). Several research groups have been cooperating in a multilaboratory replication of the Delgado results. Results described in a preliminary report (Berman et al., 1988) indicated that significant malformation increases were observed in two of the six laboratories.

Unreplicated studies have given some indications that exposure of prenatal mammals to electric fields produces deleterious effects on postnatal growth and survival (Knickerbocker et al., 1967; Marino et al., 1976, 1980; Hansson, 1981b; Sikov et al., 1987). These studies are countered by others in which rats, rabbits, or mice were exposed to 20, 50, 100, 200, or 240 kV/m and no effects on reproduction, survival, or growth and development were demonstrated (Cerretelli et al., 1979; Fam, 1980; Sikov et al., 1984; Pafkova, 1985; Rommereim et al., 1987; Portet and Cabanes, 1988).

In an evaluation of reproductive and developmental toxicology in swine, Sikov et al. (1987) observed no increased terata in progeny from the first breeding of swine exposed during pregnancy to a 60 Hz electric field. After 18 months of continued exposure the dams were rebred and their litters were examined at 100 days of gestation. At that time, malformation incidence in litters of exposed animals was significantly greater than in comparable sham-exposed litters. Similar results were obtained in litters of second generation gilts that were born in the field and bred after 18 months of exposure.

This study was followed by one of similar design (but much greater statistical power) in which rats were the experimental model. No significant differences in growth and development were observed in litters of rats exposed to 10, 65, and 130 kV/m when compared with sham-exposed controls (Rommereim et al., 1988).

In other studies a rotating magnetic field (0.5 to 15×10^{-4} T) was used to expose pregnant rats during various stages of gestation. Some differences were noted between exposed and sham-exposed offspring, including increased thyroid and testis weights in exposed pups. Also, the exposed offspring were more responsive when tested in a suppressed response paradigm (Ossenkopp et al., 1972; Persinger and Pear, 1972).

As indicated previously, conflict remains over results of studies investigating the potential for ELF electric or magnetic field exposure to affect mammalian reproduction and development. This confusion over results indicates the need for carefully designed, statistically sound experiments that will help clarify this important area of investigation.

Other Biological Functions

Bone growth and repair.   One report of animals exposed to 60 Hz electric fields (McClanahan and Phillips, 1983) indicated that bone growth per se was not affected by exposure to 100 kV/m. However, this study, as well as an additional report (Marino et al., 1979), suggested that bone fracture repair was retarded in rats and mice exposed to 5 or 100 kV/m, 60 Hz fields but not to very low (1 kV/m) field strengths. McClanahan and Phillips (1983) suggest that exposure affects the rate of healing but not the strength of the healed bone.

In contrast to the experiments with sinusoidal 60 Hz fields, research studies and clinical trials (discussed previously) have been performed in which pulsed magnetic fields were used to treat bone fractures and arthroses in humans. The weak electrical currents induced in bone tissue by magnetic field pulses may enhance fracture repair by altering intracellular concentrations of calcium ions, thus modifying cellular metabolism and stimulating growth of the osteoblasts and chondrocytes (Luben et al., 1982; Bassett, 1978).

Why 60 Hz sinusoidal electric fields cause a retardation of fracture repair, whereas pulsed magnetic fields facilitate repair, is unclear.

Cardiovascular system. Cardiovascular function has been assessed by measuring blood pressure and heart rate and performing electrocardiographic measurements. Early studies indicated as possible effects a decrease in heart rate and cardiac output in dogs exposed to 15 kV/m (Gann, 1976) and increased heart rates in chickens exposed to 80 kV/m (Carter and Graves, 1975). A more recent and comprehensive study in rats exposed to 100 kV/m showed no such effects of exposure, even when the animals were subjected to cold stress (Hilton and Phillips, 1980). Cerretelli and Malaguti (1976) reported transient increases in blood pressure in dogs exposed to 50 Hz E fields greater than 10 kV/m. Hilton and Phillips (1980) were unable to confirm a report by Blanchi et al. (1973) of electrocardiographic changes in animals exposed to 100 kV/m.

Magnetic field exposure of dogs (50 Hz, 2 T) caused a stimulation of the heart in the diastolic phase, with salvos of ectopic beats appearing in the recordings (Silney, 1985). Humans exposed to combined electric and magnetic fields (9 kV/m, 20 T) showed a longer cardiac interbeat interval than sham-exposed subjects (Graham et al., 1987).

Serum chemistry appears to be relatively unaffected by exposure to either ELF electric or magnetic fields (Marino and Becker, 1977; Mathewson et al., 1977; Ragan et al., 1979, 1983). Hematological data, however, present a more confusing picture. With electric field exposure, white blood cell count was often elevated in populations of mice and rats (Graves et al., 1979; Ragan et al., 1983). With the exception of one report by Tarakhovsky et al. (1971), all the published studies on hematological effects of magnetic field exposure have shown no field-associated effects (Beischer et al., 1973; de Lorge, 1974; Fam, 1981; Sander et al., 1982). The occasional positive or negative effects on the hematopoietic system must be carefully evaluated. Often, apparent sporadic effects are not statistically significant when the appropriate multivariate analyses are used to evaluate hematological and serum chemistry parameters.

Immunology. There is some indication that exposure of animals to electric fields does not markedly affect the immune system. In a comprehensive investigation of the humoral and cellular aspects of the immune system, Morris et al. (1979, 1982, 1983) observed no effects of exposure at very low field strengths (150 to 250 V/m) in mice or rats. In subsequent experiments at higher field exposures (100 kV/m), no effects were seen in immune system response. However, Lyle et al. (1983) reported significant decrements in the cytolytic capacity of lymphocytes exposed to radiofrequency fields modulated at 60 Hz. Further work with 60 Hz electric fields alone also resulted in a suppression of T-lymphocyte cytotoxicity (Lyle et al., 1988). A significant difference between the work reported from these two laboratories is that Morris measured lymphocyte responses from exposed animals, whereas Lyle exposed lymphocytes in culture.

In contrast to the apparent lack of strong or consistent electric field influences on the immune system, immunoresponse to mitogens and antigens appears to be significantly susceptible to ELF magnetic fields (Odintsov, 1965; Mizushima et al., 1975; Conti et al., 1983).

Carcinogenesis and mutagenesis.   No effects suggesting a direct effect of electric field exposure on mutagenesis or carcinogenesis have been observed (Mittler, 1972; Frazier et al., 1987). However, there is considerable research interest in a number of epidemiological studies that suggest a possible association between ELF magnetic field exposure and cancer (see Chapter 17). As yet, only a few published laboratory studies, conducted in animals, bear directly on this question. In a preliminary report, Leung et al. (1988) observed an increase in the number of tumors per tumor-bearing animal after exposure to 60 Hz electric fields for extended periods (approximately 180 days). The exposed and sham-exposed animals were treated with a single dose of the potent mammary tumor initiator dimethylbenz(a)anthracene at 55 days of age.

REVIEW OF CELLULAR STUDIES

The effects of electric and magnetic fields on cellular (in vitro) systems have been studied extensively in several laboratories. Such studies have great advantages in that they employ large sample sizes and permit exquisite control of experimental variables. Because single processes can be evaluated, fundamental interactions and biological mechanisms are generally most easily derived in in vitro studies. The major disadvantages of cellular work are that use of integrated systems is minimal and that exposure relationships observed in cells may be far removed from those in the whole human body. The dosimetric relationship between exposure in cellular systems and in whole animals is unclear, and extrapolation of results from less complicated systems to humans is extremely uncertain.

Many specific parameters have been examined for their responsiveness to ELF fields. These include growth and metabolism; synthesis of

DNA, RNA, and protein; cell morphology and structure; and responsiveness of cells to various stimuli, such as antigens or mitogens. An overview of in vitro work is presented in this section with specific reference to ideas on how the ELF fields effect a response in cellular systems.

Cell Viability and Growth

Growth and metabolism. Experiments in which cultured Chinese hamster ovary (CHO) cells were exposed to 3.7 V/m showed no effects on cell survival, growth, or mutation rate (Frazier et al., 1987). However, cell-plating efficiency (reflecting a possible alteration in the cell membrane) was reduced in cells exposed to 60 Hz fields at strengths greater than 0.7 V/m. At the same field strength (0.7 V/m), after several months of exposure, slime mold showed frequency-dependent effects on mitotic rate, cell respiration, and protoplasmic streaming (Marron et al., 1975; Goodman et al., 1979). These effects were observed when electric and magnetic fields were used alone or in combination. Winters (1987) reported an increase in clonogenicity of colon tumor cells in soft agar when the cells were exposed to magnetic fields of 100 μT. He observed changes in the number of transferrin receptors on the cell surface and in the susceptibility of the cells to killing by natural killer cells. The validity of his data is lessened by some unaccounted-for difficulties in methodology (Ahlbom et al., 1987).

In other work, using normal mammalian cells in culture, Nordenson et al. (1984) in Sweden reported clastogenic effects in human lymphocytes exposed to 50 Hz fields. However, Winters (1987), Basu (1987), and Rodan (1987) found essentially no changes in several measures of cell integrity and function in normal cells exposed to electric, magnetic, or mixed fields.

Thus studies of a variety of models (Greenebaum et al., 1979) have given contradictory results. Although the weight of evidence suggests that growth and metabolism in cellular systems are not generally affected by exposure to electric or magnetic fields, effects on cell division, growth, and metabolism are occasionally seen at field strengths of tenths of a volt per meter or tenths of a millitesla in the medium. However, at much higher field strengths, in the range of 10 to 100 kV/m, electrically induced cell rotation and fusion are well established (Pohl, 1978).

Genetic effects. In experiments designed to determine whether ELF fields are capable of directly damaging cellular DNA, CHO cells were exposed to 60 Hz electric and magnetic fields (1 or 38 V/m and 0.1 or 2 mT). After exposure the cells were lysed and the DNA was analyzed for breaks or cross-links. No significant differences in either parameter were detected between exposed and sham-exposed cells (Reese et al., 1988a). Similar results were obtained in human lymphocytes (Cohen et al., 1986).

As expected from these results, changes in mutation frequencies were not observed, even with extended exposure times. Since investigators could find no evidence of direct DNA damage, an examination of DNA repair mechanisms for possible genetic effects was also conducted. No evidence of altered repair of induced DNA damage was observed in mammalian cells exposed to ELF electric and magnetic fields (Reese et al., 1988b).

In contrast to the lack of ELF field effects in DNA, some investigators have observed significant changes in RNA transcription when salivary glands from fruit flies were exposed to magnetic fields (Goodman et al., 1983; Goodman and Henderson, 1986). Both sinusoidal and pulsed fields were employed, and both produced a general pattern of enhanced transcriptive activity. A degree of chromosomal specificity was indicated from the data for various signal types (pulsed versus sine-wave magnetic fields) (Goodman et al., 1987). In contrast, data from mouse or homan cells did not show increases or decreases in RNA levels after exposure to 60 Hz magnetic fields (Parker and Winters, 1988).

Membrane Effects and Activity

Experimental findings suggest that the cell membrane is the principal site of interaction between ELF fields and the interior of living systems (Adey, 1975, 1980, 1981, 1987; Bawin et al., 1978; Sheppard and Adey, 1979). These include a 10% to 20% alteration in the calcium exchange from chick or cat brain tissues exposed to ELF electric fields; either amplitude-modulated radiofrequency (RF) carrier waves or ELF sinusoidal fields (Bawin et al., 1975; Bawin et al., 1978; Blackman et al., 1982). The calcium effect is "windowed" in frequency, with maximum effects occurring at 16 Hz modulation. In the case of direct ELF exposure, Blackman et al. (1985) reported several windows in fields of less than 100 V/m in air at 15 Hz and its harmonics up to 105 Hz. A similar narrow-amplitude window limits the range in field strength. Bawin et al. (1978) found a relationship between the observed effect and the ionic composition of the bathing medium.

In the case of the ELF modulation of an RF field, the magnitude of the effective ELF field (obtained by demodulation of the RF field envelope) that acts on the calcium-binding sites depends on an unknown efficiency for a demodulation process occurring at an unidentified site. If demodulation is complete, the effective ELF field would correspond to an ELF-only field in air on the order of 100 kV/m (Adey, 1981), although with use of the RF carrier there is no significant heating of tissue (Tenforde, 1980) and no known artifact (such as spark discharges).

A calcium efflux effect is also reported for in vivo studies on cats (Budinger and Lauterbur, 1984). Possible underlying biophysical mechanisms and a relationship to the electrical properties of the brain (EEG waves) are discussed by Grodsky (1976). However, the physiological implication of the calcium efflux phenomenon is unknown.

An investigation in which invertebrate neurons from the sea hare *Aplysia* were exposed in vitro to a low-frequency electric field (Wachtel, 1979) indicated a strong frequency dependence in response to extracellular currents that included synchronization with the applied field. The neuron was most sensitive at frequencies below 1 Hz, which is close to the natural firing rate of *Aplysia* neurons, and for a particular neuronal orientation with respect to the field. Other data were reported by Sheppard et al. (1980) concerning the ELF field exposure of *Aplysia* neurons, including transient changes in the firing rate and increased variability during exposure to an electric field of 0.25 V/m RMS. Episodic synchronization between the neuron and the applied field was reported at 1.4×10^{-4} A/cm^2.

In summary, the results of in vitro studies suggest that time-varying ELF electric fields may change the properties of cell membranes and modify cell function. Several explanations have been proposed, and it seems conceivable that several parallel mechanisms exist. However, no comprehensive and experimentally confirmed theory has been proposed. Some of the effects observed on cells and tissues in vitro can also be detected in vivo.

CONCLUSION

ELF fields (less than 300 Hz) are quantified in terms of the electric field strength E (volts per meter) and the magnetic field strength H (amperes per meter) or the magnetic flux density B (tesla). Natural environmental ELF fields are normally very low, but with widespread and increasing use of electrical energy, the potential for exposure has increased considerably. Exposure from man-made sources generally ranges up to 100 V/m and from 0.1 μT to 30 μT; the higher exposures occur for short time durations. The highest occupational exposures may be on the order of tens of kilovolts per meter and tens of milliteslas. Typically, however, occupational exposures are 10 to 100 times lower than these high levels.

ELF fields are used in a variety of therapeutic and diagnostic applications, including healing of nonunion bone fractures, promotion of nerve regeneration, and acceleration of wound healing. These applications involve partial-body exposures in the range of 1 to 30 mT. Exposures to time-varying electric and magnetic fields also result from medical use of magnetic resonance devices.

Whole-body exposure to ELF electric fields may involve effects related to stimulation of sensory receptors at the body surface (hair vibration, or possible direct neural stimulation) and effects within the body caused by the flow of current. Magnetic fields appear to interact predominantly by the induction of internal current flow.

Internal current flow is described in terms of current density in tissue J (amperes per meter squared). Ohm's law permits an equivalent expression of current density in terms of internal electric field strength E (volts per meter). It is not known whether J or E is the more useful and relevant physical quantity for an understanding of the mechanisms of biological effects. Internal current densities produced by exposure to external E or B fields at practical levels (up to approximately 100 kV/m and 1 mT) are far lower than the current densities produced by contact with electrical conductors that produce various electric shock effects.

Data on neuromuscular stimulation (including respiratory tetanus and cardiac fibrillation) indicate that current densities higher than about 0.1 A/m^2 can be dangerous. Current densities near 0.01 A/m^2, particularly with long-term exposures, may cause biological effects that are important to health. At lower levels a variety of biological effects may occur; however, the health implications of exposure at such levels are not clear.

The magnitude of the internal current density is in direct proportion to the frequency for sinusoidal external E and B fields. For pulsed or other waveforms the rate of change of the field is relevant. The duration of current flow is also important. It is practical to relate observed effects to internal current density and the inducing external fields. Accurate relationships of external field and internal current density are functions of frequency, orientation of the body in the field, body size and shape, and tissue composition. Thus, from these fundamentals of interactions, possible mechanisms can be proposed and defined in terms of external unperturbed E and B field strengths, frequencies, and durations.

Although considerable advances have been made in documenting exposure conditions and defining the interaction of these fields with living systems, future research should make a greater effort to take account of the often complex characteristics of exposure, such as temporal variations and spatial nonuniformity of induced currents and fields. It is important to determine which physical parameters best represent the interaction of ELF fields with biological systems. Dosimetric considerations are essential for extrapolating data from animal and in vitro studies to human exposure conditions.

Most biological data come from experimental work conducted at electric fields of 50 and 60 Hz. Fewer studies have been conducted at lower frequencies and at frequencies between 100 and 300 Hz. An overview of the literature suggests that exposure to ELF electric and magnetic fields definitely produces biological effects, although many indices of physiological status appear relatively unaffected by exposure. Many of the biological effects reported are subtle, and evidence suggests that, at least with short-term exposure, these fields have relatively low potential hazard to biological systems.

Areas associated with the nervous system have often showed the greatest effect, including altered neuronal excitability, neurochemical changes, altered hormone levels, and changes in behavioral responses. No studies clearly demonstrate deleterious effects of ELF electric or magnetic exposure on mammalian reproduction and development, but several suggest such effects.

Knowledge about the mechanisms underlying observed biological effects is incomplete and remains a major challenge of this area of research. Further investigation is particularly needed to determine the mechanisms of effects that display nonlinear responses to field strength and frequency. A large number of models have been proposed to explain the electrochemical, cellular, and biochemical changes that occur as a result of ELF electric and magnetic field exposure. Most of these suggested models involve specific events (such as transduction and amplification) at the cell membrane. The need to define basic mechanisms of interaction has been enhanced because of emerging information on possible field associations with immunity, cancer, cell-to-cell communication, differentiation, and repair processes.

In addition to such basic information, further study is needed on the influence of electric and magnetic fields in cellular and animal systems, with emphasis on testing proposed mechanisms in systems sensitive to these fields.

REFERENCES

ADEY, W.R. (1975). Evidence for cooperative mechanisms in the susceptibility of cerebral tissue to environmental and intrinsic electric fields. In: Schmitt, F.O., Schneider, D.M., and Crothers, D.M. (eds.). Functional linkage in biomolecular systems. New York, Raven Press, pp. 325-342.

ADEY, W.R. (1980). Frequency and power windowing in tissue interactions with weak electromagnetic fields. Proc. IEEE 68:119–125.

ADEY, W.R. (1981). Tissue interactions with non-ionizing electromagnetic fields. Physiol. Rev. 61:435–514.

ADEY, W.R. (1987). Biological models of electromagnetic field interactions with tissues: a review and synthesis of recent findings. In: Andersen, L.E., Weigel, R.J., and Kelman, B.J. (eds.). Interaction of biological systems with static and ELF electric and magnetic fields. Proceedings of the 23rd Annual Hanford Life Sciences Symposium. DOE Symposium Series CONF 841041, Springfield, Va., National Technical Information Service, pp. 237–248.

AHLBOM, A., ALBERT, E.N., FRASER-SMITH, A.C., et al. (1987). Biological effects of power line fields. Final Report for New York State Power Lines Project. Albany, N.Y., Wadsworth Center for Laboratories and Research.

ANDERSON, L.E., AND PHILLIPS, R.D. (1985). Biological effects of electric fields: an overview. In: (Grandolfo, M., Michaelson, S.M., and Rindi, A. (eds.). Biological effects and dosimetry of static and ELF electromagnetic fields. New York, Plenum Publishing Corp., pp. 345–378.

ASANOVA, T.P., AND RAKOV, A.I. (1966). The state of health of persons working in electric field of outdoor 400- and 500-kV switchyards. In: Hygiene of labor and professional diseases 5. Translated by G. Knickerbocker. 1975. IEEE Power Engineering Society, Special Publication 10. Piscataway, N.J.

BANKOSKE, J.W., MCKEE, G.W., AND GRAVES, H.B. (1976). Ecological influence of electric fields. Interim Report 2, EPRI Research Project 129, EPRI Report No. EX-178. Palo Alto, Calif., Electric Power Research Institute.

BASSETT, C.A.L. (1978). Pulsing electromagnetic fields: a new approach to surgical problems. In: Buchwald, H., and Varco, R.L., (eds.). Metabolic surgery. New York, Grune & Stratton, pp. 255–306.

BASSETT, C.A.L., MITCHELL, S.N., AND GASTON, S.R. (1982). Pulsing electromagnetic field treatment in ununited fractures and failed arthrodeses. J.A.M.A. 247:623–628.

BASSETT, C.A.L., PAWLUK, R.J., AND PILLA, A.A. (1974). Acceleration of fracture repair by electromagnetic fields: a surgically noninvasive method. Ann. N.Y. Acad. Sci. 238:242–262.

BASU, P.K. (1987). Biological effects of extremely low frequency electric and magnetic fields on the ocular tissues: an in vitro study. Final Report to the New York State Power Lines Project, Albany, N.Y., Wadsworth Center for Laboratories and Research.

BAUCHINGER, M., HAUF, R., SCHMID, E., AND DRESP, J. (1981). Analysis of structural chromosome changes and SCE after occupational long-term exposure to electric and magnetic fields from 380-kV systems. Radiat. Environ. Biopys. 19:235–238.

BAWIN, S.M., KACZMAREK, L.K., AND ADEY, W.R. (1975). Effects of modulated VHF fields on the central nervous system. Ann. N.Y. Acad. Sci. 247:74–80.

BAWIN, S.M., SHEPPARD, A.R., AND ADEY, W.R. (1978). Possible mechanisms of weak electromagnetic field coupling in brain tissue. Bioelectrochem. Bioenerg. 5:67–76.

BEISCHER, D.E., GRISSETT, J.D., AND MITCHELL, R.R. (1973). Exposure of man to magnetic fields alternating at extremely low frequency, USN Report No. NAMRL-1180. Pensacola, Fla., Naval Aerospace Medical Research Laboratory.

BERMAN, E., HOUSE, D.E., KOCH, W.E., et al. (1988). Effect of pulsed magnetic fields on early chick embryos. In: 10th Annual Meeting Abstracts, Bioelectromagnetics Society, June 19–23, Stamford, Conn. Gaithersburg, Md., Bioelectromagnetics Society, p. 72.

BLACKMAN, C.F., BENANE, S.G., KINNEY, L.S., JOINES, W.T., AND HOUSE, D.E. (1982). Effects of ELF fields on calcium ion efflux from brain tissue in vitro. Radiat. Res. 92:510–520.

BLACKMAN, C.F., BENANE, S.G., RABINOWITZ, J.R., HOUSE, D.E., AND JOINES, W.T., (1985). A role for the magnetic field in the radiation-induced efflux of calcium ions from brain tissue in vitro. Bioelectromagnetics 6:327–338.

BLANCHI, C., CEDRINI, L., CERIA, F., MEDA, E., AND RE, G. (1973). Exposure of mammalians to strong 50-Hz electric fields: effect on heart's and brain's electrical activity. *Arch. Fisiol. 70*:33–34.

BONNELL, J.A., BROADBENT, D.E., LEE, W.R., MALE, J.C., NORRIS, W.T., AND STOLLERY, B.T. (1985). Can induced 50 Hz body currents affect mental functions? Presented at International Conference on Electric and Magnetic Fields in Medicine and Biology, Dec. 4–5, 1985, London.

BUDINGER, T.F., AND LAUTERBUR, P.C., (1984). Nuclear magnetic resonance technology for medical studies. *Science 226*:288–298.

CABANES, J., AND GARY, C. (1981). La perception directe du champ electrique (Direct perception of the electric field). CIGRE Report No. 233–08, International Conference on Large High Tension Electric Systems. Paris, CIGRE.

CAIN, C.S., LUBEN, R.A., AND ADEY, W.R. (1987). Pulsed electromagnetic field effects on PTH stimulated cAMP accumulation and bone resorption in mouse calvariae. *In*: Anderson, L.E., Weigel, R.J., and Kelman, B.J. (eds.). Interaction of biological systems with static and ELF electric and magnetic fields, Proceedings of the 23rd Annual Hanford Life Sciences Symposium. DOE Symposium Series CONF 841041. Springfield, Va., National Technical Information Service, pp. 269–278.

CARTER, J. H., AND GRAVES, H.B. (1975). Effects of high intensity AC electric fields on the electroencephalogram and electrocardiogram of domestic chicks: literature review and experimental results. University Park, Pennsylvania State University.

CERRETELLI, P., AND MALAGUTI, C. (1976). Research carried on in Italy by ENEL on the effects of high voltage electric fields. *Rev. Gen. Electr.* (spec. iss.):65–74.

CERRETELLI, P., VEICSTEINAS, A., MARGONATO, V., et al. (1979). 1000-kV project: research on the biological effects of 50-Hz electric fields in Italy. *In*: Phillips, R.D., et al. (eds.). Biological effects of extremely-low-frequency electromagnetic fields, Proceedings of the 18th Annual Hanford Life Sciences Symposium, CONF-781016, Springfield, Va., National Technical Information Service, pp. 241–257.

CHERNOFF, N. (1985). Reproductive and developmental effects in mammalian and avian species from exposure to ELF fields. *In*: Biological and human health effects of extremely low frequency electromagnetic fields. Arlington, Va., American Institute of Biological Sciences, pp. 227–240.

COHEN, M.M., KUNSKA, A., ASTEMBORSKI, J.A., McCULLOCH, D., AND PASKEWITZ, D.A. (1986). Effect of low-level, 60-Hz electromagnetic fields on human lymphoid cells. I. Mitotic rate and chromosome breakage in human peripheral lymphocytes. *Bioelectromagnetics 7*:415–423.

CONTI, P., GIGANTE, G.E., CIFONE, M.G., et al. (1983). Reduced mitogenic stimulation of human lymphocytes by extremely low frequency electromagnetic fields. *FEBS Lett. 162*:156–160.

CREIM, J.A., LOVELY, R.H., KAUNE, W.T., MILLER, M.C., AND ANDERSON, L.E. (1985). 60-Hz magnetic fields: do rats avoid exposure? *In*: 7th Annual Meeting abstracts,

Bioelectromagnetics Society, June 16–20, 1985, San Francisco. Gaithersburg, Md., Bioelectromagnetics Society, p. 58.

DAVIS, H.P., MIZUMORI, S.J.Y., ALLEN, H., ROSENZWEIG, M.R., BENNETT, E.L., AND TENFORDE, T.S. (1984). Behavioral studies with mice exposed to DC and 60-Hz magnetic fields. *Bioelectromagnetics* 5:147–164.

DELGADO, J.M.R., LEAL, J., MONTEAGUDO, J.L., AND GRACIA, M.G. (1982). Embryological changes induced by weak, extremely low frequency electromagnetic fields. *J. Anat.* 134:533–551.

DE LORGE, J. (1974). A psychobiological study of rhesus monkeys exposed to extremely low-frequency low-intensity magnetic fields. USN Report NAMRL-1203. NTIS No. AD A000078, Springfield, Va., NTIS.

DENO, D.W. (1977). Currents induced in the human body by high voltage transmission line electric field—measurement and calculation of distribution and dose. *IEEE Trans. Power Appar. Syst.* 96:1517–1527.

DENO, D.W., AND ZAFFANELLA, L. (1982). Electrostatic effects of overhead transmission lines and stations. *In*: Transmission line reference book, 345 kV and above, 2nd ed., Palo Alto, Calif., Electric Power Research Institute, pp. 248–280.

DOWSE, H.B. (1982). The effects of phase shifts in a 10 Hz electric field cycle on locomotor activity rhythm of *Drosophila melanogaster*. *J. Interdiscip. Cycle Res.* 13:257–264.

DUFFY, P.M. AND EHRET, C.F. (1982). Effects of intermittent 60-Hz electric field exposure: circadian phase shifts, splitting, torpor, and arousal responses in mice. *In*: Abstracts, 4th Annual Scientific Session, Bioelectromagnetics Society, June 28–July 2, Los Angeles, Gaithersburg, Md., Bioelectromagnetic Society, p. 610.

DUMANSKY, Y.D., POPOVICH, V.M., AND KOZYARIN, I.P. (1977). Effects of low-frequency (50 Hz) electromagnetic field on functional state of the human body. *Gig. Sanit.* 12:32–35.

DUMANSKY, Y.D., POPOVICH, V.M., AND PROKHVATILO, Y.V. (1976). Hygiene assessment of an electromagnetic field generated by high-voltage power transmission lines. *Gig. Sanit.* 8:19–23.

FAM, W.Z. (1980). Long-term biological effects on very intense 60-Hz electric fields on mice. *IEEE Trans. Biomed. Eng.* 27:376–381.

FAM, W.Z. (1981). Biological effects of 60-Hz magnetic field on mice. *IEEE Trans. Magnet.* 17:1510–1513.

FISCHER, G., UDERMANN, H. AND KNAPP, E. (1978). Ubt das netzfrequente wechselfeld zentrale wirkungen aus? [Does a 50-cycle alternating field cause central nervous effects?] *Zentralbl. Bakteriol. Mikrobiol. Hyg. [B]* 166:381–385.

FITTON-JACKSON, S., AND BASSETT, C.A.L., (1980). The response of skeletal tissues to pulsed magnetic fields. *In*: Richards, R.J., and Rajan, K.T. (eds.). Tissue culture in medical research (II). New York, Pergamon Press, pp. 21–28.

FOTOPOULOS, S.S., GRAHAM, C., COOK, M.R., KOONTZ, E., GERKOVICH, M.M., AND COHEN, H.D. (1987). Effects of 60-Hz fields on human neuroregulatory immunologic, hematologic, and target organ activity. *In*: Anderson, L.E., Weigel, R.J., and Kelman, B.J. (eds.). Interaction of biological systems with static and ELF electric and magnetic fields. Proceedings of the 23rd Annual Hanford Life Sciences Symposium. DOE Symposium Series CONF 841041, Springfield, Va., National Technical Information Service, pp. 455–470.

FRAZIER, M.E., SAMUEL, J.E., AND KAUNE, W.T. (1987). Viabilities and mutation frequencies of CHO-K1 cells following exposure to 60-Hz electric fields. *In*: Anderson, L.E., Weigel, R.J., and Kelman, B.J. (eds.). Interaction of biological systems with static and ELF electric and magnetic fields. Proceedings of the 23rd Annual Hanford Life Sciences Symposium. DOE Symposium Series CONF 841041, Springfield, Va., National Technical Information Service, pp. 255–268.

FREE, M.J., KAUNE, W.T., PHILLIPS, R.D., AND CHENG, H.-C. (1981). Endocrinological effects of strong 60-Hz electric fields on rats. *Bioelectromagnetics* 2:105–121.

GANN, D.W. (1976). Biological effects of exposure to high voltage electric fields: final report. Electric Power Research Institute Report RP98–02. Palo Alto, Calif., Electric Power Research Institute.

GAVALAS, R.J., WALTER, D.O., HAMMER, J., AND ADEY, W.R. (1970). Effect of low-level, low-frequency electric fields on EEG and behavior in *Macaca nemestrina*. *Brain Res.* 18:491–501.

GAVALAS-MEDICI, R., AND DAY-MAGDALENO, S.R. (1976). Extremely low frequency, weak electric fields affect schedule-controlled behavior of monkeys. *Nature* 261:256–259.

GOODMAN, E.M., GREENEBAUM, B., AND MARRON, M.T. (1979). Bioeffects of extremely low frequency electromagnetic fields: variation with intensity, waveform, and individual or combined electric and magnetic fields. *Radiat. Res.* 78:485–501.

GOODMAN, R., ABBOTT, J., AND HENDERSON, A.S. (1987). Transcriptional patterns in the X chromosome of *Sciara coprophila* following exposure to magnetic fields. *Bioelectromagnetics* 8:1–7.

GOODMAN, R., BASSETT, C.A.L., AND HENDERSON, A. (1983). Pulsing electromagnetic fields induce cellular transcription. *Science* 220:1283–1285.

GOODMAN, R., AND HENDERSON, A. (1986). Sine waves induce cellular transcription. *Bioelectromagnetics* 7:23–30.

GRAHAM, C., COHEN, H.D., COOK, M.R., PHELPS, J., GERKOVICH, M. AND FOTOPOULOS, S.S. (1987). A double-blind evaluation of 60-Hz field effects on human performance, physiology, and subjective state. *In*: Anderson, L.E., Weigel, R.J., Kelman, B.J. (eds.). Interaction of biological systems with static and ELF electric and magnetic fields. Proceedings of the 23rd Annual Hanford Life Sciences Symposium. DOE Symposium Series CONF 841041, Springfield, Va., National Technical Information Service, pp. 471–486.

GRAVES, H.B. (ed.) (1985). Biological and human health effects of extremely low frequency electromagnetic fields. Arlington, Va., American Institute of Biological Sciences.

GRAVES, H.B., CARTER, J.H., JENKINS, T., KELLMEL, D., AND POZNANIAK, D.T. (1978a). Responses of domestic chicks to 60-Hz electrostatic fields. *In*: Mahlum, D.D., Sikov, M.R., Hackett, P.L., and Andrew, F.D. (eds). Developmental toxicology of energy-related pollutants. CONF. 771017, Springfield, Va., National Technical Information Service, pp. 317–329.

GRAVES, H.B., CARTER, J.H., KELLMEL, D., COOPER, L., POZNANIAK, D.T., AND BAN-KOSKE, J.W. (1978b). Perceptibility and electrophysiological response of small birds to intense 60-Hz electric fields. *IEEE Trans. Power Appar. Syst.* 97:1070–1073.

GRAVES, H.B., LONG, P.D., AND POZNANIAK, D.T. (1979). Biological effects of 60-Hz alternating-current fields: a Cheshire cat phenomenon? *In*: Phillips, R.D. (ed.). Biological effects of extremely-low-frequency electromagnetic fields. Proceedings of the 18th Annual Hanford Life Sciences Symposium. CONF-781016, Springfield, Va., NTIS, pp. 184–197.

GREENEBAUM, B., GOODMAN, E.M., AND MARRON, M.T. (1979). Effects of extremely low frequency fields on slime mold: studies of electric, magnetic, and combined fields, chromosome numbers, and other tests. *In*: Phillips, R.D., et al. (eds.). Biological effects of extremely-low-frequency electromagnetic fields. Proceedings of the 18th Annual Hanford Life Sciences Symposium, Oct. 16–18, Richland, Wash. CONF-781016, Springfield, Va., National Technical Information Service, pp. 117–131.

GRODSKY, I.T. (1976). Neuronal membrane: a physical synthesis. *Math. Biosci.* 28:191–219.

GROZA, P., CARMACIA, R., AND BUBUIANN, E. (1978). Blood and urinary catecholamine variations under the action of a high voltage electric field. *Physiologie* 15:139–144.

HACKMAN, R.M., AND GRAVES, H.B., (1981). Corticosterone levels in mice exposed to high intensity electric fields. *Behav. Neural Biol.* 32:201–213.

HANSSON, H.-A. (1981a). Lamellar bodies in Purkinje nerve cells experimentally induced by electric field. *Exp. Brain Res.* 216:187–191.

HANSSON, H.-A. (1981b). Purkinje nerve cell changes caused by electric fields: Ultrastructural studies on long term effects on rabbits. *Med. Biol.* 59:103–110.

HAUF, R. (1974). Effect of 50 Hz alternating fields on man. *Elektrotech. Z. B26*:318–320.

HAUF, R. (1976a). Einfluss elektromagnetisches Felder auf den Menschen. [Effect of electromagnetic fields on human beings.] *Elektrotech. Z. B28*:181–183.

HAUF, R. (1976b). Influence of 50 Hz alternating electric and magnetic fields on human beings. *Rev. Gen. Electr.* Spec. Iss. (July):31–49.

HAUF, R. (1982). Electric and magnetic fields at power frequencies with particular reference to 50 and 60 Hz. *In*: Seuss, M.J. (ed.). Nonionizing radiation protection, Vol. VIII. World Health Organization No. ISBN 92–890–1101–7. WHO Regional Publications, European Series No. 10. Copenhagen, WHO Regional Office for Europe, pp. 175–198.

HILTON, D.I., AND PHILLIPS, R.D. (1980). Cardiovascular response of rats exposed to 60-Hz electric fields. *Bioelectromagnetics* 1:55–64.

HJERESEN, D.L., KAUNE, W.T., DECKER, J.R., AND PHILLIPS, R.D. (1980). Effects of 60-Hz electric fields on avoidance behavior and activity of rats. *Bioelectromagnetics* 1:299–312.

HJERESEN, D.L., MILLER, M.C., KAUNE, W.T., AND PHILLIPS, R.D. (1982). A behavioral response of swine to 60-Hz electric field. *Bioelectromagnetics* 2:443–451.

JAFFE, R.A., LASZEWSKI, B.L., AND CARR, D.B. (1981). Chronic exposure to a 60-Hz electric field: effects on neuromuscular function in the rat. *Bioelectromagnetics* 2:277–239.

JAFFE, R.A., LASZEWSKI, B.L., CARR, D.B., AND PHILLIPS, R.D. (1980). Chronic exposure to a 60-Hz electric field: effects on synaptic transmission and the peripheral nerve function in the rat. *Bioelectromagnetics* 1:131–147.

JAFFE, R.A., LOPRESTI, C.A., CARR, D.B., AND PHILLIPS, R.D. (1983). Perinatal exposure to 60-Hz electric fields: effects on the development of the visual-evoked response in the rat. *Bioelectromagnetics* 4:327–339.

KAUNE, W.T. (1981). Power-frequency electric fields averaged over the body surfaces of grounded humans and animals. *Bioelectromagnetics* 2:403–406.

KAUNE, W.T. (1985). Coupling of living organisms to ELF electric and magnetic fields. *In*: Biological and human health effects of extremely low frequency electromagnetic fields. Arlington, Va., American Institute of Biological Sciences, pp. 25–60.

KAUNE, W.T., AND FORSYTHE, W.C. (1985). Current densities measured in human models exposed to 60-Hz electric fields. *Bioelectromagnetics* 6:13–32.

KAUNE, W.T., AND FORSYTHE, W.C. (1988). Current densities induced in swine and rat models by power-frequency electric fields. *Bioelectromagnetics* 9:1–24.

KAUNE, W.T., KISTLER, L.M., AND MILLER, M.C. (1987). Comparison of the coupling of grounded and ungrounded humans to vertical 60-Hz electric fields. *In*: Anderson, L.E., Weigel, R.J., and Kelman, B.J. (eds.). Interaction of biological systems with static and ELF electric and magnetic fields. Proceedings of the 23rd Annual Hanford Life Sciences Symposium. DOE Symposium Series CONF 841041, Springfield, Va., National Technical Information Service, pp. 185–196.

KAUNE, W.T., AND PHILLIPS, R.D. (1980). Comparison of the coupling of grounded humans, swine and rats to vertical, 60-Hz electric fields. *Bioelectromagnetics* 1:117–129.

KAUNE, W.T., AND PHILLIPS, R.D. (1985). Dosimetry for extremely low frequency electric fields. *In*: Grandolfo, M., Michaelson, S.M., and Rindi, A. (eds.). Biological effects and dosimetry of non-ionizing radiation: static and ELF electromagnetic fields. New York, Plenum Publishing Corp., pp. 145–165.

KAUNE, W.T., PHILLIPS, R.D., HJERESEN, D.L., RICHARDSON, R.L., AND BEAMER, J.L. (1978). A method for the exposure of minature swine to vertical 60-Hz electric fields. *IEEE Trans. Biomed. Eng.* 25:276–283.

KAVALIERS, M., OSSENKOPP, K.-P., AND HIRST, M. (1984). Magnetic fields abolish the enhanced nocturnal analgesic response to morphine in mice. *Physiol. Behav.* 32:261–264.

KNICKERBOCKER, G.G., KOUWENHOVEN, W., AND BARNES, H. (1967). Exposure of mice to strong AC electric field—an experimental study. *IEEE Trans. Power Appar. Syst.* 86:498–505.

KOROBKOVA, V.A., MOROZOV, Y.A., STOLAROV, M.S., AND YAKUB, Y.A. (1972). Influence of the electric field in 500- and 750-kV switchyards on maintenance staff and means for its protection. International Conference on Large High Tension Electric Systems. Paris, CIGRE.

KOZYARIN, I.P. (1981). Effects of low frequency (50-Hz) electric fields on animals of different ages. *Gig. Sanit. 8*:18–19.

KRUEGER, W.F., BRADLEY, J.W., GIAROLA, A.J., AND DARUVALLA, S.R. (1972). Influence of low-level electric and magnetic fields on the growth of young chickens. *Biomed. Sci. Instrum. 9*:183–186.

KUHNE, B. (1978). Einfluss electrischer felder auf lebende organismus. *Prakt. ARZT. 15.*

LEUNG, F.C., ROMMEREIM, D.N., STEVENS, R.G., WILSON, B.W., BUSCHBOM, R.L., AND ANDERSON, L.E. (1988). Effects of electric fields on rat mammary tumor development induced by 7,12-dimethylbenz(a)anthracene. *In:* 10th Annual Meeting abstracts, Bioelectromagnetics Society, June 19–23, 1988, Stamford, Conn., Gaithersburg, Md., Bioelectromagnetics Society, p. 2.

LOVELY, R.H. (1988). Recent studies in the behavioral toxicology of ELF electric and magnetic fields. *In:* O'Connor, M.E., and Lovely, R.H. (eds.). Electromagnetic fields and neurobehavioral function. New York, A.R. Liss, Inc., p. 2.

LOVSUND, P., OBERG, P.A., AND NILSSON, S.E.G. (1979). Influence on vision of extremely low frequency electromagnetic fields. *Acta Ophthalmol. 57*:812–821.

LOVSUND, P., OBERG, P.A., NILSSON, S.E.G., AND REUTER, T. (1980). Magnetophosphenes: a quantitative analysis of thresholds. *Med. Biol. Eng. Comput. 18*:326–334.

LUBEN, R.A., CAIN, C.D., CHEN, M.C.-Y., ROSEN, D.M., AND ADEY, W.R. (1982). Effects of electromagnetic stimuli on bone and bone cells in vitro: inhibition of responses to parathyroid hormone by low-energy low-frequency fields. *Proc. Natl. Acad. Sci. U.S.A. 79*:4180–4184.

LYLE, D.B., AYOTTE, R.D., SHEPPARD, A.R., AND ADEY, W.R. (1988). Suppression of T-lymphocyte cytotoxicity following exposure to 60-Hz sinusoidal electric fields. *Bioelectromagnetics 9*:303–313.

LYLE, D.B., SCHECHTER, P., ADEY, W.R., AND LUNDAK, R.L. (1983). Suppression of T-lymphocyte cytotoxicity following exposure to sinusoidally amplitude-modulated fields. *Bioelectromagnetics 4*:281–292.

MAHLUM, D.D., SIKOV, M.R., HACKETT, P.L., AND ANDREW, F.D. (1978). Developmental toxicology of energy-related pollutants. CONF 771017, Springfield, Va., NTIS.

MANTELL, B. (1975). Untersuchungen uber die Wirkung eines magnetischen Wechselfeldes 50 Hz auf den menschen. [Investigations into the effects on man of an alternating magnetic field at 50 Hz.] Ph.D. Dissertation, Freiburg University, Freiburg, Federal Republic of Germany.

MARINO, A.A., AND BECKER, R.O. (1977). Biological effects of extremely low-frequency electric and magnetic fields: a review. *Physiol. Chem. Phys. 9*:131–147.

MARINO, A.A., BECKER, R.O., AND ULLRICH, B. (1976). The effects of continuous exposure to low frequency electric fields on three generations of mice: a pilot study. *Experientia 32*:565–566.

MARINO, A.A., BERGER, T.J., AUSTIN, B.P., BECKER, R.O., AND HART, F.X. (1977). In vivo bioelectrochemical changes associated with exposure to extremely low frequency electric fields. *Physiol. Chem. Phys. 9*:433–441.

MARINO, A.A., CULLEN, J.M., REICHMANIS, M., AND BECKER, R.O. (1979). Fracture healing in rats exposed to extremely low-frequency electric fields. *Clin. Orthop.* *145*:239–244.

MARINO, A.A., REICHMANIS, M., BECKER, R.O., ULLRICH, B., AND CULLEN, J.M. (1980). Power frequency electric field induces biological changes in successive generations of mice. *Experientia 36*:309–311.

MARRON, M.T., GOODMAN, E.M., AND GREENEBAUM, B. (1975). Mitotic delay in the slime mold *Physarum polycephalum* induced by low intensity 60- and 75-Hz electromagnetic fields. *Nature 254*:66–67.

MATHEWSON, N.S., OOSTA, G.M., LEVIN, S.G., DIAMOND, S.S., AND EKSTROM, M.E. (1977). Extremely low frequency (ELF) vertical electric field exposure of rats: a search for growth, food consumption and blood metabolite alterations. Armed Forces Radiobiology Research Institute, Defense Nuclear Agency, Bethesda, Md., ADA 035954, Springfield, Va., NTIS.

McCLANAHAN, B.J., AND PHILLIPS, R.D. (1983). The influence of electric field exposure on bone growth and fracture repair in rats. *Bioelectromagnetics 4*:11–20.

MICHAELSON, S.M. (1979). Analysis of studies related to biologic effects and health implications of exposure to power frequencies. *Environ. Prof. 1*:217–232.

MITTLER, S. (1972). Low frequency electromagnetic radiation and genetic abberrations, Final Report, Northern Illinois University, AD-749959, Springfield, Va., NTIS.

MIZUSHIMA, Y., AKAOKA, I., AND NISHIDA, Y. (1975). Effects of magnetic field on inflammation. *Experientia 21*:1411–1412.

MOOS, W.S. (1964). A preliminary report on the effects of electric fields on mice. *Aerospace Med. 35*:374–377.

MORRIS, J.E., AND PHILLIPS, R.D. (1982). Effects of 60-Hz electric fields on specific humoral and cellular components of the immune system. *Bioelectromagnetics 3*:341–348.

MORRIS, J.E., AND PHILLIPS, R.D. (1983). (Erratum) Effects of 60-Hz electric fields on specific humoral and cellular components of the immune system. *Bioelectromagnetics 4*:294.

MORRIS, J.E., AND RAGAN, H.A. (1979). Immunological studies with 60-Hz electric fields. *In*: Phillips, R.D., et al. (eds.). Biological effects of extremely-low-frequency electromagnetic fields. Proceedings of the 18th Annual Hanford Life Sciences Symposium. CONF 781016, National Technical Information Service, Springfield, Va.

MOSE, J.R. (1978). Problems of housing quality. *Zentralbl. Bakteriol. Mikrobiol.* [B] *166*:292–304.

(1977). National Academy of Sciences. Biologic effects of electric and magnetic fields associated with proposed Project Seafarer, report of the Committee on Biosphere Effects of Extremely-Low-Frequency Radiation. Washington D.C., National Research Council.

NORDENSON, I., HANSSON MILD, K., NORDSTROM, S., SWEINS, A., AND BIRKE, E. (1984). Clastogenic effects in human lymphocytes of power frequency electric fields: in vivo and in vitro studies. *Radiat. Environ. Biophys. 23*:191–201.

NORTON, L.A. (1982). Effects of pulsed electromagnetic field on a mixed chondroblastic tissue culture. *Clin. Orthop. 167*:280–290.

ODINTSOV, Y.N. (1965). The effect of a magnetic field on the natural resistance of white mice to *Listeria* infection. *Tomsk Voprosy Epidemiol. Mikrobiol. Immunol. 16*:234–238.

OLCESE, J., REUSS, S., AND VOLLRATH L. (1985). Evidence for the involvement of the visual system in mediating magnetic field effects on pineal melatonin synthesis in the rat. *Brain Res. 333*:382–384.

OSSENKOPP, K.-P., KOLTEK, W.T., AND PERSINGER, M.A. (1972). Prenatal exposure to an extremely low frequency-low intensity rotating magnetic field and increases in thyroid and testicle weight in rat. *Dev. Psychobiol. 5*:275–285.

PAFKOVA, H. (1985). Possible embryotropic effect of the electric and magnetic component of the field of industrial frequency. *Pracov. Lek. 37*:153–158.

PARKER, J.E., AND WINTERS, W.D. (1988). Expression of gene specific RNA in cultured cells exposed to cyclic 60 Hz magnetic fields. *In*: 10th Annual Meeting abstracts, June 19–23, 1988, Stamford, Conn., Gaithersburg, Md., Bioelectromagnetics Society, p. 27.

PERSINGER, M.A. (1969). Open-field behavior in rats exposed prenatally to a low intensity-low frequency, rotating magnetic field. *Dev. Psychobiol. 2*:168–171.

PERSINGER, M.A., AND FOSTER IV, W.S. (1970). ELF rotating magnetic fields: prenatal exposures and adult behavior. *Arch. Meteorol. Geophys. Biol. Ser. B 18*:363–369.

PERSINGER, M.A., AND PEAR, J.J. (1972). Prenatal exposure to an ELF-rotating magnetic field and subsequent increase in conditioned suppression. *Dev. Psychobiol. 5*:269–274.

PHILLIPS, R.D., CHANDON, J.H., FREE, M.J., et al. (1978). Biological effects of 60-Hz electric fields on small laboratory animals. Annual Report, DOE Report No. HCP/T1830-3. Washington, D.C., Department of Energy.

PHILLIPS, R.D., AND KAUNE, W.T. (1977). Biological effects of static and low-frequency electromagnetic fields: an overview of United States literature. EPRI Special Report No. EA-490-SR. Palo Alto, Calif., Electric Power Research Institute.

POHL, H.A. (1978). Dielectrophoresis: the behaviour of matter in non-uniform electric fields. London, Cambridge University Press.

POLK, C., AND POSTOW, E. (1986). Handbook of biological effects of electromagnetic fields. Boca Raton, Fla., CRC Press.

PORTET, R.T., AND CABANES, J. (1988). Development of young rats and rabbits exposed to a strong electric field. *Bioelectromagnetics 9*:95–104.

QUINLAN, W.J., PETRONDAS, D., LEBDA, N., PETTIT, S., AND MICHAELSON, S.M. (1985). Neuroendocrine parameters in the rat exposed to 60-Hz electric fields. *Bioelectromagnetics 6*:381–389.

RAGAN, H.A., BUSCHBOM, R.L., PIPES, M.J., PHILLIPS, R.D., AND KAUNE, W.T. (1983). Hematologic and serum chemistry studies in rats and mice exposed to 60-Hz electric fields. *Bioelectromagnetics 4*:79–90.

RAGAN, H.A., PIPES, M.J., KAUNE, W.T., AND PHILLIPS, R.D. (1979). Clinical pathologic evaluations in rats and mice chronically exposed to 60-Hz electric fields. *In*: Phillips, R.D., et al. (eds.). Biological effects of extremely-low-frequency electromagnetic fields. Proceedings of the 18th Annual Hanford Life Sciences Symposium. CONF-781016, Springfield, Va., National Technical Information Service, pp. 297–325.

REED, T.J., AND GRAVES, H.B. (1984). Effects of 60-Hz electric fields on embryo and chick development, growth, and behavior, Vol. 1. Final Report, EPRI Project 1064–1. Palo Alto, Calif., Electric Power Research Institute.

REESE, J.A., JOSTES, R.F. AND FRAZIER, M.E. (1988a). Exposure of mammalian cells to 60-Hz magnetic or electric fields: analysis for DNA single-strand breaks. *Bioelectromagnetics* 9:237–248.

REESE, J.A., JOSTES, R.F., MORRIS, J.E., AND FRAZIER, M.E. (1988b). Single-strand break repair in human lymphocytes exposed to 60-Hz AC electromagnetic fields. *In*: 10th Annual Meeting abstracts, June 19–23, 1988, Stamford, Conn., Gaithersburg, Md., Bioelectromagnetics Society, p. 39.

REUSS, S., AND OLCESE, J. (1986). Magnetic field effects on the rat pineal gland: role of retinal activation by light. *Neurosci. Lett.* 64:97–101.

RODAN, G.A. (1987). Effect of 60 Hz electric and magnetic fields on neural and skeletal cells in culture. Final report to New York State Power Lines Project, Albany, N.Y., Wadsworth Center for Laboratories and Research.

ROGERS, W.R., FELDSTONE, C.S., GIBSON, E.G., POLONIS, J.J., SMITH, H.D., AND CORY, W.E. (1987). Effects of high-intensity, 60-Hz electric fields on operant and social behavior of nonhuman primates. *In*: Anderson, L.E., Weigel, R.J., and Kelman, B.J. (eds.). Interaction of biological systems with static and ELF electric and magnetic fields. Proceedings of the 23rd Annual Hanford Life Sciences Symposium. DOE Symposium Series, CONF 841041, Springfield, Va., National Technical Information Service, pp. 365–378.

ROMMEREIM, D.N., KAUNE, W.T., BUSCHBOM, R.L., PHILLIPS, R.D., AND SIKOV, M.R. (1987). Reproduction and development in rats chronologically exposed to 60-Hz electric fields. *Bioelectromagnetics* 8:243–258.

ROMMEREIM, D.N., ROMMEREIM, R.L., ANDERSON, L.E., AND SIKOV, M.R. (1988). Reproductive and teratologic evaluation in rats chronically exposed at multiple strengths of 60-Hz electric fields. *In*: 10th Annual Meeting abstracts, June 19–23, 1988, Stamford, Conn., Gaithersburg, Md., Bioelectromagnetics Society, p. 37.

ROSENBERG, R.S., DUFFY, P.H., SACHER, G.A., AND EHRET, C.F. (1983). Relationship between field strength and arousal response in mice exposed to 60-Hz electric fields. *Bioelectromagnetics* 4:181–191.

SANDER, R., BRINKMANN, J., AND KUHNE, B. (1982). Laboratory studies on animals and human beings exposed to 50-Hz electric and magnetic fields. *In*: International Conference on Large High Voltage Electrical Systems (abstracts), No. 36–01. Paris, CIGRE.

SEDEL, L., CHRISTEL, P., DURIEZ, J., et al. (1981). Resultats de la stimulation par champ electromagnetique de la consolidation des pseudarthroses. *Rev. Chir. Orthop.* 67:11–23.

SEMM, P. (1983). Neurobiological investigations on the magnetic sensitivity of the pineal gland in rodents and pigeons. *Comp. Biochem. Physiol.* 76A:683–689.

SEUSS, M. (ed.). (1984). Environmental health criteria 35: extremely low frequency (ELF) fields. Geneva, World Health Organization.

SHEPPARD, A.R., AND ADEY, W.R. (1979). The role of cell surface polarization in biological effects of extremely low frequency fields. *In*: Phillips, R.D., et al. (eds.). Biological effects of extremely-low-frequency electromagnetic fields. Proceedings of the 18th Annual Hanford Life Sciences Symposium. NTIS CONF-781016, Springfield, Va., National Technical Information Service, pp. 147–158.

SHEPPARD, A.R., AND EISENBUD, M. (1977). Biologic effects of electric and magnetic fields of extremely low frequency. New York, New York University Press.

SHEPPARD, A.R., FRENCH, E., AND ADEY, W.R. (1980). ELF electric fields alter neuronal excitability in *Aplysia* neurons. *Bioelectromagnetics* 1:227.

SIKOV, M.R. (1985). Reproductive and developmental alterations associated with exposure of mammals to ELF (1–300 Hz) electromagnetic fields. *In*: Assessments and viewpoints on the biological and human health effects of extremely low frequency (ELF) electromagnetic fields. Washington D.C., American Institute of Biological Sciences, pp. 295–311.

SIKOV, M.R., MONTGOMERY, L.D., SMITH, L.G., AND PHILLIPS, R.D. (1984). Studies on prenatal and postnatal development in rats exposed to 60-Hz electric fields. *Bioelectromagnetics* 5:101–112.

SIKOV, M.R., ROMMEREIM, D.N., BEAMER, J.L., BUSCHBOM, R.L., KAUNE, W.T., AND PHILLIPS, R.D. (1987). Developmental studies of Hanford miniature swine exposed to 60-Hz electric fields. *Bioelectromagnetics* 8:229–242.

SILNEY, J. (1979). Effects of electric fields on the human organism. Institut zur Enforschung Electrischer Unfalle, Cologne, Medizinisch - Technischer Berichte, p. 39.

SILNEY, J. (1981). Influence of low-frequency magnetic field on the organism. *Proc. EMG*, Zurich, pp. 175–180, Proceed. 4th Symposium on Electromagnetic Compatibility, Mar. 10–12, 1981.

SILNEY, J. (1985). The influence thresholds of the time-varying magnetic field in the human organism. *In*: Bernhardt, J. (ed.). Proceedings of the Symposium on Biological Effects of Static and ELF Magnetic Fields. Neuherberg, May 13–15, 1985, BGA-Schriftenreibe, Munchen, MMV Medizin Verlag.

SMITH, R.F., AND JUSTESEN, D.R. (1977). Effects of a 60-Hz magnetic field on activity levels of mice. *Radio Sci.* 12:279–285.

STERN, S., LATIES, V.G., STANCAMPIANO, C.V., COX, C., AND DE LORGE, J.O. (1983). Behavioral detection of 60-Hz electric fields by rats. *Bioelectromagnetics* 4:215–247.

STOLLERY, B.T. (1987). Human exposure to 50 Hz electric currents. *In*: Anderson, L.E., Weigel, R.J., and Kelman, B.J. (eds.). Interaction of biological systems with static and ELF electric and magnetic fields. Proceedings of the 23rd Annual Hanford Life Sciences Symposium. DOE Symposium, Series CONF 841041, Springfield, Va., National Technical Information Service, pp. 445–454.

SULZMAN, F.M., AND MURRISH, D.E. (1987). Effects of electromagnetic fields on primate circadian rhythms. Report to the New York State Power Lines Project, Albany, N.Y., Wadsworth Center for Laboratories and Research.

SZUBA, M., AND NOSOL, B. (1985). Duration of conscious reaction in those exposed to electric field of 50 Hz frequency. *Med. Pracy* 36:21–26.

TAKASHIMA, S., ONARAL, B., AND SCHWAN, H.P. (1979). Effects of modulated RF energy on the EEG of mammalian brains: effects of acute and chronic irradiations. *Radiat. Environ. Biophys.* 16:15–27.

TARAKHOVSKY, M.L., SAMBROSKAYA, Y.P., MEDVEDEV, B.M., ZADEROZHNAYA, T.D., OKHRONCHUK, B.V., AND LIKHTENSHTEIN, E.M. (1971). Effects of constant and variable magnetic fields on some indices of physiological function and metabolic processes in albino rats. *Fiziol. Zh. RSR–17*:452–459. (English translation *JPRS 62865*:37–46.)

TENFORDE, T.S. (1980). Thermal aspects of electromagnetic field interactions with bound calcium ions at the nerve cell surface. *J. Theoret. Biol.* 83:517–521.

TENFORDE, T.S. (1985). Biological effects of ELF magnetic fields. *In*: Biological and human health effects of extremely low frequency electromagnetic fields. Arlington, Va., American Institute of Biological Sciences, pp. 79–128.

TENFORDE, T.S. (1986). Interaction of time-varying ELF magnetic fields with living matter. *In*: Polk, C., and Postow, E. (eds.). Handbook of biological effects of electromagnetic fields. Boca Raton, Fla., CRC Press, pp. 197–228.

TENFORDE, T.S., AND BUDINGER, T.F. (1985). Biological effects and physical safety aspects of NMR imaging and in vivo spectroscopy. *In*: Thomas, S.R. (ed.). NMR in medicine: instrumentation and clinical applications. New York, American Association of Physicists in Medicine.

TENFORDE, T.S., AND KAUNE, W.T. (1987). Interaction of extremely low frequency electric and magnetic fields with humans. *Health Phys.* 53:585–606.

UBEDA, A., LEAL, J., TRILLO, M.A., JIMENEZ, M.A., AND DELGADO, J.M.R. (1983). Pulse shape of magnetic field influences chick embryogenesis. *J. Anat.* 137:513–536.

VASQUEZ, B.J., ANDERSON, L.E., LOWERY, C.I., AND ADEY, W.R. (1988). Diurnal patterns in brain biogenic amines of rats exposed to 60-Hz electric fields. *Bioelectromagnetics* 9:229–236.

VEICSTEINAS, A., MARGONATO, V., CONTI, R., AND CERRETELLI, P. (1987). Effect of 50-Hz electric field exposure on growth rate of chicks. *In*: Anderson, L.E., Weigel, R.J., and Kelman, B.J. (eds.). Interaction of biological systems with static and ELF electric and magnetic fields. Proceedings of the 23rd Annual Hanford Life Sciences Symposium. DOE Symposium Series CONF 841041, Springfield, Va., National Technical Information Service, pp. 341–346.

WACHTEL, H. (1979). Firing pattern changes and transmembrane currents produced by extremely low frequency fields in pacemaker neurons. *In*: Phillips, R.D., et al. (eds.). Biological effects of extremely-low-frequency electromagnetic fields. Proceedings of the 18th Annual Hanford Life Sciences Symposium. CONF-781016, Springfield, Va., National Technical Information Service, pp. 132–146.

WEIGEL, R.J., JAFFE, R.A., LUNDSTROM, D.L., FORSYTHE, W.C., AND ANDERSON, L.E.

(1987). Stimulation of cutaneous mechanoreceptors by 60-Hz electric fields. *Bioelectromagnetics* 8:337–350.

WEIGEL, R.J., AND LUNDSTROM, D.L. (1987). Effect of relative humidity on the movement of rat vibrissae in a 60-Hz electric field. *Bioelectromagnetics* 8:107–110.

WELKER, H.A., SEMM, P., WILLIG, R.P., COMMENTZ, J.C., WILTSCHKO, W., AND VOLL-RATH, L. (1983). Effects of an artificial magnetic field on serotonin *N*-acetyltransferase activity and melatonin content of the rat pineal. *Exp. Brain Res.* 50:426–432.

WEVER, R. (1971). Influence of electric fields on some parameters of circadian rhythms in man. *In*: Menaber, M. (ed.). Biochronometry, Washington, D.C., National Academy of Sciences, pp. 117–132.

WILSON, B.W., ANDERSON, L.E., HILTON, D.I., AND PHILLIPS, R.D. (1981). Chronic exposure to 60-Hz electric fields: effects on pineal function in the rat. *Bioelectromagnetics* 2:371–380.

WILSON, B.W., ANDERSON, L.E., HILTON, D.I., AND PHILLIPS, R.D. (1983). (Erratum) Chronic exposure to 60-Hz electric fields: effects on pineal function in the rat. *Bioelectromagnetics* 4:293.

WILSON, B.W., CHESS, E.K., AND ANDERSON, L.E. (1986). 60-Hz electric field effects on pineal melatonin rhythms: time course for onset and recovery. *Bioelectromagnetics* 7:239–242.

WINTERS, W.D. (1987). Biological functions of immunologically reactive human and canine cells influenced by in vitro exposure to 60-Hz electric and magnetic fields. Report to New York State Power Lines Project, Albany, N.Y., Wadsworth Center for Laboratories and Research.

WOLPAW, J.R., SEEGAL, R.F., DOWMAN, R.I., AND SATYA-MURTI, S. (1987). Chronic effects of 60 Hz electric and magnetic fields on primate central nervous system function. Final Report to the New York State Power Lines Project, Albany, N.Y., Wadsworth Center for Laboratories and Research.

10

Biological Effects of Radiofrequency Electromagnetic Fields

STEPHEN F. CLEARY

Assessment of health hazards and beneficial applications of radiofrequency (RF) electromagnetic (EM) radiation must be based on a detailed and thorough understanding of biological effects. To the uninitiated reader it may come as a surprise that, although this area has been actively researched for more than three decades, many basic issues regarding the biological effects of RF radiation remain unresolved. Historical and fundamental explanations for this situation are the subject of this chapter. Chapters 11 to 16 cover specific topics related to the biological effects of RF radiation. These topics either represent physiologically relevant effects that have been induced in mammalian systems by RF exposure or illustrate characteristic aspects of the interaction of RF fields with such systems.

HISTORICAL PERSPECTIVE

Guided by the experimental observations of Faraday, Oersted, and Ampere, Maxwell theoretically described EM radiation in the middle of the nineteenth century. Toward the end of that century Hertz experimentally verified Maxwell's predictions by generating and detecting radiative EM fields. Implications of these findings were clear to researchers such as Marconi and deForest, who engineered the development of wireless communication by RF radiation around the turn of the century. Since then, RF environmental intensities in the United States and other technologically oriented societies have increased exponentially because of an increasing number of RF generators and applications and higher-power outputs. As a consequence of the development of radar during World War II, and subsequent military and civilian deployment of radar devices, intensities in the microwave segment of the RF spectrum (30 MHz to 300 GHz) have been added to the RF background. At various times during the development of RF applications, the potential for adverse effects of exposure in humans was recognized by physicists and engineers, primarily as a result of occupational overexposure. However, the true nature of the exposure problem was not fully appreciated until relatively recently.

During the early era of the development of RF communications systems, D'Arsonval, a physician, used low-frequency and RF electrical currents to investigate the electrophysiological properties of nerves and muscles. D'Arsonval detected distinct differences in the effects of low- and high-frequency EM fields on tissue preparations, one of which was that RF fields induced tissue heating. Believing that heating was thera- peutically beneficial, D'Arsonval and others applied RF fields to the treat- ment of various human ailments, including cancer (Rowbottom and Suss- kind, 1984). Diathermy (the general term used to describe tissue heating) has been the principal therapeutic application of RF and microwave ra- diation (see Chapter 18 and Cleary, 1983). Diagnostic medical applica- tions of RF radiation are being investigated, as discussed by Iskander (Chapter 19).

Although most researchers studying the medical applications and biological effects of RF radiation had limited contact with physicists and engineers who were developing communications and radar systems, work- ers in both fields were aware of adverse biological effects. Since in both instances exposures were generally of short duration and at intensities sufficient to cause significant tissue heating, the hypothesis emerged that biological effects of RF were principally indirect or nonspecific ther- mal effects. Theoretical support for this hypothesis was provided by appli- cation of thermodynamics and Debye dielectric dispersion theory to the interaction of RF radiation with biological systems (Schwan, 1957). The primary mechanisms of interaction of RF radiation with biological systems were thought to be induced dipolar orientation and ionic conduction, relaxation phenomena that were not associated with resonant absorption, the occurrence of which could result in frequency-specific RF effects.

Cleary (1973) arrived at a similar conclusion by comparing activation energies for various biochemical events, such as hydrogen bond breakage or ionization, with the quantized energy of 2.45 GHz microwave radiation, which is on the order of 10^{-4} eV. Photon energies of microwave and lower-frequency radiation were so small compared with biochemical acti- vation energies that it was difficult to understand how low-intensity or nonthermal RF intensities could affect living systems. Thus, on the basis of available information about the structure, function, and energetics of biological systems, there were no mechanisms to explain how RF radiation could alter such systems, other than by thermally induced alterations. It was assumed that by limiting the intensity (or power density) of incident RF fields to levels that did not induce significant tissue heating (1° C or less), adverse effects would be averted. This reasoning, together with data on the effects of RF radiation on experimental animals, resulted in the recommendation of a maximum safe exposure intensity of 10 mW/ cm^2, independent of RF frequency (Schwan and Li, 1956; U.S.A. Standards Institute, 1966). Although this exposure standard did not depend on radiation frequency per se, or on modulation of the RF field, some researchers were aware that such factors might be important in relating RF exposure to effects in biological systems (see, for example, Tomberg, 1961 and Anne et al., 1961).

Experimental evidence supporting thermal damage as the mechanism responsible for RF radiation damage of experimental animals and humans was provided by studies of acute lethality and cataract formation. A number of studies conclusively demonstrated that an absorbed RF dose of about 30 J/gm in experimental animals resulted in body core temperature elevations on the order of 5° to 6° C, followed by rapid death. Postmortem pathologic examination indicated hyperpyrexia as the cause of death. Although a cause-and-effect relationship between acute RF exposure, tissue heating, and death was demonstrated, detailed comparison of the exposure conditions involved in these experiments suggested that factors other than RF intensity or exposure duration were involved (Cleary, 1983a).

Acute exposure studies involving experimental animals, as well as reported occupational overexposures of microwave workers, provided examples of RF-induced thermal damage to lens tissue. Indeed, cataracts are the best-documented type of irreversible RF damage in humans. Not surprisingly, microwave-caused cataract formation was the subject of numerous investigations in early research on the biological effects of RF radiation. Typically cataract induction was studied in animals such as New Zealand white rabbits, with exposure techniques generally involving near-zone RF fields that resulted in localized exposure of ocular regions. (Carpenter et al., 1974; Appleton et al., 1975; Guy et al., 1975). At intensities of 100 to 300 mW/cm^2, 2.45 GHz microwave radiation caused detectable lens opacification in rabbits as soon as 24 hours after exposure. Experimental studies such as these, as well as theoretical studies, indicated that acute microwave-induced heating of the mammalian lens to 43° C or higher results in cataracts (Cleary, 1980).

As in the acute lethality studies, factors other than RF-induced heating per se appeared to be involved in cataract induction. For example, when the effects of ocular heating by other thermal modalities were compared with RF heating, heating rates and thermal gradients were found to have a marked effect on cataract formation (Carpenter et al., 1977). Comparison of the sensitivity of different species of experimental animals to microwave cataractogenesis revealed significant differences that were attributed to anatomical configuration (Kramer et al., 1978), as well as radiation frequency (Hagan and Carpenter, 1975). Furthermore, studies involving exposure of rabbits to repeated subcataractogenic microwave doses suggested the cumulation of lens damage at induced tissue temperatures lower than those involved in single-exposure cataractogenesis (Carpenter et al., 1974). Data inconsistent with, and in some instances contradictory to, the thermal hypothesis of RF bioeffects emerged from a number of other studies conducted in the 1960s and 1970s, principally by scientists in the Soviet Union and other Eastern European nations (Letavet and Gordon, 1962). Characteristically such studies involved effects of RF radiation on the central nervous, immunological, or endocrine systems of experimental animals (or in some instances occupationally exposed humans) with long-term exposure to low intensities of RF radiation (Cleary, 1977). The weight of accumulated evidence suggested the need for reassessing the biological effects of RF radiation, especially in view of the increasing potential for human exposure owing to elevations in occupational and environmental RF intensities and the introduction of microwave ovens into homes across the nation.

REASSESSMENT: THE SPECIFIC ABSORPTION RATE HYPOTHESIS

Until the 1970s most U.S. data pertaining to the effects of RF radiation on experimental animals suggested the involvement of tissue heating. Typically such studies were conducted with microwave frquencies at relatively high intensities (on the order of 10 mW/cm^2) and exposure was limited to a few hours. Data analysis revealed an expected dependence of the outcome on the biological end point, but in addition a pattern emerged that indicated dependence on physical exposure parameters such as the relationship between the size of the animal and the wavelength of the radiation, as well as the orientation to the RF field vectors. Thus attention was focused on physical aspects of coupling of RF fields to experimental animals and humans, a concept previously considered by Anne et al. (1961), who investigated field coupling (relative absorption cross section) to spherical dielectric models theoretically and to spherical tissue models experimentally.

Anne's and subsequent studies provided theoretical and experimental evidence that the amount of coupling to RF fields and the internal distribution of absorbed energy were functions of the size, shape, orientation, and dielectric properties (for example, dielectric constant and conductivity) of human or other animal bodies. Gandhi (1975), for example, applied antenna theory to an animal body, modeled as a lossy dielectric, to show that the amount of RF absorption is a function of wavelength. Because of the body's antenna-like properties, the absorption efficiency is at a maximum for a 1.75 m tall human weighing 70 kg at a wavelength of 4.4 m (frequency 68 MHz) (Gandhi, 1975). In contrast, the so-called whole-body resonant frequency for a 5.4 cm long, 15 gm mouse is about 2.5 GHz. The resonant frequency, as well as the efficiency of field coupling, has been shown both theoretically and experimentally to depend on the orientation of the long axis of a body to the polarity of the RF field. In general, maximum coupling occurs when the long axis is parallel to the RF electric field vector (E).

Consideration of frequency- and polarity-dependent RF field coupling to animal and human bodies provided a ready explanation for previously unexplained variations in biological responses and indicated the need for a parameter other than incident field intensity, or power density, to characterize the biological effects of RF radiation. Hence, the concept of a mass-averaged rate of RF energy absorption in a body, referred to as the specific absorption rate (SAR), was introduced to provide a means of dose, or dose rate, normalization.

At a resonant frequency of 77 MHz, a homogeneous prolate spheroidal model of a human would have an SAR of 0.022 W/kg for each incident watt per square meter, whereas a model of a mouse at its resonant frequency of 2.5 GHz would have an SAR of 0.12 W/kg for each watt per square meter (Durney et al., 1978). Under whole-body resonance conditions, therefore, RF field coupling to a mouse is about 5 times more efficient than to a human. The magnitude of the difference in SAR for resonant field coupling between different mammalian species is additional evidence of the complex nature of RF absorption. The difference is due in part to frequency-dependent differences in tissue conductivity, which accounts for approximately twice as much RF energy being absorbed at 2.5 GHz as at 77 MHz. The remaining difference in SAR, approximately 300%, must therefore be due to such factors as body shape, which indicates the complexities involved in interspecies extrapolation of RF bioeffects data. A further indication of species-dependent differences in SAR is provided by comparing the SARs of two species that differ significantly in size and shape. At 2.5 GHz, for instance, the SAR of a mouse (0.12 W/kg for each watt per square meter) is approximately 30 times greater than that of a human (0.004 W/kg for each watt per square meter).

Tissue dose normalization in terms of the frequency-dependent SAR offers a mean of interspecies extrapolation of bioeffects data. This is important in assessing human health effects of RF radiation for two reasons. First, most data have been derived from studies of experimental animals, primarily mice, rats, and rabbits, with limited quantitative data for human exposure effects. Second, most animal studies have been conducted in the 2 to 3 GHz frequency region (primarily 2.45 GHz). In principle the interspecies or interfrequency extrapolation of exposure effects data can be done with the SAR concept, but in practice difficulties have been encountered. For the preceding example of an RF frequency of 2.5 GHz, for instance, extrapolation in terms of SAR suggests that, if a specific exposure effect, such as an alteration in blood chemistry, were induced in a mouse by an incident power density of 2.5 mW/cm^2, 75 mW/cm^2 (that is, 30 times 2.5 mW/cm^2) would induce an equivalent response in a human. Whereas, in this hypothetical situation, equivalent responses might occur in the two species exposed to these two power densities for certain exposure durations, exposure for an hour or more could be tolerated by a mouse but would probably be fatal for a human exposed to 75 mW/cm^2. In addition to absorbed dose, physiological differences in species must be taken into account (Cleary, 1983b).

If it is assumed that RF-induced exposure effects are solely of thermal origin (a questionable assumption, as discussed below), interspecies differences in thermal physiology must be taken into consideration. Factors such as comparative rates of basal metabolic heat generation or thermoregulatory mechanisms are interspecies variables that could significantly affect extrapolation of exposure effects. For example, the average resting metabolic rate of an adult 15 gm mouse is 10 W/kg, compared with 1.26 W/kg for a 20- to 24-year-old human. In addition, humans dissipate heat by the evaporative heat loss mechanism of sweating, which is not available to mice. The thermal neutral zone is 24° to 31° C for humans and 30° to 33° C for mice. However, the maximum critical air temperature is 37° C for a mouse and 32° C for a normal adult human. Although conceptually such species-dependent differences in thermal physiology could be factored into the extrapolation of RF exposure effects, practical methods for doing so are not generally available.

In addition to the fact that the efficiency of RF field coupling depends on the wavelength of the radiation and the size, shape, and orientation of the absorbing body, the internal distribution of absorbed energy also depends on wavelength and the dielectric properties of tissue. When the free-space wavelength of the RF radiation is significantly smaller than the absorbing body and the dimensions of organs or tissue layers are of the same magnitude as the wavelength in tissue, complex modes of internal energy absorption occur because of reflections and standing waves. Such nonuniform energy distributions are referred to as EM hot spots. Thus, depending on the wavelength and intensity of the RF radiation and on the animal species, significant nonuniform internal heating patterns called thermal hot spots can occur. Such hot spots could result in atypical physiological alterations and therefore must be considered in the interspecies extrapolation of RF bioeffects.

Nonuniform RF absorption in models of laboratory animals or humans has been the subject of theoretical and experimental studies with models of animals or humans (Shapiro et al., 1971; Johnson and Guy, 1972; Tell, 1972; Neuder, 1979; Olsen and Griner, 1987). The results of such studies indicate that hot spots of significant magnitude may occur in model systems. D'Andrea and colleagues (1985) detected electromagnetic hot spots in the brain, rectum, and tail of rat carcasses exposed to 360 or 2450 MHz RF radiation. Exposure to 2450 GHz radiation caused the localized SAR in rat tails to exceed the whole-body-averaged SAR by a factor of 18, whereas at a frequency of 360 MHz the SAR at this site was 50 times greater than the whole-body SAR (D'Andrea et al., 1985). To determine the effect of thermoregulatory mechanisms in rats in limiting localized tissue temperature elevations by convective cooling by blood circulation, D'Andrea et al. (1987) studied RF-induced localized tissue temperature elevations in anesthetized rats. Irradiation for 10 to 16 minutes with 2450, 700, or 360 MHz RF radiation at whole-body-averaged SARs of 2, 6, or 10 W/kg resulted in immediate postexposure localized temperature elevations in regions that had previously exhibited high EM hot spots (that is, elevated SARs). Temperatures in the rectum and tail were significantly higher in anesthetized rats exposed to 360 MHz. Tail temperatures were also higher in rats exposed to 2.45 GHz than in those exposed to 700 MHz. These effects occurred at whole-body-averaged SARs of 6 W/kg at 360 MHz and 10 W/kg at 2.45 GHz. Exposure also induced brain temperature elevations of a smaller magnitude than tail or rectal temperature increases.

D'Andrea et al. (1987) discussed the potential significance of these data relative to rat thermal physiology. They noted that at an environmental temperature of 24° C, which is below thermoneutrality for a rat, the colonic temperature is 37.5° C, whereas the tail temperature is approximately equal to the ambient air temperature. Since vasodilation in the tail is a primary thermoregulatory mechanism in the rat, RF-induced localized heating of the tail could significantly impair overall thermoregulation, an effect that would be both species and wavelength specific. Obviously, extrapolating the effects of exposure of rats to RF radiation at a frequency that induces thermal hot spots in the tail to effects at the same or other frequency in tailless animals would be of undetermined validity.

The results of studies demonstrating the induction of frequency-dependent EM and thermal hot spots in experimental animals suggest that effects of RF radiation-induced heat stress would differ from heat stress induced by other heating modalities. Studies of experimental animals in which microwave-induced heat stress effects were compared with effects of exposure to elevated environmental temperatures suggest both qualitative and quantitative differences in responses (Cleary, 1977).

Assessments of the potentially harmful effects of nonuniform RF absorption must also involve consideration of another mechanism of avoiding adverse tissue heating: behavioral thermoregulation. Perhaps the most obvious example of direct behavioral thermoregulation is avoidance, as when an animal sensing a condition of adverse thermal stress moves to a more tolerable environment. Carroll et al. (1980) exposed rats to potentially lethal intensities of 918 MHz RF radiation (that is, to intensities resulting in SARs of up to 60 W/kg). Even though exposure induced rectal temperature elevations of up to 41° C, the rats in this study did not learn to avoid exposure by escaping from the RF field. In contrast, all the unexposed rats motivated by electric foot shock rapidly learned to avoid that noxious stimulus. The authors concluded that whole-body hyperthermia induced by RF, under the conditions of their experiment, lacked the painful or directional sensory stimulus to induce escape from the field. In this context it may be noted that, in mammals, thermally sensitive nerve end-organs are located in the dermis where absorption of infrared or "thermal" radiation normally occurs. If, as in the case of absorption of lower-frequency, more penetrating microwave radiation, significant absorption occurs in tela subcutanea or deeper-lying muscle tissue, atypical thermal stimuli and responses may occur. Not unexpectedly, therefore, RF-induced heating may elicit both physiological and behavioral responses that are not concordant with effects of other thermal sources.

The need to consider absorption characteristics of RF radiation in the interspecies extrapolation of bioeffects is further illustrated by Cleary (1983b), who hypothesized a local RF exposure effect. For example, exposure to 2.5 GHz radiation has a tissue-depth distribution of absorbed energy that depends on the skin, subcutaneous fat, and muscle thicknesses, as well as surface contours (Tell, 1972). If, for the sake of simplicity, anatomical differences in the skin and surface contours of mice and humans are ignored, it can be assumed that the radiation will be absorbed exponentially with depth. At 2.5 GHz the penetration depth, or the thickness of tissue required to reduce the incident RF field strength by 86%, is approximately 2 cm (Durney et al., 1978). The 2 cm penetration depth of 2.5 GHz radiation is thus of the same order of magnitude as the thickness of a mouse, so absorption occurs throughout the mouse's body. In a human exposed to the same RF field, absorption is effectively localized in a 2 cm thick surface layer (in a plane-wave field, the surface facing the RF source). Physiological responses to whole-body RF irradiation of the mouse could differ significantly from those induced in a human superficially exposed to the same radiation frequency.

The preceding discussion summarizes some of the uncertainties involved in using the SAR to extrapolate RF bioeffects across species and across frequencies. These uncertainties derive from physiological and anatomical differences between animals, which in many instances have been difficult to account for because of limited data, and from frequency-dependent variations in RF field coupling and internal distribution of absorbed energy. The latter class of uncertainties can be countered by advanced methods of theoretical modeling and measurement, such as the joint frequency-intensity extrapolation method, which takes into account both field coupling and internal SAR distributions (Durney et al., 1978; Cleary, 1988). Uncertainties stemming from differences between animals will require further experimental investigations, including basic physiological research and specific RF bioeffects studies. One approach to elucidating the direct effects of RF on living systems has been to investigate cellular responses in vitro, with exposure under well-controlled conditions. The results of cellular effects studies, which are providing valuable insights about RF exposure effects, are discussed later in this chapter under the heading "Emerging Issues."

DIRECT RADIOFREQUENCY FIELD EFFECTS

The preceding discussions of historical developments and the SAR concept have implied that bioeffects are primarily an indirect consequence of RF energy absorption. As such, RF effects would be classified as nonstochastic, threshold phenomena, even though quantitative dose-response relationships and thresholds have not been well defined in most cases. This premise has been the basis for standards or guidelines to prevent or limit deleterious occupational or environmental RF exposure effects, as discussed in the following section.

Unquestionably, exposure to intense RF radiation fields can cause morbidity or mortality in humans and other living systems under conditions associated with tissue heating. Prime examples of nonstochastic RF thermal effects, as discussed previously, are cataractogenesis and rapid death from hyperpyrexia. As noted, however, even for these end points, thermal causality has not been fully established. Data from recently published studies of RF effects, including cancer induction and various other cellular alterations, provide evidence of possible direct RF field effects on biological systems. Direct RF field effects are potentially significant in assessing bioeffects because they introduce the possibility of low–field intensity thresholds, frequency specificity and dependence on the instantaneous induced electric or magnetic field strength per se. Such concepts as time and spatial averaging of RF energy absorption in a body, as well as the assumption that effects are independent of radiation frequency (other than in terms of macroscopic field coupling and nonuniform internal energy distributions discussed previously), must be reexamined as pertinent data appear.

SPECIFIC ABSORPTION RATE EXPOSURE ASSESSMENTS AND SAFETY GUIDELINES

Despite inherent limitations regarding interspecies and interfrequency extrapolation of RF bioeffects data, the SAR concept has provided a more adequate means of comparing and categorizing data than the use of incident RF field intensity or power density. The marked dependence of

RF absorption on wavelength and the size, shape, and orientation of a body, such as an experimental animal (as indicated by Durney et al., 1978, and others) indicates the need for a method of normalizing exposure effects in terms of dose rate or dose. The SAR has provided a means for such normalization, even in instances in which the SAR was not determined in the original study.

Experimental techniques of accurate SAR determinations have become generally available to researchers only in the past decade, and in some instances their deployment in experiments has proved costly or difficult (Cleary, 1988). Consequently, a significant number of studies, especially those conducted more than 10 years ago, did not involve estimation of SARs. However, given basic information about the RF exposures such as incident power density, wavelength, and the species, size, and weight of the experimental animal, it is possible to determine SARs retrospectively using the methods described by Durney et al. (1978). Correlation of reported bioeffects with SAR, using such methods of estimation, has been used in a number of instances to determine safe RF exposure levels. The basic approach has been to obtain a measured value of SAR from a given experimental study, or to calculate it from the data provided, and to associate the occurrence or nonoccurrence of a bioeffect with the SAR. Based on the theoretically predicted frequency dependence of SAR, frequency-dependent safe exposure levels or guidelines have been developed, as described in Chapter 2.

Application of the SAR concept to the bioeffects data base led Committee C95.1 of the American National Standards Institute (ANSI, 1982) and Scientific Committee 53 of the National Council on Radiation Protection and Measurements (NCRP, 1986) to conclude that the threshold for alteration of RF-exposed mammals was a whole-body-averaged SAR of approximately 4 W/kg. When a safety margin of 10 was applied, a fundamental SAR exposure criterion of 0.4 W/kg was established for frequencies from 3 MHz to 100 GHz. Whereas the ANSI recommendation applies to all human exposure, the NCRP recommended lower SARs for population exposure than for occupational exposure (NCRP, 1986).

Scientists at the Health Effects Research Laboratory (Elder and Cahill, 1984) of the Environmental Protection Agency used an approach similar to those of ANSI (1982) and NCRP (1986) to assess the biological effects of RF radiation. The general conclusions of this critical review are presented here to provide an overview of this field and as background material for topics discussed in detail in the following chapters.

Significant effects in laboratory animals that occur at SARs of 4 to 8 W/kg are:

1. Temporary sterility in male rats exposed at an SAR = 5.6 W/kg for 4h/day for 20 days (Berman et al., 1980).

2. Bradycardia in rats after whole-body exposure (SAR = 6.5 W/kg) (Phillips et al., 1975b). Exposure of the head of the rabbit at an SAR of 3 W/kg caused tachycardia (Birenbaum et al., 1975).

Potentially significant biological effects that have been reported at SARs < 4 W/kg include the following:

1. The decrease in behavioral response rates cited in ANSI (1982) were based on studies done at ambient temperatures of 20 to 25° C. Gage (1979b) has shown that similar changes in behavior occur at lower SARs when exposures are conducted at higher ambient temperature: that is, at 22° C the effective SAR was 3 W/kg, whereas at 28° C SARs of 1 and 2 W/kg were effective.
2. Although RF radiation does not appear to be a primary carcinogenic agent (cancer inducer), there is evidence from one laboratory that RF radiation acts as a cancer promoter or cocarcinogen in three different tumor systems in mice at an SAR of 2 to 3 W/kg (Szmigielski et al., 1980, 1982).
3. A decrease in the number of Purkinje cells in the brain of rats exposed at an SAR of 2 W/kg was reported by Albert et al. (1981a).
4. Endocrine gland function and blood chemistry changes are similar to those observed during heat stress and are generally associated with SARs > 1 W/kg. . . .
5. Effects on the hematologic and immunologic systems occur at SARs ≥ 0.5 W/kg and appear to result from some form of thermal involvement due to absorbed RF energy. . . .
6. Changes in cellular energy metabolism in the rat brain have been reported at an SAR of 0.1 W/kg; the data support the conclusion that the effect is frequency specific (Sanders et al., 1980).
7. Results of studies of amplitude-modulated (AM) radio-waves, particularly AM frequencies near or at 16 Hz, have shown changes in calcium-ion efflux from chick brain tissues in vitro. The effect has been shown to be frequency and intensity specific and to occur at SARs as low as 0.0013 W/kg (Blackman et al., 1979, 1980a,b). In 1984 Dutta et al. reported that 16-Hz AM microwave radiation caused changes in calcium-ion efflux from human brain cells in culture at an SAR of 0.5 W/kg.*

Table 10-1 (adapted from Elder and Cahill, 1984) summarizes reported biological effects of RF radiation that occurred as a result of exposure at SARs less than 10 W/kg.

On the basis of a critical review of RF bioeffects using the SAR concept, scientists at HERL made the following conclusions:

---

* From Elder, J. A., and Cahill, D. F. (eds.) (1984). Biological effects of radiofrequency radiation. Report No. EPA-600/8-83-026F, Research Triangle Park, N.C., Health Effects Research Laboratory, Environmental Protection Agency.

TABLE 10-1   **Representative Reported Biological Effects of Radiofrequency Radiation and Associated Range and Mean Specific Absorption Rates**

Bioeffect	SAR range (W/kg)	Mean SAR (W/kg)
Behavior	0.4–7	2.5
Central nervous system	0.0001–12.5	1.8
Hematology/ immunology	0.4–11.8	4.3
Hormones	1.0–5.0	4.8
Drug potentiation	0.2–1.0	0.6
Mutations/chromosome aberrations	0.05–5.0	2.5
Neurotransmitter levels	6.0	6.0
Fertility	5.6	5.6
Clinical chemistry	1.6–4.0	2.8
Cardiovascular system	3.0–8.0	5.8

Modified from Elder, J. A., and Cahill, D. F. (eds.) (1984). Biological effects of radiofrequency radiation. Report No. EPA-600/8–83–026F, Research Triangle Park, N.C., Health Effects Research Laboratory, Environmental Protection Agency.

In summary, the data currently available on the relation of SAR to biological effect show evidence for biological effects at an SAR of about 1 W/kg. This value is lower by a factor of 4 than 4 W/kg, the value above which reliable evidence of hazardous effects was found by ANSI (1982) following a review of the literature in February 1979. The above conclusion is based on:

1. the findings that more thermally stressful conditions result in lower threshold SARs for behavioral changes similar to those changes determined by ANSI (1982) to be the most sensitive measures of biological effects.
2. the effects on endocrine gland function, blood chemistry, hematology, and immunology that appear to result from some form of thermal involvement due to absorbed RF energy.
3. data from one laboratory showing that RF radiation can act as a cancer promoter or cocarcinogen and results from another laboratory describing changes in brain cellularity.

The experimental evidence suggests that the central nervous system is particularly sensitive to RF radiation. Two other areas of research that may prove to be highly significant are calcium-ion efflux and brain energy metabolism.*

It may be concluded that bioeffects data normalization using the SAR concept has provided a systematic means of cause-effect categorization. Obvious, highly significant differences in the sensitivity of organs and organ systems of experimental animals to RF exposure emerge from such approaches. Although quantitative data on human exposure effects is limited, the reported sensitivity of humans to RF exposure appears to be in general agreement with the conclusions based on experimental data, for example, that the mammalian central nervous system is maximally sensitive. The extent to which overall physiological differences between species affect the validity of SAR-dependent cause-effect comparisons is not evident at present. The RF bioeffects data base consists primarily of results of short-term exposures to microwave radiation, most prominently at a frequency of 2.45 GHz. The effects of this limitation cannot be assessed, but as discussed in the following section, there are indications of significant differences in the sensitivity of mammalian systems to long-term exposure to low-intensity RF radiation. The now well-documented biphasic or "windowed" intensity and modulation rate effects of RF and lower-frequency EM fields suggests currently unknown mechanisms of effects on living systems.

EMERGING ISSUES

Many of the issues and questions that emerged from assessments of RF bioeffects by ANSI (1982), HERL (Elder and Cahill, 1984), and NCRP (1986) remain unanswered, in part because of decreased research efforts in this area, perhaps owing to a shift in interest to the effects of extremely low-frequency (ELF), low-intensity electric and magnetic fields. ELF field effect studies have revealed unexpected sensitivities of living systems, including humans (see Chapter 14).

A number of recent studies have reported an association between exposure to 60 Hz electric fields and cancer induction. In a case-control study, for example, a significantly higher proportion of primary brain tumor deaths (mainly from gliomas and astrocytomas) occurred among electricians, electrical or electronic engineers, and utility company servicemen. The increased relative incidence of brain tumors was related to

---

* From Elder, J. A., and Cahill, D. F. (eds.) (1984). Biological effects of radiofrequency radiation. Report No. EPA-600/8–83–026F, Research Triangle Park, N.C., Health Effects Research Laboratory, Environmental Protection Agency.

exposure level, and the average age at death was significantly younger for workers exposed to electric fields (Lin et al., 1985). Other studies have indicated a possible association between occupational exposure to 60 Hz fields and incidence of brain tumors (Mancuso, 1982; Preston-Martin et al., 1982; Milham, 1979). Increased incidence of leukemia has also been reported to occur among electricians (Milham, 1982; Wright et al., 1982; Coleman et al., 1983; McDowall, 1983). An increased incidence of all types of cancer was reported to occur in children (Wertheimer and Leeper, 1979; Tomenius et al., 1982) and adults (Wertheimer and Leeper, 1982) exposed to magnetic or electric fields from 60 Hz electric power lines. Although epidemiological studies of these types seldom determine exposure levels accurately, the weight of evidence suggests a cause-effect relationship between cancer induction and long-term exposure to 60 Hz electric or magnetic fields.

Other effects of ELF fields include altered calcium ion binding to brain tissue (Bawin and Adey, 1980) and synaptosomes (Lin-Liu and Adey, 1982); noradrenaline release from neurons (Dixey and Resin, 1982); potassium ion fluxes in Chinese hamster ovary cells (Stevenson and Tobey, 1985); and transcriptional activity of cells (Goodman and Henderson, 1986). The common finding of these experimental and epidemiological studies is that living systems are for some unknown reason sensitive to low-intensity ELF fields. The outcomes appear to result primarily from a direct field interaction, not as an indirect consequence of heating caused by energy absorption.

The apparent sensitivity of biological systems to weak ELF electric or magnetic fields raises new questions about the effects of higher-frequency RF fields. Although it is somewhat doubtful that a common mechanism is involved in ELF and RF bioeffects (Cleary, 1987), the results of ELF studies indicate the need to reconsider the effects of low-intensity RF exposure on living systems. That few such RF effects have been reported may relate more to the dearth of studies involving chronic low-intensity exposure than to the absence of effects.

In view of the seriousness of the disease, the results of ELF studies, and results of a few studies of RF effects, the possibility of an association between cancer and RF exposure should be carefully examined. The potential carcinogenic potential of RF radiation has been suggested by experimental findings indicating tumor promotion (Szmigielski et al., 1982; Kunz et al., 1985), increased incidence of leukemia in experimental animals (Prausnitz and Susskind, 1962), and the promotion of cell transformation in vitro (Balcer-Kubiczek and Harrison, 1985). Milham (1988) has reported that amateur radio operator licensees have a statistically significant excess mortality from acute myeloid leukemia, multiple myeloma, and possibly certain types of malignant lymphomas, a pattern consistent with that observed among electrical workers. The ubiquitous presence and ever-increasing levels of RF radiation in our environment, together with a possible association with cancer promotion and other health effects, firmly establishes the need for additional biological effects research.

REFERENCES

ALBERT, E.N., SHERIF, M.F., AND PAPADOPOULOS, N.J. (1981a). Effects of non-ionizing radiation on the Purkinje cells of the uvula in squirrel monkey cerebellum. *Bioelectromagnetics* 2:241–246.

ANNE, A., SAITO, M., SALATI, O.M., AND SCHWAN, H.P. (1961). Relative microwave absorption cross sections of biological significance. *In*: Peyton, M.F. (ed.). Biological effects of microwave radiation. New York, Plenum Publishing Corp., pp. 153–176.

ANSI (1982). American National Standards Institute. American national standard C95.1, safety levels with respect to human exposure to radio frequency electromagnetic fields, 300 kHz to 100 GHz, New York, Institute of Electrical and Electronic Engineers, Inc.

APPLETON, B., HIRSCH, S.E., AND BROWN P.V.K. (1975). Investigation of single-exposure microwave ocular effects of 3000 MHz. *Ann. N.Y. Acad. Sci.* 247:125–135.

BALCER-KUBICZEK, E.K., AND HARRISON, C.H. (1985). Evidence for microwave carcinogenesis *in vitro*. *Carcinogenesis* 6:859–864.

BAWIN, S.M., AND ADEY, S. (1976). Sensitivity of calcium binding in cerebral tissue to weak environmental electrical fields oscillating at low frequency. *Proc. Natl. Acad. Sci. U.S.A.* 73:1999–2003.

BERMAN, E., CARTER, H.B., AND HOUSE, D. (1980). Tests of mutagenesis and reproduction in male rats exposed to 2450-MHz (CW) microwaves. *Bioelectromagnetics* 1:65–76.

BIRENHAUM, L., KAPLAN, I.T., METLAY, W., ROSENTHAL, S.W., AND ZARET, M.M. (1975). Microwave and infra-red effects on heart rate, respiration rate and subcutaneous temperature of the rabbit. *J. Microwave Power* 10:3–18.

BLACKMAN, C.F., ELDER, J.A., WEIL, C.M., BENANE, S.G., EICHINGER, D.C., AND HOUSE, D.E. (1979). Induction of calcium-ion efflux from brain tissue by radiofrequency radiation: effects of modulation frequency and field strength. *Radio Sci.* 14(suppl. 6):93–98.

BLACKMAN, C.F., BENANE, S.G., ELDER, J.A., HOUSE, D.E., LAMPE, J.A., AND FAULK, J.M. (1980a). Induction of calcium-ion efflux from brain tissue by radiofrequency radiation: effect of sample number and modulation frequency on the power-density window. *Bioelectromagnetics* 1:35–43.

BLACKMAN, C.F., BENANE, S.F., JOINES, W.T., HOLLIS, M.A., AND HOUSE, D.E. (1980b). Calcium-ion efflux from brain tissue: power-density versus internal field-intensity dependencies at 50 MHz RF radiation. *Bioelectromagnetics* 1:277–283.

CARPENTER, R.L., FERRI, E.S., AND HAGAN, G.L. (1974). Assessing microwaves as a hazard to the eye—progress and problems. *In*: Proceedings of an International Symposium on Biological Effects and Health Hazards of Microwave Radiation. Warsaw, Polish Medical Publishers, pp. 178–185.

CARPENTER, R.L., HAGAN, G.J., AND DONOVAN, G.L. (1977). Are microwave cataracts thermally caused? *In*: Symposium on Biological Effects and Measurements of RF and Microwaves. HEW Pub. No. (FDA) 77–8026, Rockville, Md., pp. 352–379.

CLEARY, S.F. (1973). Uncertainties in the evaluation of the biological effects of microwave and radiofrequency radiation. *Health Phys. 25*:387–404.

CLEARY, S.F. (1977). Biological effects of microwave and radiofrequency radiation. *In*: Straub, C.P. (ed.). CRC critical review in environmental control. Boca Raton, Fla., CRC Press, pp. 121–166.

CLEARY, S.F. (1980). Microwave cataractogenesis. *Proc. IEEE 68*:49–55.

CLEARY, S.F. (1983a). Bioeffects of microwave and radiofrequency radiation. *In*: Storm, F.K. (ed.). Hyperthermia in cancer therapy. Boston, G.K. Hall, pp. 545–566.

CLEARY, S.F. (1983b). Microwave radiation effects on humans. *Bioscience 33*:269–273.

CLEARY, S.F. (1987). Cellular effects of electromagnetic radiation. *IEEE Eng. Med. Biol.*, March, pp. 26–30.

CLEARY, S.F. (1988). Biological effects of nonionizing radiation. *In*: Webster, E. (ed.). Encyclopedia of medical devices and technology, Vol. 1, New York, John Wiley & Sons.

COLEMAN, M., BELL, J., AND SKEET, R. (1983). Leukemia incidence in electrical workers (Letter). Lancet *1*:982–983.

D'ANDREA, J.A., EMMERSON, R.Y., BAILEY, C.M., OLSEN, R.G., AND GANDHI, O.P. (1985). Microwave radiation absorption in the rat: frequency dependent SAR distribution in body and tail. *Bioelectromagnetics 6*:199–206.

D'ANDREA, J.A., EMMERSON, R.Y., DEWITT, J.R.D., AND GANDHI, O.P. (1987). Absorption of microwave radiation by the anesthetized rat: electromagnetic and thermal hotspots in body and tail. *Bioelectromagnetics 8*:385–396.

DIXEY, R., AND REIN, G. (1982). ^{3}H-noradrenaline release potentiated in a clonal nerve cell by low-intensity pulsed magnetic fields. *Nature 296*:253–256.

DURNEY, C.H., JOHNSON, C.C., BARBER, P.W., et al. (1978). Radiofrequency radiation dosimetry handbook, 2nd ed. USAF School of Aerospace Medicine, Brooks Air Force Base, Tex., Contract No. SAM-TR-78–22.

DUTTA, S.K., SUBRAMONIAM, A., GHOSH, B., AND PARSHAD, R. (1984). Microwave radiation-induced calcium ion efflux from human neuroblastoma cells in culture. *Bioelectromagnetics 5*:71–78.

ELDER, J.A., AND CAHILL, D.F. (eds.). (1984). Biological effects of radiofrequency radiation. Report No. EPA-600/8–83–026F, Research Triangle Park, N.C., Health Effects Research Laboratory, Environmental Protection Agency.

GAGE, M.I. (1979). Microwave irradiation and ambient temperature interact to alter rate behavior following overnight exposure. *J. Microwave Power 14*:389–398.

GANDHI, O.P. (1975). Conditions of strongest electromagnetic power deposition in man and animals. *IEEE Trans. Microwave Theory and Tech. 23*:1021–1029.

GOODMAN, R., AND HENDERSON, A.S. (1986). Sine waves enhance cellular transcription. *Bioelectromagnetics 7*:23–29.

GUY, A.W., LIN, J.C., KRAMAR, P.O., AND EMERY, A.F. (1975). Effect of 2450-MHz radiation on the rabbit eye. *IEEE Trans. Microwave Theory Tech. 23*:492–498.

HAGAN, G.J., AND CARPENTER, R.L. (1975). Relative cataractogenic potencies of two microwave frequencies. *In*: Proceedings of the URSI/USNC Annual Meeting, Boulder, Colo., Washington, D.C., National Academy of Sciences, pp. 143–155.

JOHNSON, C.C., AND GUY, A.W. (1972). Non-ionizing electromagnetic wave effects in biological materials and systems. *Proc. IEEE 60*:692–718.

KRAMER, P.O., HARRIS, C., EMERY, A.F., AND GUY, A.W. (1978). Acute microwave irradiation and cataract formation in rabbits and monkeys. *J. Microwave Power 11*:135–136.

KUNZ, L.L., JOHNSON, R.B., THOMPSON, D., CROWLEY, J., CHOU, C.K., AND GUY, A.W. (1985). Effects of long-term low-level radiofrequency radiation exposure on rats. USAF School of Aerospace Medicine. Report No. SAM-TR-85–11, Vol. 8, Brooks Air Force Base, Tex.

LETAVET, A.A., AND GORDON, Z.V. (eds.) (1962). The biological action of ultrahigh frequencies. (English translation.) JPRS: 12471, Washington, D.C. U.S. Joint Publications Research Service.

LIN, R.S., DISCHINGER, P.C., CONDE, J., AND FARREL, K.P. (1985). Occupational exposure to electromagnetic fields and brain tumors: an observed association. *J. Occup. Med. 27*:413–419.

LIN-LIU, S., AND ADEY, W.R. (1982). Low frequency amplitude modulated microwave fields change efflux rates from synaptosomes. *Bioelectromagnetics 3*:309–322.

MANCUSO, T.B. (1982). Epidemiological study of tumors of the central nervous system in Ohio. *Ann. N.Y. Acad. Sci. 381*:17–39.

McDOWALL, M.E. (1983). Leukemia mortality in electrical workers in England and Wales (Letter). *Lancet 1*:246.

MILHAM, S. (1979). Mortality in aluminum reduction plant workers. *J. Occup. Med. 21*:475–480.

MILHAM, S. (1982). Mortality from leukemia in workers exposed to electrical and magnetic fields (Letter). *N. Engl. J. Med. 307*:249.

MILHAM, S. (1988). Increased mortality in amateur radio operators due to lymphatic and hematopoietic malignancies. *Am. J. Epidemiol. 127*:50–54.

NCRP (1986). National Council on Radiation Protection and Measurements. Biological effects and exposure criteria for radiofrequency electromagnetic fields, Report No. 86, Washington, D.C.

NEUDER, S.M. (1979). Electromagnetic fields in biological media. II. The SCAT program, multilayered spheres, theory and applications. DHEW Pub. No. (FDA) FDA-79–8072, Washington, D.C., U.S. Government Printing Office.

OLSEN, R.G., AND GRINER, T.A. (1987). Specific absorption rate in models of man and monkey at 225 and 2000 MHz. *Bioelectromagnetics* 8:377–384.

PHILLIPS, R.D., HUNT, E.L., CASTRO, R.D., AND KING, N.W. (1975). Thermoregulatory, metabolic and cardiovascular response of rats to microwaves. *J. Appl. Physiol.* 38:630–635.

PRAUSNITZ, S., AND SUSSKIND, C. (1962). Effect of chronic microwave irradiation on mice. *IRE Trans. Biomed. Electron.* 9:104–108

PRESTON-MARTIN, S., HENDERSON, B.E., AND PETERS, J. (1982). Descriptive epidemiology of central nervous system neoplasms in Los Angeles County. *Ann. N.Y. Acad. Sci.* 381:202–208.

ROWBOTTOM, R., AND SUSSKIND, C. (1984). Electricity and medicine: history of their interaction. San Francisco, San Francisco Press.

SANDERS, A.P., SCHAEFER, D.J., AND JOINES, W.T. (1980). Microwave effects on energy metabolism of rat brain. *Bioelectromagnetics* 1:171–181.

SCHWAN, H.P. (1957). Electrical properties of tissue and cell suspensions. *Adv. Biol. Med. Phys.* 5:147–209.

SCHWAN, H.P., AND LI, K. (1956). Hazards due to total body irradiation by radar. *Proc. IRE* 41:1572–1581.

SHAPIRO, A.R., LUTOMIRSKI, R.F., AND YURA, H.T. (1971). Induced fields and heating within a cranial structure irradiated by EM plane waves. *IEEE Trans. Microwave Theory Tech.* 19:187–197.

STEVENSON, A.P., AND TOBEY, R.A. (1985). Potassium ion influx measurements on cultured Chinese hamster cells exposed to 60-Hz electromagnetic fields. *Bioelectromagnetics* 6:189–198.

SZMIGIELSKI, S., SZYDZRINSKI, A., PIETRASZEK, A., AND BIELEC, M. (1980). Acceleration of cancer development in mice by long-term exposition to 2450-MHz microwave fields. *In*: Berteaud, A.J., and Servantie, B. (eds.). URSI International Symposium Proceedings, Ondes electromagnetiques et biologie, Paris, pp. 165–169.

SZMIGIELSKI, S., SZYMDZINSKI, A., PIETRASZEK, A., BIELEC, M., JANIAK, M., AND WREINBEL, J.K. (1982). Accelerated development of spontaneous and benzopyrene-induced skin cancer in mice exposed to 2450-MHz microwave radiation. *Bioelectromagnetics* 3:179–191.

TELL, R.A. (1972). Reference data for radiofrequency emission hazard analysis. Report No. ORP/DIS 72–3, Washington, D.C., Environmental Protection Agency.

TOMBERG, V.T. (1961). Specific thermal effects of high frequency fields. *In*: Peyton, M.F. (ed.). Biological effects of microwave radiation. New York, Plenum Publishing Co. pp. 221–228.

TOMENIUS, L., HELLSTROM, L., AND ENANDER, B. (1982). Electrical construction and 50 Hz magnetic field at the dwelling of tumor cases (0–18 years of age) in the county of Stockholm. Presented at the International Symposium on

Occupational Health and Safety Mining and Tunnelling, Prague, June 21–25, 1982.

U.S.A. Standards Institute. 1966. Safety level of electromagnetic radiation with respect to personnel. C95.1, New York.

WERTHEIMER, N., AND LEEPER, E. (1979). Electrical wiring configurations and childhood cancer. *Am. J. Epidemiol. 109*:273–284.

WERTHEIMER, N., AND LEEPER, E. (1982). Adult cancer related to electrical wires near the home. *Int. J. Epidemiol. 11*:343–355.

WRIGHT, W.E., PETERS, J.M., AND MACK, T.M. (1982). Leukemia in workers exposed to electrical and magnetic fields (Letter). *Lancet 2*:1160–1161.

11

Thermo-physiological Effects of Electromagnetic Radiation

ELEANOR R. ADAIR

Long before the demonstration of certain subtle biological consequences of exposure to low-intensity electromagnetic (EM) radiation (so-called athermal effects), well-defined consequences of tissue heating were recognized and quantified. Much of this early research was conducted by Michaelson (1983) and his colleagues and involved microwave power densities in excess of 100 mW/cm^2. Generally, when the rate of energy absorption during exposure to such fields exceeds the rate of energy dissipation, the body temperature rises. Thus the deep body temperature of experimental animals was shown to rise at a rate proportional to the intensity of the imposed field; if the field was sufficiently intense, death from hyperthermia could result unless the field was extinguished in timely fashion. At sublethal levels, daily exposure was shown to produce a tolerance to particular exposure conditions that took the form of a gradually reduced elevation in body temperature with time; this phenomenon is akin to acclimatization to warm environments. Adequate hydration during exposure to EM radiation was found to help prevent excessive increases in body temperature, presumably because evaporative heat loss was enhanced. In addition, the role of the environmental temperature became evident, with cool environments fostering efficient thermoregulation during exposure and warm environments hindering it. In sum, the thermophysiological responses of organisms exposed to EM radiation appeared to resemble the responses to vigorous exercise or hot environments.

Most early studies quantified little more than changes in deep body temperature, and often that was measured after the exposure had terminated because special nonperturbing thermometers for use in radiofrequency fields were not yet available. The little study by Nielsen and Nielsen (1965) was one of the first to evaluate individual responses of metabolic heat production, thermal conductance, and sweating, as well as changes in body temperature, in humans who were either passively heated by diathermy or actively generating metabolic heat through exercise. When the energy generated in the body was the same, irrespective of how the energy was introduced, the thermoregulatory responses were identical. This result confirmed the hypothesis that the fate of energy introduced into the body by exposure to EM radiation is no different from that of energy produced by the body itself.

During the past two decades much has been learned about specific thermophysiological responses to EM radiation. These facts form the bulk of this chapter. However, in recent years research interest has shifted away from apparently dull "thermal" to more exciting "athermal" biological effects. This situation is unfortunate because many questions, vital to standards setting as well as to our general knowledge of bioeffects, remain unresolved. For example, the complications for thermoregulation of a febrile state in an organism exposed to nonionizing EM radiation have never been explored. Similarly, little is known of the synergism that may occur when an exposed organism is under the influence of alcohol or other drugs known to interfere with the normal physiological processes that regulate the body temperature. Some scientists have concluded, on flimsy evidence, that warm and humid environments exacerbate the risk of hyperthermia imposed on humans by exposure to EM radiation (Elder and Cahill, 1984). Also, certain categories of humans (such as infants, the aged, and the infirm) are considered more susceptible than others to the ravages of such exposure (Environmental Protection Agency, 1986). Tragically, no data that can be brought to bear on any of these questions have been generated. Much of what we do know of thermophysiological changes induced by exposure to EM radiation is summarized in this chapter.

FUNDAMENTALS OF THERMOREGULATION

"Warm-blooded," or endothermic, organisms are capable of generating heat in their bodies through metabolic processes. When endotherms are exposed to EM radiation, frictional heat can also be generated passively in body tissues as the water molecules oscillate at the frequency of the imposed electric field. To avoid a rise in body temperature, the body must transfer excess heat to the environment by radiation, conduction, and convection (the avenues of dry heat loss) or by the evaporation of water from the skin or respiratory tract or both. The efficiency of heat transfer depends on the physical characteristics of the environment, particularly on the air temperature. In general, if more heat is generated in the body than can be dissipated to the environment, the body temperature rises; if more heat is lost by the body to the environment than can be generated, the body temperature falls.

The local temperature of many body tissues is sensed by specialized nerve cells located both in the skin and deep body structures as well as in neural centers such as the brainstem, medulla, and spinal cord. Afferent signals from these receptors are probably integrated in the medial preoptic/anterior hypothalamic region of the brainstem, often called the central thermostat, and the integrated signal is compared with an internal reference or set point. If a load error occurs (that is, actual temperature different from set temperature), an effector command is generated to energize an appropriate autonomic response that will restore the body temperature to the set level. The particular thermoregulatory response mobilized in any given environment, as well as its vigor, may be predicted on the basis of a thermoregulatory profile that is unique to each species. The thermoregulatory profile delineates how specific effector responses of metabolic heat production, thermal conductance, and evaporative heat loss vary with ambient temperature. Thus it can conveniently be used to estimate the consequences of additional heat generated passively in the body during exposure to EM radiation. This analytical method has recently been explored in depth to gain insight into the probable response of humans irradiated by EM waves (Adair, 1987b). To date, the most revealing investigations into the thermophysiological effects of EM radiation in any species consider both the thermoregulatory profile of the exposed organism and the environmental conditions under which the exposure takes place, in addition to the characteristics of the radiation itself.

Figure 11-1, a schematic thermoregulatory profile of a typical endotherm, illustrates graphically how the principal autonomic responses of heat production and heat loss depend on the ambient temperature (T_a). The responses are considered to be steady state rather than transient, and the air is considered to have minimal movement and water content. Three distinct zones can be defined in terms of the prevailing autonomic adjustment. Below the lower critical temperature (LCT), thermoregula-

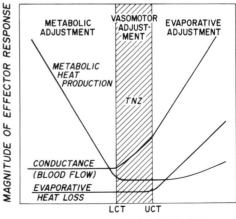

Figure 11-1 Schematic thermoregulatory profile of typical endothermic organism to illustrate dependence of principal types of autonomic responses on prevailing ambient temperature. *LCT*, Lower critical temperature; *UCT*, upper critical temperature; *TNZ*, thermoneutral zone.

tion is achieved by changes in metabolic heat production, other responses remaining at minimal strength. As T_a falls further and further below LCT, heat production increases proportionately. The profile predicts that at cool T_a, EM energy absorbed by an endotherm will spare the metabolic system in proportion to the field strength and will not affect other autonomic responses (for details see Adair, 1987b).

At T_a above the LCT, metabolic heat production is at the species-typical, resting level, evaporative heat loss is minimal, and thermoregulation is achieved by changes in thermal conductance. Conductance is a measure of heat flow from the body core to the skin and reflects the vasomotor state of the peripheral blood vessels. As vasoconstricted vessels begin to dilate, warm blood is brought from the body core to the surface so that heat may be lost to the environment by radiation and convection. These vasomotor adjustments take place within a species-typical range of T_a called the thermoneutral zone (TNZ). Thus, if an endotherm at thermoneutrality is exposed to EM radiation, augmented vasodilation may occur so that excess heat generated in deep tissues may be quickly brought to the surface for dissipation to the environment.

At the upper limit of the TNZ, called the upper critical temperature (UCT), the endotherm is fully vasodilated and dry heat loss is maximal. A further increase in T_a mobilizes heat loss by evaporation, either from the skin (sweating) or from the respiratory tract (panting). Humans and certain other mammals sweat copiously to achieve thermoregulation in hot environments. If these species are exposed to EM radiation at T_a above the UCT, their evaporative heat loss increases in proportion to the field strength. However, other mammals, especially rodents, neither sweat nor pant and must depend on behavioral maneuvers, such as spreading saliva or urine on the fur, to achieve some degree of thermoregulation when heat stressed. Opportunities for behavioral thermoregulation are vital when these species undergo exposure to EM radiation at T_a above the UCT.

Any organism may adopt thermoregulatory behavior as an alternative strategy for dealing with the thermalizing effects of exposure to EM radiation. Changes in certain behaviors can alter the physical characteristics of the air-skin interface and thereby maximize the efficiency of heat transfer. Examples are the selection of a more favorable thermal environment, the resetting of a thermostat, and the addition or subtraction of body insulation. These thermoregulatory behaviors also minimize the involvement of autonomic responses of heat production and heat loss, conserve bodily stores of energy and fluid, and produce a state of maximal thermal comfort. Because behavioral responses may be quickly mobilized and are of high gain, they should be considered in any discussion of the thermophysiological consequences of exposure to EM radiation.

THRESHOLDS FOR RESPONSE MOBILIZATION

For any given species, under any given exposure conditions, an intensity of an imposed EM field can be determined that will reliably initiate or alter whatever thermophysiological response is appropriate to the prevailing environmental conditions; this intensity can be designated the threshold for response mobilization. Intensities above this threshold level will also alter the response, usually to a degree that is intensity dependent (Adair, 1981). Much recent research into thermophysiological effects has involved determination of these thresholds in laboratory animals. Once determined, such thresholds may be evaluated for their applicability to the human condition, a fundamental goal of this research. The task becomes far easier if the thermoregulatory profile of the particular animal studied has been considered in the design and conduct of the research. It is then useful to catalogue thresholds for response mobilization in terms of the prevailing autonomic adjustment, whether metabolic, vasomotor, or evaporative.

Metabolic Compensation for Electromagnetic Heating

As Figure 11-1 shows, the metabolic heat production (M) of an endotherm equilibrated to a T_a well below the LCT will be elevated by an amount directly proportional to T_a. During brief (a few minutes to ½ hour), far-field exposure to EM radiation, the elevated M of nonhuman primates will be reduced by an amount proportional to the field strength or the specific absorption rate (SAR) (Adair and Adams, 1982; Candas et al., 1985; Lotz and Saxton, 1987). As a result of this response adjustment the internal body temperature is usually regulated with precision within the limits normal for the species. Similar results have been demonstrated in rodents after a period of whole-body EM irradiation in either a multimodal cavity (Phillips et al., 1975) or a waveguide (Ho and Edwards, 1977, 1979). A threshold SAR must be surpassed before a reliable reduction in M occurs; this species-dependent threshold probably varies with T_a (Adair, 1987b). If only part of the body is exposed to the EM field, the magnitude of the response change reflects the total absorbed energy as though it were integrated over the whole body (Adair, 1988). It is not yet known whether the threshold for a given species also varies with frequency, thereby reflecting different patterns of tissue heating. It has been demonstrated that rhesus monkeys, exposed to the resonant frequency (225 MHz), limit the storage of heat in the body by reducing M, but this reduction is often insufficient to prevent a rise in deep body temperature during the exposure (Lotz and Saxton, 1987). Whether frequency or species underlies this finding has not been determined.

Vasomotor Changes during Electromagnetic Exposure

When an endotherm is briefly exposed to EM radiation at a T_a just below the LCT (Figure 11-1), the stage is set to initiate the peripheral vasomotor response as soon as M has been reduced to the resting level (Adair, 1987a). In laboratory animals the vessels of the tail and the ears usually vasodilate before those of the extremities. Generally, once the field strength is sufficient to induce vasodilation (threshold), the response occurs rapidly at field onset and the magnitude or degree of vasodilation is a direct function of the SAR (Adair and Adams, 1980a; Gordon et al., 1986) or the total heat load (Gordon, 1983b). Extinction of the EM field induces rapid vasoconstriction. Exposure to infrared fields of comparable intensity fails to induce dilation of the tail in squirrel monkeys (Adair and Adams, 1980a), indicating that noncutaneous thermosensors may mediate activation of this thermoregulatory response. There is solid experimental evidence that both the threshold and the magnitude of the vasomotor response depend on the imposed frequency (Lotz, personal communication). The closer the frequency to whole-body resonance, the less energy required to induce vasodilation at a given T_a and the greater the response magnitude at a given SAR.

Peripheral vasodilation can also occur spontaneously during the course of a prolonged EM exposure that is carried out at a T_a below the LCT (Ward and Spiegel, 1984; Candas et al., 1985; Lotz and Saxton, 1987). Vasodilation is mobilized because the internal body temperature slowly rises during the exposure, eventually surpassing a threshold for initiation of the response. Indeed, changes in the caliber of blood vessels deep in the body, as well as in the periphery, accompany EM exposure and the rate of blood flow increases dramatically whenever the temperature of the heated tissue exceeds 42° to 43° C (Sekins, 1981). This phenomenon forms the basis of the treatment of localized malignancies by microwave hyperthermia, achieved with arrays of EM devices (Guy and Chou, 1983). Healthy tissue is better perfused with blood than is cancerous tissue; thus it is possible to heat tumors to levels (45° C and above) that kill cells while normal tissue is protected by a significant increase in local blood flow.

Changes in Evaporative Heat Loss during Electromagnetic Exposure

When the peripheral blood vessels of an endotherm are fully vasodilated, dry heat loss from the body nears its maximum. To prevent significant heat storage and a resultant rise in body temperature, the body must initiate heat loss by evaporation. As shown in Figure 11-1, this occurs when T_a equals UCT; it also occurs at T_a within the TNZ during exposure to EM fields at SARs sufficiently high to produce full vasodilation (Adair, 1987b). Because cellular processes in the body speed up as tissue temperature rises, a small increase in heat production, coincident with initiation of evaporation, also occurs at high T_a (Figure 11-1). Any attempt to predict the evaporative capability of a particular endotherm in the presence of EM fields must consider the thermoregulatory profile, the type of evaporative response available (panting or sweating), or whether there may not be such capability, as is the case with rodents. Fortunately, humans have an extraordinary capability to lose body heat through sweating when T_a rises above 30° to 31° C or the deep body temperature exceeds 37° C (Wenger, 1983).

Thermoregulatory sweating from the foot of a squirrel monkey equilibrated to a T_a just below the UCT can be reliably initiated by exposure to 2450 MHz continuous wave microwaves at a SAR equivalent to about 20% of the animal's resting heat production (Adair, 1985b). The threshold energy required to elicit a criterion sweating response is linearly related to the T_a at which the EM exposure takes place. Like heat production, the magnitude of the sweating response depends on the integration of absorbed EM energy over the whole body, not energy deposited in some locus such as the "central thermostat" of the hypothalamus. Indeed, thermoregulatory sweating occurs when a microwave field is present, even when the hypothalamus is artificially cooled to prevent its temperature from rising (Adair, 1988).

Sweating from the calf of a rhesus monkey, when the animal is exposed to 225 MHz microwaves in thermoneutral environments of 26° and 32° C, is reported to occur at somewhat higher SARs, closer to the equivalent of 80% of the animal's resting heat production (Lotz and Saxton, 1986). In the cooler environment, peripheral vasodilation preceded the onset of sweating, as predicted by the thermoregulatory profile. However, sweating in thermoneutral environments, like reduced M in cooler environments (Lotz and Saxton, 1987), failed to prevent a substantial rise in deep body temperature of the rhesus monkey during exposure at the resonant frequency. Clearly, further study is required to determine the consequences for thermoregulation of exposure at frequencies resonant to different body sizes.

Gordon (1982) has reported a much higher threshold for initiation of evaporative heat loss in microwave-exposed mice. In these experiments a mouse was irradiated in a waveguide and the increase in relative humidity of the air flowing through the waveguide was taken as a measure of heat lost by evaporation of body water. As previously noted, mice neither pant or sweat but are said to increase respiratory frequency somewhat when heat stressed (Gordon, 1983a) in addition to spreading saliva over the fur. None of these responses could be observed, nor could the body temperature be recorded, to provide evidence that the animals were indeed thermoregulating normally. Since the T_a during the experiments was 22° C, well below the TNZ for the mouse, changes in M, not changes in evaporative heat loss, would first be anticipated during EM exposure. The latter should occur only after M was reduced to resting level and the peripheral vasculature of the animal was fully vasodilated. With this perspective the high evaporative threshold reported for the mouse may be more easily understood (Adair et al., 1983).

THERMOREGULATORY RESPONSES TO SUPRATHRESHOLD INTENSITIES

Hierarchy of Thermoregulatory Responses

The range of response magnitudes across which an EM exposure has an effect (for example, on metabolic heat production) depends on the prevailing T_a (Adair, 1987b). Whatever the T_a (below the LCT), an SAR can be found that will reduce heat production to its resting level. In the steady state when heat storage is zero, this SAR (in watts per kilogram) should be equal to the amount by which heat production is elevated above the normal resting level (also in watts per kilogram). This prediction was verified for the squirrel monkey exposed to 2450 MHz at low field strengths (Adair and Adams, 1982) and later reconfirmed at higher field strengths during partitional calorimetric studies of the same species (Adair, 1985a, 1987a). On the other hand, Lotz and Saxton (1987, 1988) did not always find a steady-state reduction in heat production of similar magnitude to the imposed SAR when the rhesus monkey was exposed to the resonant frequency (225 MHz) at a T_a of 20° and 26° C; often heat storage was evidenced by an elevated deep body temperature in these experiments. However, damping of apparent pulses in M, during EM exposure, was a novel finding that was hypothesized to reflect changes in circulating catecholamine levels (Lotz and Saxton, 1988). It is still not clear whether exposure to the resonant frequency per se somehow overwhelms the thermoregulatory system even at low SARs (Lotz, 1985) or whether some artifact in the experimental arrangement conspired against the efficient mobilization of appropriate heat loss responses. To date, these results remain unreplicated in the rhesus monkey or any other species.

Figure 11-1 predicts that when M is reduced to the resting level by EM exposure at an appropriately high SAR, the second response in the hierarchy, altered thermal conductance, will be mobilized. In practice, vasodilation of the extremities such as the tail or foot of an experimental animal is usually indexed by an abrupt rise in the skin temperature of the dilating extremity. This prediction has been verified in two species;

the tail vessels of cold-exposed squirrel monkeys (Candas et al., 1985) or rhesus monkeys (Lotz and Saxton, 1987, 1988) vasodilate actively after M has been reduced to the resting level by microwave exposure. As a consequence, the body temperature continues to be regulated at a near-normal level.

If the strength of an EM field continues to increase, the next response in the normal hierarchy, evaporative heat loss, should be mobilized as soon as vasodilation is complete. This further prediction has been verified in partitional calorimetric studies of squirrel monkeys exposed to 2450 MHz microwaves at high SARs in cool environments (Adair, 1987a). For example, exposure at 9 W/kg in a 20° C environment was found to mobilize all the thermoregulatory responses in the hierarchy sequentially; first, the elevated heat production was reduced to resting level, then tail vasodilation, followed by foot vasodilation, and finally sweating was initiated. All of these responses served to regulate the internal body temperature at a near-normal level throughout the 90-minute microwave exposure. Consecutive response mobilization of this type was perhaps responsible for the triphasic response of body temperature measured by Michaelson et al. (1961) in dogs exposed to intense microwave fields. It surely explains the initiation of evaporative cooling in mice exposed to microwaves in a cool waveguide (Gordon, 1982). However, the implications of these findings for humans is reassuring: the full hierarchy of responses available for thermoregulation will be mobilized in turn to counter any significant tissue heating that accompanies EM exposure.

Potential for Response Adaptation

The question of the possibility for adaptation of thermophysiological responses during chronic exposure to EM fields is an interesting one about which we know relatively little. Most investigations have involved acute exposures at durations from a few minutes to a few hours per test session. Only a few studies have been undertaken that feature chronic exposure of experimental animals to microwave fields. In the most complex of these studies, conducted at the University of Washington, no change in metabolic rate, among a host of other physiological variables, was detected in rats chronically exposed to microwaves 21 hours a day for more than 2 years (Johnson et al., 1984). It has been suggested that a reduced metabolic rate might explain the absence of change in whole-body growth rate with decreased food consumption that was measured in adult rats repeatedly exposed to microwaves for 10 hours a day at an SAR of 3.2 W/kg (Lovely et al., 1983). Another study (Adair et al., 1985) was designed to examine the potential for adaptation of the thermoregulatory responses of squirrel monkeys during chronic microwave exposure (40 hours a week for 15 weeks) at controlled T_a of 25°, 30°, and 35° C. The most reliable effect appeared to be a small reduction in body mass of microwave-exposed animals that was not accompanied by a reduction in heat production.

A significant body of literature describes the thermophysiological adaptation of humans to warm environments and to work and exercise in the heat (Goldman, 1983). Such response changes as reduced M, lowered skin temperature, altered vasomotor thresholds, a significant drop in deep body temperature during exercise, and augmented sweating rates should also accompany chronic exposure to EM fields. Unfortunately, the requisite carefully controlled experiments are costly, time consuming, and unlikely to be carried out on either animals or humans; on the other hand, epidemiological studies lack measurements of the particular environmental and biological variables necessary to confirm the potential for thermoregulatory adaptation by chronic exposure to EM fields.

Tolerance of high-intensity EM fields was demonstrated to develop with time in dogs repeatedly exposed to 2800 MHz pulsed fields (Michaelson, 1983). This type of adaptation took two forms: a gradual reduction in the elevation of deep body temperature on successive days and a lengthening of tolerable exposure duration. Recent partitional calorimetric studies on squirrel monkeys, exposed for 90-minute periods to 2450 MHz continuous wave microwaves, have determined the SAR at which thermal balance can be maintained in cool, neutral, and warm environments (Adair, 1987a). The SARs tolerated (9 W/kg at $T_a = 20°$ C; 6.75 W/kg at $T_a = 26°$ C; 3 W/kg at $T_a = 32°$ C) are related in curvilinear fashion to both T_a and the animal's average skin temperature. Most important, they may be directly understood in terms of the normal thermoregulatory profile of the squirrel monkey.

SOME THERMOPHYSIOLOGICAL BENEFITS OF ELECTROMAGNETIC EXPOSURE

The thermophysiological basis for the use of microwave hyperthermia as an adjunct to the treatment of localized malignancies has already been mentioned; this application of EM fields must be considered a substantial benefit to humankind. Despite the continuing climate of apprehension about the safety of human exposure to very low-intensity electric and magnetic fields, basic research and industrial activity have proceeded along several other avenues that promise comparable benefits. Some of these deserve mention here because they have provided considerable new knowledge about certain thermophysiological consequences of EM exposure.

Behavioral Thermoregulation and Thermal Comfort

Humans and other endotherms continually seek a comfortable thermal environment, one that provides maximal satisfaction and minimal physiological strain. When we set the thermostat, open the window, or put on clothing, we are responding to a need for thermal comfort. The maintenance of thermal homeostasis underlies this need; as we have seen, a stable body temperature maximizes conservation of the body's energy and fluid stores.

The comfortable environment for resting endotherms is often thermally neutral; that is, it falls within the TNZ (Figure 11-1). Sometimes, as after heavy exercise, a cool environment feels comfortable; at other times, as after prolonged cold exposure, a warm environment may feel comfortable. Thus the deep body temperature, as well as the skin temperature, exerts a strong bias on sensations of thermal comfort. Extensive human research (Fanger, 1973) indicates that the thermal environment selected or preferred is that which maximizes comfort and facilitates thermoregulation. Thus the study of thermal comfort in any environment, including those in which EM fields are present, embodies study of behaviors that accomplish effective thermoregulation.

In cold environments, metabolic heat must ordinarily be supplemented by exogenous energy sources to maximize thermal comfort. Similarly, in warm environments, sources of convective cooling eliminate the necessity for excessive heat loss by evaporation. Most organisms readily learn to manipulate radiant or convective sources, or position themselves strategically near such sources, to thermoregulate efficiently (Cabanac, 1983). In any ambient temperature, the more intense the source of heating or cooling is, the less it will be energized. Also, the more the ambient temperature deviates from that preferred, the more the source of heating or cooling will be energized. If the body temperature is perturbed (as by exercise), the preferred ambient (skin) temperature will be oppositely altered (Cabanac et al., 1971). In laboratory animals, heating or cooling a thermode implanted in the preoptic area of the hypothalamus (site of the "internal thermostat") will cause the animal to select a cooler or warmer environment, respectively. The greater the displacement of local preoptic temperature from its neutral level, the greater the shift in preferred environmental temperature (Adair et al., 1970). Local temperature changes in other parts of the central nervous system (such as the medulla and spinal cord) can often stimulate equivalent behavioral changes.

Changes in behavior ensure the maintenance of a stable body temperature or the rapid restabilization of a body temperature that has been perturbed. An appropriate shift in the thermal gradient between skin and environment, or between body core and skin, accomplishes the regulation.

Research during the last decade has confirmed that laboratory animals energize or orient around a source of EM energy in the environment as if it were a source of radiant or convective heat. Lizards bask in the radiation from a microwave antenna and thereby regulate their body temperature effectively (D'Andrea et al., 1978). Rats, trained to press a lever for infrared heat in a cold environment, suppress lever pressing in inverse proportion to the strength of a superimposed microwave field (Stern et al., 1979). Mice select a cooler part of a thermal gradient as the imposed microwave field inside a waveguide becomes more intense (Gordon, 1983b). A discrete power density threshold governs such behavioral changes (Adair and Adams, 1980b), and the behavior, once initiated, persists until the microwave field is extinguished (Adair and Adams, 1983). Rhesus monkeys learn to press a lever for intermittent pulses of 6.4 GHz microwaves when they are cold (Marr et al., 1988). Similarly, squirrel monkeys can be trained to turn a source of microwaves on and off; the duration of voluntary microwave exposure is inversely proportional to the field strength (Bruce-Wolfe and Adair, 1985). Always, the change in thermoregulatory behavior regulates the body temperature at a level close to normal. All evidence indicates that a state of thermal comfort is achieved simultaneously.

If only part of the body (such as the head or trunk) is exposed to microwaves, the change in selected ambient temperature is governed by an integrated energy deposition over the whole body, not by energy deposited in some specific locus such as the brain. Indeed, the hypothalamic "thermostat" appears to play no more vital a role in thermoregulation during microwave exposure than do other thermosensitive regions of the body (Adair, 1988), which reinforces current views of the neurophysiological control of thermoregulation.

In the steady state the environmental temperature selected by a microwave-exposed animal is a linear function of the imposed field strength. Figure 11-2 shows this relationship for trained squirrel monkeys exposed unilaterally to a homogeneous 2450 MHz continuous wave microwave field inside an anechoic chamber (Adair, 1987a). As demonstrated by Berglund (1983), the function in Figure 11-2 represents the conditions that provide a constant level of thermal comfort or operative temperature (T_o). Because the relationships between T_o, comfort, and thermoregulation are well understood for humans, Berglund was able to predict the effect of microwave energy on human thermal comfort over a wide range of ambient conditions. The concept of microwave heating for comfort, recently proposed by Pound (1980), appears to have great potential for improving the thermal environment in many situations and perhaps for saving energy as well (Adair and Berglund, 1985).

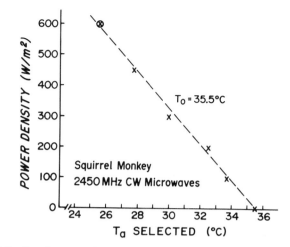

Figure 11-2   Steady-state air temperature chosen by sedentary squirrel monkeys exposed unilaterally to homogeneous microwave field at different power densities. T_o, operative temperature; T_a, air temperature.

Thermal Effects in Magnetic Resonance Imaging

Exposure of patients to the magnetic resonance imaging (MRI) environment may produce heating of body tissue related to the changing fields of the gradient and radiofrequency coils. The potential thermalization is exaggerated in instruments that operate at the upper range of frequencies. Although two reports (Gremmel et al., 1984; Sperber et al., 1984) indicated body temperature changes in both humans and mice exposed to stationary magnetic fields, Tenforde (1986) was unable to confirm these results in rodents subjected to large uniform magnetic fields and strong magnetic field spatial gradients.

Few experimental data are related directly to the problem of radiofrequency heating during MRI because of the difficulty and inconvenience of making the appropriate measurements in the clinic. Schaefer et al. (1985) reported that the colonic temperature of anesthetized unshorn sheep, exposed for 17 minutes in a body coil at an SAR of 2 to 4 W/kg, rose less than 0.6° C during the scanning procedure. Other unpublished observations, together with evidence of an anecdotal nature, indicate that, although thermoregulatory responses such as sweating may be mobilized during MRI, the deep body temperature will rise very little.

In a different approach to this problem, a simple computer model of human thermoregulation, based on the concept of body heat balance and the thermoregulatory profile, has been adapted to predict the thermoregulatory consequences of exposure to the MRI environment (Adair and Berglund, 1986). Based on knowledge of thermoregulatory processes and how heat is exchanged between a person and the environment, the model predicts physiological heat loss responses in real time as a function of selected ambient temperature (T_a), air movement (v), and rate of whole-body radiofrequency energy deposition (SAR). Assuming a criterion elevation in deep body temperature (ΔT_{co}) of 0.6° C, a T_a of 20° C, and a v of 0.8 m/sec, a 70 kg pajama-clad patient could undergo a MRI exposure of infinite duration at an SAR of 5 W/kg. Lowering T_a or increasing v permits a rise in SAR for a given ΔT_{co}. The limiting response appears to be the rate of peripheral blood flow, although sweating can play a significant role in preventing an excessive rise in T_{co}.

A more recent modeling effort (Adair and Berglund, 1989) has examined the effects of cardiovascular impairment on physiological heat loss responses during MRI by imposing restrictions on peripheral blood flow. The results indicate that, under the conditions that normally prevail in the clinic, patients with such impairment should undergo scans of 20 minutes or less at SARs of 3 W/kg or less to ensure that the body temperature does not rise more than 1° C during the procedure. In general, under any given ambient conditions, the thermoregulatory response to radiofrequency energy deposited in the body during MRI is similar to that which would be expected during an increase in metabolic heat production (for example, during exercise). This is the same conclusion reached by Nielsen and Nielsen in 1965.

Microwave Incubation of Infant Mammals and Rewarming from Hypothermia

The proposal by Pound (1980) that microwaves be used for the comfort heating of humans, conceived in the aftermath of the energy crisis, may not be realized for decades because of present concerns for the potential hazards attending such exposure. However, microwave heating for therapy, for rapid rewarming of hypothermia victims, and for incubation of newborn mammals is being vigorously explored on many fronts. Given a frequency that will allow penetration of the EM energy well below the surface of an organism, rapid heating of the body can be accomplished far more efficiently than with radiant or convective sources. Buffler (1988) described the standard practice of immersing a hypothermic newborn lamb for hours in a hot water bath as tedious and marginally successful. Furthermore, such prolonged soaking removes the animal's scent so that the mother rejects it afterward. Heated shelters for sheep are expensive and therefore little used. Instead, Buffler proposes rewarming the lamb rapidly with microwave energy to enhance its survival and ensure its acceptance by the mother.

Flocks of chicks have been successfully incubated with microwaves on a demand basis beginning on the seventh day of life (Morrison et al., 1986). In a cool environment (16° C), either 2450 MHz microwaves or infrared heat was provided when a chick pecked at a wall panel. The birds used both sources of thermal energy efficiently for periods as long as 22 days. No differences in growth rate between infrared- and microwave-heated chicks were evident, nor were there any visible detriments in health or overall behavior in the microwave-exposed birds. Similar techniques are being developed for the microwave warming of newborn piglets (Morrison, personal communication).

The potential for microwave incubation of newborn rats is being explored in my laboratory, with emphasis on changes that may occur in thermoregulatory ability when immature rats are repeatedly exposed to microwave fields. The goal of this research is to determine the optimal conditions (SAR and T_a) for the incubation of rats from 2 to 18 days of age; after such incubation the exposed animals will be allowed to grow to maturity, mate, and produce young, while being tested for a wide variety of biological end points. Although protracted periods away from the mother for microwave exposure reduce growth in developing rats, supplemental feedings can compensate for loss of body mass. To date, no hazardous consequences of acute or repeated exposure to microwaves at low SARs have been found (Spiers and Adair, 1987; Spiers and Baummer, 1986) and it seems certain that optimal conditions for microwave incubation will be easily determined and implemented. It is only a short step, then, to the consideration of a microwave incubation system for premature infants, who are so susceptible to the dehydrating and burning characteristics of conventional convective and radiant incubators.

Profoundly hypothermic, anesthetized rhesus monkeys have been successfully rewarmed to normal body temperature by radiofrequency radiation treatment with an induction coil (Olsen and David, 1984; Olsen et al., 1987). Deep body temperatures as low as 20° C, the point of cardiovascular collapse, were returned to the normal level within 2 hours, and no deleterious aftereffects were observed over a period of 9 months following the treatments. Analyses of blood samples showed characteristic elevations of serum enzymes on the day after treatment, but this occurred whether the rewarming was done slowly with a heating pad or rapidly by EM radiation. The ultimate goal of this research is an EM resuscitation system for hypothermic humans. Apart from the necessity of controlling for skin burns by closely monitoring the dose rate and the skin temperature, there seems to be little doubt that this method of rewarming can have great utility in the future.

CONCLUSION

The thermoregulatory capabilities of endothermic organisms exposed to thermalizing levels of EM fields have been described in terms of the normal hierarchy of responses available to these species. In most cases, experimental data confirm that during such exposure the deep body temperature is regulated with precision at a level close to normal and responses are mobilized in orderly fashion. Some evidence, awaiting confirmation, indicates that exposure to a frequency near whole-body resonance may provide a special case in which hyperthermia is more likely to occur than during exposure to other frequencies. In general, under any given ambient conditions, the thermoregulatory response to absorbed EM energy is similar to that which would be expected during exercise or exposure to warm environments. Innovative uses of EM energy for the heating of body tissues, either localized or whole body, are being explored to realize the many biological benefits of nonionizing EM radiation.

REFERENCES

ADAIR, E.R. (1981). Microwaves and thermoregulation. *In*: Mitchell, J.C. (ed.). Aeromedical review USAF Radiofrequency Radiation Bioeffects Research Program—a review. USAF Report No. SAM-TR-81-30, December, USAF School of Aerospace Medicine, Brooks Air Force Base, Tex., pp. 145–158.

ADAIR, E.R. (1985a). Microwave radiation and thermoregulation. USAF Report No. USAFSAM-TR-85-3, May, USAF School of Aerospace Medicine, Brooks Air Force Base, Tex.

ADAIR, E.R. (1985b). Thermal physiology of RFR interactions in animals and humans. *In*: Mitchell, J.C. (ed.). Proceedings of a workshop on radiofrequency radiation bioeffects. USAF Report No. SAM-TR-85-14, April, USAF School of Aerospace Medicine, Brooks Air Force Base, Tex., pp. 37–54.

ADAIR, E.R. (1987a). Microwave challenges to the thermoregulatory system. USAF Report No. USAFSAM-TR-87-7, USAF School of Aerospace Medicine, Human Services Division (AFSC), Brooks Air Force Base, Tex.

ADAIR, E.R. (1987b). Thermophysiological effects of electromagnetic radiation. *IEEE Eng. Med. Biol. 6*:37–41.

ADAIR, E.R. (1988). Microwave challenges to the thermoregulatory system. *In*: O'Connor, M.E., and Lovely, R.H. (eds.). Electromagnetic waves and neurobehavioral function. New York, Alan R. Liss, pp. 179–201.

ADAIR, E.R., AND ADAMS, B.W. (1980a). Microwaves induce peripheral vasodilation in squirrel monkey. *Science 207*:1381–1383.

ADAIR, E.R., AND ADAMS, B.W. (1980b). Microwaves modify thermoregulatory behavior in squirrel monkey. *Bioelectromagnetics 1*:1–20.

ADAIR, E.R., AND ADAMS, B.W. (1982). Adjustments in metabolic heat production by squirrel monkeys exposed to microwaves. *J. Appl. Physiol. 52*:1049–1058.

ADAIR, E.R., AND ADAMS, B.W. (1983). Behavioral thermoregulation in the squirrel monkey: adaptation processes during prolonged microwave exposure. *Behav. Neurosci. 97*:49–61.

ADAIR, E.R., AND BERGLUND, L.G. (1985). Comfort heating with microwaves: an idea whose time may have come. *In*: Fanger, P.O. (ed.). CLIMA 2000, Vol. 4, Copenhagen, VVS Kongres/VVS Messe, pp. 115–120.

ADAIR, E.R., AND BERGLUND, L.G. (1986). On the thermoregulatory consequences of NMR imaging. *Magn. Reson. Imaging 4*:321–333.

ADAIR, E.R., AND BERGLUND, L.G. (1989). Thermoregulatory consequences of cardiovascular impairment during NMR imaging in warm/humid environments. *Magn. Reson. Imaging. 7*:25–37.

ADAIR, E.R., CASBY, J.U., AND STOLWIJK, J.A.J. (1970). Behavioral temperature regulation in the squirrel monkey: changes induced by shifts in hypothalamic temperature. *J. Comp. Physiol. Psychol. 72*:17–27.

ADAIR, E.R., SPIERS, D.E., RAWSON, R.O., ET AL. (1985). Thermoregulatory consequences of long-term microwave exposure at controlled ambient temperature. *Bioelectromagnetics 6*:339–364.

ADAIR, E.R., SPIERS, D.E., WENGER, C.B., AND STOLWIJK, J.A.J. (1983). Technical note: on changes in evaporative heat loss that result from exposure to nonionizing electromagnetic radiation. *J. Microwave Power 18*:209–211.

BERGLUND, L.G. (1983). Characterizing the thermal environment. *In*: Adair, E.R. (ed.). Microwaves and thermoregulation. New York, Academic Press, pp. 15–31.

BRUCE-WOLFE, V., AND ADAIR, E.R. (1985). Operant control of convective cooling and microwave irradiation by squirrel monkeys. *Bioelectromagnetics 6*:365–380.

BUFFLER, C.R. (1988). Whole body microwave heating of humans and livestock. *Harvard Graduate Soc. Newsl., Summer*:11–13.

CABANAC, M. (1983). Thermoregulatory behavioral responses. *In*: Adair, E.R. (ed.). Microwaves and thermoregulation. New York, Academic Press, pp. 307–357.

CABANAC, M., CUNNINGHAM, D.J., AND STOLWIJK, J.A.J. (1971). Thermoregulatory set point during exercise: a behavioral approach. *J. Comp. Physiol. Psychol. 76*:94–102.

CANDAS, V., ADAIR, E.R., AND ADAMS, B.W. (1985). Thermoregulatory adjustments in squirrel monkeys exposed to microwaves at high power densities. *Bioelectromagnetics 6*:221–234.

D'ANDREA, J.A., CUELLAR, O., GANDHI, O.P., LORDS, J.L., AND NIELSEN, H.C. (1978). Behavioral thermoregulation in the whiptail lizard (*Cnemidorphorus tigris*) under 2450 MHz CW microwaves. *In*: Biological effects of electromagnetic waves. Abstracts URSI General Assembly, Helsinki, Finland, p. 88.

ELDER, J.A., AND CAHILL, D.F. (eds.) (1984). Biological effects of radiofrequency radiation. EPA Report No. EPA 600/8–83–026F. NTIS accession number PB85–120–848. Washington, D.C., Environmental Protection Agency.

Environmental Protection Agency (1986). Federal radiation protection guidance: proposed alternatives for controlling public exposure to radiofrequency radiation; notice of proposed recommendations. *Fed. Register 51*, No. 146, July 30.

FANGER, P.O. (1973). Thermal comfort. New York, McGraw-Hill Book Co.

GOLDMAN, R.F. (1983). Acclimation to heat and suggestions, by inference for microwave radiation. *In*: Adair, E.R. (ed.). Microwaves and thermoregulation. New York, Academic Press, pp. 275–282.

GORDON, C.J. (1982). Effects of ambient temperature and exposure to 2450-MHz microwave radiation on evaporative heat loss in the mouse. *J. Microwave Power 18*:377–383.

GORDON, C.J. (1983a). Behavioral and autonomic thermoregulation in mice exposed to microwave radiation. *J. Appl. Physiol. 55*:1242–1248.

GORDON, C.J. (1983b). Influence of heating rate on control of heat loss from the tail in mice. *Am. J. Physiol. 244*:R778-R784.

GORDON, C.J., LONG, M.D., AND FEHLNER, K.S. (1986). Temperature regulation in the unrestrained rabbit during exposure to 600 MHz radiofrequency radiation. *Int. J. Radiat. Biol. 49*:987–997.

GREMMEL, H., WENDHAUSEN, H., AND WUNSCH, F. (1984). Biologische Effekte statischer Magnetfelder bei NMR-Tomographie am Menschen. *Wiss. Mitt.*, University of Kiel, Radiologische Klinik, Kiel, Federal Republic of Germany.

GUY, A.W., AND CHOU, C.-K. (1983). Electromagnetic heating for therapy. *In*: Adair, E.R. (ed.). Microwaves and thermoregulation. New York, Academic Press, pp. 57–93.

HO, H.S., AND EDWARDS, W.P. (1977). Oxygen-consumption rate of mice under differing dose rates of microwave radiation. *Radio Sci. 12*:131–138.

HO, H.S., AND EDWARDS, W.P. (1979). The effect of environmental temperature and average dose rate of microwave radiation on the oxygen-consumption rate of mice. *Radiat. Environ. Biophys. 16*:325–338.

JOHNSON, R.B., KUNZ, L.L., THOMPSON, D., CROWLEY, J., CHOU, C.-K., AND GUY, A.W. (1984). Effects of long-term low-level radiofrequency radiation exposure on rats. Vol. 7. Metabolism, growth, and development. USAF Report No. USAFSAM-TR-84-31, September. USAF School of Aerospace Medicine, Brooks Air Force Base, Tex.

LOTZ, W.G. (1985). Hyperthermia in radiofrequency exposed rhesus monkeys: a comparison of frequency and orientation effects. *Radiat. Res. 102*:59–70.

LOTZ, W.G., AND SAXTON, J.L. (1986). Influence of radiofrequency exposure on sweating and body temperature in rhesus monkeys. BEMS Eighth Annual Meeting abstracts, Gaithersburg, Md., Bioelectromagnetic Society. p. 79.

LOTZ, W.G., AND SAXTON, J.L. (1987). Metabolic and vasomotor responses of rhesus monkeys exposed to 225-MHz radiofrequency energy. *Bioelectromagnetics 8*:73–89.

LOTZ, W.G., AND SAXTON, J.L. (1988). Thermoregulatory responses in the rhesus monkey during exposure at a frequency (225 MHz) near whole-body resonance. *In*: O'Connor, M.E., and Lovely, R.H. (eds.). Electromagnetic fields and neurobehavioral function. New York, Alan R. Liss, pp. 203–218.

LOVELY, R. H., MIZUMORI, S.J.Y., JOHNSON, R.B., AND GUY, A.W. (1983). Subtle consequences of exposure to weak microwave fields: are there nonthermal effects? In: Adair, E.R. (ed.). Microwaves and thermoregulation. New York, Academic Press, pp. 401–429.

MARR, M.J., DE LORGE, J.O., OLSEN, R.G., AND STANFORD, M. (1988). Microwaves as reinforcing events in a cold environment. In: O'Connor, M.E., and Lovely, R.H. (eds.). Electromagnetic fields and neurobehavioral function. New York, Alan R. Liss, pp. 219–234.

MICHAELSON, S.M. (1983). Thermoregulation in intense microwave fields. In: Adair, E.R. (ed.). Microwaves and thermoregulation. New York, Academic Press, pp. 283–295.

MICHAELSON, S.M., THOMSON, R.A.E., AND HOWLAND, J.W. (1961). Physiologic aspects of microwave irradiation of mammals. Am. J. Physiol. 244:351–356.

MORRISON, W.D., McMILLEN, I., BATE, L.A., OTTEN, L., AND PEI, D.C.T. (1986). Behavioral observations and operant procedures using microwaves as a heat source for young chicks. Poultry Sci. 65:1516–1521.

NIELSEN, B., AND NIELSEN, M. (1965). Influence of passive and active heating on the temperature regulation of man. Acta Physiol. Scand. 64:323–331.

OLSEN, R.G., AND DAVID, T.D. (1984). Hypothermia and electromagnetic rewarming in the rhesus monkey. Aviat. Space Environ. Med. 55:111–117.

OLSEN, R.G., BALLINGER, M.B., DAVID, T.D., AND LOTZ, W.G. (1987). Rewarming of the hypothermic rhesus monkey with electromagnetic radiation. Bioelectromagnetics 8:183–193.

PHILLIPS, R.D., HUNT, E.L., CASTRO, R.D., AND KING, N.W. (1975). Thermoregulatory, metabolic and cardiovascular responses of rats to microwaves. J. Appl. Physiol. 38:630–635.

POUND, R.V. (1980). Radiant heat for energy conservation. Science 208:494–495.

SCHAEFER, D.J., BARBER, B.J., GORDON, C.J., ZAWIEJA, D.C., ZIELONKA, J.S., AND HECKER, J. (1985). SAR studies in magnetic resonance imaging. BEMS Seventh Annual Meeting abstracts. Gaithersburg, Md., Bioelectromagnetics Society, p. 90.

SEKINS, K.M. (1981). Microwave hyperthermia in human muscle: an experimental and numerical investigation of the temperature and blood flow occurring during 915 MHz diathermy. Ph.D. Dissertation, University of Washington, Seattle.

SPERBER, D., OLDENBOURG, E., AND DRANSFELD, K. (1984). Magnetic field induced temperature change in mice. Naturwissenschaften 71:100–101.

SPIERS, D.E., AND ADAIR, E.R. (1987). Thermoregulatory responses of the immature rat following repeated postnatal exposures to 2450-MHz microwaves. Bioelectromagnetics 8:283–294.

SPIERS, D.E., AND BAUMMER, S.C. (1986). Thermoregulatory responses in the immature rat during acute exposure to 2450 MHz microwaves. BEMS 8th Annual Meeting abstracts, BEMS, Gaithersburg, Md., Bioelectromagnetics Society, p. 4.

STERN, S., MARGOLIN, L., WEISS, B., LU, S.-T., AND MICHAELSON, S. (1979). Microwaves: effect on thermoregulatory behavior in rats. Science 206:1198–1201.

TENFORDE, T.S. (1986). Thermoregulation in rodents exposed to high-intensity stationary magnetic fields. *Bioelectromagnetics* 7:341–346.

WARD, T.R., AND SPIEGEL, R.J. (1984). Thresholds of microwave-induced vasodilation in the squirrel monkey. BEMS Sixth Annual Meeting abstracts. Gaithersburg, Md., Bioelectromagnetics Society, p. 37.

WENGER, C.B. (1983). Circulatory and sweating responses during exercise and heat stress. *In*: Adair, E.R. (ed.). Microwaves and thermoregulation. New York, Academic Press, pp. 251–274.

12

Auditory Perception of Pulsed Microwave Radiation

JAMES C. LIN

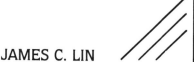

The microwave auditory phenomenon has been widely recognized as one of the most interesting biological effects of microwave radiation. Short rectangular pulses of microwave energy impinging on heads of animals and humans have been shown to elicit auditory responses. In recent years, considerable efforts have been devoted to the study of this interesting phenomenon. A great deal has been learned concerning mechanism and mode of interaction. The response is believed to stem from thermoelastic expansion of tissue in the head, which absorbed the pulsed microwave energy. Specifically, when a microwave pulse impinges on the head, the absorbed energy is converted into heat, which produces a small but rapid rise in temperature. This temperature rise, occurring in a very short time, generates rapid thermoelastic expansion of tissue in the head, which launches a propagating acoustic wave of pressure detected by hair cells in the cochlea of the inner ear.

The audition of the microwave pulses is a unique exception to the energy normally encountered by humans in auditory perception. Although the hearing apparatus responds to acoustic or sound pressure waves in the audiofrequency range, the hearing of microwave pulses involves electromagnetic (EM) waves whose frequency ranges from hundreds of megahertz to tens of gigahertz. Since EM waves are seen but not heard, the report of auditory sensation of microwave pulses was quite surprising and initially its authenticity was widely questioned.

The earliest report of the auditory perception of microwave pulses was provided anecdotally by radar operators during World War II. They described an audible sound, a click or buzz that occurred at the repetition rate of radar while they stood in front of the antenna. These reports of microwave auditory effect were documented by Frey (1961, 1962, 1963, 1967), who began by interviewing and testing under controlled conditions a number of people who had reported the sensation. Frey's papers were met with skepticism until Guy et al. (1973) confirmed his observations. The mechanism of microwave auditory effect remained obscure for more than a decade. Frey had hypothesized that the microwave auditory effects involved direct electrical stimulation of the cochlear nerve or neurons at more central sites along the auditory pathway. This route has since been shown not to be involved; instead, the absorption of microwave pulses launches a traveling thermoelastic wave of pressure that propagates to the cochlear to evoke the auditory sensation.

This chapter first summarizes psychophysical, physiological, and behavioral observations on animals and humans and includes a review of theoretical studies of physical mechanisms for the conversion of microwave pulses to auditory signals. The measurements of displacement and pressure made in phantom modeling materials and animal tissues are described together with a comparison between theoretical predictions and experimental results. The discussion concludes with comments on the probability that the microwave auditory effect might become a health risk and on the potential use of microwave pulse–induced thermoelastic pressure waves in noninvasive imaging of biological tissues.

The objective of this chapter is to present in a succinct manner what is actually known about the microwave auditory effect. In reviewing the accumulation of experimental data and advances in theoretical development, I tried to select results that are of major importance and lasting significance.

PSYCHOPHYSICAL STUDIES ON HUMANS

Human subjects whose heads were irradiated with rectangular pulses of microwave energy, with peak incident power densities as low as 250 mW/cm^2, perceived an audible sound. The sensation appeared as a click, knock, buzz, or chirp depending on such factors as peak power, pulse width, and repetition frequency of the incident microwave radiation, and it usually was perceived as originating within or near the head. The frequencies of microwaves ranged from 200 to 3000 MHz, and the pulse width varied from 1 to 1000 μs.

Although an ideal, noise-free laboratory condition is not a requirement for perception (Frey, 1962, 1963), when earplugs, microwave anechoic chambers, or sound isolation rooms were used to attenuate ambient noise, the subjects indicated an apparent increase in the loudness of microwave-induced sound (Frey, 1961; Frey and Messenger, 1973; Guy et al., 1973, 1975). Indeed, the threshold energy density required in some cases decreased by more than 6 dB when earplugs were applied (Guy et al., 1973, 1975). The sensation occurred instantaneously, and rotation of the head in the microwave field did not change the loudness of perceived sound (Frey, 1962, 1963).

Subjects with air-conduction hearing loss (50 dB) but with good bone conduction could hear the microwave-induced sound at about the same incident power density as normal subjects could. In contrast, subjects with normal air-conduction hearing but poor bone conduction for frequencies above 5 kHz usually had difficulty perceiving pulse-modulated microwave energy. The incident power required to elicit a response from a subject with sensorineural conduction impairment near 3.5 kHz was approximately 4 times that required for a subject with normal hearing (Guy et al., 1973, 1975). In a sound-matching experiment, it was found that subjects had difficulty matching the microwave-induced sound to sinusoidal audiofrequency signals (Tyazhelov et al., 1979). Subjects perceived the best match of the microwave-induced sound with high-frequency noise above 5 kHz.

Since the first report that pulse-modulated microwave radiation induces an auditory sensation in humans, several investigators have attempted to assess the thresholds for sensation as a function of microwave parameters. Table 12-1 shows the thresholds for microwave-induced auditory effect obtained from a subject with normal hearing seated approximately 30 cm in front of a horn antenna in a shielded room lined with microwave-absorbing material. Microwave pulses 1 to 32 μs wide at 2450 MHz could be heard at peak incident power from 1 to 40 W/cm² at the threshold of sensation as distinct clicks, and short pulse trains could be heard as chirps with a tone that corresponded to the pulse repetition frequency (Guy et al., 1973, 1975). The threshold energy density per pulse and the specific absorption (SA) or energy absorption per pulse stayed the same for 1 to 10 μs pulses. For pulse widths greater than 10 μs, however, these threshold values exhibited definite oscillations. Similarly, Frey and Messenger (1973) found that the perceived loudness for pulse widths between 10 and 70 μs first increased and then decreased when the peak power density was held constant while energy density per pulse was allowed to increase with the pulse width. This indicated that the perceived loudness is a function of peak power density rather

TABLE 12-1   Threshold for Microwave-Induced Auditory Effect in Human Subjects (45 dB Background Noise, 2450 MHz)

Pulse width (μs)	Peak power (W/cm²)	Energy density/ pulse (μJ/cm²)	Peak SAR* (W/g)	Pulse (mJ/g)
1	40.00	40	16.00	16
2	20.00	40	8.00	16
4	10.00	40	4.00	16
5	8.00	40	3.20	16
10	4.00	40	1.60	16
15	2.33	35	0.93	14
20	2.15	43	0.86	17
32	1.25	40	0.50	16

* Based on absorption in equivalent spherical model of the head.

than energy density per pulse and led to the conclusion that a band of optimal pulse widths exists. As discussed later, this conclusion is compatible with the thermoelastic theory of microwave auditory effect.

Loudness of perception as a function of pulse width for human subjects exposed to pulse-modulated 800 MHz microwave fields was determined in 18 men and women with normal high-frequency auditory acuity (Tyazhelov et al., 1979). The pulses were 5 to 150 μs wide, and the repetition rates varied from 50 to 20,000 pulses per second (pps). The threshold for sensation at a repetition rate of 8000 pps is shown in Figure 12-1. Perceived loudness is inversely related to threshold of sensation. As the widths of pulses of constant peak power density were gradually increased from 5 to 150 μs a complex oscillatory loudness function was observed. The loudness increased as pulse width increased from 5 to 50 μs, then diminished with further increase of pulse widths from 70 to 100 μs, and then increased again with longer pulse widths. The character of the loudness curve is consistent with data reported by Frey and Messenger (1973) and Guy et al. (1973, 1975).

Interestingly, Tyazhelov et al. (1979) noted that the pitch (frequency) of sound induced by microwave pulses less than 50 μs wide persisted as the subject's head along with the body was lowered into saline water, while the loudness diminished roughly in proportion to the depth of immersion. With complete immersion the auditory sensation disappeared. For pulse widths larger than 50 μs even partial immersion resulted in

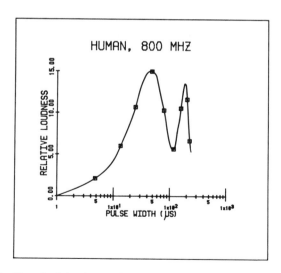

Figure 12-1 Perceived loudness of microwave auditory effect as function of pulse width for human subjects, calculated from data given in Tyazhelov et al. (1979). Note that perceived loudness is inversely proportional to threshold of sensation.

loss of perception. Furthermore, in beat frequency experiments these authors found that matching of sound induced by a microwave pulse (10 μs, 8000 pps) to a phase-shifted 8 kHz sinusoidal sound wave resulted in loss of auditory perception.

DETECTION BY LABORATORY ANIMALS

The previous section showed that under certain conditions humans can perceive pulse-modulated microwave energy. Because the auditory perception involves a discrimination response, a common concern in studies involving human subjects is avoided: the possibility of subjective responses. However, confirmatory data in lower animals substantially enhance the acceptance of a microwave-induced auditory sensation.

That microwave pulses are acoustically perceptible and can serve as a discriminatory auditory cue in behavioral situations is supported by the work of several investigators. Food-deprived laboratory rats were trained to make a nose-poking response to obtain food only during presentation of an acoustic cue (7.5 kHz acoustic pulse, 3 μs wide, 10 pps). After the behavior was conditioned to an acoustic stimulus, 918 MHz microwave pulses (from a square-aperture antenna at a peak power density of 15 W/cm^2, 10-μs, 10 pps) were surreptitiously substituted for the acoustic stimulus. As shown in Figure 12-2, the animals demonstrated a continued ability to perform correctly (85% to 90% level) on the discriminative task when presented with either the acoustic or the microwave cue (Johnson et al., 1976). This clearly suggested an auditory component in the pulsed microwave control of this behavior.

In a like fashion, rats tested in a two-compartment shuttle box, in which one compartment was exposed to 33 W/cm^2 of 2880 MHz microwave pulsed at 100 pps with a puse width of 3 μs, and the other was shielded, spent significantly more time in the shielded side (Hjeresen et al., 1979). When a high-frequency (37.5 kHz tone) acoustic stimulus was exchanged for the microwave pulses, rats exhibited a preference for the acoustically "quiet" side. In addition, the amount of side-to-side traversing activity was greater in rats exposed either to microwave pulses or to acoustic stimuli in both sides of the box than in unexposed control animals. The simultaneous presentation of a broad-band "pink" acoustic noise (20 to 40 kHz) and pulsed microwaves produced no statistically significant difference in side preference between experimental and control groups. In contrast, in all cases the number of traverses made by exposed rats were significantly greater than those of unexposed control rats. These results indicate that the pulsed microwave stimulus and the acoustic tone stimulus can result in similar behavior patterns and support the

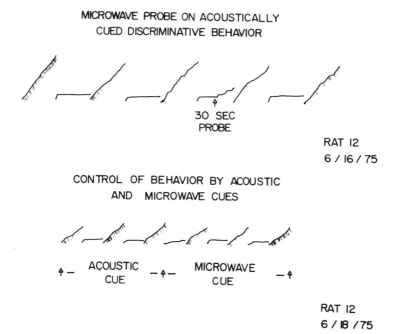

Figure 12-2 Cumulative performance record showing discriminative control of behavior by microwave and acoustic pulses. (From Johnson, R.B., et al. [1976]. Discriminative control of appetitive behavior by pulse microwave radiation in rats. *In:* Biological effects of electromagnetic waves. Selected papers of the USNC/URSI Annual Meetings, Boulder, Colo., Oct. 20–23, 1976, HEW Pub. No. [FDA] 77-8010, *1*, pp. 238–247.)

contention that rats acoustically detected the microwave pulses and generalized the microwave-induced sound and conventional acoustic cues.

ELECTROPHYSIOLOGICAL RECORDINGS

Behavioral investigations have suggested that microwave pulses interact with the auditory system and are perceived by laboratory rats in the same manner as conventional acoustic pulses. It should be noted, however, that behavioral studies rely on inference rather than direct measurement of the anatomical or physiological entities involved in microwave pulse interaction with the auditory system. They should therefore be complemented by direct observations in identifying the anatomical or physiological substrates. Such observations, which would contribute to definition of the characteristics, mechanisms, and site of transduction of this phenomenon, have been made through direct neurophysiological investigations.

On numerous sites along the auditory pathway, electrodes may be inserted to record electrical potentials arising in response to acoustic pulse stimulation. If the electrical potentials elicited by microwave pulses exhibited characteristics akin to those evoked by conventional acoustic pulses, this would vigorously support the behavioral findings that pulsed microwaves are acoustically perceptible. Furthermore, if microwave-evoked potentials were recorded from each of those loci, this would lend further support to the contention that microwave auditory phenomena are mediated at the periphery, as is the sensation of a conventional acoustic stimulus.

A large amount of accumulated electrophysiological evidence demonstrates that auditory responses are elicited by microwave pulses and that these responses are similar to those evoked by conventional acoustic pulses. Recordings have been made from the surface of the vertex and from the central auditory system itself (Lin, 1978, 1980, 1981; Chou et al., 1982).

Brainstem-Evoked Responses

The auditory brainstem-evoked responses, as recorded from the vertex with surface electrodes, represent the volume conduction of electrical events that occur in the auditory brainstem nuclei within the first 8 ms after onset of an acoustic stimulus. The resemblance of brainstem potentials evoked by microwave and acoustic pulses from the vertex of a cat scalp is shown in Figure 12-3. To facilitate visual comparison, stimulus artifacts have been omitted; only the responses are plotted. Microwave-evoked responses are always seen immediately after delivery of stimuli, without the familiar propagation delay associated with acoustic waves that must travel at a much slower speed in air. The responses are not exactly the same because of the considerably higher frequency content in microwave-induced sound compared with the acoustic pulse stimulus. Similarly, comparable brainstem auditory responses have been recorded from cats (Cain and Rissman, 1978; Lin et al., 1978, 1979), guinea pigs (Chou et al., 1975; Chou and Guy, 1979) and rats (Chou et al., 1985). These results show that the same pathway through the central auditory nervous system is activated by both microwave and acoustic pulses.

Furthermore, as shown in Figure 12-4, when the external auditory meatus of guinea pigs was blocked by cotton balls soaked in mineral oil, the amplitude of microwave-evoked brainstem potentials remained unaltered. Filling the middle ear cavity with mineral oil, which impeded ossicular movement, had no effect on microwave-evoked responses. Furthermore, disablement of both tympanic membrane and middle ear ossi-

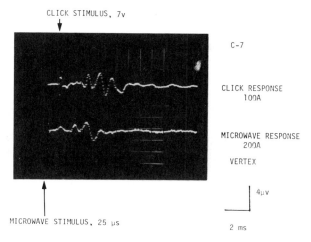

CLICK STIMULUS, 7v

C-7

CLICK RESPONSE
100A

MICROWAVE RESPONSE
200A

VERTEX

4µv

MICROWAVE STIMULUS, 25 µs

2 ms

Figure 12-3 Brainstem potentials evoked by microwave and acoustic pulses.

cles led only to a reduced brainstem potential (Chou and Galambos, 1979). This indicated that the middle ear was not the route primarily used by microwave-induced sound and that the decrease in brainstem potential probably derived from a small relative motion between the stapes and the cochlear oval window. In contrast, destroying the cochlea by perforating the round window would completely abolish the response (Taylor and Ashleman, 1974; Chou and Galambos, 1979).

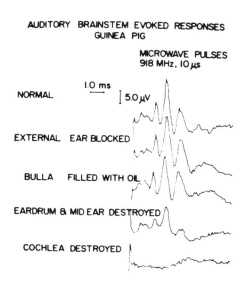

AUDITORY BRAINSTEM EVOKED RESPONSES
GUINEA PIG

MICROWAVE PULSES
918 MHz, 10 µs

1.0 ms

NORMAL

5.0 µV

EXTERNAL EAR BLOCKED

BULLA FILLED WITH OIL

EARDRUM & MID EAR DESTROYED

COCHLEA DESTROYED

Figure 12-4 Effect of middle ear manipulation on microwave pulse–evoked auditory brainstem potential in guinea pig. (From Chou, C.K., and Galambos, R. [1979]. *J. Microwave Power* 14:321–326.)

Central Auditory Pathway

Microwave-evoked neural electrical activities have been recorded from five levels of the central auditory system: primary auditory cortex, medial geniculate nucleus, inferior colliculus nucleus, lateral lemniscus nucleus, and superior olivary nucleus. Microwave energy was applied to the head with horn antennas, aperture radiators, and direct contact applicators operating between 900 and 3000 MHz. Rectangular pulses with pulse widths of 1 to 32 μs were presented at repetition rates of 1 to 100 pps and at peak incident power densitites on the order of 1 W/cm^2.

Recordings from electrodes placed on the primary auditory cortexes of anesthetized cats (Taylor and Ashleman, 1974) and guinea pigs (Chou et al., 1976a) after surgical removal of overlying soft tissue and bony structures showed remarkable similarity between microwave pulse– and acoustic pulse–evoked signals (Figure 12-5). The acoustic stimuli were rectangular pulses 10 μs in duration. Essentially identical activities also were recorded from the medial geniculate nucleus (Guy et al., 1973, 1975; Chou et al., 1976a,b; Lin et al., 1978), from the inferior colliculus nucleus (Cain and Rissman, 1978; Lin et al., 1978, 1979), from the lateral lemniscus nucleus (Lin et al., 1978, 1979), and from the superior olivary nucleus of cats (Lin et al., 1978, 1979) in response to both microwave and acoustic pulse stimulation (Figure 12-6).

By modifying the surgical procedure used to record electrical activities from the central auditory elements, Taylor and Ashleman (1974) recorded compound action potentials from the auditory branch of the eighth cranial nerve and from the cochlear round window of cats. As

AUDITORY CORTEX

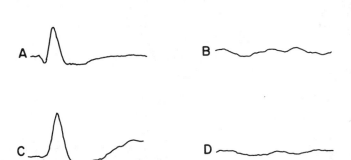

Figure 12-5 Cortical response in cat to acoustic (**A** and **B**) and microwave (**C** and **D**) pulses before and after cochlear ablation. (From Taylor, E.M., and Ashleman, B.T. [1974]. *Brain Res.* 74:201–208.)

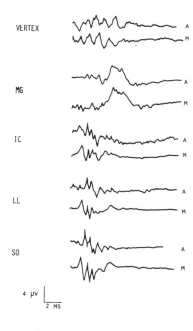

Figure 12-6 Acoustic and microwave pulse–evoked responses in brainstem of cats. *MG*, Medial geniculate; *IC*, inferior colliculus; *LL*, lateral lemniscus; *SO*, superior olive. (From Lin, J.C., et al. [1979]. *J. Microwave Power* 14:291–296.)

can be seen from Figure 12-7, the classical components of the auditory nerve action potentials are present in both the microwave and acoustic cases. These results suggest that the site of initial interaction of pulse-modulated microwave energy with the auditory system is at or outside the cochlea.

This interpretation finds support in systematic studies of responses from brainstem nuclei after successive production of coagulative lesions in the central auditory loci (Lin et al., 1978, 1979). The effect of brainstem lesions on electrical potentials recorded from the lateral lemniscus nucleus in response to microwave pulse stimulation is shown in Figure 12-8.

RECORDINGS FROM AUDITORY NERVE

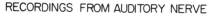
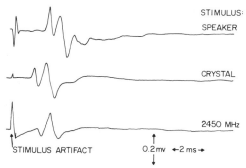

Figure 12-7 Auditory nerve response of cat irradiated with acoustic and microwave pulses. (From Lin, J.C. [1978]. Microwave auditory effects and applications. Springfield, Ill., Charles C Thomas, Publisher.)

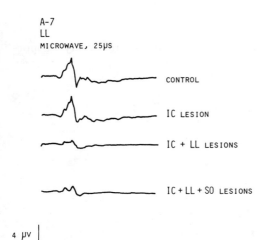

A-7
LL
MICROWAVE, 25μS

CONTROL

IC LESION

IC + LL LESIONS

IC + LL + SO LESIONS

4 μV

2 MS

Figure 12-8 Effect of brainstem lesions on evoked potentials from lateral lemniscus (*LL*). *IC*, Inferior colliculus; *SO*, superior olive.

Lesions in proximal nuclei (inferior colliculus) had negligible influence on the response recorded from the lateral lemniscus nucleus. However, the response disappeared after lesions were made in the distal nucleus (superior olive), thus confirming the peripheral nature of the primary site of transduction.

Neural responses at the periphery to 915 MHz microwave pulses have been studied in cats by recording extracellular action potentials of individual neurons, or "units," in the eighth nerve and in the cochlear nucleus with glass microelectrodes. Post–stimulus time histograms (PSTHs) of the firing of eighth nerve auditory fibers and cochlear nucleus units show time-locked microwave responses having patterns similar to those for acoustic clicks (Lebovitz and Seaman, 1977a,b). For small microwave pulse amplitudes, the microwave response depends monotonically on pulse amplitude but nonmonotonically on pulse duration (Lebovitz and Seaman, 1977a,b; Seaman and Lebovitz, 1987). The results of single-unit studies not only support a microwave interaction site at or peripheral to the cochlea, but are also consistent with the thermoelastic expansion theory, as shown later in the chapter.

It should be noted that the specific absorption rate (SAR) and SA thresholds per pulse of 6 W/kg and 0.5 to 4 mJ/kg, respectively, for single-unit responses are the lowest found in previously reported studies. Moreover, auditory units with lower characteristic frequencies (a few kilohertz) appeared to be more responsive to microwave pulses than were units with higher characteristic frequencies. This finding seems inconsistent with the theoretical prediction of a high-frequency response in cats and guinea pigs (Lin, 1978) and also in disagreement with the cochlear microphonic data obtained from animals (Chou et al., 1975, 1976a,b). However, the single-unit experiments used pulses longer than 20 μs. Since the frequency bandwidth of microwave-induced sound is inversely proportional to pulse width, longer pulses would indeed give rise to predominantly lower-frequency signals. Furthermore, the results of Tyazhelov et al. (1979) showed that two observers with a high-frequency auditory limit of 10 kHz could not sense shorter microwave pulses but were able to perceive the longer pulses. Thus the results of single-unit recordings in cats are consistent with both theory and human experience when the pulse widths are long.

These electrophysiological activities recorded from central and peripheral portions of the auditory system imply that microwave and acoustic pulses affect the auditory system in the same manner and suggest that a similar mode of perception is operating both in the microwave and the acoustic cases. This interpretation has been augmented by the observations in systematic studies of loci involved through production of lesions in ipsilateral auditory nuclei and bilateral ablation of the cochlea, the known first stage of transduction for acoustic energy. Successive lesion production in the inferior colliculus, lateral lemniscus, and superior olivary nuclei resulted in a drastic reduction of response amplitudes recorded from these nuclei. The effect of cochlear disablement was abolishment of all potentials recorded from three levels of the auditory nervous system (primary auditory cortex, brainstem nuclei, eighth nerve) evoked by both microwave and acoustic energy. These data indicate that the site of initial interaction of pulse-modulated microwave energy with the auditory system is distal to the cochlea.

Cochlear Microphonics

A peripheral interaction should involve displacement of the tissues in the head with resultant dynamic effect in the cochlear fluids and nervous system consequences that have been well described for the acoustic case. However, cochlear microphonics, the signature of mechanical distortion of cochlear hair cells, eluded investigators for a long time. This led to the persistent speculation that microwave pulses, in contrast to conventional acoustic pulses, might not act on any receptor before acting directly on the inner ear apparatus.

The existence of cochlear microphonics has been elegantly demonstrated in cats and guinea pigs (Chou et al., 1975, 1976a,b, 1982) with cylindrical waveguide cavities that efficiently coupled impinging microwave energy into the heads of experimental animals. Figure 12-9 illustrates the evoked potentials recorded from the round window of a guinea pig. The cochlear microphonic preceded the well-defined N_1 and N_2 auditory nerve responses and immediately followed the microwave pulse arti-

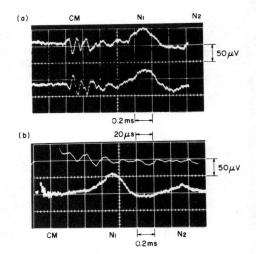

Figure 12-9 Cochlear microphonics recorded from round window of guinea pig. **A,** Acoustic pulse stimulation. **B,** Microwave pulse stimulation including time expansion of initial 200 μs. (From Chou, C.K., et al. [1975]. *J. Microwave Power 10*:361–367.)

fact. After death of the animal, whether by anoxia or by drug overdose, microwave-evoked nerve responses disappeared before the cochlear microphonic. Similar disappearance occurred for acoustically evoked cochlear microphonics. Thus the microwave auditory phenomenon is accompanied by mechanical disturbance of hair cells and is mediated by an electromechanical interaction initiated distal to the cochlea.

MECHANISM OF INTERACTION

Several transduction mechanisms involving mechanical displacement of the cranium for microwave-induced auditory sensation have been suggested (Foster and Finch, 1974; Sharp et al., 1974; Guy et al., 1975; Lin, 1976a, 1978). A comparison of the most likely candidates revealed that thermoelastic expansion is the most effective mechanism, since pressure generated by thermoelastic stress in brain tissues may be one to three orders of magnitude greater than the other possible mechanisms (Table 12-2). A detailed mathematical analysis of the acoustic signals generated in the heads of animals and humans exposed to plane-wave microwave pulses has been developed by considering an equivalent spherical head consisting only of brain matter (Lin, 1976b, 1977a,b, 1978). It suggested that the minuscule (10^{-6} °C) but rapid (10 μs) rise of temperature in the head as a result of microwave energy absorption creates thermoelastic expansion of tissue matter, which then launches an acoustic wave of pressure that travels to the cochlea and is detected by the hair cells there.

The mathematical analysis has been generalized through a thermo-

TABLE 12-2 Comparison of Three Physical Mechanisms of Acoustic Energy Production in Semi-Infinite Models of Biological Materials Exposed to Short Microwave Pulses*

Material	Electrostriction/ radiation pressure	Thermoelastic stress/radiation pressure	Thermoelastic stress/ electrostriction
Brain	10.67	1301	122
Muscle	15.67	1290	82
Water	26.00	1225	47

* Given as the relative amplitude waves generated by impinging 2450 MHz microwave pulses.

dynamic formulation that has given rise to a set of nonlinear differential equations (Guo et al., 1984). If isotropic elastic properties of the medium- and small-amplitude waves are assumed, the fundamental equations governing the behavior of microwave-induced thermoelastic pressure waves may be reduced to a simple linear equation similar to that used in the above-mentioned solution.

Acoustic Frequency

The thermoelastic theory (Lin, 1976b, 1977a,b, 1978) describes the acoustic waves (frequency, pressure, and displacement) generated in the head as functions of brain size and characteristics of impinging and absorbed microwave energies. It shows that there are an infinite number of resonant frequencies, each corresponding to a mode of vibration of the brain-equivalent sphere. The frequency of vibration was found to be independent of microwave absorption pattern; it was only a function of the equivalent radius and acoustic properties of the brain. Specifically, the frequencies of vibration under the two boundary conditions are given by

$$f_{cm} = \frac{(k_m a)v}{2a\pi}, \qquad \begin{array}{l} k_m a = 4.49, 7.73. 10.9, \ldots \\ \text{for constrained surface} \end{array} \tag{1}$$

$$f_{sm} = \frac{mv}{2a}, \qquad \begin{array}{l} m = 1, 2, 3, \ldots. \\ \text{for stress-free surface} \end{array} \tag{2}$$

where v is the velocity of acoustic wave propagation and a is the radius of the brain-equivalent sphere (Lin, 1977a,b). The fundamental frequencies of vibration are given by:

$$f_{c1} = 0.72 \ v/a \quad \text{for constrained surface} \tag{3}$$

or

$$f_{s1} = 0.50 \ v/a \quad \text{for stress-free surface} \tag{4}$$

These results suggest that the frequency of sound perceived by a subject is the same regardless of the frequency of the impinging microwave.

It is observed readily from Eq. 1 to 4 that the frequency of sound is a function only of equivalent radius of the head and of brain tissue acoustic properties. It does not depend at all on characteristics of microwave absorption. Clearly, the acoustic pitch perceived by a given subject is the same regardless of the frequency of the impinging microwave radiation.

The fundamental frequencies computed using the data given in Table 12-3 are shown in Figure 12-10. The frequency varies inversely with radius; the smaller the radius, the higher the frequency. The fundamental frequency predicted by the constrained-surface formulation is about 50% higher than that computed from the stress-free expression. Since the head is not perfectly spherical and the surface may best be described as semirigid, the actual values for the fundamental frequency of sound may reside somewhere between the two curves shown in Figure 12-10.

Pressure and Displacement

The explicit expressions for the acoustic waves generated in a spherical model of the head as irradiated by rectangular pulses (t_0 = pulse width) of microwave energy have been presented elsewhere (Lin, 1976b, 1977a,b, 1978). Briefly, it was shown that the pattern of absorbed energy inside a head-equivalent sphere may be approximated by the spherically symmetrical function $\sin(N\pi r/a)/(N\pi r/a)$ for many combinations of sizes and frequencies, where r is the radial variable, a is the radius of the sphere, and N is the number of standing wave–like oscillations in the absorption pattern.

On the basis of the symmetry of the absorption pattern and the

---

TABLE 12-3 Thermoelastic Properties of Brain Matter Used for Computation

Specific heat, c_h	0.88 cal/g $-$ ° C (0.21 J/g $-$ ° C)
Density, ρ	1.05 g/cm^3
Coefficient of linear thermal expansion, α	4.1 × 10^{-5}/° C
Lame's constant, λ	2.24 × 10^{10} dyn/cm^2
Lame's constant, μ	10.52 × 10^3 dyn/cm^2
Bulk velocity of propagation, c_1	1.46 × 10^5 cm/s

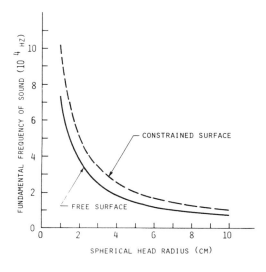

Figure 12-10 Fundamental frequencies of microwave pulse–induced sound inside brain-equivalent sphere.

assumption that thermal conduction does not take place within the short period of time under consideration, the inhomogeneous thermoelastic equation of motion was solved for the acoustic wave parameters under both stress-free and constrained-surface conditions. In particular, it was found that under the stress-free assumption the displacement is given by

$$u_f = u_0\, Qt + \sum_{m=1}^{\infty} A_m j_1(k_m r)(\sin\omega_m t/\omega_m), \qquad 0 \leq t \leq t_0 \tag{5}$$

$$u_f = u_0\, Qt_0 + \sum_{m=1}^{\infty} A_m j_1(k_m r)[(\sin\omega_m t)/\omega_m$$
$$- \sin\omega_m (t - t_0)/\omega_m], \qquad t \geq t_0 \tag{6}$$

where j_1 denotes Bessel function of the first kind and t_0 is the width of the pulse. The radial pressure is

$$\sigma_f = 4\mu u_0\, St + \sum_{m=1}^{\infty} A_m k_m M_m(\sin\omega_m t/\omega_m), \qquad 0 \leq t \leq t_0 \tag{7}$$

$$\sigma_f = 4\mu u_0 St_0 + \sum_{m=1}^{\infty} A_m k_m M_m[(\sin\omega_m t)/\omega_m$$
$$- \sin\omega_m (t - t_0)/\omega_m], \qquad t \geq t_0 \tag{8}$$

where

$$u_0 = (I_0/\rho c_h)[\beta/(\lambda + 2\mu)] \tag{9}$$

$$Q = (a/N\pi)j_1(N\pi r/a) \pm [4\mu/(3\lambda + 2\mu)][r/(N\pi)^2] \tag{10}$$

$$S = \pm(1/N\pi)^2 - j_1(N\pi r/a)/(N\pi r/a) \tag{11}$$

$$M_m = [(\lambda + 2\mu)j_0(k_m r) - 4\mu j_1(k_m r)/(k_m r)] \tag{12}$$

$$A_m = \mp 2u_0 a/(N\pi)^2\{[4\mu/(3\lambda + 2\mu)][j_2(k_m a)/(k_m a) \\ - k_m a j_0(k_m a)/[(k_m a)^2 - (N\pi)^2]\}/\{[j_1(k_m a)]^2 - j_0(k_m a)j_2(k_m a)\} \tag{13}$$

and β, λ and μ represent thermoelastic properties of tissue for $k_m a = m\pi$. In cases where $m\pi = N\pi$, Eq. 13 reduces to

$$A_m = -u_0 a/(N\pi)[1 + 24u/(3\lambda + 2\mu)(1/N\pi)^2] \tag{14}$$

The upper sign in Eq. 10 to 13 and in subsequent expressions denotes $N = 1,3,5, \ldots$, and the lower sign denotes $N = 2,4,6, \ldots$.
The radial displacement for constrained surfaces is given by

$$u = u_0 Dt + \sum_{m=1}^{\infty} A_m j_1(k_m r)(\sin\omega_m t/\omega_m), \qquad 0 < t < t_0 \tag{15}$$

$$u = u_0 Dt_0 + \sum_{m=1}^{\infty} A_m j_1(k_m r)[\sin\omega_m t/\omega_m \\ - \sin\omega_m(t - t_0)/\omega_m], \qquad t > t_0 \tag{16}$$

and the pressure is

$$\sigma = u_0 Gt + \sum_{m=1}^{\infty} A_m k_m H_m(\sin\omega_m t/\omega_m), \qquad 0 < t < t_0 \tag{17}$$

$$\sigma = u_0 Gt_0 + \sum_{m=1}^{\infty} A_m k_m H_m[\sin\omega_m t/\omega_m \\ - \sin\omega_m(t - t_0)/\omega_m], \qquad t > t_0 \tag{18}$$

where

$$D = (1/N\pi)[aj_1(N\pi r/a) \mp (r/N\pi)], \tag{19}$$

$$G = -(4\mu a/N\pi r)j_1(N\pi r/a) \mp (1/N\pi)^2(3\lambda + 2\mu) \tag{20}$$

$$H_m = (\lambda + 2\mu)j_0(k_m r) - (4\mu/k_m r)j_1(k_m r) \tag{21}$$

$$A_m = \pm 2u_0 a(1/N\pi)^2\{(1/k_m a)j_2(k_m a) \pm k_m a j_0(k_m a)/[(k_m a)^2 \\ - (N\pi)^2]\}/\{[j_1(k_m a)]^2 - j_0(k_m a)j_2(k_m a)\} \tag{22}$$

It should be noted that the displacement and pressure under both stress-free and constrained-surface conditions would experience a transient buildup, which increases almost linearly with time and lasts for the duration of the pulse width. In addition, there would be an infinite series of harmonic contributions to the displacement and pressure inside the brain-equivalent sphere. Both these quantities are proportional to peak power density and therefore would increase monotonically with peak power absorption or SAR. The dependence on pulse width is more involved and nonmonotonic in general. For short pulses ($\omega_m t_o \ll 1$), however, the thermoelastic pressure wave in the head model is nearly proportional to the product of power density and pulse width or energy density per pulse.

Extensive numerical computations have shown that, although the resultant waveforms are qualitatively similar, both pressures and displacements computed on the basis of the constrained-surface formulation are consistently higher than those calculated with the stress-free expressions. The following presentation is therefore specifically related to the constrained-boundary expressions given by Eq. 15 to 22.

Figures 12-11 and 12-12 show the pressure and displacement at $r = 0$, 1, and 2 cm for a sphere of 2 cm radius that simulates the head of a guinea pig under 2450 MHz radiation. In this case the approximate microwave absorption pattern is obtained by setting $N = 3$. These waveforms are evaluated for $t_0 = 10$ μs. The pressure is highest at the center of the head and has a maximum value of 4.08 dyn/cm^2 for a peak absorption rate of 1 W/g (which corresponds to a power density of 445 mW/cm^2 of incident radiation [Johnson and Guy, 1972]) at the end of the pulse and then oscillates around a constant average value in the absence of elastic damping. As expected, the displacement is zero both at the center and at the surface of the sphere for the constrained-boundary condition. The peak displacement at $r = 1$ cm is about 2.16×10^{-13} m. A high-frequency component is superimposed on the fundamental frequency, which correlates perfectly with that shown in Figure 12-10.

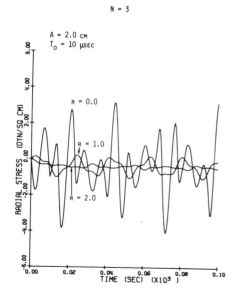

Figure 12-11 Sound pressure generated in 2 cm radius, brain-equivalent sphere exposed to 2450 MHz microwave at peak absorption rate of 1 W/g.

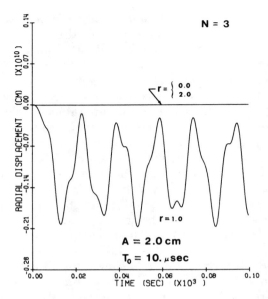

Figure 12-12 Displacement produced in 2 cm radius, brain-equivalent sphere (see Figure 12-11).

The peak pressure and displacement at $r = 0$, 1.5, and 3 cm for a 3 cm sphere, which simulates the head of a cat exposed to 2450 MHz radiation, are illustrated in Figures 12-13 and 12-14. In this case the approximate microwave absorption pattern is obtained by setting $N = 6$. Again, the pressure is highest at the center and has a value of 3.69 dyn/cm^2 for a peak absorption rate of 1 W/g or 589 mW/cm^2 of incident radiation. The displacement in the model of the cat's head is about 1.51×10^{-13} m. The fundamental frequency of oscillation obtained from Figure 12-13 agrees well with that given in Figure 12-10.

For a 5 cm sphere that simulates the head of an infant exposed to 915 MHz radiation, the peak pressure at the center is 9.61 dyn/cm^2 as shown in Figures 12-15 and 12-16. This curve was obtained by letting $N = 3$ in the approximated microwave absorption pattern. The displacement in this case is approximately 9.34×10^{-13} m for a peak absorption of 1 W/g and an incident power density of 1.25 W/cm^2. As before, the pulse width is assumed to be 10 μs. Again, good agreement is found between the fundamental frequency of mechanical oscillation and that predicted in Figure 12-10 for a 5 cm sphere.

Figures 12-17 and 12-18 present the pressure and displacement in a 7 cm sphere that simulates the head of an adult human irradiated by

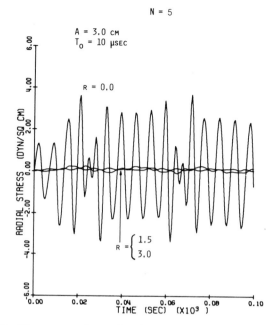

Figure 12-13 Microwave pulse–induced sound pressure in 3 cm radius, brain-equivalent sphere (see Figure 12-11).

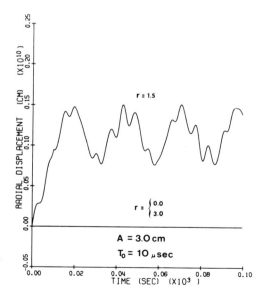

Figure 12-14 Microwave pulse–induced displacement in 3 cm radius, brain-equivalent sphere (see Figure 12-11).

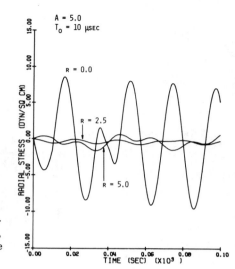

Figure 12-15 Microwave pulse–generated sound pressure in 5 cm radius, brain-equivalent sphere (see Figure 12-11).

915 MHz microwaves. Again, the pulse width is 10 μs and the peak absorption is 1 W/g, which corresponds to 2.18 W/cm^2 of incident plane-wave power. The calculated peak pressure is 6.82 dyn/cm^2, and the displacement is about 3.97×10^{-13} m.

　　Table 12-4 is a summary of peak pressures and displacements in four animals irradiated by 10 μs pulses at the same level of absorbed

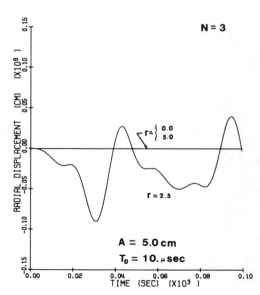

Figure 12-16 Microwave pulse–generated displacement in 5 cm radius, brain-equivalent sphere (see Figure 12-11).

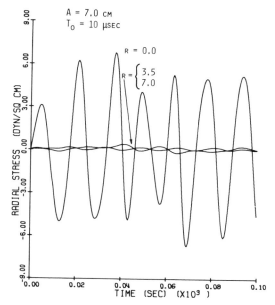

Figure 12-17   Microwave pulse–produced sound pressure in 7 cm, brain-equivalent sphere (see Figure 12-11).

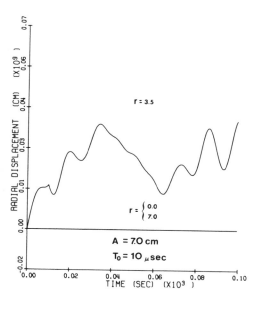

Figure 12-18 Microwave pulse–produced displacement in 7 cm radius, brain-equivalent sphere (see Figure 12-11).

TABLE 12-4   Peak Pressure and Displacement in Spherical Head Models Irradiated with 10 µs Rectangular Microwave Pulses at a Peak Adsorption Rate of 1 W/g

Sphere radius (cm)	Microwave frequency (MHz)	Species	Pressure (dyn/cm²)	Displacement (10^{-11} cm)	Incident power (mW/cm²)
2	2450	Guinea pig	4.08	2.16	445
3	2450	Cat	3.69	1.51	589
5	918	Human infant	9.61	9.34	1282
7	918	Human adult	6.82	3.97	2183

energy. The incident power density and the frequency differ according to the species involved. Although the pulse width and peak absorption rate are the same in each case, the pressure and displacement differ considerably.

The computed pressure as a function of pulse width is shown in Figures 12-19 and 12-20 for a 3 cm radius sphere exposed to 2450 MHz radiation and for a 7 cm radius sphere exposed to 915 MHz radiation, respectively. The curves are evaluated at an absorbed microwave energy density rate of 1000 kW/kg. The microwave-induced pressure peaks around 2 µs for the first case and around 5 µs for the second case and falls off rapidly for shorter pulse widths in both cases. Its decrease for

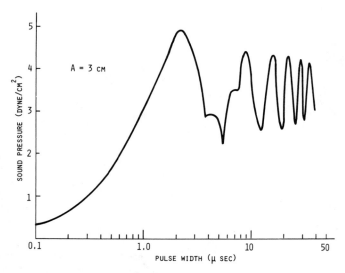

Figure 12-19 Computed pressure as function of pulse width for 3 cm radius, brain-equivalent sphere exposed to 2450 MHz microwave.

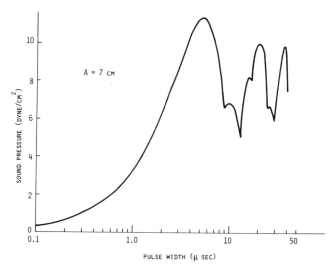

Figure 12-20 Computed pressure as function of pulse width for 7 cm radius, brain-equivalent sphere exposed to 915 MHz microwave.

longer pulse widths is characterized by some oscillating behavior. Therefore these values can be considered the optimum pulse width required for efficient conversion of pulsed microwave to acoustic energy in the head. These numerical results are qualitatively similar to the free-surface formulation, although the detailed dependence on pulse width differs somewhat for the two boundary conditions.

MEASUREMENT OF ACOUSTIC PRESSURE

In an attempt to elucidate the mechanism responsible for the microwave auditory effect, Sharp et al. (1974) found that carbon-impregnated polyurethane microwave absorber acted as a transducer from microwave energy to acoustic energy. They reported that, if the microwave absorber was placed between the observer and the source of pulsed microwave in an anechoic chamber, the apparent locus of the audible click moved from the observer's head to the absorber. Using a microphone and sound level meter, they were able to detect sounds produced by microwave pulses in absorbers as small as 4 mm square by 2 mm thick. Having examined the preceding evidence and available literature on the conversion of EM to acoustic energy by the surface heating of a liquid (White, 1963; Gournay, 1966), Foster and Finch (1974) suggested the conversion of absorbed microwave pulses to acoustic energy through thermal expansion as a likely mechanism for the microwave auditory effect. They observed that microwave pulses in water produced hydrophone-detectable transient acoustic pressures within the audible frequency range of 200 Hz to 20 kHz, with peak amplitude well above the expected threshold for perception by bone conduction. In addition, they used a large polystyrene container filled with 0.15 N potassium chloride solution at 25° C, which was exposed to 2450 MHz microwave pulses at a constant energy density per pulse of 800 mJ/m^2 while the pulse width was varied from 2 to 25 μs in a microwave anechoic chamber. For pulses shorter than 20 μs, peak pressure stayed nearly constant. However, the peak pressure was directly proportional to the peak power density for longer pulses.

Pressure Waves in Spherical Head Models

There have also been hydrophone measurements of microwave-induced pressure signals in spherical head models filled with brain-equivalent dielectric materials. The spherical models were composed of hemispherical voids carefully machined in 20.3 × 20.3 × 7.6 cm blocks of foamed polystyrene and filled with brain-equivalent phantom materials. The foamed polystyrene provided a stress-free boundary of the brain model. The phantom material has electromagnetic, mechanical, and thermal properties similar to those of brain tissues. It is made from a gelling agent, finely granulated polythylene powder, sodium chloride, and water and has a sonic propagation speed of 1600 m/s at room temperature (Olsen and Lin, 1981).

A spherical, barium titanate, piezoelectric hydrophone, 1 cm in diameter, was placed in the center of the model. Its output signal was displayed on an oscilloscope and photographed on film. The microwave pulses (1.1 GHz and 4 kW peak power) were applied to the spherical models with an open-ended model no. WR-650 waveguide placed in contact with the foam molds.

A typical series of experiments began with the application of a single microwave pulse to elicit an acoustic response. The "ringing" in the response after microwave irradiation gave the approximate fundamental mode frequency. Also, during the single-pulse irradiations an optimum pulse width that produced the highest-amplitude response was determined. Brief pulse trains, or bursts, consisting of three microwave pulses were then applied to the spherical model. The pulse repetition frequency was equal to the fundamental mode frequency. For each pulse train combination, the maximum postartifact hydrophone output voltage was recorded and graphed as a function of pulse repetition frequency. Figure 12-21 shows the output voltage of the hydrophone as a function of pulse repetition frequency for the 6 cm diameter model. A pulse repetition frequency of 25.5 kHz gave the highest acoustic pressure amplitude, indicating a resonant frequency of about 25.5 kHz.

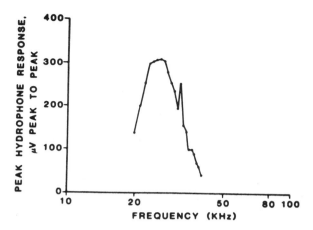

Figure 12-21 Amplitude of hydrophone response in 3 cm radius, spherical head model irradiated with 10 μs wide, 1.1 GHz microwave pulses at different frequencies.

In the 10 cm diameter sphere a single pulse produced a 16 kHz ringing signal with maximum acoustic pressure occurring at a microwave pulse width of 14 μs, which indicates a resonant frequency at 16 kHz. This is also revealed in the response "tuning curve," shown in Figure 12-22, which peaked at 16 kHz. In the 14 cm diameter model, single-pulse irradiation yielded a ringing frequency of slightly above 10 kHz, and a pulse width of 35 μs produced maximum acoustic response. Figure

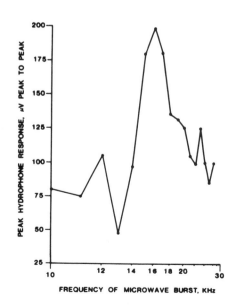

Figure 12-22 Amplitude response curve of 5 cm radius, brain-equivalent sphere irradiated with 10 μs wide, 1.1 GHz microwave pulses at indicated frequencies.

12-23 shows the results of irradiating the 14 cm model with various combinations of three-pulse bursts. Clearly a pulse repetition frequency of 11.5 kHz gave the highest-pressure amplitude, indicating a resonant frequency of around 11.5 kHz.

The preceding results demonstrate that microwave pulses can indeed generate measurable acoustic pressures in spherical models of human and animal heads. Furthermore, they show that appropriately selected pulse repetition frequencies stimulate acoustic resonance that can elevate the microwave-induced acoustic pressure by several fold. For example, the acoustic signal produced by a three-pulse burst was increased by threefold over the response to a single pulse. In general, the hydrophone response gradually increases from a low value to a peak amplitude at the resonant frequency and then falls off rapidly as the pulse repetition frequency further increases.

The measured resonant frequencies of pressure waves in the spherical models compared favorably with those predicted by the thermoelastic theory based on a homogeneous brain-equivalent sphere with stress-free boundaries (Figure 12-24). Specifically, measured resonant frequencies for 6, 10, and 14 cm diameter brain spheres were 25.5, 16, and 11.5 kHz, respectively. The corresponding fundamental frequencies of sound pressures calculated from the thermoelastic theory were 26.6, 16, and 11.4 kHz, respectively. The slight discrepancy at 6 cm (about 4%) probably occurred because the spherical brain had to be disengaged (with consequent changes in shape and dimensions) from the polystyrene foam to increase microwave coupling efficiency.

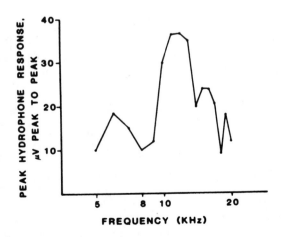

Figure 12-23 Amplitude response curve of 7 cm radius, brain-equivalent sphere irradiated with 10 μs wide, 1.1 GHz microwaves at different repetition frequencies.

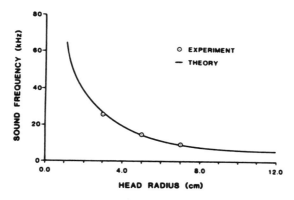

Figure 12-24 Comparison of measured and predicted frequencies of micro-wave-induced pressure waves in brain-equivalent spherical head models.

Pressure Waves in Animal Heads

Although these results lend support for the predicted thermoelastic signals inside the head, similar confirmation in animal preparations would be desirable. Pressure waves have been measured in brains of rats, cats, and guinea pigs irradiated with pulsed 2.450 and 5.655 GHz microwaves (Olsen and Lin, 1981, 1983). Pressure waves were sensed by a small disk hydrophone element composed of lead zirconate-titanate material electroplated on each side. The disk elements were 3.18 mm in diameter and 0.51 mm thick. The hydrophone signals were amplified and displayed on an oscilloscope.

Results of frequency response experiments in cats are shown in Figure 12-25. A peak in hydrophone outputs was observed at 39 kHz. Indeed, a sound wave near this frequency was expected on the basis of experimental data obtained in the study of microwave-induced cochlear microphonics (Chou et al., 1976b). Additional information concerning the nature of hydrophone signals was provided through on-line spectral analysis in rat experiments. The hydrophone output signals resembled those recorded from cats and guinea pigs, and the corresponding spectrum of each recording showed a rich harmonic content consisting of many modes of vibration (Olsen and Lin, 1983). That the records of the various subjects were not identical was not surprising because the transducer radiation pattern was not omnidirectional and because precise positioning of the device in terms of stereotaxic position and disk orientation was not attempted in these initial experiments.

Measurements of propagating pressure waves were made in brains of cats irradiated with pulsed microwaves (Lin et al., 1988). Single pulses of microwave (2 μs at 2.45 GHz) were produced with a microwave genera-

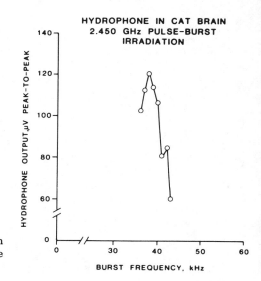

Figure 12-25 Frequency response from cat measured with small hydrophone transducer implanted in brain.

tor, which was controlled by an external pulse-forming circuit. The pulses were applied to the surface of the head with a direct-contact applicator (15 mm in diameter). The peak incident power of pulsed microwave was 15 kW. A hydrophone transducer was used to detect the pressure wave. The cylindrical lead zirconate-titanate ceramic element was enclosed in a waterproof Neoprene sheath (2 × 4 mm) and had a response of −130 dB (reference 1 V/μbar) for the pertinent range of frequencies (1 to 400 kHz). The directivity pattern was circular in the transverse plane at both 80 and 400 kHz. The hydrophone transducer was inserted stereotaxically through a matrix of holes drilled on the skull into the brain tissue of cats and advanced precisely to desired locations with a micromanipulator. Microwave-induced pressure waves detected by the transducer were conditioned with a high-gain amplifier and a bandpass filter having cutoff frequencies at 1 kHz and 1 MHz. The first 100 μs of response was displayed on an oscilloscope and photographed on film. In addition, a fast Fourier transform of the response was obtained with a digital oscilloscope.

Some typical hydrophone output waveforms are shown in Figure 12-26. Hydrophone responses detected in brain tissue at the same depth (27 mm) through five midline holes (separated by 1 cm) are shown in Figure 12-26, A. Signals detected at the same five holes but along a straight line from the applicator are shown in Figure 12-26, B. The time delay associated with wave propagation is obvious. The hydrophone outputs obtained at a single location but several depths in brain tissue and at the same depth but three separate locations are shown in Figure 12-26, C and D, respectively. The time delay between traces in these figures is not as evident, since the measurement points are at approxi-

CAT #1314 1V/div, 10μS/div 2450MHz MW 15KW 2μSec

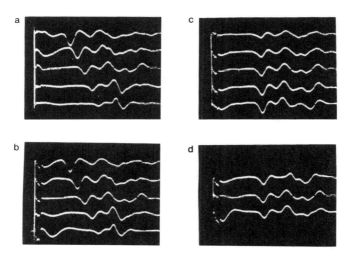

Figure 12-26 Representative recordings from hydrophone implanted inside cat brain.

mately the same distance from the center of the applicator and are located on the same wavefront. These results confirm the propagating nature of microwave-induced acoustic pressure waves in the cat brain.

A representative frequency response is shown in Figure 12-27. A distinct fundamental component occurred at 40 kHz, the predicted fundamental mode of a 5 cm diameter brain sphere (Lin, 1978). The measured frequency response showed, in addition, several higher-order components as suggested by prior theoretical and experimental investigations (Lin, 1977a,b; Olsen and Lin, 1983). The thermoelastic theory prescribed a frequency response that was a simple function of the head size and speed of pressure wave propagation independent of power deposition pattern.

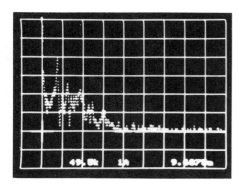

Figure 12-27 Frequency spectrum of microwave pulse–induced thermoelastic pressure wave in cat brain. Horizontal scale is 49.5 kHz per division.

TABLE 12-5 Speed of Thermoelastic Pressure Wave Propagation in Cat Brain Derived from Time-Delay Measurements

Distance (cm)	No. of samples	Speed (mean ± SD, m/s)
2.5–3.0	4	1463.75 ± 4.79
3.5–4.0	11	1532.78 ± 22.12
4.0–4.5	6	1554.92 ± 10.79
4.5–5.0	13	1498.03 ± 22.52
5.0–5.5	23	1531.33 ± 15.40
5.5–6.0	7	1531.09 ± 21.58
TOTAL	64	1522.77 ± 28.45

Thus it is interesting to observe the comparable frequency responses of Olsen and Lin's study and predictions based on a spherical head with symmetrical power deposition that peaked at the center.

The speed of thermoelastic pressure wave propagation in the cat brain may be derived from the measured time delay and known distance traveled. As given in Table 12-5, the mean speed of propagation was 1522.77 m/s. This was based on an ensemble of 64 measurements made at six different sets of distances. This number is slightly higher than that used in earlier calculations. The amplitude attenuation follows the well-known exponential law and has an attenuation coefficient of 0.56 Np/m. This value is higher than the 0.11 Np reported in the literature for ultrasound propagation in brain tissue (Dunn et al., 1969). Speed of propagation and attenuation coefficient are both functions of frequency and temperature in general. These experimental results indicate a microwave-induced pressure wave propagating in the cat brain with a speed of 1523 m/s. This speed of pressure wave propagation is close to that of conventional acoustic wave propagation in brain. These results lend further support to the notion that a thermoelastic pressure wave is induced in heads of humans and animals exposed to pulsed microwaves.

COMPARISON OF MEASURED AND PREDICTED CHARACTERISTICS

The acoustic pressure measurements described in the previous section for various-size spherical head models filled with brain-equivalent materials and for heads of rats, cats, and guinea pigs irradiated with pulsed microwave energy not only showed the existence of thermoelastic pressure waves but also indicated a unique acoustic frequency response that corresponded to a size-dependent mechanical resonance in the head as predicted by the thermoelastic theory of interaction. Although this helps to advance the theory, its credibility as the primary mechanism of interaction would be enhanced by corroborative observation from behavioral and physiological experimentation.

Figure 12-28 illustrates measured cochlear microphonic frequency in cats and guinea pigs (Chou et al. 1975, 1976a,b) and predicted fundamental acoustic frequency. It also includes the well-documented requirement for human perception of pulsed microwaves: the ability to hear sonic energy above 8 kHz (Cain and Rissman, 1978; Tyazhelov et al. 1979). Clearly there is agreement between observed and calculated sound frequency. Furthermore, the theory suggests that the frequency of sound perceived by a subject exposed to microwave pulses is the same regardless of the frequency of impinging microwaves and is independent of the pattern of absorbed energy. This is supported by the report that the same cochlear microphonics were produced by 918 and 2450 MHz in radiation (Chou et al. 1976a). Moreover, evoked brainstem potential measurements made by moving a small contact applicator around the head of a cat (Lin et al., 1982) showed remarkable preservation of amplitude and temporal relations (Figure 12-29).

Another body of support exists for the theory that predicted a sound pressure that initially increased with pulse width but soon reached a peak and then gradually oscillated to a lower value with further increases in pulse width. Several studies provided evidence from cats (Lin, 1980, 1981; Lin et al., 1982), guinea pigs (Chou and Guy, 1979), and humans (Tyazhelov et al., 1979). Figure 12-30 shows the calculated sound pressure amplitude and the variation of microwave-induced auditory brainstem

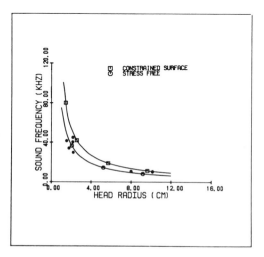

Figure 12-28 Comparison of experimental and theoretical fundamental frequency of sound induced in mammalian heads by pulsed microwaves.

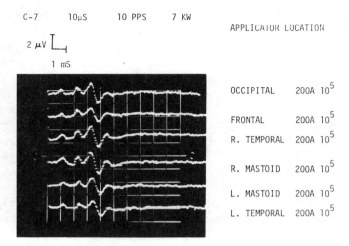

Figure 12-29 Brainstem potential evoked by microwave pulses delivered through small contact applicator positioned at different points of cat's head.

response in cats with the width of impinging microwave pulses while the peak power and repetition rate are kept constant (Lin, 1980). Similar relationships between relative loudness or sound pressure in guinea pigs and pulse width are given in Figure 12-31. This is equivalent to the observation that increasing the pulse width decreases the SAR required

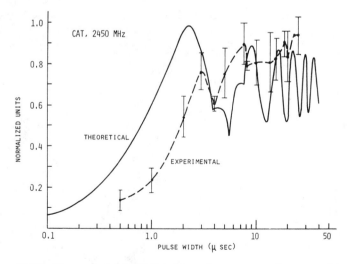

Figure 12-30 Comparison of calculated sound pressure and measured amplitude of brainstem evoked response in cats as function of microwave pulse width.

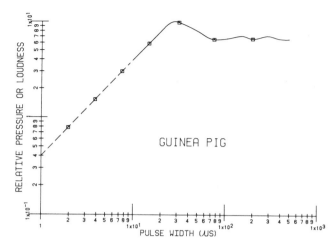

Figure 12-31 Sound pressure variation in head of guinea pig irradiated with microwave pulse of different widths; calculations from measured specific absorption rate threshold required to elicit auditory brainstem response (after Chou, C.K., and Guy, A.W. [1979]. *Radio Sci. 14*[suppl. 6]:193–197.)

to elicit a threshold auditory brainstem response. The characteristics of these curves are remarkably similar. The sound pressure, loudness, or brainstem response increased and then decreased as suggested by the theory. Furthermore, this nonmonotonic dependence of the response on pulse width was also seen in some single auditory neurons of cats (Lebovitz and Seaman, 1977a,b), especially for long pulse widths. Measurements in human subjects are presented in Figure 12-1. The calculated sound pressure at a comparable frequency is shown in Figure 12-20. The nonlinear dependence on pulse width is as evident as the similarity between these curves. The slight difference between the pulse widths at which sound pressure or loudness reached a maximum probably stemmed from a difference in microwave frequency and the actual and assumed head geometry and radii or circumferences. In general, sound pressure peaks at wider pulse widths for larger head radii (Lin, 1977a,b, 1978). Thus an impressive array of evidence substantiates the thermoelastic mechanism of microwave-induced auditory effect.

An experiment by Tyazhelov et al. (1979) showed that the pitch (frequency) of sound induced by microwave pulses of widths less than 50 μs persisted as the subject's head was lowered into a saline-filled tank, while the loudness diminished roughly in proportion to the depth of immersion. On complete immersion, auditory sensation disappeared. For pulse widths longer than 50 μs even partial immersion resulted in loss of perception. This was interpreted as being at odds with the thermoelastic theory. However, there is an explanation that seems to fit the data.

The theory suggests that the frequency of sound (pitch) evoked by microwave pulses is the same regardless of absorbed energy distribution and that the amplitude of sound (loudness) increases in proportion to the rate of energy absorption. Moreover, the amplitude of sound or loudness rises, peaks, and then falls as the pulse width increases from a low to a high value. Thus, as the subject's head was lowered into water, the absorbed energy and its distribution would have changed (decreased), but the acoustic property would have remained unaltered. (Since skull and water differ by a large margin, immersion would not alter the acoustic characteristic by an appreciable amount.) Therefore the perceptual quality of microwave-induced sound persisted while the loudness diminished in proportion to the depth of immersion. The reason for the disappearance of auditory sensation on complete immersion is that the impinging microwave energy was greatly attenuated by water before reaching the head. The small fraction that did reach the head was probably below the threshold of perception. The observation that even partial immersion resulted in loss of perception for pulse widths greater than 50 μs could be resolved by recalling that 50 μs was reported as being the optimum pulse width for auditory perception by the subjects. Hence, microwaves pulses of widths greater than 50 μs would not be so effective in eliciting an acoustic sensation and could easily be disrupted when the head was lowered partially into water. Clearly these findings would strengthen rather than weaken the thermoelastic theory of microwave auditory effect.

Tyazhelov et al. (1979) found in their beat frequency experiment that matching of microwave pulses (10 μs, 8000 pps) to a phase-shifted 8 kHz sinusoidal sound input resulted in loss of auditory perception, as the thermoelastic theory would suggest. However, cancellation also occurred when a 5000 pps train of pulses was properly phased with a 10 kHz sound signal. Seemingly some modification is necessary to account for this finding. It may turn out that the discrepancy was related to harmonic generation by the audio equipment.

The thermoelastic theory is apparently adequate to characterize the more salient aspects of the auditory effect occurring in heads of humans and animals exposed to pulsed microwaves. The existing theoretical calculations are based on assumptions made for mathematical simplicity. These assumptions include a head-equivalent homogeneous sphere filled only with brain tissue, exposure of the head model in isolation from its adjoining body, and absence of attenuation of the acoustic pressure wave in brain tissue. In fact, the precise dependence of the microwave auditory effect on parameters of the impinging radiation and the exact amplitude and frequency of the induced thermoelastic pressure wave inside the head can be determined only by rigorously solving the governing differential equation, which is highly nonlinear in general. Nevertheless, it should be mentioned that the simple theory is applicable to a host of physiological and psychophysical observations, as well as physical measurements made in phantom models. That it may be incomplete and thus require further extension to account for certain additional experimental findings or to satisfy the demands of scientific exactness should not detract from its fundamental role in explaining the microwave auditory phenomenon.

CONCLUSION

The preceding discussion of microwave auditory phenomena emphasizes demonstration of auditory responses and delineation of interactive mechanisms. This attention is warranted, since the effect is very different from that associated with responses to continuous wave irradiation—so much so, that it implies the possibility of significant neurophysiological interaction. The results described in this chapter document collectively that the auditory systems of animals and humans respond to pulsed microwaves. They leave little likelihood that microwave auditory phenomena arise from direct interaction of microwave pulses with the cochlear nerve or neurons at higher structures along the central auditory pathway. Rather, the pulsed microwave energy initiates a thermoelastic wave of pressure in brain tissue that travels to activate the inner ear receptors. Indeed, studies of the phenomenas' characteristics have reached the point that it is possible to specify with some precision the relationship between microwave parameters such as microwave frequency, peak power, pulse width and repetition rate, and induced sound pressure frequency, as well as perceived pitch and loudness. However, two highly pertinent questions remain. Do microwave auditory phenomena pose a health risk to an individual? Under what conditions does pulsed microwave exposure become a hazard?

The problem can be approached, in principle, from the equivalency of microwave and acoustic pulse-evoked responses and from the perspective of sound exposure of humans (Lin, 1980). The known effects of sound exposure can be divided into two types: auditory effects (effects of sound exposure on hearing) and nonauditory effects (the general physiological and psychological reactions). Unfortunately, there are few data regarding the effect on hearing of exposure to microwave pulses. The relationship between the sound exposure in air and microwave-induced hearing is unknown.

The nonauditory effects of sound exposure are quite subtle compared with the responses of the hearing apparatus. The reactions are in many aspects similar to general stress responses that can be elicited by such stimuli as pain and motion stress. Annoyance is the most widely reported nonauditory effect of sound exposure. In fact, criteria for limiting community noise are often based on the presence of annoyance reactions among exposed population groups (Rylander et al., 1976; Ahrlin and Ohrstrom, 1978; Krichagin, 1978). Although annoyance reaction has not been explicitly evaluated in humans, as mentioned earlier several studies have shown that laboratory rats find the microwave auditory effect sufficiently aversive that they actively avoid the exposure. Presumably, microwave-induced sound annoyed the animals, much as acoustic noise and impulses are annoying to humans.

Although it is unlikely that microwave auditory effects at threshold incident power density constitute a hazard, thermoelastic pressures generated by exposure at levels significantly higher than threshold are undoubtedly harmful to humans (Lin, 1989). However, neither the physiological nor the behavioral data are sufficient at present to permit a complete analysis of this problem. Studies that would be useful are behavioral investigations of animals exposed to pulsed microwaves, including effects on performance, and morphological examinations of the hearing apparatus, cerebral cells, and vasculature of exposed animal subjects.

An interesting and potentially useful application of microwave-induced thermoelastic pressure waves has been introduced in recent years (Caspers and Conway, 1982; Olsen, 1982; Olsen and Lin, 1983; Lin and Chan, 1984; Su and Lin, 1987; Chan and Lin, 1988). Reports have suggested the use of these waves as an imaging modality for biological tissue. In one system, designed to digitally acquire and process thermoelastic pressure waves to yield projections of body tissues, a two-dimensional array of piezoelectric transducers is positioned next to a particular body region and a pulsed microwave source beams a pulse or short sequence of pulses to the opposite side of the body (Olsen and Lin, 1983; Lin and Chan, 1984). A prototype system with a 20 × 20 array of piezoelectric transducers and a microcomputer-based, two-dimensional data acquisition and processing system has provided projections of phantom models of bone, muscle, and other tissue-equivalent materials with a spatial resolution better than 1 cm. A representative image of two 0.9 cm diameter test tubes filled with muscle- and fat-equivalent materials separated by a distance of 0.9 cm inside a water phantom is shown in Figure 12-32. Since materials inside the test tubes are homogeneous, the intensity difference in this threshold image depicts the difference in attenuation through each test tube (Chan and Lin, 1988). Computer-assisted tomographic images can be obtained by allowing either the phantom object or the source-receiver apparatus (gantry system) to rotate. Such a system is under development, and some preliminary results (Su and Lin, unpublished) suggest that filtered back-projection of 16 views can render cross-sectional images with sufficient resolution to permit imaging of absorption and thermoelastic expansion. Since thermoelastic wave formation is a

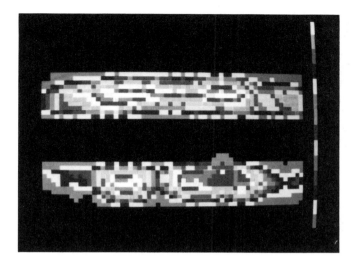

Figure 12-32 Thermoelastic image of fat- and muscle-equivalent phantom in water tank.

temperature-dependent process, a thermoelastic imaging system might be designed to yield estimates of temperature distribution inside biological bodies.

REFERENCES

AHRLIN, V., AND OHRSTROM, E. (1978). Medical effects of environmental noise on humans. *J. Sound Vibrat. 59*:79–87.

CAIN, C.A., AND RISSMAN, W.J. (1978). Mammalian auditory response to 3.0 GHz microwave pulses. *IEEE Trans. Biomed. Eng. 25*:288–293.

CASPERS, F., AND CONWAY, J. (1982). Measurement of power density in a lossy material by means of electromagnetically induced acoustic signals for non-invasive determination of spatial thermal absorption in connection with pulsed hyperthermia. *In*: Proceedings of the 12th European Microwave Conference, Helsinki, Finland, pp. 565–568.

CHAN, K.H., AND LIN, J.C. (1988). Microwave-induced thermoelastic tissue imaging. Presented at the Engineering in Medicine and Biology Society 10th Annual International Conference. New Orleans.

CHOU, C.K., GALAMBOS, R., GUY, A.W., AND LOVELY, R.H. (1975). Cochlear microphonics generated by microwave pulses. *J. Microwave Power 10*:361–367.

CHOU, C.K., GUY, A.W., and GALAMBOS, R. (1976a). Microwave-induced auditory response: cochlear microphonics. *In*: Johnson, C.C., and Shore, M.L. (eds.). Biological effects of electromagnetic waves 1. HEW Pub. No. FDA, 77-8010, pp. 89–103.

CHOU, C.K., GUY, A.W., AND GALAMBOS, R. (1976b). Microwave-induced cochlear microphonics in cats. *J. Microwave Power* 11:171–173.

CHOU, C.K., AND GALAMBOS, R. (1979). Middle-ear structures contribute little to auditory perception of microwave. *J. Microwave Power* 14:321–326.

CHOU, C.K., AND GUY, A.W. (1979). Microwave-induced auditory responses in guinea pigs: relationship of threshold and microwave-pulse duration. *Radio Sci. 14(suppl. 6)*:193–197.

CHOU, C.K., GUY, A.W., AND GALAMBOS, R. (1982). Auditory perception of radio-frequency electromagnetic fields. *J. Acoust. Soc. Am.* 71:1321–1334.

CHOU, C.K., YEE, K.C., AND GUY, A.W. (1985). Auditory response in rats exposed to 2,450 MHz electromagnetic fields in a circularly polarized waveguide. *Bioelectromagnetics* 6:323–326.

DUNN, F., EDMONDS, P.D., AND FRY, W.J. (1969). Absorption and dispersion of ultrasound in biological media. *In*: Schwan, H.P. (ed.). Biological engineering. New York, McGraw-Hill Book Co., pp. 205–332.

FOSTER, K.R., AND FINCH, E.D. (1974). Microwave hearing: evidence for thermoacoustic auditory stimulation by pulsed microwaves. *Science* 185:256–258.

FREY, A.H. (1961). Auditory system response to RF energy. *Aerospace Med.* 32:1140–1142.

FREY, A.H. (1962). Human auditory system response to modulated electromagnetic energy. *J. Appl. Physiol.* 17:689–692.

FREY, A.H. (1963). Some effects on human subjects of ultra-high-frequency radiation. *Am. J. Med. Electron.* 2:28–31.

FREY, A.H. (1967). Brain stem evoked response associated with low-intensity pulsed UHF energy. *J. Appl. Physiol.* 23:984–988.

FREY, A.H., AND MESSENGER, R. (1973). Human perception of illumination with pulsed UHF electromagnetic energy. *Science* 181:356–358.

GUO, T.C., GUO, W.W., AND LARSEN, L.E. (1984). Microwave-induced thermoelastic effect in dielectrics and its coupling to external medium-A thermodynamic formulation. *IEEE Trans. Microwave Theory Tech.* 32:835–843.

GOURNAY, L.S. (1966). Conversion of electromagnetic to acoustic energy by surface heating. *J. Acoust. Soc. Am.* 40:1322–1330.

GUY, A.W., CHOU, C.K., LIN, J.C., AND CHRISTENSEN, D. (1975). Microwave-induced acoustic effects in mammalian auditory systems and physical materials. *Ann. N.Y. Acad. Sci.* 247:194–218.

GUY, A.W., TAYLOR, E.M., ASHLEMAN, B., AND LIN, J.C. (1973). Microwave interaction with the auditory systems of humans and cats. *In*: Proceedings of the IEEE International Microwave Symposium, Boulder, Colo., pp. 231–232.

HJERESEN, D.L., DOCTOR, S.K., AND SHELTON, R.L. (1979). Shuttlebox side preference as mediated by pulsed microwave and conventional auditory cues. *In*: Proceedings of Symposium on Electromagnetic Fields in Biological Systems, International Microwave Power Institute, 78CHI438-1 MTT, Ottawa, pp. 194–214.

JOHNSON, C.C., AND GUY, A.W. (1972). Nonionizing electromagnetic wave effects in biological materials and systems. *Proc. IEEE* 60:692–718.

JOHNSON, R.B., MYERS, D.E., GUY, A.W., LOVELY, R.H., AND GALAMBOS, R. (1976). Discriminative control of appetitive behavior by pulse microwave radiation in rats, in biological effects of electromagnetic waves. Selected papers of the USNC/URSI Annual Meetings, Boulder, Colo., Oct. 20–23, 1976, HEW Pub. No. (FDA) 77-8010, *1*, pp. 238–247.

KRICHAGIN, V.J. (1978). Health effects of noise exposure. *J. Sound Vibrat.* 59:65–71.

LEBOVITZ, R.M., AND SEAMAN, R.L. (1977a). Microwave hearing: the response of single auditory neurons in the cat to pulsed microwave radiation. *Radio Sci.* 12(*suppl.* 6):229–236.

LEBOVITZ, R.M., AND SEAMAN, R.L. (1977b). Single auditory unit responses to weak pulsed microwave radiation. *Brain Res.* 126:370–375.

LIN, J.C. (1976a). Microwave auditory effect—a comparison of some possible transduction mechanisms. *J. Microwave Power* 11:77–87.

LIN, J.C. (1976b). Theoretical analysis of microwave-generated auditory effects in animals and man. *In:* Biological effects of electromagnetic waves, HEW Pub. No. (FDA) 77-8010, Washington, D.C., pp. 36–48.

LIN, J.C. (1977a). Further studies on the microwave auditory effects. *IEEE Trans. Microwave Theory Tech.* 29:938–943.

LIN, J.C. (1977b). On microwave-induced hearing sensation. *IEEE Trans. Microwave Theory Tech.* 25:605–613.

LIN, J.C. (1978). Microwave auditory effects and applications. Springfield, Ill., Charles C Thomas, Publisher.

LIN, J.C. (1980). The microwave auditory phenomenon. *Proc. IEEE* 68:67–73.

LIN, J.C. (1981). The microwave hearing effect. *In:* Illinger, K.H. (ed.). Biological effects of nonionizing radiation. ACS Symposium Series 157, Washington, D.C., American Chemical Society, pp. 317–330.

LIN, J.C. (1989). Pulsed radiofrequency field effects in biological systems. *In:* Lin, J.C. (ed.). Electromagnetic interaction with biological systems. New York, Plenum Publishing Corp., pp. 165–177.

LIN, J.C., AND CHAN, K.H. (1984). Microwave thermoelastic tissue imaging-system design. *IEEE Trans. Microwave Theory Tech.* 32:854–860.

LIN, J.C., MELTZER, R.J., AND REDDING, F.K. (1978). Microwave-evoked brain stem auditory responses. *Proc. San Diego Biomed. Symp.* 17:461–465.

LIN, J.C., MELTZER, R.J., AND REDDING, F.K. (1979). Microwave-evoked brain stem potentials in cats. *J. Microwave Power* 14:291–296.

LIN, J.C., MELTZER, R.J., AND REDDING, F.K. (1982). Comparison of measured and predicted characteristics of microwave-induced sound. *Radio Sci.* 17(*suppl.* 5):159S–163S.

LIN, J.C., SU, J.L., AND WANG, Y. (1988). Microwave-induced thermoelastic pressure wave propagation in the cat brain. *Bioelectromagnetics* 9:141–147.

OLSEN, R.G. (1982). Generation of acoustic images from the absorption of pulsed microwave energy. *In:* Powers, J.P. (ed.). Acoustic imaging. New York, Plenum Publishing Corp., pp. 53–59.

OLSEN, R.G., AND LIN, J.C. (1981). Microwave pulse-induced acoustic resonances in spherical head models. *IEEE Trans. Microwave Theory Tech.* 29:1114–1117.

OLSEN, R.G., AND LIN, J.C. (1983). Acoustic imaging of a model of a human hand using pulsed microwave irradiation. *Bioelectromagnetics* 4:397–400.

OLSEN, R.G., AND LIN, J.C. (1983). Microwave-induced pressure waves in mammalian brains. *IEEE Trans. Biomed. Eng.* 30:289–294.

RYLANDER, R., SORENSEN, S., AND KAJLAND S. (1976). Traffic noise exposure and annoyance reactions. *J. Sound Vibrat.* 47:237–242.

SEAMAN, R.L., AND LEBOVITZ, R.M. (1987). Auditory unit responses to single-pulse and twin-pulse microwave stimuli. *Hear. Res.* 26:105–116.

SHARP, J.C., GROVE, H.M., AND GANDHI, O.P. (1974). Generation of acoustic signals by pulsed microwave energy. *IEEE Trans. Microwave Theory Tech.* 22:583–584.

SU, J.L., AND LIN, J.C. (1987). Thermoelastic signatures of tissue phantom absorption and thermal expansion. *IEEE Trans. Biomed. Eng.* 34:178–182.

TAYLOR, E.M., AND ASHLEMAN, B.T. (1974). Analysis of the central nervous involvement in the microwave auditory effect. *Brain Res.* 74:201–208.

TYAZHELOV, V.V., TIGRANIAN, R.E., KHIZHNIAK, E.P., AND AKOEV, I.G. (1979). Some peculiarities of auditory sensations evoked by pulsed microwave fields. *Radio Sci.* 14(suppl. 6):259–263.

WHITE, R.M. (1963). Generation of elastic waves by transient surface heating. *J. Appl. Physics* 34:3559–3567.

13

Behavioral Effects of Electromagnetic Fields

JOHN A. D'ANDREA
JOHN O. de LORGE

Electromagnetic (EM) energy in the microwave portion of the spectrum has many diverse applications. Industrial uses include the welding of plastics, various annealing processes, and the drying of fabrics. In the telecommunications industry, ground and satellite links that use microwaves are expanding rapidly. The use of radar for military and civilian purposes also continues to increase. In medicine, microwave sources have utility both as diagnostic tools and as a therapeutic adjunct to produce hyperthermia. The wide use of microwave energy has meant a concomitant increase in the inadvertent exposure of workers in all these occupations and thus has caused some apprehension about adverse health effects. As the number of microwave emitters increases, so does the power output of many of these devices. Consequently, knowledge of the interaction of microwave energy with the human body has been important in understanding and defining hazards and formulating radiation safety standards. To evaluate the potential for health risks, scientists from a variety of disciplines have endeavored to provide a data base from which rational evaluations of health risks can be made.

A variety of behavior alterations in animals exposed to microwave radiation have been reported in recent years. Much of this research has been reviewed in several publications: the behavioral effects of microwave irradiation (Monahan and D'Andrea, 1985), the interaction of organisms (ranging from fishes to humans) with EM fields (O'Connor and Lovely, 1988), the influence of microwaves on thermoregulatory behavior (Adair, 1983), and the interaction of microwaves with psychoactive drugs (Lai et al., 1987). Newer research has provided different insights on the previous data. In this chapter we attempt to review and integrate findings reported in the scientific literature, to identify behavioral effects, behavioral thresholds, and the interaction between microwave field characteristics and the organism, and finally to resolve some issues important in assessing health risks.

The views expressed in this article are those of the authors and do not reflect the official policy or position of the Department of the Navy, the Department of Defense, or the U.S. Government.

BEHAVIORAL DESCRIPTIONS

Behavior can be viewed as a complex stream of activity comprising many components. Moving through the environment, getting food, escaping predators, and reproducing are only a few of these activities. However, the complexity of behavior does not mean that it is beyond rational analysis. Behavior must first be broken down and described in units suitable for experimental study. Hinde (1970) provided several descriptions of behavioral classification. Although the descriptive categories are not mutually exclusive, they have been useful in practice. Essentially, behavior is described by two methods. The first is the patterning and degree of muscular contractions. Grouped together, these patterns allow descriptions of such behaviors as scratching, sniffing, walking, and sleeping. For the purposes of this chapter these are called innate patterns. The second method has been termed description by consequence (Hinde, 1970). A rat pressing a lever does not refer simply to a predefined set of muscular contraction patterns necessary to press the lever, but also to the consequence, which in this case is closure of a microswitch. This is understood by the fact that some rats press the lever with the left paw, others with the right paw, and some perhaps with the chin. The advantage of this method of description is that several different patterns of muscular activity may be described objectively in terms of some action on or with respect to the environment. For our purposes these patterns are termed learned patterns. Although the two behavioral descriptions, innate and learned, provide a means for classifying behavior, they are not mutually exclusive and must be recognized as only methods of description.

In the last two decades, behavioral assessment has proved useful in delineating the effect of microwave radiation on living organisms. Behavior alterations after microwave exposure have been reported for the two categories of behavior. Additional descriptions of each type of behavior are offered in the following paragraphs.

Innate Behavior

Behaviors natural to an animal species are often said to be innate. For rodents, a species often used in microwave research, all types of motor activity such as locomotion, sniffing, grooming, scratching, and nest building are innate. Many such motor acts, occurring individually or in combination, constitute an animal's normal and spontaneous behavioral repertoire. Development of methods to quantify these innate behaviors has been difficult. Two approaches have been followed in recent years. The classical approach is *direct observation* to quantify individual and well-defined components of behavior. In the area of microwave bioeffects research, study of locomotor behavior with an open field test apparatus has been conducted most frequently. In this procedure the rat is placed in a large arena and a variety of innate motor behaviors are scored by one or more observers. Ambulation over grid squares painted on the floor of the arena and frequency of upward rearing by the rat are commonly recorded behaviors. Other observational techniques use time lapse photography of rats confined in small Plexiglas observation boxes (Norton, 1973). The film record is then scored for as many as 15 innate behaviors. The major drawback to the observational method of measuring innate behavior has been the large amount of time necessary to score behavior either directly or from the film record. This approach is labor intensive and can be used only with a few animals and a limited number of experimental treatments.

The second approach to quantifying innate behaviors uses many different *automated techniques* to record components of behavior. These techniques measure an animal's behavior either directly (by means of photocells, touch detectors, or ultrasonic detectors) or indirectly by monitoring the animal's living space (tilt cages, stablimeter cages, exercise wheels). Each automated device measures different individual components of behavior. Thus a better understanding of behavior may be gained by measuring innate behaviors in several automated devices and also using direct observational techniques.

Learned Behavior

Two traditional means are used to describe learned behavior. Certain classes of stimuli are known to elicit responses. A tap on the patellar tendon elicits a knee-jerk response, and light flashed in the eye elicits a pupillary contraction. These motor responses following the stimulus are known as *respondents*. The most famous respondent is the salivary response of a hungry dog on seeing food (Pavlov, 1927). Respondent behaviors are susceptible to classical or pavlovian conditioning in which neutral stimuli paired with the stimulus eventually elicit the respondent in the absence of the original eliciting stimulus.

Behaviors that are natural to a species and do not require an eliciting stimulus are also susceptible to conditioning. In this case the delivery of a stimulus close in time to the behavior may increase the probability of subsequent performance of that behavior. If it does, the stimulus is referred to as a *reinforcer*, and the process, known as instrumental conditioning, can be operationally defined as the arrangement of the environment so that certain motor acts are more likely to occur than others. This kind of behavior is established by arranging for the experimental animal to alter or affect its environment in some way by a response known as an *operant*. Researchers have conditioned a large variety of operants, such as lever pressing, pecking a lighted key, or breaking a photobeam. When the operant response occurs at an appropriate time, it changes the environment in some way by producing a reinforcer such as food or water or escaping electric shock (Honig and Staddon, 1977). Often visual or auditory exteroceptive stimuli are used as a signal of impending events. The arrangement of how stimuli and operant responses produce a reinforcer and interact with the particular operant is the reinforcement schedule. The arrangement and sequencing of stimuli and reinforcers is a schedule that produces schedule-controlled behavior. To gain control and minimize the effect of extraneous variables, investigators often rely on schedule-controlled behavior. When some aspects of the animal's environment are arranged according to the reinforcement schedule, control over feeding schedules, housing conditions, and so on, the effect of extraneous variables can be minimized and their interaction with microwave absorption reduced. Control over the extraneous variables is essential, especially for subsequent successful replications of the experiment.

EXPERIMENTAL DESIGN AND EXPOSURE METHODOLOGY

When an animal is exposed to a microwave field, the primary consequence is tissue heating. However, a microwave-induced behavioral effect is more than simply the transduction of electromagnetic to thermal energy. It is the interaction of the state of the organism and microwave energy absorption. The state of the organism includes its history, current ongoing behavior, and present environment. The history of the animal, the type and frequency of past experiences, dictates outcome behavior relative to the current environmental state (both external and internal) of the animal.

Research in the area of exposure to microwave fields can be divided arbitrarily into two categories: short-term and long-term exposure. Each category has been used to assess effects on both innate and learned behavior. Short-term exposures are typically 60 minutes or less and are given only once a day. Long-term exposures are given for 7 to 10 hours a day, ostensibly to mimic the human workday. Short-term exposures are generally used to identify health risks associated with intense microwave exposure and ensuing thermal effects, which overwhelm the natural thermoregulatory capability of the experimental animal. Long-term experiments are used to investigate the cumulative effects of exposure over weeks and months at relatively low microwave field power densities. In long-term studies the experimental animal's thermoregulatory capability prevents a deviation of body temperature from the normal range.

SHORT-TERM EXPOSURE STUDIES

A thermal burden from microwave exposure can cause behavioral and other effects, some of which may be detrimental to the organism. Justesen (1979) evaluated behavioral effects of short-term microwave exposure. Several classes of behavior were operationally defined and used by the author to categorize behavioral effects: convulsions, endurance, work stoppage, work perturbation, aversion, and perception. For the most part the categories assume that effects are the product of intensity and duration of exposure. As these increase, the effects produced proceed from perception and possibly aversion to the other extreme of the thermal insult, grand mal convulsions usually followed by death.

Thermal Effects and Behavior

Recent investigations of the behavioral effects of microwaves have acknowledged their thermal nature and have attempted to capitalize on this aspect. Modak et al. (1981) found that single pulses of 2450 MHz microwave radiation incapacitate mice when intense energy is used. The motor activity of mice exposed to single 15 or 25 ms pulses decreased immediately after exposures and remained low for at least 5 minutes. The longer pulse had a more lasting effect. Body temperature increased $2°$ and $4°$ C, respectively, at the two pulse durations with energy doses of 14.25 and 18.70 J. Higher-power and longer pulses produced high brain temperatures with convulsions and loss of consciousness in rats (Guy and Chou, 1982). The latter study used 918 MHz with pulse widths of 1 µs to 360 ms at power levels of 2 to 10 kW.

The effects of body temperature increases and thermoregulatory behavior have been extensively investigated. Behavioral changes are reliably associated with concomitant changes in body temperature. Using rats, squirrel monkeys, and rhesus monkeys, de Lorge (1983) demonstrated that disruption of an operant response was associated with body temperature increases greater than $1°$ C.

Adair and Adams (1983) showed that behavioral thermoregulation during short exposures (10 minutes) can be affected in squirrel monkeys even at relatively low power densities (6 to 8 mW/cm^2). At lower power densities (1 to 5 mW/cm^2), however, repeated exposures do not produce reliable alterations in thermoregulatory behavior (Adair et al., 1985).

Increases in ambient temperature have been used to study the thermal nature of microwave radiation. Gage and Guyer (1982) found that responses in rats exposed for 15½ hours at 8 and 14 mW/cm^2 were disrupted and that the effect was enhanced by increasing the ambient temperature.

Decreasing the ambient temperature of the environment allows the positive reinforcing nature of microwave radiation to surface. Even though Justesen (1983) and his colleagues have argued that microwaves are poor-quality stimuli, Bruce-Wolf and Adair (1985) found that squirrel monkeys learn to respond for an exposure to 2450 MHz irradiation paired with a 30° C air circulation alternating with a 10° C air circulation alone. The monkeys responded less frequently at 30 mW/cm^2 than at 20 and 25 mW/cm^2, indicating that they could discriminate between small differences in power densities. Several other studies have demonstrated more conclusively that rats (Vitulli et al., 1986, 1987) and rhesus monkeys (Marr et al., 1988) maintained in very cold environments learn an operant response with microwaves as the positive reinforcer. As Justesen et al. (1988) stated, the stimulus attributes of microwave radiation rely on their thermal characteristics and hence are vague; nevertheless, under appropriate conditioning regimens, microwave irradiation can be a positive reinforcer and allow schedules of reinforcement to exert their control. As pointed out by Marr et al. (1988), such demonstrations are not easily accomplished. The demonstration of microwave radiation as a positive reinforcer depends on the animal species, its inherent reaction to cold, microwave frequency, power density, pulse length, paired stimuli, and schedule of reinforcement.

Wasserman et al. (1984, 1985) developed a unique approach to study the effects of microwaves on behavior. They found that house finches and blue jays demonstrate stressful behavior and spend less time in microwave fields of 25 and 50 mW/cm^2 (2450 MHz), whereas fields of 10 mW/cm^2 have no effect. Again, responses were not observed at levels at which thermal effects were not produced.

Microwave Absorption Characteristics and Behavior

Behavioral studies to investigate short-term exposures have been useful in delineating the effects of specific characteristics of the microwave field and corroborating analytical and dosimetric predictions. The thermal aspects of such characteristics as frequency-dependent absorption, animal shape and size, and localized hot spots in the animal have been investigated.

To determine the effect of frequencies at and near the predicted whole-body resonant frequency, D'Andrea et al. (1977) trained male rats to press a lever on a simple variable-interval schedule of reinforcement for a food pellet reward. This schedule typically produces high response rates and proved to be very sensitive to microwave exposures at 400, 500, 600, and 700 MHz. The rats pressed a lever in Plexiglas cages while the 20 mW/cm^2 exposures were given on different days and in random order. The primary dependent variable was the time of microwave exposure necessary to cause the rats' response rates to drop below 33%

of baseline rates (time to work stoppage). Rats exposed to 600 MHz had the quickest time to work stoppage; lower and higher frequencies required longer exposure times. The results confirmed previous analytical predictions that whole-body resonance was an important factor in determining the behavioral response to microwaves (Gandhi, 1974; Johnson, 1974).

In a series of studies, de Lorge (1976, 1980, 1984; de Lorge and Ezell, 1980) investigated the disruption of learned behavior by examining microwave frequency and animal size (actually animal species) interactions. In the study by de Lorge and Ezell (1980), rats exposed to 1.28 and 5.6 GHz radiation were trained to press a lever during 40-minute sessions. After extensive training, various intensities of 5.6 GHz radiation (7.5 to 48.5 mW/cm^2) and 1.28 GHz radiation (5.5 to 15 mW/cm^2) were tested for their performance-disrupting abilities. The higher the power density, the greater the work disruption. At 5.6 GHz, all eight rats had their behavior disturbed at 38.5 mW/cm^2 and higher and seven of eight rats showed behavioral changes at 26 mW/cm^2 and higher. At 1.28 GHz, all rats were behaviorally disrupted at 15 mW/cm^2 and significant change was seen even at 10 mW/cm^2. Different power densities affected the animals at different frequencies. The authors attributed this to the thermal consequence of different specific absorption rate (SAR) spatial distributions in the animals. These SAR variations were confirmed by measurements in foamed polystyrene models containing simulated muscle tissue. An article (de Lorge, 1983) summarizing this series examined the issue of extrapolation of microwave effects based on animal size and behavioral disruption.

Although de Lorge observed no microwave effects that were not thermal, he concluded that some thermal effects on behavior are not easily extrapolated from simple heat deposition in an animal. An animal exposed to microwaves on one body side at a relatively high frequency may simply move away from a response lever to be exposed from a different direction. The animal may not stop working at this time. If exposed dorsally, however, the animal might stop working much sooner. A very high lever in an operant box might orient the animal differently from a lever placed in a lower position. Animals have learned to deal with surface (infrared) exposure much better than with deep heat, so they might withstand much greater SARs at 6 GHz than at 600 MHz merely because of innate cooling behaviors.

D'Andrea et al. (1985) discovered microwave radiation–induced hot spots in the tails and rectums of rat carcasses exposed to 360 and 2450 MHz but not to 700 MHz. The hot spots exceeded the whole-body average SAR by 50 and 18 times for 360 and 2450 MHz exposures, respectively. Regions of intense energy absorption were generally believed to be of little consequence because convective heat transfer via the circulatory system presumably largely equilibrates thermalized energy. The maximal thermal effect of SAR hot spots would then be reflected in generalized, rather than localized, hyperthermia. However, D'Andrea et al. (1987) determined that blood flow in anesthetized rats did not entirely ameliorate some thermal hot spots. In a recent set of experiments, D'Andrea et al. (1988) used a novel behavioral paradigm to investigate the behavioral consequences of thermal hot spots in awake rats. Groups of rats were tested during a baseline period to determine the naturally preferred end of a long Plexiglas cage. In the first experiment rats were placed in the Plexiglas cage, one end of which, when occupied by a rat, commenced microwave radiation exposure; occupancy of the other end terminated exposure. Exposure to 360, 700, or 2450 MHz microwave radiation was contingent on occupancy of the preferred end. The microwave field power density was adjusted for each frequency to yield equivalent whole-body SARs of 1, 2, 6, and 10 W/kg. During 360 and 2450 MHz exposures, occupancy of the preferred end was significantly lower than during 700 MHz exposures. In a second experiment with this procedure, semichronic exposures (6 hours a day, 8 to 28 days) revealed that the whole-body SAR threshold for reduced exposure of 2450 MHz microwaves was between 2.1 and 2.8 W/kg.

LONG-TERM EXPOSURE STUDIES

Numerous reports of biological and behavioral effects from the Soviet Union and other Eastern bloc countries have heightened controversy about the existence of low-level exposure effects (Dumanski and Shandala, 1974; Rudnev et al., 1978). The reported effects in albino rats include lowered reactivity to electric footshock, altered blood levels of cholinesterase and sulfhydryl groups, increased urinary output of 17-ketosteroids, and deficits of performance in the shuttlebox. Low-level exposure effects have been consistently identified during the past two decades as an area that needs further investigation (Johnson, 1973). Although some studies have focused on long-term exposures, many more have investigated short-term exposure to high-intensity fields.

A major obstacle in conducting a long-term exposure experiment is the problem of exposing large numbers of laboratory animals to microwaves for extended periods. The difficulty is in providing both an acceptable living environment for the animals and uniform microwave exposures for all subjects in the experiment. For example, the use of an anechoic chamber and standard horn antenna to expose a large group of animals would produce different energy couplings as a function of number of animals in the group, distance between the animals, and orientation of the animals to the microwave fields (Gandhi et al., 1979). Furthermore, it is hard to provide food and water to the animals without causing large pertubations in the microwave fields by the food and water apparatus. Numerous exposure systems have been designed to solve the problems. D'Andrea et al. (1979) used a monopole-above-ground system to expose groups of rats intermittently up to 8 hours a day to uniform plane-wave fields. Food and water were not placed in the chamber. The circular waveguide exposure system, developed by Guy and Chou (1976), provides uniform subject exposure and has the added advantage of continuous monitoring of SAR during microwave exposure for each subject. The system also allows food and water to be given to the animal with minimal impact on the microwave fields.

Despite the difficulties of conducting long-term exposure experiments, some progress has been made in determining behavioral effects and identifying thresholds for low-level exposures. A summary of recent long-term exposure studies is shown in Table 13-1. The studies are arranged in order of ascending radiation frequency and, within each frequency class, in order of descending whole-body SAR.

Frequency-Specific Behavioral Thresholds

Since frequency-specific behavioral thresholds have been identified with short-term exposure experiments (D'Andrea et al., 1977), it seems reasonable to evaluate the long-term studies by radiation frequency. However, Table 13-1 shows that a firm threshold of behavioral effect cannot be estimated. Only a range within which a threshold may lie can be specified, both because of the varied experimental procedures used by different investigators and because of the few long-term experiments conducted at each radiation frequency.

Moe et al. (1976) exposed male Wistar rats in circularly polarized waveguides (Guy and Chou, 1976) to 918 MHz radiation at 10 mW/cm^2 for 10 hours a night for 3 weeks. The resulting whole-body SAR was 3.61 W/kg, and the cumulative total exposure time was 210 hours. Natural behaviors of eating, drinking, grooming, resting, and activity were scored at 11 PM, 3 AM, and 7:30 AM. If a resting behavior was observed, the behavior was subdivided into stretched-out or curled-up position. The exposed group showed lower activity levels and spent most of the rest time in a stretched-out position. Food intake and blood glucose level were also significantly lower for the exposed group than for the sham-exposed group. The authors suggested that the lowered food intake and stretched-out or prone position meant that the rats were coping with the added thermal loading provided by the microwave exposure.

D'Andrea et al. (1980) exposed 20 male Long-Evans rats in a monopole-above-ground exposure chamber to plane-wave 915 MHz radiation at 5 mW/cm^2 for 8 hours a day, 5 days a week, for 16 weeks. The resulting whole-body SAR was 2.46 W/kg at the outset of the study, and the total

TABLE 15-1 Long-Term Microwave Exposure Experiments

Citation	Frequency (MHz)	SAR (W/kg)	Power density (mW/cm²)	Exposure duration (h)	Exposure mode	Behavior test	Behavioral effect
Moe et al. (1976)	918	3.61	10.00	210	CW	Observation of behavior	Decrease activity level
						Serum glucose	Decrease blood glucose
						Food intake	Decrease food intake
D'Andrea et al. (1980)	915	2.46	5.00	640	CW	Stablimetric platform	Increase activity level
						Activity wheel	None
Lovely et al. (1983)	918	2.00	5.00	1200	CW	Food intake	Decrease food intake
Lovely et al. (1977)	918	0.90	2.50	910	CW	Observation of behavior	None
Lebovitz (1981)	1300	6.70	17.20	90	PW	Lever press—mult(FR/timeout)	None/decreased rate
	1300	3.60	9.20	135	PW	Lever press—mult(FR/timeout)	None/decreased rate
	1300	1.50	3.90	120	PW	Lever press—mult(FR/timeout)	None/None
Lebovitz (1983)	1300	6.70	17.20	15	PW	Lever press—mult(FR/timeout)	Decreased rate (both)
	1300	5.80	15.20	15	CW	Lever press—mult(FR/timeout)	Decreased rate (both)
	1300	3.60	9.20	15	CW	Lever press—mult(FR/timeout)	None/decreased rate
	1300	3.60	9.20	15	PW	Lever press—mult(FR/timeout)	None/decreased rate
Lovely et al. (1983)	2450	3.20	5.00	1200	CW	Food intake	Decrease food intake
Mitchell et al. (1977)	2450	2.30	—	550	CW	Lafayette activity platform	Increase activity level
						Lever press—(mult/FR/timeout)	None/increased rate
						Sidman avoidance—lever press	None
D'Andrea et al. (1979)	2450	1.23	5.00	640	CW	Stablimetric platform	Decrease activity level
						Activity wheel	None
D'Andrea et al. (1986a)	2450	0.70	2.50	630	CW	Footshock sensitivity	Decreased
						Lever press—IRT	Increase rate
						Open field	Increased activity (delayed)
						Active avoidance shuttlebox	Increased latency
Johnson et al. (1983)	2450	0.40–0.15	0.48	15,750	PW	Open field	None
D'Andrea et al. (1986b)	2450	0.14	0.50	630	CW	Footshock sensitivity	None
						Lever press—IRT	Increase rate
						Open field	None
						Active avoidance shuttlebox	Increased latency
DeWitt et al. (1987)	2450	0.14	0.50	630	CW	Footshock sensitivity	None
						Lever press—IRT	Decrease rate
						Open field	None
						Active avoidance shuttlebox	None

CW, Continuous wave; PW, pulsed wave; *mult(FR/timeout)*, multiple fixed ratio time out schedule; *IRT*, interresponse time.

cumulative exposure was 640 hours. An additional 20 rats were given sham exposures in a chamber similar to the monopole-above-ground exposure chamber. After each 8-hour or sham exposure the rats were housed overnight in Wahmann rodent activity cages. Food and water intakes, as well as activity on a stablimetric platform, were assessed at 4-week intervals. Blood samples were collected at 4-week intervals and assayed for hematocrit, red and white blood cell counts, plasma and red blood cell cholinesterase levels, and plasma sulfhydryl levels. Urine samples were also collected at 4-week intervals and assayed for 17-ketosteroid levels. In contrast to Moe et al. (1976), D'Andrea et al. (1980) found an increase in activity, although it was not statistically significant.

Lovely et al. (1983) exposed different groups of adult male rats to 915 MHz microwaves for 10 hours a night for 16 weeks. The exposures to microwaves at 5 mW/cm^2 produced a whole-body SAR of 2 W/kg. Food and water intakes were monitored periodically. In addition, serum electrolyte, glucose, urea nitrogen, corticosterone, and carbon dioxide levels were assayed from blood samples collected at different times during the microwave and sham exposures. A significant reduction of food intake was observed during the long-term microwave exposure. Since body mass was not affected during the study, the authors concluded that the reduced food intake was a metabolic compensation for the energy absorbed from the microwave field.

Lovely et al. (1977) exposed male rats to 918 MHz microwaves at 2.5 mW/cm^2 for 10 hours each night over a 13-week period. The total cumulative exposure in the cylindrical waveguides was 910 hours at a whole-body SAR of 0.9 W/kg. The procedures in this study generally followed those used by Moe et al. (1976). Measures of food and water intake, as well as one- and two-bottle saccharin solution intake (to measure possible radiation-induced malaise), produced no differences between sham- and microwave-exposed rats. In addition, several serum chemistry measures, including serum corticosterone, did not show any radiation-induced stress.

At 918 MHz it is reasonable to assume that the threshold for behavioral effects lies within the range 0.9 to 2 W/kg. Lovely et al. (1977) exposed rats at an SAR of 0.9 W/kg and reported no effect on behavior, whereas Lovely et al. (1983) reported a significant decrease in food intake at 2 W/kg. At SARs of 2.46 and 3.61 W/kg, alterations of activity level and food intake were also reported, which supports the threshold range of 0.9 to 2 W/kg, since effects continue to be observed at SARs greater than 2 W/kg (Moe et al., 1976; D'Andrea et al., 1980).

Lebovitz (1981) exposed female rats to circularly polarized 1300 MHz pulsed microwaves (600 pps, 1 µs pulse durations) for 3 hours a day, 5 days a week for 6 to 9 weeks. The rats were trained in the circular waveguides to press levers on a multiple fixed-ratio (FR) timeout schedule of reinforcement. Food pellets were delivered during FR responding in the presence of a discriminative stimulus (light) and were withheld during responding in absence of the light. When behavioral responding had stabilized, the rats were exposed to microwaves at whole-body SARs of 1.5 to 6.7 W/kg. At an SAR of 1.5 W/kg, microwave exposure had no significant effect on behavioral performance. The exposures at 3.6 and 6.7 W/kg produced decrements of responding during the timeout components of the schedule. This effect was more pronounced at the higher SAR. During the light-discriminated FR components a slight reduction in FR response rates was observed.

In a similar study Lebovitz (1983) compared continuous wave (CW) and pulsed wave (PW) microwave exposures at similar whole-body SARs in adult male rats exposed for 3 hours a day. Rats were trained to stable performance on the multiple FR and timeout schedule. Subsequent microwave exposure was given during behavioral performance at SARs of 5.8 and 6.7 W/kg for CW and PW microwaves, respectively. Response rates on both the FR and timeout components were equally reduced by the different microwave exposures and were associated with body temperature elevations of 0.5° to 1° C. At an exposure SAR of 3.6 W/kg, responses on the timeout components dropped significantly, irrespective of CW or PW irradiation.

Studies conducted by Lebovitz (1981, 1983) at 1300 MHz suggest that a threshold for behavioral effects at this frequency must lie between 1.5 and 3.6 W/kg. At SARs of 3.6 W/kg rats showed a decreased rate of lever pressing during the timeout components of a multiple FR/timeout schedule of reinforcement. This effect was not observed at an SAR of 1.5 W/kg.

Lovely et al. (1983) exposed different groups of adult male rats to 2450 MHz microwaves for 10 hours a night for 16 weeks. The exposures to microwaves at 5 mW/cm^2 produced whole-body SARs of 3.2 W/kg. Food and water intakes were monitored periodically. A significant reduction in food intake was observed during the long-term microwave exposure. Since body mass was not affected during the study, the authors concluded that the reduced food intake was a metabolic compensation for the energy absorbed from the microwave field.

Mitchell et al. (1977) exposed female Sprague-Dawley rats to 2450 MHz microwave radiation, 5 hours a day, 5 days a week, for 22 weeks. The exposures were conducted in a multimode cavity and produced SARs of 2.3 W/kg. Locomotor activity was periodically measured with an activity platform. Both food reward and electric shock avoidance were used as reinforcement to train rats to press levers. Significant increases in locomotor activity were observed during the weeks of exposure. In addition, rats trained to press levers for food reward with visual discriminative stimuli showed disrupted differential responses on this task. In contrast, performance on the shock avoidance task using a Sidman avoidance paradigm (Sidman, 1966) was not affected by microwave exposure.

D'Andrea et al. (1979) intermittently exposed adult male rats to 2450 MHz microwaves for 640 hours at a field intensity of 5 mW/cm^2. The exposures were given 8 hours a day, 5 days a week, for 16 weeks at an average SAR of 1.23 W/kg. Several behavioral end points were measured repeatedly. Locomotor behavior measured overnight by an activity wheel did not differentiate exposed from sham-exposed rats. Locomotor behavior measured with a stablimetric platform did show less activity in the exposed rats than in the sham-exposed rats.

D'Andrea et al. (1986a) exposed adult male rats to 2450 MHz microwave radiation at 2.5 mW/cm^2 for 7 hours a day, 7 days a week, for a total of 630 hours in a monopole-above-ground radiation chamber. A variety of health status and behavioral measures were assayed before, during, and after microwave exposure. For example, body mass and food intake were sampled weekly and were not affected by microwave exposure. However, sensitivity of the rats to electric footshock significantly decreased during the weeks of irradiation. Behavioral measures taken at the end of 14 weeks of microwave exposure included open field activity, shuttlebox avoidance performance, and schedule-controlled lever pressing for food. All of these measures significantly differentiated microwave- from sham-exposed rats.

Johnson et al. (1983) reported a long-term study in which rats were exposed to 2450 MHz microwaves at a field power density of 0.48 mW/cm^2 and periodically tested for activity changes in an open field apparatus. The average SAR ranged from 0.15 to 0.4 W/kg during the lengthy exposure of 25 months. The authors found no significant differences between microwave- and sham-exposed rats on the open field test.

D'Andrea et al. (1986b) exposed adult male rats to 2450 MHz microwave radiation at 0.5 mW/cm^2 for 7 hours a day for up to 98 days. The microwave exposure produced an SAR of 0.14 W/kg. A variety of behaviors were assayed periodically during the weeks of exposure. Sensitivity to electric footshock and open field behavior did not differentiate microwave- from sham-exposed rats. However, the exposed rats did show increased latencies to respond in an active avoidance shuttlebox task and increased lever-pressing rates on an operant task.

In a study similar to that of D'Andrea et al. (1986b), DeWitt et al. (1987) exposed male adult rats to 2450 MHz microwave radiation at 0.5 mW/cm^2 for 7 hours a day for up to 98 days. The microwave exposure produced an SAR of 0.14 W/kg. A variety of behaviors were periodically assayed during the weeks of exposure. In this study, sensitivity to electric footshock, open field behavior, and the active avoidance shuttlebox task did not differentiate microwave- from sham-exposed rats. However, exposed rats did show increased lever pressing on the operant task, as found earlier by D'Andrea et al. (1986b).

The studies at 2450 MHz present a large range within which to locate a threshold. For example, at the high end, Lovely et al. (1983) present convincing evidence that chronic exposure at 3.2 W/kg decreases food intake significantly. Mitchell et al. (1977) discovered that an SAR of 2.3 W/kg increased activity level and response rate during timeout on a lever-pressing task but had no effect on a Sidman avoidance task. At SARs of 1.23 W/kg and 0.7 W/kg, D'Andrea et al. (1979, 1986a) discovered a variety of effects. Decreased and increased activity, increased footshock sensitivity, increased lever-pressing rate on an interresponse time (IRT) schedule, and increased latency to respond in a shuttlebox avoidance task were reported. At a whole-body SAR of 0.14 W/kg, ambiguous and contradictory results were obtained by D'Andrea et al. (1986b) and DeWitt et al. (1987). In the earlier study, increased lever pressing on an IRT schedule and increased latency to respond in a shuttlebox avoidance task were reported (D'Andrea et al., 1986b). In the latter study, DeWitt et al. (1987) used behavioral procedures identical to those in the previous study but failed to find the increased latency in the shuttlebox task and discovered decreased response rates for the microwave-exposed rats on the lever-pressing task. The authors concluded that at an SAR of 0.14 W/kg most behavioral measures (food and water intake, open field behavior) failed to discriminate microwave- from sham-exposed rats, and the contradictory findings for the measures that did discriminate the two groups should not be surprising at threshold levels of microwave treatment. The long-term exposure study conducted by Johnson et al. (1983) also did not discover significant effects with the open field test at an SAR of 0.4 W/kg. Based on the results of these studies, it is possible to specify that a threshold for significant behavioral effects at 2450 MHz is between 0.4 and 0.7 W/kg.

CONCLUSION

Short-term exposure to microwave radiation may result in behavioral changes. The minimum colonic temperature rise associated with significant behavioral changes in rodents and nonhuman primates is close to 1° C (de Lorge, 1984). Under normal ambient conditions the SAR associated with this temperature rise is approximately 4 W/kg; it is less under high ambient temperature and relative humidity. The behavioral changes include alterations in trained performance, motor behavior, and behavioral thermoregulation. Microwave exposure can result in thermal stress reactions and in less time spent in the microwave field. On the other hand, under low ambient temperature the thermal reinforcing properties of microwave radiation maintain schedule-controlled behavior and actually result in more time spent in the microwave field.

Long-term exposure to microwave radiation at low-field power densities also leads to behavioral changes. In this case colonic temperature rise is not expected, since the absorbed energy is easily dissipated by the rodent's thermoregulatory capabilities. The behavioral changes include alterations in trained performance and motor behavior. These changes are microwave frequency specific and occur at SARs of 0.9 to 2 W/kg at 915 MHz, 1.5 to 3.6 W/kg at 1300 MHz, and 0.4 to 0.7 W/kg at 2450 MHz. The differences resulting from radiation frequency may reflect heterogeneous energy absorption in the rodent body. This effect may be especially true for 2450 MHz, which has been predicted as a head resonant frequency for the rodent (Hagmann et al., 1979), although D'Andrea et al. (1985) have shown that hot spots also exist in the tails of rats at this frequency. Although mechanisms for the low-exposure experiments cannot be specified, the results mandate further research with species other than rats to better predict the effects of long-term, low-level exposures on human behavior. While the behavioral studies reported to date provide information useful in delineating hazards of microwave exposure, new and powerful microwave generators dictate that additional research is needed. The effects of exposure to high–peak power microwave pulses with short pulse durations are unknown. Pulses of 20 to 85 ns in duration and peak powers of 10 to 50 kW/cm^2 are now available. Although peak powers are high, the SARs associated with exposure to single pulses or even low pulse repetition rates (fewer than 10 pps) are so small as to be undetectable. Further research is necessary to determine whether behavioral effects will result from such exposures.

REFERENCES

ADAIR, E.R., AND ADAMS, B.W. (1983). Behavioral thermoregulation in the squirrel monkey: adaptation processes during prolonged microwave exposure. *Behav. Neurosci.* 97:49–61.

ADAIR, E.R., SPIERS, D.W., RAWSON, R.O., ADAMS, B.W., AND SHELDON, D.K. (1985). Thermoregulatory consequences of long-term microwave exposure at controlled ambient temperatures. *Bioelectromagnetics* 6:339–363.

BRUCE-WOLF, V., AND ADAIR, E.R. (1985). Operant control of convective cooling and microwave irradiation by the squirrel monkey. *Bioelectromagnetics* 6:365–380.

D'ANDREA, J.A., DEWITT, J.R., EMMERSON, R.Y., BAILEY, C., STENSAAS, S., AND GANDHI, O.P. (1986a). Intermittent exposure of rats to 2450 MHz microwaves at 2.5 mW/cm^2: behavioral and physiological effects. *Bioelectromagnetics* 7:315–328.

D'ANDREA, J.A., DEWITT, J.R., GANDHI, O.P., et al. (1986b). Behavioral and physiological effects of chronic 2,450 MHz microwave irradiation of the rat at 0.5 mW/cm^2. *Bioelectromagnetics* 7:45–46.

D'ANDREA, J.A., DEWITT, J.R., PORTUGUEZ, L.M., AND GANDHI, O.P. (1988). Reduced exposure to microwave radiation by rats: frequency specific effects. *In*: O'Connor, M.E., and Lovely, R. (eds.). Electromagnetic fields and neurobehavioral function. New York, Alan R. Liss, pp. 289–308.

D'ANDREA, J.A., EMMERSON, R.Y., BAILEY, C.M., OLSEN, R.G., AND GANDHI, O.P. (1985). Microwave radiation absorption in the rat: frequency-dependent SAR distribution in body and tail. *Bioelectromagnetics* 6:199–206.

D'ANDREA, J.A., EMMERSON, R.Y., DEWITT, J.R., AND GANDHI, O.P. (1987). Absorption of microwave radiation by the anesthetized rat: electromagnetic and thermal hotspots in body and tail. *Bioelectromagnetics* 8:385–396.

D'ANDREA J.A., GANDHI O.P., AND LORDS J.L. (1977). Behavioral and thermal effects of microwave radiation at resonant and nonresonant wavelengths. *Radio Sci.* 12(suppl. 6):251–256.

D'ANDREA, J.A., GANDHI, O.P., LORDS, J.L., DURNEY, C.H., JOHNSON, C., AND ASTLE, L. (1979). Physiological and behavioral effects of chronic exposure to 2450 MHz mirowaves. *J. Microwave Power* 14:351–362.

D'ANDREA, J.A., GANDHI, O.P., LORDS, J.L., et al. (1980). Physiological and behavioral effects of prolonged exposure to 915 MHz microwaves. *J. Microwave Power* 15:123–125.

DE LORGE, J.O. (1976). Behavior and temperature in rhesus monkeys exposed to low level microwave irradiation. NAMRL-1222, Naval Aerospace Medical Research Laboratory, Pensacola, Fla. (AD A021769).

DE LORGE, J. (1980). The effects of microwaves on animal behavior. *In*: Berteaud, A.J., and Servantie, B. (eds.). Proceedings of an International Conference Ondes Electromagnetique et Biologie [Electromagnetic waves and biology]. Jouy En Josas, France, URSI, CNFRS, pp. 171–176.

DE LORGE, J.O. (1983). The thermal basis for disruption of operant behavior by microwaves in three animal species. *In*: Adair, E.R. (ed.). Microwaves and thermoregulation. New York, Academic Press, pp. 379–400.

DE LORGE, J.O. (1984). Operant behavior and colonic temperature of *Macaca mulatta* exposed to radio frequency fields at and above resonant frequencies. *Bioelectromagnetics* 5:233–246.

DE LORGE, J.O., AND EZELL, C.S. (1980). Observing-responses of rats exposed to 1.28 and 5.62 GHz microwaves. *Bioelectromagnetics* 1:183–198.

DEWITT, J.R., D'ANDREA, J.A., EMMERSON, R.Y., AND GANDHI, O.P. (1987). Behavioral effects of chronic exposure to 0.5 mW/cm^2 of 2450 MHz microwaves. *Bioelectromagnetics* 8:149–157.

DUMANSKI, J.G., AND SHANDALA, M.G. (1974). The biologic action and hygienic significance of electromagnetic fields of superhigh and ultrahigh frequencies in densely populated areas. *In*: Proceedings of an International Symposium on Biologic Effects and Health Hazards of Microwave Radiation, Warsaw, Oct. 15–18, 1973, Warsaw, Polish Medical Publishers, pp. 289–293.

GAGE, M.I., AND GUYER, W.M. (1982). Interaction of ambient temperature and microwave power density on schedule-controlled behavior in the rat. *Radio Sci. 17*(suppl. 5):179–184.

GANDHI, O.P. (1974). Polarization and frequency effects on whole animal energy absorption of RF energy. *Proc. IEEE 62*:1171–1175.

GANDHI, O.P., HAGMANN, M.J., AND D'ANDREA, J.A. (1979). Partbody and multibody effects on absorption of radio frequency electromagnetic energy by animals and by models of man. *Radio Sci. 14*(suppl. 6):15–22.

GUY, A.W., AND CHOU, C.K. (1976). System for quantitative chronic exposure of a population of rodents to UHF fields. *In*: Johnson, C.C., and Shore, M.L. (eds.). Biological effects of electromagnetic waves. Vol. II. Selected papers of the USNC/URSI Annual Meeting, Oct. 20–23, 1975, Boulder, Colo. HEW Pub. No. (FDA) 77–8011, Washington, D.C., U.S. Government Printing Office, pp. 389–422.

GUY, A.W., AND CHOU, C.K. (1982). Effects of high intensity microwave pulse exposure of rat brain. *Radio Sci. 17*(suppl. 5):169–178.

HAGMANN, M.J., GANDHI, O.P., D'ANDREA, J.A., AND CHATTERJEE, I. (1979). Head resonance: numerical solutions and experimental results. *IEEE Trans. Microwave Theory Tech. 27*:809–813.

HINDE, R.A. (1970). Animal behavior: a synthesis of ethology and comparative psychology. New York, McGraw-Hill Book Co.

HONIG, W.K., AND STADDON, J.E.R. (1977). Handbook of operant behavior. Englewood Cliffs, N.J., Prentice-Hall, Inc.

JOHNSON, C.C. (1973). Research needs for establishing a radio frequency EMR safety standard. *J. Microwave Power 8*:367–388.

JOHNSON, C.C. (1974). ANSI Committee C-95 comments on research needs for establishing a radio frequency EMR safety standard. *J. Microwave Power 9*:219–220.

JOHNSON, R.B., SPACKMAN, D., CROWLEY, J., et al. (1983). Effects of long-term low-level radiofrequency radiation exposure on rats. Vol. 4. Open-field behavior and corticosterone. USAFSAM-TR-83–42, USAF School of Aerospace Medicine, Brooks Air Force Base, Tex.

JUSTESEN, D.R. (1979). Behavioral and psychological effects of microwave radiation. *Bull. N.Y. Acad. Med. 55*:1058–1078.

JUSTESEN, D.R. (1983). Sensory dynamics of intense microwave irradiation: a comparative study of aversive behaviors by mice and rats. *In*: Adair, E.R., (ed.). Microwaves and thermoregulation. New York, Academic Press, pp. 203–227.

JUSTESEN, D.R. (1988). Microwave and infrared radiations as sensory, motivational, and reinforcing stimuli. *In*: O'Connor, M.E., and Lovely, R.H. (eds.). Electromagnetic fields and neurobehavioral function. New York, Alan R. Liss, pp. 235–264.

LAI, H., HORITA, A., CHOU, C.D., AND GUY, A.W. (1987). A review of microwave irradiation and actions of psychoactive drugs. *IEEE Eng. Med. Biol.* 6:31–36.

LEBOVITZ, R.M. (1981). Prolonged microwave irradiation of rats: effects on concurrent operant behavior. *Bioelectromagnetics* 2:169–185.

LEBOVITZ, R.M. (1983). Pulse modulated and continuous wave microwave radiation yield equivalent changes in operant behavior of rodents. *Physiol. Behav.* 30:891–898.

LOVELY, R.H., MIZUMORI, S.J.Y., JOHNSON, R.B., AND GUY, A.W. (1983). Subtle consequences of exposure to weak microwave fields: are there nonthermal effects? *In*: Adair, E.R. (ed.). Microwaves and thermoregulation. New York, Academic Press, pp. 401–429.

LOVELY, R.H., MYERS, D.E., AND GUY, A.W. (1977). Irradiation of rats by 915 MHz microwaves at 2.5 mW/cm^2: delineating the dose-response relationship. *Radio Sci.* 12:139–146.

MARR, M.J., DE LORGE, J.O., OLSEN, R.G., AND STANFORD, M. (1988). Microwaves as reinforcing events in a cold environment. *In*: O'Connor, M.E. and Lovely, R.H. (eds.). Electromagnetic fields and neurobehavioral function. New York, Alan R. Liss, pp. 219–234.

MITCHELL, D.S., SWITZER, W.G., AND BRONAUGH, E.L. (1977). Hyperactivity and disruption of operant behavior in rats after multiple exposures to microwave-radiation. *Radio Sci.* 12:263–271.

MODAK, A.T., STAVINOHA, W.B., AND DEAM, A.P. (1981). Effect of short electromagnetic pulses on brain acetylcholine content and spontaneous motor activity of mice. *Bioelectromagnetics* 2:89–92.

MOE, K.E., LOVELY, R.H., MYERS, D.E., AND GUY, A.W. (1976). Physiological and behavioral effects of chronic low level microwave radiation in rats. *In*: Johnson, C.C., and Shore, M.L. (eds.). Biological effects of electromagnetic waves. Vol. I. Selected papers of the USNC/URSI Annual Meeting, Oct. 20–23, 1975, Boulder, Colo., HEW Pub. No. (FDA) 77–8011, Washington, D.C., U.S. Government Printing Office, pp. 248–256.

MONAHAN, J.C., AND D'ANDREA, J.A. (eds.) (1985). Behavioral effects of microwave radiation absorption, HHS Pub. No. FDA 85–8238.

NORTON, S. (1973). Amphetamine as a model for hyperactivity in the rat. *Physiol. Behav.* 11:181–186.

O'CONNOR, M.E., AND LOVELY, R.H. (eds.) (1988). Electromagnetic fields and neuro-behavioral function. New York, Alan R. Liss.

PAVLOV, I.P. (1927). Conditioned reflexes. (Translated by G.V. Anrep.) London, Oxford University Press. (Reprinted 1960, New York, Dover.)

RUDNEV, M., BOKINA, A., EKSLER, N., AND NAVAKATIKYAN, M. (1978). The use of evoked potential and behavioral measures in the assessment of environmental insult. *In*: Otto, D.A. (ed.). Multidisciplinary perspectives in event-related brain potential research. Washington, D.C., Environmental Protection Agency, Office of Research and Development, pp. 444–447.

SIDMAN, M. (1966). Avoidance behavior. *In*: Honig, W.K. (ed.). Operant behavior: areas of research and application. New York, Appleton-Century-Crofts, pp. 448–498.

VITULLI, W.F., LAMBERT, K., BROWN, S.W., AND QUINN, J.M. (1987). Behavioral effects of microwave reinforcement schedules and variations in microwave intensity on albino rats. *Percept. Motor Skills* 65:787–795.

VITULLI, W.F., MOTT, J.M., QUINN, J.M., LOSKAMP, K.L., AND DODSON, R.S. (1986). Behavioral thermoregulation with microwave radiation of albino rats. *Percept. Motor Skills* 62:831–840.

WASSERMAN, F.E., DOWD, C., BYMAN, D., SCHLINGER, B.A., BATTISTA, S.P., AND KUNZ, T.H. (1984). The effects of microwave radiation on avian dominance behavior. *Bioelectromagnetics* 5:331–339.

WASSERMAN, F.E., DOWD, C., BYMAN, D., SCHLINGER, B.A., BATTISTA, S.P., AND KUNZ, T.H. (1985). Thermoregulatory behavior of birds in response to continuous wave 2.45-GHz microwave irradiation. *Physiol. Zool.* 58:80–90.

14

Cellular Effects of Radiofrequency Electromagnetic Fields

STEPHEN F. CLEARY

RATIONALE FOR CELL STUDIES

Difficulties encountered in interpreting the biological effects of radiofrequency (RF) electromagnetic radiation are discussed in detail in this chapter. Principally problems are related to the complex nature of RF field coupling to mammals and nonuniformities in the internal distribution of absorbed energy. Dosimetric and densitometric complexities have precluded the determination of direct dose-response relationships that would provide an adequate basis for interspecies or interfrequency extrapolation of data. Inherent physiological complexity of mammalian systems adds to the uncertainty.

An issue of central importance in RF bioeffects research is mechanisms of interaction. Although there is ample evidence that intense RF radiation has indirect heating effects on living systems, evidence of direct effects and their possible mechanisms is inadequately documented. For example, the question of whether biological effects of low-intensity RF fields depend on radiation frequency or instantaneous tissue-induced electric or magnetic fields remains unanswered. One reason for this is uncertainty in the measurement or prediction of internally induced fields, but even if such information were available, detection of direct exposure effects would be difficult for physiological reasons. An organism such as a mammal comprises a number of discrete but interactive organs and organ systems. Thus, to determine the direct effects of RF exposure on a component organ, an investigator must account for both direct and indirect effects on all other components of the organism. Since this has not been possible, direct interactions of RF radiation with living systems such as laboratory animals or humans have not been documented. However, direct RF exposure effects can be investigated at the cellular or subcellular level in vitro. This approach significantly reduces the problem of physiological complexity, since individual, essentially noninteracting units, namely living mammalian cells or cell components, may be exposed under conditions of precise environmental control. RF cell exposure systems provide a practical means of exposing cells to a wide range of RF frequencies and field strengths, under essentially isothermal conditions, permitting the detection of direct exposure effects (Cleary, et al., 1982, 1985a,b; Liu and Cleary, 1988).

This chapter also reviews the cellular effects of RF radiation to consider evidence for its direct effects. What follows is not a comprehensive review of RF cellular effects; some cell studies have found no RF-induced alterations, but such results, unless pertinent to the evidence presented for direct RF field effects, are not reviewed here. A more comprehensive discussion of cellular effects of RF radiation can be found in the review by Allis (in Elder and Cahill, 1984).

LIMITATIONS OF CELL STUDIES

Investigation of in vitro cell responses to RF radiation affords a unique means of detecting direct exposure effects and gaining insight into their mechanisms. Although in some instances in vitro cell studies can be conducted under conditions that simulate in vivo conditions, duplication of the in vivo cell environment is not possible. The extent to which differences in cell environment affect responses to RF radiation depends on the cell type; cells that are functionally dependent on interactions with other cells in vivo are potentially more sensitive to such perturbations. Thus, whereas cells such as erythrocytes may be relatively unaffected by in vitro conditions of altered environment, cells such as neurons may be more significantly affected. The effects of using transformed (and hence abnormal) cell lines in research must also be taken into consideration. In addition, in vitro cell studies cannot include the influence of the wide variety of in vivo cell interactions. It may thus be concluded that investigations of the cellular effects of RF radiation are necessary for basic understanding of such phenomena but insufficient to determine health effects in highly integrated mammalian systems.

ERYTHROCYTES

Erythrocytes afford a convenient system for cell biological studies because of their availability, ease of handling, stability in vitro, and structural and functional simplicity relative to other types of mammalian cells. These characteristics have been exploited extensively in cell biology, especially in the areas of energy metabolism and membrane transport, and a large body of background information exists in these areas. Since in vivo and in vitro studies have suggested the cell membrane as a likely site of interaction of RF radiation (Liu et al., 1979), effects on erythrocyte plasmalemma permeability have been the subject of a number of investigations (Cleary, 1987).

Previous in vitro studies have shown that erythrocyte plasmalemma permeability depends on temperature, so this variable must be carefully controlled in studies of RF exposure effects. Under conditions of precise temperature control, Liu et al. (1979) exposed human, canine, and rabbit red blood cells to continuous wave (CW) 2.45, 3, and 3.95 GHz microwaves. Variation of the specific absorption rate (SAR) up to 200 W/kg was used to expose cell suspensions at various temperatures in the range 26° to 44° C. Microwave exposure caused dose-dependent increases in cell potassium ion (K^+) efflux, sodium ion (Na^+) influx, hemoglobin release, and osmotic lysis. However, sham exposure of cells to conventional (hot water) heating at the same temperatures as microwave-exposed red blood cells resulted in similar effects on membrane permeability, which suggests no direct microwave effect (Liu et al., 1979). Olcerst et al. (1980), on the other hand, reported apparently contradictory effects of 2.45 MHz CW radiation on rabbit red blood cell permeability. Exposure to SARs of 100, 190, and 390 W/kg (approximate internal electric field strengths of 353, 487, or 700 V/m, respectively) caused statistically significant effects on passive Na^+ and rubidium ion (Rb^+) efflux, but only at temperatures of 8° to 11°, 22.5°, and 36° C. The pronounced temperature dependence of the microwave effect on erythrocyte cation permeability provided an explanation for differences in the results of Liu et al. (1979) and Olcerst et al. (1980), since exposures were not conducted at the same temperatures in these studies. On the basis of well-documented temperature-dependent alterations in erythrocyte membranes, including cation fluxes, Cleary et al. (1982) suggested the involvement of membrane phase transitions in microwave-induced permeability changes. Subsequent studies provided additional evidence in support of this hypothesis.

Statistically significant increases in K^+ release from rabbit erythrocytes exposed under specific conditions to 8.42 GHz microwaves were reported by Cleary et al. (1982). There were no differences in K^+ release from cells exposed or sham exposed to various combinations of SAR and temperature in the ranges of 21 to 90 W/kg and 20° to 30° C, respectively. However, cells exposed to an SAR of 22 W/kg (electric field strength of 100 V/m) at 24.6° C exhibited enhanced K^+ release, but not at higher or lower SARs or temperatures. The effect was greater in cells exposed in whole (heparinized) blood than in cells exposed in isotonic saline solution, and K^+ release was consistently greater from cells exposed to pulsed microwaves than from those exposed to CW 8.42 GHz microwaves. The authors suggested that the specificity of the effect was related to the interaction of microwave radiation with membrane cation transport processes at the membrane phase transition temperature. The experimental conditions were such that both active and passive membrane transport processes might have been involved in the effect observed.

Liburdy and Penn (1984) and Liburdy and Vanek (1985) extended the studies of Olcerst et al. (1980) and demonstrated altered Na^+ permeability in rabbit erythrocytes exposed to 2.45 GHz microwaves in a specific temperature range of 17.7° to 19.5° C. In this temperature range there was a dose-dependent linear increase in Na^+ permeability up to a field strength of 600 V/m, above which no further increase was detected. The electric field strength threshold for the induction of altered Na^+ permeability was approximately 150 V/m. In addition to changes in membrane Na^+ permeability, Liburdy and Penn (1984) and Liburdy and Vanek (1985) reported associated phenomena of membrane protein shedding, dependence on oxygen tension, and effects of membrane cholesterol and antioxidants (ascorbic acid or mercaptoethanol). These and earlier findings indicate that microwave-induced plasmalemma alterations depend partly on the extracellular environment and may be global rather than restricted to specific membrane transport sites or processes.

The involvement of the extracellular environment in microwave-induced cellular alterations had been suggested previously by Cleary et al. (1982), who found significantly greater effects of microwave radiation on erythrocyte cation fluxes and hemoglobin release in whole cell suspensions than on cells suspended in physiological saline solution. Liburdy and Penn (1984) and Liburdy and Vanek (1985) also reported enhancement of microwave effects on Na^+ permeability in the presence of plasma. Studies of the effects of pulsed square-wave electric fields on the induction of K^+ and hemoglobin permeability alterations of rabbit red blood cells exposed in whole blood, compared with 1:1 cell suspensions in isotonic buffered saline solution, revealed a similar effect of the cell environment (Cleary et al. 1979). Mechanisms for enhanced microwave or pulsed electric field effects on erythrocyte permeability in whole blood are uncertain. The effect does not appear to depend on the presence of leukocytes or serum electrolytes but may be due to proteins or lipoproteins, although a specific effector has not been identified (Cleary et al., 1982).

The results of studies of the interaction of microwave radiation with membrane transport processes at phase transition temperatures provide evidence for direct effects of such radiation on cells. Insight regarding a possible mechanism for this effect was provided by Allis and Sinha-Robinson (1987). Human erythrocyte membranes were exposed to 2.45 GHz CW microwaves at an SAR of 6 W/kg (field strength approximately 87 V/m) at 1° C temperature increments between 23° and 27° C. Spectrophotometric assays of Na^+/K^+ adenosine triphosphatase (ATPase) activity during microwave exposure revealed a 35% inhibition of enzyme activity, which occurred only at 25° C. There was a marginally significant effect of microwave radiation on the ouabain-insensitive Ca^{+2} ATPase activity. The authors ruled out the involvement of microwave-induced heating, since heating would have increased rather than decreased enzyme activity. The results of Allis and Sinha-Robinson (1987) are in agreement with those of Fisher et al. (1982), who reported a 40% decrease in ouabain-sensitive Na^+ efflux from human erythrocytes at 23° and 24° C exposed to 2.45 GHz microwaves at an SAR of 3 W/kg (electric field strength 44 V/m).

Allis and Sinha-Robinson (1987) concluded that the transition in activity of the enzyme Na^+/K^+ ATPase that occurs at 25° C results either from protein-lipid interaction at their interface within the erythrocyte membrane or directly within the enzyme per se. They proposed that 2.45 GHz microwave radiation interacts with the enzyme or the enzyme-lipid transition state in a manner that suppresses the enzyme activity, resulting in decreased active Na^+ and K^+ transport across the membrane. This effect is consistent with altered cation fluxes in erythrocytes exposed to microwave radiation at specific temperatures as reported by Cleary et al. (1982) and Fisher et al. (1982). Qualitatively similar effects on Na^+, K^+, or Rb^+ transport were reported by Olcerst et al. (1980), Liburdy and Penn (1984), and Liburdy and Vanek (1985), who studied passive rather than active cation transport. This suggests that microwave radiation may interact with more than one site in the membrane to affect cation transport. Reported differences in the temperature or temperature range at which microwave radiation affects erythrocyte cation transport may be due to differences in the temperature dependence of active and passive transport processes, as well as interspecies and intraspecies differences in membrane composition that are well known to affect membrane transport functions (Claret et al., 1978; Roelofsen, 1981). Differences in erythrocyte membrane composition, as well as temperature-dependent differences in activation energy for active and passive plasmalemma cation transport, may account for the variance in the minimum microwave field strengths from 44 V/m (Fisher et al., 1982) to 353 V/m (Olcerst et al., 1980), reported to elicit the effect.

The results of the preceding studies indicate a direct, molecular level interaction between microwave radiation and specific erythrocyte membrane components. The extent to which microwave-induced alteration in red blood cell cation transport depends on radiation frequency is difficult to determine, since the majority of the studies were conducted at 2.45 GHz. However, because Cleary et al. (1982) reported similar results following red blood cell exposure to 8.42 GHz microwave radiation, the effect is probably not frequency specific, at least in the range 2.45 to 8.42 GHz. There is evidence that lower-frequency RF radiation does not induce qualitatively or quantitatively similar effects on mammalian erythrocytes (Cleary, 1987).

Cleary et al. (1985a) reported a field strength–dependent hemolytic effect of CW radiofrequency radiation on rabbit erythrocytes. Erythrocytes in whole heparinized rabbit blood were hemolyzed after 2 hours exposure to 50 or 100 MHz fields at field strengths of 400 V/m or greater. To induce similar effects from exposure to 10 MHz RF radiation, field strengths of 900 V/m were necessary. Since the exposure temperature was controlled to 22.5° ± 0.2° C, Cleary et al. concluded that the hemolytic effect was not due to heating per se or to temperature gradients. In addition to the lower hemolytic field strength thresholds for 50 and 100 MHz than for 10 MHz, no RF frequency affected cellular K^+ or Na^+ concentrations. Comparison of the results of this study with previous studies conducted at 8.42 GHz under similar experimental conditions with the same assay procedures (Cleary et al., 1982) led the authors to conclude that RF radiation, at the frequencies investigated, appeared to have different effects on rabbit red blood cells from those of higher-frequency microwave radiation (Cleary et al., 1985a).

The results of Serpersu and Tsong (1983) provide additional evidence in support of the hypothesis that RF radiation affects erythrocyte membranes by direct frequency– and electric field strength–dependent interactions. These authors, who investigated the effect of RF radiation on Rb^+ uptake in human erythrocytes, found increased uptake, which peaked at 2 kV/m and a frequency of 1 kHz. The effect was detected at 3° and 20° C, and there was no alteration in Na^+ transport. Under these conditions, RF-stimulated Rb^+ uptake was totally inhibited by ouabain, which led the authors to conclude that the effect involved a direct electromagnetic field interaction with the membrane cation transport enzyme Na^+/K^+ ATPase. The authors agreed with Allis and Sinha-Robinson (1987) that the stimulatory effect was due to a frequency- and amplitude-dependent, RF electromagnetic field–induced, conformational change in Na^+/K^+ ATPase molecules in the red blood cell membrane. In contrast to the results of Allis and Sinha-Robinson, who found that 2.45 GHz microwave exposure at a field strength of 87 V/m inhibited Na^+/K^+ ATPase activity, Serpersu and Tsong detected a stimulation of enzyme activity caused by exposure at a lower frequency (1 kHz) and significantly higher field strength (2 kV/m). Although these experiments were also conducted at different temperatures, which may partially explain the markedly different outcomes, the results provide additional evidence of direct frequency-dependent effects of RF radiation on cells.

The effect of RF radiation on erythrocyte membrane fluidity has also been investigated. Allis and Sinha (1981), for example, studied the internal viscosity of human red blood cell membranes during exposure to 1 GHz CW microwave radiation at SARs of 0.6, 2, and 154 W/kg, in the temperature range 15° to 40° C. The activation energy for motion of the fluorescent membrane probe was not detectably altered by microwave exposure, and there was no evidence of a lipid phase transition. Kim et al. (1985) also used fluorescent membrane probes to investigate the effects of 340 or 900 MHz RF radiation on erythrocytes and erythrocyte ghosts. RF exposure decreased membrane lipid viscosity, altered the structural state of lipid-protein contact regions, and decreased protein shielding of lipids, effects that corresponded to indirect, thermally induced alterations. Ortner et al. (1981) also reported structural changes in membrane proteins and lipids that were related to radiation-induced temperature elevations. These results suggest that, in the studies mentioned, RF-induced alterations in cation fluxes across red blood cell membranes at phase transition temperatures probably resulted from direct interaction with membrane macromolecules or macromolecular complexes, such as Na/K^+ ATPase, rather than generalized changes in membrane lipids or fluidity.

Finally, erythrocytes have been used to investigate effects of RF exposure on cell surface charge density, as measured by electrophoretic mobility. The possibility that RF exposure may induce such effects was suggested by Wilkins and Heller (1963), who reported RF effects on the electrophoretic mobility of several colloids. Ismailov (1977), who exposed human erythrocytes to 1 GHz microwave radiation, found exposure duration–dependent increases and decreases in electrophoretic mobility immediately after exposure. A dose-dependent maximum increase in mobility of 23% occurred 30 minutes after exposure at 37° C. Bamberger et al. (1981) exposed human erythrocytes to the same microwave frequency at 37° C at approximate SARs of 75 to 150 W/kg, compared with 45 W/kg used by Ismailov (1977). The cell concentration was 100 times larger in the study by Bamberger et al. (1981) than in that by Ismailov (1977). Bamberger et al. (1981) could not detect an effect of microwave exposure on electrophoretic mobility, which leaves open the question of RF-induced effects on cell surface charge density.

LEUKOCYTES

Exposure of leukocytes in vitro to CW and amplitude-modulated RF fields indicates that only certain cell functions are affected. Lyle et al. (1983), for instance, reported significant inhibition of allogenic cytotoxicity of the target cell MPC-11 by murine cytotoxic T lymphocytes when the assay was conducted during exposure to a 450 MHz RF field at an incident intensity of 1.5 mW/cm^2, sinusoidally amplitude modulated at 60 Hz. A similar effect was detected when T lymphocytes were exposed to the RF field before assay, suggesting to the authors that the effect was a direct field interaction with cytolytic T lymphocytes. RF-induced cytolytic activity was a reversible effect; T lymphocytes recovered full activity in $12\frac{1}{2}$ hours. Maximum suppression of T-cell cytotoxicity occurred from exposure to 450 MHz fields modulated at 60 Hz relative to 40, 16, or 3 Hz modulation. The unmodulated (CW) 450 MHz carrier wave had no effect on cytotoxicity. It was concluded that the recognition phase of the cytolytic effect was affected by amplitude-modulated RF radiation.

Suggested mechanisms for effects on T-cell cytotoxicity include field inter-action with glycoprotein target cell receptor molecules in the T-lymphocyte membrane and modulation of critical calcium ion flux (Lyle et al., 1983).

Membrane-related alteration of human lymphocytes by RF radiation has been reported to occur at other modulation frequencies as well. Byus et al. (1984) exposed human tonsil lymphocytes to 450 MHz fields with a peak intensity of 1 mW/cm^2, sinusoidally amplitude modulated at fre-quencies between 3 and 100 Hz for periods of up to 60 minutes. Total non–cyclic adenosine monophosphate (cAMP)–dependent protein kinase activity of the lymphocytes decreased to less than 50% of control levels after 15- to 30-minute exposures at a modulation frequency of 16 Hz, with a smaller decrease after exposure at 60 Hz. After 45 to 60 minutes of continuous RF exposure the protein kinase activity returned to control levels, indicating a "time window" response. There were no exposure-related effects on cAMP-dependent protein kinase activity, which suggests that the effect was related to a transient induction of a persistent but reversible molecular state in specific components of the lymphocyte trans-ductive system (Byus et al., 1984).

Sultan et al. (1983a,b) investigated the effects of RF and microwave radiation on another lymphocyte function, capping of plasma membrane antigen-antibody complexes. B lymphocytes were exposed for 30 minutes to 2.45 GHz microwave radiation at an SAR of 45 W/kg at 37°, 41°, and 42.5° C, or to 147 MHz RF radiation amplitude modulated by a 9, 16, or 60 Hz sine wave at a maximum SAR of approximately 2 W/kg and at temperatures of 37° or 42° C. For nonirradiated control lymphocytes there was a significant temperature-dependent decrease in capping but no difference between exposed and sham-exposed cells at any tempera-ture. Also, there was no significant difference between control cells and cells exposed to 2.45 GHz microwaves during capping when the sample temperatures were both 38.5° C (Sultan et al., 1983a).

Lloyd et al. (1986) investigated the effects of 20-minute exposure of human blood in vitro to 2.45 GHz microwaves at SARs of 4 to 200 W/kg. During exposure the blood temperature increased from 37° to 40° C. Analysis of cultured blood lymphocytes revealed no radiation-induced increase in chromosomal damage. Finally, Cleary et al. (1989a) investi-gated the effects of isothermal (37° ± 0.2° C) in vitro RF and microwave exposure on mitogenesis in human peripheral lymphocytes. At SARs in the range of 10 to 50 W/kg, a 2-hour exposure to CW 2.45 GHz microwave radiation caused an increase in phytohemagglutinin-stimulated mitogen-esis 3 days after exposure. Simultaneous exposure of blood aliquots to 27 MHz of CW RF radiation at the same temperature, at SARs of 50 W/kg or greater, resulted in statistically significant suppression of mito-genesis 3 days after exposure.

Ottenbreit et al. (1981) reported that 2.45 GHz CW microwave radiation at SARs of 250 W/kg or greater inhibited the proliferative capacity of human neutrophil precursor colony-forming unit cells (CFU-C) after 15-minute exposures at 7°, 22°, 37°, or 41° C. The irreversible effect was dose dependent and not related to exposure temperature or to the state of the cell cycle. The authors noted that CFU-C requires the addition of exogenous glycoprotein stimulators for cell growth. Since the glycoproteins are known to interact with neutrophil membrane receptors, Ottenbreit et al. suggested that microwave exposure alters membrane receptors, making them unresponsive to stimulatory factors. A similar mechanism of interaction could explain the RF-induced suppression of phytohemagglutinin-stimulated mitogenesis reported by Cleary et al. (1987b).

The effect of 100 MHz RF radiation on phagocytic activity of rabbit neutrophils was investigated by Cleary et al. (1985b). Cells were exposed in vitro for 30 minutes to CW or amplitude-modulated (20 Hz) 100 MHz RF radiation at SARs of 120 to 341 W/kg (electric field strengths of 250 to 410 V/m). Exposure at 37° ± 0.2° C had no detectable effect on neutrophil viability or phagocytosis.

BRAIN AND NEURAL CELLS

Persistent indications that the mammalian central nervous system is perhaps the most sensitive tissue for RF-induced alterations has provided the rationale for in vitro studies of effects on brain tissue and brain and neural cells. Not surprisingly, in vitro brain cell sensitivities to RF exposure are among the highest reported.

Wachtel et al. (1975) and Seaman and Wachtel (1978) investigated the effects of 1.5 and 2.45 GHz CW and pulse-modulated microwaves on the firing rate of isolated neurons from the marine gastropod *Aplysia*. Atypical alterations were detected in cells exposed to microwave radiation of SARs between 1 and 100 W/kg. In 13% of the *Aplysia* pacemaker cells, microwave irradiation reversed the normal temperature dependence on firing rate; the rate decreased or fell to zero in response to microwave-induced temperature elevations. The rapid component of the response, which occurred within 1 second after commencement of microwave exposure, was always associated with a decrease in firing rate, whereas increased temperature increased the rate. These authors concluded that, at an SAR of approximately 1 W/kg, about 0.1% of the absorbed microwave energy was converted into a polarizing current across the membrane, which resulted in altered firing rates. This effect, which results from a direct effect of microwave radiation on a neural cell in vitro, has been reported by other workers.

Arber (1976) reported hyperpolarization of the resting potential of neurons of the mollusk *Helix pomatia* as a result of a 1-hour exposure to 2.45 GHz CW microwaves at an SAR of approximately 15 W/kg. By treating the neurons with ouabain after exposure, Arber demonstrated that the altered hyperpolarization was partly due to inhibition of Na/K$^+$ ATPase. Arber's finding was interesting in light of a subsequent report by Allis and Sinha-Robinson (1987) of a similar direct microwave effect on this cation transport enzyme in the erythrocyte membrane in vitro. Yamaura and Chichibu (1967) reported effects of 11 GHz microwave radiation at an SAR of 100 W/kg on crayfish and prawn ganglia firing rates. During exposure the firing rate decreased rapidly. Immediately after exposure the rate increased to greater than normal before reverting to preexposure levels. Elevated temperature caused an increase in firing rate as reported by Wachtel et al. (1975) and Seaman and Wachtel (1978).

Pickard and Barsoum (1981) exposed single giant algal cells from *Chara braunii* and *Nitella flexilis* to 250 msec, pulse-modulated, 0.1 to 10 MHz RF radiation. Fast and slow increments in membrane resting potential were induced by RF exposure. Whereas the authors attributed the slow component to RF-induced temperature rise, the fast component, which was inversely dependent on RF frequency, vanished at 10 MHz. Pickard and Barsoum (1981) suggested that the fast component was due to rectification of the RF field by the cell membrane, an effect predictable on the basis of membrane dielectric properties. Subsequent studies by Barsoum and Pickard (1982), using similar experimental methods but extending RF frequencies to 20 to 300 MHz, failed to detect membrane rectification, again in agreement with dielectric theory applied to cell membranes. In addition to studying RF effects on *Chara* membrane resting potentials, Liu et al. (1982) investigated the effects of CW, pulse-modulated, and sinusoidally amplitude-modulated, S-band microwave radiation on amplitude of the action potential, rise and decay time of the action potential, conduction velocity, and excitability. Cells maintained at 22° ± 0.1° C during exposure showed no consistent or statistically significant microwave-dependent alteration, in basic agreement with the results of Pickard and Barsoum (1981) and Barsoum and Pickard (1982).

Sanders et al. (1984) compared the relative effects of microwave and RF radiation on rat brain energy metabolism. Technically, since these studies were conducted with brain tissue per se rather than cell preparations, they should not be considered in this section. However, because of the nature of the conclusion relative to the direct effects of RF radiation on cells, they are included. A dose-dependent increase in nicotinamide adenine dinucleotide (NADH) fluorescence was detected after a 2-minute exposure to 200 or 591 MHz CW radiation at a threshold electric field strength of 3 to 5 V/m. Exposure of rat brain tissue to the same intensity of 2.45 GHz CW microwave radiation had no detectable effect. Exposure to 200 or 591 MHz RF radiation decreased brain tissue adenosine triphosphate (ATP); 2.45 GHz exposure had no effect. Measurement of the energy metabolite creatine phosphate (CP) revealed a suppression only in response to 591 MHz radiation but not 200 or 2450 MHz. The authors proposed that RF irradiation induced a frequency-dependent direct effect on specific mitochondrial enzymes or on electron transport proteins involved in maintenance of brain cell ATP pools. The authors suggested that the mechanism for the effect was RF-induced dipole oscillations involving the divalent metal ion at the active site during either catalytic or transport activity. This hypothesis is qualitatively similar to that advanced by Allis and Sinha-Robinson (1987) to explain an RF effect on Na^+/K^+ ATPase activity in the erythrocyte membrane, as discussed previously. Sanders et al. (1985) presented additional experimental evidence supporting their hypothesis in a study of the effects of CW, sinusoidal amplitude-modulated, and pulsed square wave–modulated 591 MHz radiation on brain energy metabolism.

Statistically significant decreases in incorporation of ^{3}H-thymidine and ^{3}H-uridine in human glioma cells (LN71) in vitro were detected by Cleary et al. (1989b) 3 or 5 days after a 2-hour exposure at $37° \pm 0.2°C$ to 27 MHz CW RF radiation at an electric field strength of 160 V/m or greater. Simultaneous exposure of glioma to 2.45 GHz microwave radiation under identical conditions but at lower electric field strengths (less than 1.3 V/cm) resulted in increased ^{3}H-thymidine uptake 3 days after exposure. These data indicate a persistent field strength–dependent effect of isothermal RF exposure on cellular DNA and RNA synthesis (Cleary et al., 1989b).

WINDOW EFFECTS

Additional evidence of the sensitivity of mammalian brain cells to RF and lower-frequency electromagnetic fields has resulted from a series of investigations of effects on Ca^{++} binding to chick brains in vitro. These studies revealed that weak amplitude-modulated electromagnetic fields induce alteration in Ca^{++} binding under specific exposure conditions that involve intensity and modulation frequency "windows." In some instances the location of these windows was found to depend on magnetic fields with intensities equivalent to geomagnetic fields.

Bawin and Adey (1976) reported a reduction in the release of $^{45}Ca^{++}$ from chick and cat cerebral tissue exposed in vitro to 1, 6, 16, 32, or 75 Hz sinusoidal electric fields. Threshold applied electric field strengths of 10 and 56 V/m were detected for chick and cat brain tissue, respectively. Smaller field-induced releases occurred at 5 and 100 V/m. The maximum reduction in $^{45}Ca^{++}$ release, which was about 12% to 15%, occurred at 6 and 16 Hz.

Frequency and amplitude windows for field-induced release of

$^{45}Ca^{++}$ from chick cerebral tissue have also been reported to result from exposure to VHF and UHF fields amplitude modulated at ELF frequencies. Exposure of chick brain tissue to 0.8 mW/cm², 147 MHz RF radiation, sinusoidally amplitude modulated, resulted in a statistically significant increase in $^{45}Ca^{++}$ efflux at frequencies from 6 to 16 Hz and in a decreased efflux in response to fields modulated from 20 to 35 Hz (Bawin et al., 1975). Blackman et al. (1979) reported similar effects of sinusoidally modulated 147 MHz RF fields on chick brain tissue, again detecting a modulation frequency windowed response between 9 and 16 Hz. Effects of these modulated RF fields on calcium efflux were significant only at incident power densities of approximately 1 mW/cm². A similar power density window was detected for chick brain tissue exposed to 450 MHz RF radiation sinusoidally modulated at 16 Hz (Bawin et al., 1978). In this series of experiments, increased $^{45}Ca^{++}$ efflux occurred only at 0.1 and 1 mW/cm², but not at 0.05 or 5 mW/cm². Tissue electric field strengths that induced calcium release were on the order of 10 V/m. Blackman et al. (1985) determined that the extremely low-frequency (ELF) alternating magnetic field component was involved in $^{45}Ca^{++}$ release from chick brain tissue and that the effectiveness of the field at a given frequency depended on the local static geomagnetic field intensity. Liboff (1985) suggested that the interaction of alternating and static magnetic fields with charged ions such as Ca^{++} may be explained theoretically as cyclotron resonance. Additional evidence in support of cyclotron resonance as a mechanism for the effects of ELF electric or magnetic fields on living systems was provided by behavioral studies with rats (Thomas et al., 1986) and diatoms (Smith et al., 1987).

The mechanisms for the ELF field–induced release of Ca^{++} from brain or other tissues remain uncertain. The field-induced efflux of calcium from brain tissue appears to occur at sites on membrane surfaces, rather than from intracellular calcium pools (Lin-Liu and Adey, 1982). Although the physiological consequences of such windowed phenomena have not been determined, it is well known that calcium ions are involved in membrane transductive coupling in various neurobiological, immunological, and endocrinological systems. Consequently, if such windowed responses are induced in vivo by exposure to low intensity by ELF fields, the potential exists for physiological perturbations of undetermined significance.

OTHER CELLULAR EFFECTS

Studies using other cell types and dependent variables have provided additional evidence of varied cellular responses to RF radiation. Peters et al. (1979), for example, reported effects on the cell cycle in vitro, including cell type–specific inhibition of proliferation after exposure to 2.45 GHz microwave radiation. Microwave exposure altered the growth of synchronized L60T cells if exposure occurred during the mitotic (M) and intermitotic (G_1) phases. Exposure of asynchronous L60T cell cultures at four successive 4-hour intervals, as the cultures entered the M and G_1 phases of the mitotic cycle, caused a pronounced suppression of proliferation.

Balcer-Kubiczek and Harrison (1985) used in vitro methods to study the carcinogenicity of RF radiation. They exposed C3H/10T½ mouse embryo fibroblasts in vitro to 4.4 W/kg pulsed 2.45 GHz microwave radiation for 24 hours. Latent transformation damage was induced, as revealed by the action of the tumor promoter 1,2,-O-tetradecanoyl-phorbol-1,3-acetate (TPA). The ability of microwave radiation to promote cell transformation in vitro is of interest in view of the reports by Szmigielski et al. (1980, 1982) and Kunz et al. (1985) of tumor promotion by microwaves in vivo.

CONCLUSION

Investigations of the cellular effects of RF radiation in vitro provide definite evidence of direct, frequency-dependent, and field strength–dependent alterations of various types of mammalian cells. These effects cannot be attributed to heating per se. Examples of such effects reviewed here include altered active and passive membrane cation transport, frequency-dependent increase or decrease in the activity of Na^+/K^+ ATPase, inhibition of allogenic T lymphocytes, decrease in non-cAMP-dependent protein kinase activity, effects on neutrophil precursor membrane receptors, altered firing rates and resting potentials of neurons, frequency-dependent effects on brain cell energy metabolism, alteration in DNA and RNA synthesis in glioma cells, mitogenic effects on human lymphocytes, cell cycle–specific effects on proliferation, and promotion of cell transformation.

The variety of cellular effects induced by RF exposure, as well as differences in the exposure conditions (frequency, field strength, modulation, and so on), suggest multiple macromolecular interaction mechanisms. The only generalization that appears justified at this time is that these effects involve RF interactions with cell membranes, most prominently the plasma membrane. Continued research at the cellular level promises a more complete understanding of the biological effects of exposure to RF electromagnetic radiation.

REFERENCES

ALLIS, J.A., AND SINHA, B.L. (1981). Fluorescence depolarization studies of red cell membrane fluidity: the effect of exposure to 1.0-GHz microwave radiation. *Bioelectromagnetics* 2:13–22.

ALLIS, J.W., AND SINHA-ROBINSON, B.L. (1987). Temperature-specific inhibition of human red cell Na^+/K^+ ATPase by 2,450-MHz microwave radiation. *Bioelectromagnetics* 8:203–212.

ARBER, S.L. (1976). Effect of microwaves on resting potential of giant neurons of mollusk *helix pomatia*. *Electronnaya Obrabotka Materialov* 6:78–79.

BALCER-KUBICZEK, E.K., AND HARRISON, G.H. (1985). Evidence for microwave carcinogenesis in vitro. *Carcinogenesis* 6:859–864.

BAMBERGER, S., KEILMANN, F., STORCH, F., ROTH, G., AND RUHENSTROTH-BAUER, G. (1981). Experimental results contradicting claimed 1009-MHz influence on erythrocyte mobility. *Bioelectromagnetics* 2:85–88.

BARSOUM, Y.H., AND PICKARD, W.F. (1982). Effects of electromagnetic radiation in the range 20–300 MHz on the vacuolar potential of Characean cells. *Bioelectromagnetics* 3:193–201.

BAWIN, S.M., AND ADEY, W.R. (1976). Sensitivity of calcium binding in cerebral tissue to weak environmental electric fields oscillating of low frequency. *Proc. Natl. Acad. Sci. U.S.A.* 73:1999–2003.

BAWIN, S.M., ADEY, W.R., AND SABBOT, I.M. (1978). Ionic factors in release of $^{45}Ca^{2+}$ from chicken cerebral tissue by electromagnetic fields. *Proc. Natl. Acad. Sci. U.S.A.* 75:6314–6318.

BAWIN, S.M., KACZMAREK, L.K., AND ADEY, W.R. (1975). Effects of modulated VHF fields on the central nervous system. *Ann. N.Y. Acad. Sci.* 247:74–81.

BLACKMAN, C.F., BENANE, S.G., RABINOWITZ, J.R., HOUSE, D.E., AND JONES, W.T. (1985). A role for the magnetic field in the radiation-induced efflux of calcium ions from brain tissue *in vitro*. *Bioelectromagnetics* 6:327–337.

BLACKMAN, C.F., ELDER, J.A., WEIL, C.M., BENANE, S.G., EICHINGER, D.C., AND HOUSE, D.E. (1979). Induction of calcium-ion efflux from brain tissue by radio frequency radiation: effects of modulation frequency and field strength. *Radio Sci.* 4(suppl.):93–98.

BYUS, C.V., LUNDAK, R.L. FLETCHER, R.M., AND ADEY, W.R. (1984). Alterations in protein kinase activity following exposure of cultured human lymphocytes to modulated microwave fields. *Bioelectromagnetics* 5:341–351.

CARROL, D.R., LEVINSON, D.M., JUSTESEN, D.R., AND CLARKE, R.L. (1980). Failure of rats to escape from a potentially lethal microwave field. *Bioelectromagnetics* 1:101–115.

CLARET, M., GARAY, R., AND GIRAUD, F. (1978). The effect of membrane cholesterol on the sodium pump in red blood cells. *J. Physiol.* 274:247–263.

CLEARY, S.F. (1987). Cellular effects of electromagnetic radiation. *IEEE Eng. Med. Biol. Magazine* 6:26–30.

CLEARY, S.F., GARBER, F., AND LIU, L.M. (1982). Effects of X-band microwave exposure on rabbit erythrocytes. *Bioelectromagnetics* 3:453–466.

CLEARY, S.F., LIU, L.M., AND GARBER, F. (1985a). Erythrocyte hemolysis by radiofrequency fields. *Bioelectromagnetics* 6:313–322.

CLEARY, S.F., LIU, L.M., AND GARBER, F. (1985b). Viability and phagocytosis of neutrophils exposed *in vitro* to 100 MHz radiofrequency radiation. *Bioelectromagnetics* 6:53–60.

CLEARY, S.F., LIU, L.M., AND MERCHANT, R. (1989a). Lymphocyte proliferation modulated in vitro by isothermal radiofrequency radiation exposure. *Bioelectromagnetics* (in press).

CLEARY, S.F., LIU, L.M., AND MERCHANT, R. (1989b). Glioma proliferation modulated in vitro by isothermal radiofrequency radiation exposure. *Rad. Res.* (in press).

CLEARY, S.F., LIU, L.M., NICKLESS, F., AND SMITH, G. (1979). Effects of pulsed DC fields on mammalian blood cells. *In*: Taylor, L.S., and Cheung, A.W. (eds.). The mechanisms of microwave biological effects. College Park, University of Maryland, p. 16.

ELDER, J.A. AND CAHILL, D.F. (eds.) (1984). Biological effects of radiofrequency radiation. Report No. EPA-600/8-83-026 F. Research Triangle Park, N.C., Health Effects Research Laboratory, Environmental Protection Agency.

FISHER, P.D., POZNARSKY, M.J., AND VOSS, W.A.G. (1982). Effect of microwave radiation (2450 MHz) on the active and passive components of $^{24}Na^+$ efflux from human erythrocytes. *Radiat. Res.* 92:411–422.

ISMAILOV, E.S. (1977). Effect of ultrahigh frequency electromagnetic radiation on the electrophoretic mobility of erythrocytes. *Biofizika* 22:493–498. (Translated in *Biophysics* 22:510–516, 1978.)

KIM, Y.A. FOMENKO, B.S. AGAFONOVA, T.A., AND AKOEV, I.G. (1985). Effects of microwave radiation (340 and 900 MHz) on different structural levels of erythrocyte membranes. *Bioelectromagnetics* 6:305–312.

KUNZ, L.L., JOHNSON, R.B., THOMPSON, D., CROWLEY, J., CHOU, C.K., AND GUY, A.W. (1985). Effects of long-term low-level radiofrequency radiation exposure on rats. USAF School of Aerospace Medicine, Report No. SAM-TR-85-11, Vol. 8, Brooks Air Force Base, Tex.

LIBOFF, A.R. (1985). Geomagnetic cyclotron resonance in living cells. *J. Biol. Phys.* 13:99–102.

LIBURDY, R.P., AND PENN, A. (1984). Microwave bioeffects in the erythrocyte are temperature and pO_2 dependent: cation permeability and protein shedding occur at the membrane phase transition. *Bioelectromagnetics* 5:283–291.

LIBURDY, R.P., AND VANEK, P.F. (1985). Microwaves and the cell membrane. II. Temperature, plasma, and oxygen mediate microwave-induced membrane permeability in the erythrocyte. *Radiat. Res.* 102:190–205.

LIN-LIU, S., AND ADEY, W.R. (1982). Low frequency amplitude modulated microwave fields change calcium efflux rates from synaptosomes. *Bioelectromagnetics* 3:309–322.

LIU, L.M., AND CLEARY, S.F. (1988). Effects of 2.45 GHz microwaves and 100

MHz radiofrequency radiation on liposome permeability at the phase transition temperature. *Bioelectromagnetics 9*:249–257.

LIU, L.M., GARBER, F., AND CLEARY, S.F. (1982). Investigation of the effects of continuous-wave, pulse- and amplitude-modulated microwaves on single excitable cells of Chara corallina. *Bioelectromagnetics 3*:203–212.

LIU, L.M., NICKLESS, F.G., CLEARY, S.F. (1979). Effects of microwave radiation on erythrocyte membranes. *Radio Sci. 14*:109–115.

LLOYD, D.C., SAUNDERS, R.D., MOQUET, J.E., AND KOWALCZUK, C.I. (1986). Absence of chromosomal damage in human lymphocytes exposed to microwave radiation with hyperthermia. *Bioelectromagnetics 7*:235–237.

LYLE, D.B., SCHECHTER, P., ADEY, W.R., AND LUNDALE, R.L. (1983). Suppression of T-lymphocyte cytotoxicity following exposure to sinusoidally amplitude-modulated fields. *Bioelectromagnetics 4*:281–292.

OLCERST, R.B., BELMAN, S., EISENBUD, M., MUMFORD, W.W., AND RABINOWITZ, J.R. (1980). The increased passive efflux of sodium and rubidium from rabbit erythrocytes by microwave radiation. *Radiat. Res. 82*:244–256.

ORTNER, M.J., GALVIN, M.J., CHIGNELL, C.F., AND McREE, D.I. (1981). A circular dichroism study of human erythrocytes ghost proteins during exposure to 2450 MHz microwave radiation. *Cell Biophys. 3*:335–347.

OTTENBREIT, M.J., LIN, J.C., INOUE, S., AND PETERSON, W.D. (1981). In vitro microwave effects on human neutrophil precursor cells (CFU-C). *Bioelectromagnetics 2*:203–215.

PETERS, W.J., JACKSON, R.W., AND IWANO, K. (1979). Effects of controlled electromagnetic radiation on the growth of cells in tissue culture. *J. Surg. Res. 27*:8–13.

PICKARD, W.F., AND BARSOUM, Y.H. (1981). Radiofrequency bioeffects at the membrane level: separation of thermal and athermal contributions in the Characeae. *J. Membr. Biol. 61*:39–54.

ROELOFSEN, B. (1981). The (non)specificity in the lipid-requirement of calcium and sodium plus potassium-transporting adenosine triphosphatases. *Life Sci. 29*:2235–2247.

SANDERS, A.P., JOINES, W.T., AND ALLIS, J.W. (1984). The differential effects of 200, 591, and 2450 MHz radiation on rat brain energy metabolism. *Bioelectromagnetics 5*:419–433.

SANDERS, A.P., JOINES, W.T., ALLIS, J.W. (1985). Effects of continuous-wave, pulsed, and sinusoidal-amplitude-modulated microwaves on brain energy metabolism. *Bioelectromagnetics 6*:89–97.

SEAMAN, R.L., AND WACHTEL, H. (1978). Slow and rapid responses to CW and pulsed microwave radiation by individual *Aplysia* pacemakers. *J. Microwave Power 13*:77–86.

SERPERSU, E.H., AND TSONG, T.Y. (1983). Stimulation of a ouabain-sensitive Rb^+ uptake in human erythrocytes with an external electric field. *J. Membr. Biol. 74*:191–201.

SMITH, S.D., McLEOD, B.R., LIBOFF, A.R., AND COOKSEY, K. (1987). Calcium cyclotron resonance and diatom mobility. *Bioelectromagnetics 8*:215–227.

SULTAN, M.F., CAIN, C.A., AND TOMPKINS, W.A.F. (1983a). Effects of microwaves and hyperthermia on capping of antigen-antibody complexes on the surface of normal mouse B lymphocytes. *Bioelectromagnetics 4*:115–122.

SULTAN, M.F., CAIN, C.A., AND TOMPKINS, W.A.F. (1983b). Immunological effects of amplitude modulated radiofrequency radiation: B lymphocyte capping. *Bioelectromagnetics 4*:157–165.

SZMIGIELSKI, S., SZUDZINSKI, A., PIETRASZEK, A., AND BIELEC, M. (1980). Acceleration of cancer development in mice by long-term exposition to 2450-MHz microwave fields. *In:* Berteaud, A.J., and Servantie, B. (eds.). International symposium Proceedings of an Ondes Electromagnetiques et Biologie, (URSI, CNFRS) Jouy en Josas, France, June 30–July 4, 1980, pp. 165–169.

SZMIGIELSKI, S., SZUDZINSKI, A., PIETRASZEK, A., BIELEC, M., JANIAK, M., AND WREMBEL, J.K. (1982). Accelerated development of spontaneous and benzopyrene-induced skin cancer in mice exposed to 2450-MHz microwave radiation. *Bioelectromagnetics 3*:179–191.

THOMAS, J.R., SCHROT, J., LIBOFF, A.R. (1986). Low-intensity magnetic fields alter operant behavior in rats. *Bioelectromagnetics 7*:349–357.

WACHTEL, H., SEAMAN, R., AND JOINES, W. (1975). Effects of low-intensity microwaves on isolated neurons. *Ann. N.Y. Acad. Sci. 247*:46–62.

WILKINS, D.J., AND HELLER, J.H. (1963). Effect of radio-frequency fields on the electrophoretic mobility of some colloids. *J. Chem. Physics 39*:3401–3405.

YAMAURA, I., AND CHICHIBU, S. (1967). Super-high frequency electric field and crustacean ganglionic discharges. *Tohoku J. Exp. Med. 93*:249–259.

15

Teratogenesis: Nonionizing Electromagnetic Fields

MARY ELLEN O'CONNOR

This chapter focuses on the teratogenic studies associated with exposure to nonionizing electromagnetic (NEM) fields. Some of the methodological issues in the study of teratogenic effects are introduced, as well as some special considerations required to evaluate teratogens. Studies conducted with frequencies in the microwave portion of the NEM spectrum and extremely low-frequency (ELF) fields are included. Studies concentrating on both the electric and magnetic components of the ELF field are discussed. This chapter is not a comprehensive literature review but does include a summary of the teratogenic potential of these fields and some suggestions for further research directions.

PRINCIPLES AND METHODS OF TERATOLOGY

When an abnormality is observed at birth, it is seldom possible to determine whether the defect is the result of genetic flaws or environmental influences. When the defect is apparently the result of environmental influences, it is considered teratogenic. Humans have several well-known genetic defects such as Down's syndrome. Environmental agents, such as ionizing radiation, and certain drugs, including thalidomide and even alcohol, can interfere with the development of an organism that was normal at conception. The effects of environmental agents range from skeletal deformities to more complex conditions such as the fetal alcohol syndrome (FAS). FAS includes a variety of physical and functional defects. Other agents can cause less severe and less obvious alterations. For example, cigarette smoking during pregnancy results in smaller fetuses that have lower survival rates than larger, heavier infants. Although the potential for an environmental agent to be a teratogen can sometimes be determined by epidemiological observations in human populations, teratogenic agents are more commonly identified in laboratory studies of nonhuman organisms.

Several principles must be considered in the design and evaluation of laboratory studies to determine teratogenic potential of an agent. One of the most essential is the time in the organism's development at which the agent is introduced. Prenatal development is divided into stages from conception to birth. The appearance of the major organ systems and the rate of growth are different throughout the stages. A single teratogen can produce totally different effects if applied at different stages of development. Some teratogens affect only specific systems. If a teratogen is harmful only to a specific system, it may have no apparent effect if the exposure occurs at a stage when this system is not undergoing critical development or growth.

Other critical parameters include dose, dose rate, the species under investigation, and maternal effects. Some teratogens produce defects only in certain species. Thalidomide produces severe defects in mice, cats, and humans but not in rats. Unfortunately, the laboratory testing of thalidomide was conducted in rats, and its ability to induce severe birth defects in humans was not discovered until the drug was in use. Current federal research guidelines indicate that federally funded teratogenic investigations should include more than one species or strain over multiple generations. Very few investigations on NEM fields meet this requirement. It is possible to compare continuous research projects from a single laboratory or similar studies from several independent laboratories. Maternal effects are also important. The studies in this chapter report effects in small laboratory mammals, particularly mice and rats, and in chicken embryos. The exposure of the chicken eggs obviously results in more independent and direct exposure of the developing organism than similar studies on mammalian organisms inside the maternal, also exposed, organism.

These special considerations do not necessarily have to be treated as research problems. Indeed, the prenatal organism can be considered a model system for bioeffects research (O'Connor, 1985). The fact that organ systems develop at different times and rates can be used to target a specific system. In addition, the sensitivity of the organism can be used to explore weak effects that might not appear in adult, fully developed organisms. The rapid changes in the relatively short time from conception to birth, in contrast to postnatal development through puberty and adulthood, can be used to investigate effects that might occur only after repeated or continuous exposure.

Most reports of teratogenic effects do not discuss possible underlying mechanisms of action other than heat. The cellular processes involved in development, such as induction, proliferation, migration, aggregation, and differentiation, have been described. However, the molecular basis for embryological development is not known at present (Edelman, 1984). Without knowing the molecular basis for normal development, researchers can only speculate on mechanisms for disruption of this development.

EFFECTS FOLLOWING EXPOSURE TO MICROWAVE FIELDS

Experimental Observations

The most widely investigated part of the NEM spectrum is the radiofrequency (RF), particularly microwave, portion. However, most of the studies are confined to a few representative frequencies, particularly 2450 MHz (O'Connor, 1980). Plane continuous wave (CW) fields have been investigated more than pulsed fields, and the majority of studies used a single acute exposure. Resorptions and reduced fetal body mass in mice and rats are the most frequently reported teratogenic effects, and these appear to be thermally induced (Rugh et al., 1974; Lary et al., 1983; O'Connor, 1985; NCRP, 1986).

Maternal lethality and temperature increase. Early studies of C3H/HeJ mice and Holtzman rats suggested that teratogenic effects occur only at exposure levels high enough to increase maternal lethality significantly (Chernovetz et al., 1975, 1977, 1978). However, another series of studies exposed rats at several RF frequencies with continuous monitoring of maternal colonic temperature so that no maternal lethality occurred (Lary et al., 1982a,b; 1983). These rats were compared with a yoked group of rats raised to the same colonic temperatures in a circulating water bath. The authors concluded that the threshold for observing effects is not lethality but rather colonic temperature. The colonic temperature required to cause death is approximately 42° C (O'Connor, 1985), whereas the apparent threshold for teratogenic effects is approximately 40° C (Berman et al., 1978; Lary et al., 1982a,b; 1983).

Embryopathic and teratogenic effects have been claimed to occur at levels that do not significantly increase maternal colonic temperature (Berman et al., 1978). Exencephaly was observed in mice exposed for 100 minutes to 2450 MHz CW fields at intensities ranging from 1 to 28 mW/cm^2 (equivalent specific absorption rate [SAR] of 22 W/kg). The abnormal fetuses were clustered in the highest exposure levels, but exposed and nonexposed fetuses did not differ significantly unless the data for three exposure groups were pooled. The postexposure rectal temperatures of the maternal subjects were not higher than the preexposure temperatures, which has been cited as evidence for nonthermal effects. However, the studies were conducted with CF-1 mice. Recent research comparing female Long-Evans rats and female CF-1 mice exposed to 2450 MHz radiation at SARs of 2, 4, 6, and 8 W/kg for durations of 1 to 6 hours showed totally different temperature profiles for the two species (O'Connor and Strattan, in press). The rat colonic temperatures increased during the exposures, but the colonic temperatures of the mice decreased. The thermoregulatory efficiency of mice prevented increased colonic temperatures even after 6 hours of exposure at a rate of 8 W/kg. Colonic temperature increase is not a good measure of the thermal nature of exposure, and the lack of an increase in this measure should not be used to label exposure conditions as athermal.

Prolonged exposure studies.   As mentioned previously, most of the earlier studies used short-term exposure sessions. However, O'Connor and Strattan (1985) exposed both CF-1 mice and albino guinea pigs for longer periods. The pregnant mice received no radiation (sham) or 10 or 30 mW/cm^2 for 6 hours daily from gestational day 1 through day 18. The ambient temperature in the exposure chamber was 22° C, since this temperature had been used in previous studies reporting teratogenic effects (for example, Berman et al., 1978). No differences were observed between the exposed and nonexposed groups. Although the differences were not statistically significant, the sham animals had the lowest fetal body and brain mass, more resorption, and more abnormal fetuses than any other group. The investigators hypothesized that a 6-hour exposure, as compared with several minutes at an ambient temperature of 22° C might induce slight cold stress in the mouse. Additional mice received sham exposure or 30 mW/cm^2 with the ambient chamber temperature at 20° or 25° C. Colony control animals were maintained for all of the groups. At 25° C both the sham- and microwave-exposed fetuses had lower fetal body mass than the colony controls. The microwave-exposed fetuses were also significantly smaller than the sham exposed. The fetal brain mass was the same for the colony control and sham-exposed groups but was significantly reduced in the microwave-exposed fetuses. At 20° C the only significant difference observed was an increased fetal brain mass in the sham-exposed litters. Embryopathic effects at these levels of irradiation also appear to depend on the ambient temperature in the chamber.

Pregnant albino guinea pigs were exposed on days 18 through 25 of gestation for 60 minutes at a power density of 47 mW/cm^2. The design parameters of the study were based on reports of teratogenic effects from hyperthermia in guinea pigs (Edwards and Wanner, 1977). Fetal body mass was higher in the sham-exposed than the cage control animals. Body mass did not differ for male fetuses, but the female sham fetuses had larger body masses than either the cage control or microwave-exposed groups, which did not differ from each other.

One interesting aspect of these studies is the inclusion of the cage (that is, colony) control groups. The authors reported that the results might have been interpreted quite differently without the cage control subject data. For example, if the colony or cage control subjects were excluded from the statistical analysis for the initial mouse data at 22° C, the analysis would show significantly smaller fetal body mass in the sham subjects. Without data showing that the microwave-exposed subjects were similar in size to the cage controls, the difference between microwave- and sham-exposed fetuses might have been attributed to enhanced fetal growth after microwave exposure rather than ambient temperature. Without the cage control comparisons in the guinea pig study, the microwave-exposed fetuses would have appeared to have both reduced body and brain mass. Nearly all subsequent teratogenic studies have included cage control comparisons.

Behavioral teratology studies. In addition to focusing on skeletal or organ deformities, investigators have asked whether prenatal microwave exposure or a combination of prenatal and postnatal exposure could produce functional (that is, behavioral) changes. These studies were prompted by some early Soviet reports of physiological and behavioral effects from long-term exposure to extremely low levels of microwave radiation (Dodge, 1969; Dodge and Glaser, 1977). Attempts to replicate and extend some of these behavioral observations resulted in mixed conclusions (Chernovetz et al., 1975; Johnson et al., 1977; Lovely et al., 1983; Jensh et al., 1983b, 1984b). Johnson et al. (1977) exposed rats to 918 MHz microwave radiation in a circularly polarized waveguide (Guy et al., 1979) for 8 hours daily throughout the gestation period. The maternal subjects were permitted to deliver the pups, which were observed for development of reflexes. Additional studies were performed to assess postweaning function such as activity level and avoidance behavior (Lovely et al., 1983). No main effects of microwave exposure were statistically evident. Some differences were reported between individual cells in experimental subgroupings (such as prenatally and postnatally exposed cross-fostered females), but without main effects these results are inconclusive.

Jensh and associates (1983a,b, 1984a,b) exposed pregnant Wistar rats to 2450 and 6000 MHz microwave radiation. Some of the subjects were sacrificed for morphological observations of the uterine contents, and others delivered their pups, which were used for postnatal psychophysiological analysis. The 2450 MHz exposures were conducted at 20 mW/cm^2 for 6 hours daily throughout pregnancy (SAR approximately 4 W/kg). No morphological effects were observed. Behavioral tests were conducted between 60 and 90 days of age, after which time the prenatally exposed subjects were bred for teratogenic analysis of their offspring. Although a variety of behavioral measures were used, the only significant differences were in activity, with the irradiated females more active than irradiated males and more active than either the male or female control rats.

A slightly different protocol was used for the 6000 MHz exposures. The maternal subjects were exposed at 35 mW/cm^2 (SAR approximately

7 W/kg) for 8 hours daily throughout the pregnancy. Investigators divided the subjects into two groups to perform both morphological analysis at term and postnatal behavioral tests. In addition, after the pups were weaned, the exposed maternal subjects were rebred and then killed on the twenty-second gestational day for maternal blood and organ analysis, as well as teratological examination of their uterine contents. For the 6000 MHz exposures the irradiated fetuses exhibited growth retardation at term and several of the psychophysiological measures were significant. The fetuses from the rebred mothers had reduced fetal weight at term. The pups that had been prenatally exposed exhibited differences in eye opening, postnatal growth to the fifth week, water T-maze performance, and activity in an open field test. The authors concluded that exposure at these levels may result in subtle, long-term neurophysiological alterations that are not detectable with conventional morphological teratogenic procedures. Although this may be true, their conclusion is based on a very small number of litters within the subcells used for statistical analysis.

Another study also investigated prenatal microwave exposure at 2450 MHz with postnatal analysis of psychomotor development and behavior (O'Connor, 1988). The maternal subjects were exposed for 6 hours daily from day 1 through day 18 or 19 of gestation at power levels of 30 mW/cm^2. Both sham-exposed and colony cage control groups were maintained. The offspring were observed and tested with 14 independent psychomotor development and behavioral tests. Of all the measures, the only one that resulted in significant differences was thermal preference. When placed in a thermal gradient the prenatally microwave-exposed pups preferred the cooler section of the alleyway. This observation was used to develop the hypothesis that prenatal microwave exposure might result in functional differences specifically associated with thermal cues.

In a second investigation the prenatally exposed pups were tested for thermal seizure susceptibility, huddle formation at three ages, and exploratory behavior in an open field test with and without a concomitant injection of caffeine. No significant differences were observed in the exploratory behavior study. In the seizure study the microwave-exposed group's latency to seizure was significantly greater at day 2 of age than that of either the sham-exposed or cage control group. Another group tested at day 10 of age had increased latencies for all three conditions, but latencies in the microwave-exposed group did not increase as much as in either the sham-exposed or colony control groups.

The huddle size was significantly smaller in 5-day-old microwave-exposed pups. Huddle size was remeasured in 10- and 15-day-old pups. As expected, the huddles consistently decreased in size as the pups aged, but the differences were much greater for the sham-exposed and cage control groups than for the microwave-exposed group. The results of the study were reported to support the general hypothesis that prenatal microwave exposure might specifically alter postnatal development of thermoregulatory behaviors.

An attempt to repeat the huddle and seizure studies in pups whose mothers were exposed to 2450 MHz CW at 10 W/kg for 1 or 3 hours daily from days 12 through 18 of gestation did not produce any significant results (O'Connor and Strattan, in press).

Conclusions

The microwave portion of the RF NEM radiation spectrum has been fairly well investigated, particularly at 2450 MHz. Both high-level acute effects and lower-level chronic effects have been studied. Exposures at levels that raise the maternal colonic temperature to a point that obviously imposes a thermal burden on the animal result in teratogenic effects in the offspring. Effects have sometimes been observed at lower, but not necessarily nonthermal, levels, but they do not appear particularly robust. The most frequently reported effect is reduced fetal body mass. A number of behavioral teratology studies have been conducted, but the reported effects have been inconsistent and indicate that microwave radiation is not a strong behavioral teratogen. Studies have not been conducted across the RF spectrum of frequencies, few studies have observed the effects of pulsed fields, exposure to multiple frequencies has not been investigated, and the number of species investigated is limited.

EXTREMELY LOW-FREQUENCY ELECTRIC FIELD STUDIES

There have been fewer teratogenic investigations in the ELF region of the NEM spectrum than in the microwave region. Although some earlier work is cited here, the extensive electric field studies conducted at Battelle Research Institute on miniature swine (Sikov et al., 1987) and rats (Rommereim et al., 1987; Anderson, personal communication) are featured.

Experimental Studies

Prenatal exposure to electric fields has been investigated in darkling beetles (D'Ambrosio et al., 1980), chickens (Graves et al., 1979), and mice and rats (Knickerbocker, 1967; Marino et al., 1976; Seto et al., 1984; Sikov et al., 1984; Rommereim et al., 1987). The predominant frequency studied was 60 Hz. Positive effects reported include reduced egg production (Krueger et al., 1975), decreased body weight in male offspring of exposed mice (Knickerbocker, 1967), and decreased body weight in rats (Marino et al., 1976).

The first multigenerational study was reported by Seto et al. (1984). Rats had long-term exposure to a 60 Hz field at 80 kV/m unperturbed intensity across four generations. The exposure facility was designed so that observations could be made in the blind and the investigators could control ambient electric and magnetic fields, corona and ozone, acoustic noise, drinking water tube shock, and electric field uniformity. No statistically significant differences were observed between sham and exposed subjects. The statistical power of the investigation was calculated, and the authors concluded that it was sufficient to determine that no effects had occurred.

An extensive study was conducted on several generations of Hanford miniature swine with an attempted replication in rats (Rommereim et al., 1987; Sikov et al., 1987). The swine were exposed continuously through two generations at a frequency of 60 Hz and an intensity of 30 kV/m. Some evidence of slow breeding in the second generation and also some fetal abnormalities occurred. The second teratogenic analysis resulted in the observation of some abnormalities but not of the same type observed in the first analysis. Because the effects had no pattern, the authors suggested three possible explanations for the observed changes: caused by exposure, random variation, or an experimental effect not directly related to exposure. The group sizes were small, the effects were inconsistent, and an infection and treatment of the Fo sows occurred in the 3- to 10-month period before their second breeding at 18 months.

Because of the difficulties in interpreting the results of the preceding study and the expense associated with swine, a second study was undertaken with rats (Rommereim et al., 1987). Some statistically significant effects were observed, but they were also inconsistent and different from the ones observed in the swine study. The authors concluded that rats are not an adequate model for swine and that the lack of any biological pattern in the relatively few effects indicates that they were expressions of random events. An attempt to follow through on this study with rats has resulted in a few statistically significant but inconsistent effects (L. Anderson, personal communication).

Conclusions

It would appear that the electric field associated with 60 Hz current is not teratogenic. Several species have been tested, and in a few of the studies exposures occurred across several generations. A few statistically significant effects were observed, but the type of effects differed between studies of the same species and even within a single multigenerational study.

EXTREMELY LOW-FREQUENCY MAGNETIC FIELD STUDIES

In 1982 a group of investigators in Spain reported that ELF pulsed magnetic fields induced embryological changes in developing chicken embryos (Delgado et al., 1982). This observation received considerable attention and led to several attempts at replication throughout the world. The earliest attempts, such as that by Maffeo et al. (1984), tended to have negative results, and the ensuing controversy prompted the Office of Naval Research (ONR) in cooperation with the Environmental Protection Agency (EPA) to initiate an extensive study in six independent laboratories in the United States, Canada, and Europe. This collective study is referred to as the Henhouse Project.

Experimental Studies

Delgado et al. (1982) exposed Leghorn chicken eggs to rectangular waves of 0.5 msec pulse duration generated by a magnetic field of 10, 100, or 1000 Hz at intensities of 0.12, 1.2, and 12 μT. After 48 hours the eggs were opened, observed microscopically for gross form, and rated for stage of development (Hamburger and Hamilton, 1951). Significant differences in abnormality were reported between exposed and control embryos, with the cephalic nervous system being the most likely to be disrupted. There were no effects at 10 Hz, and at both 100 Hz and 1000 Hz the effects occurred at 1.2 μT but not at the lower or higher intensity. The authors concluded that fields of 100 Hz at 1.2 μT affect chicken embryogenesis, delaying it at a very early stage and limiting development to the formation of the three primitive layers. The results were described as occurring at both frequency and intensity windows. Changes in glycosaminoglycans were observed, and the authors suggested that exposure to these fields could change the electrostatic properties of glycosaminoglycans, which are found associated with embryonic cell membranes and are involved in morphogenesis and cell differentiation.

A subsequent investigation (Ubeda et al., 1983, 1985) used four different pulse shapes at 100 Hz and intensities of 0.4 to 104 μT. The 100 μsec pulse rise time at intensities of 1 and 13.9 μT produced changes, but no alterations were observed at the lower or higher intensities. At 1 μT the changes were observed in the truncal nervous system, whereas at 13.9 μT the changes were in the circulatory system and the foregut. The authors noted again that the effects seemed to depend on certain frequency and intensity windows.

The first reported replication to appear (Maffeo et al., 1984) did not produce significant results. The imposed magnetic fields were reported to be comparable in amplitude, pulse rise time, pulse length, and pulse frequency to the first study reported by the Spanish group. The eggs were of the same variety but were from different suppliers. Leal et al. (1986) later suggested that the horizontal component of the earth's magnetic field may play a role. Specifically, it was suggested that the orientation of the eggs, long axis in the horizontal plane in the east-west magnetic orientation, was critical to the success of the experiment.

Discrepancies in the results prompted the beginning of the Henhouse Project. The results of this 4-year study are discussed later in the chapter (Berman et al., 1988). However, other investigators were also attempting to follow up on these studies. Juutilainen et al. (1986) exposed chick embryos during their first 52 hours of development to 100 Hz fields with sinusoidal, square and pulsed waveforms at average field strengths of 0.1 to 80 A/m. Some significant differences were observed, but frequency and intensity windows were not observed. The effects indicated a threshold-type dependence on field strength, with no effects observed below 1 A/m and a constant percentage of abnormalities above this level. Another study appeared to support this threshold dependence (Juutilainen and Saali, 1986). Further investigations from this laboratory indicated dependence on incubation temperature and storage procedures (Juutilainen, 1986) and suggested a relationship between field strength and abnormal development (Juutilainen et al., 1987).

Small laboratory mammals have also been investigated with regard to prenatal exposure to magnetic fields (Frolen et al., 1987; Tribukait et al., 1987). Tribukait et al. (1987) reported an increased occurrence of external malformations is C3H mice exposed at 15 μT to sawtooth pulse waveforms at 20 kHz. The 15 μT, 20 kHz conditions with sawtooth pulse waveforms were used by Frolen et al. (1987) to study CBA/S mice. This study resulted in significantly more dead fetuses and a higher frequency of resorption in the exposed group, but not greater abnormalities. The exposed fetuses also weighed more than the controls.

As indicated earlier, the Henhouse Project was begun in 1984. The aim of the project was to conduct six independent studies with procedures that were as close as possible to identical. Each laboratory was equipped with incubators fabricated at and distributed from an EPA laboratory. The eggs were exposed to unipolar pulsed magnetic fields with pulse durations of 500 μs and pulse rise and fall times of 2 μs, at intensities of 1 μT and a frequency of 100 Hz. Eggs were evaluated for fertility, and embryos for developmental stage, normal structure, and maturity. Two of the six laboratories showed a significant increase in the proportion of abnormal embryos in the exposed group, three reported more abnormalities in the exposed group without reaching statistical significance, and one had fewer abnormalities in the exposed group. The data were combined, and both exposure and laboratory were significant for the proportion of abnormal embryos, as was the interaction of the two. The authors concluded that, in general, the results of the Henhouse Project support the earlier positive results (Berman et al., 1988).

Conclusions

Clear discrepancies in the data have yet to be accounted for. However, the number of studies that have reported positive results and the general trends observed in the Henhouse Project indicate that ELF pulsed magnetic fields can induce alterations in embryogenesis in chickens and possibly mice. The failure to reach statistical significance in some (although not all) studies suggests that the effect is not robust. The specific conditions of the different laboratories responsible for the significant interaction have not been identified. Further attempts merely to replicate what appear to be minimum effects do not seem justified. Attempts to identify the underlying mechanism should be the focus of further research.

CONCLUSION

Much more effort has been directed at investigating teratogenic potential of NEM energy in the RF portion than in the ELF portion of the spectrum. RF, particularly microwaves, can induce teratogenic effects when the exposure is of an intensity to place a thermal burden on the maternal subject and thus the uterine contents. The most frequently encountered effects are reduction in fetal body mass and increased number of resorptions rather than some specific abnormality in a specific organ system. Effects that are the result of nonthermalizing exposure conditions are difficult to discuss, partly because of the difficulty in defining exactly what conditions should be considered nonthermal. Whether relatively low levels can induce functional problems that are demonstrated postnatally has not been determined conclusively.

ELF fields have not been as widely researched. However, the majority of studies investigating the electric components of such fields generally reported negative results. The situation with regard to the magnetic component of the fields is considerably different. Several reports of alterations in developing chick embryos and mouse fetuses have appeared. Discrepancies in the results of the studies from different laboratories are not yet understood.

REFERENCES

BERMAN, E., CARTER, H.B., AND KINN, J.B. (1978). Observations of mouse fetuses after irradiation with 2.45 GHz microwaves. *Health Phys. 35*:791–801.

BERMAN, E., HOUSE, D.E., KOCH, W.E., et al. (1988). The Henhouse Project: effect of pulsed magnetic fields on early chick embryos. *In*: Bioelectromagnetics Society Meeting Abstracts, Frederick, Md., Bioelectromagnetics Society.

CHERNOVETZ, M.E., JUSTESEN, D.R., KING, N.W., AND WAGNER, J.E. (1975). Teratology, survival, and reversal learning after irradiation of mice by 2450-MHz microwave energy. *J. Microwave Power* 10:391–409.

CHERNOVETZ, M.E., JUSTESEN, D.R., AND LEVINSON, D.M. (1978). Acceleration and deceleration of fetal growth of rats by 2450-MHz microwave radiation. *In*: Stuchly, S. (ed.). Proceedings of the 1978 Symposium on Electromagnetic Fields in Biological Systems. Edmonton, Alberta, Canada, International Microwave Power Institute, pp. 175–193.

CHERNOVETZ, M.E., JUSTESEN, D.R., AND OKE, A.F. (1977). A teratological study of the rat: microwave and infrared radiations compared. *Radio Sci.* 12:191–197.

D'AMBROSIO, G., MEGLIO, F.D., FERRARA, G., AND TRANFAGLIA, A. (1980). Entomological experiments on the teratogenic effect of electromagnetic fields. *Alta Frequenza* 49:115–159.

DELGADO, J.M.R., LEAL, J., MONTEAGUDO, J.L., AND GRACIA, M.G. (1982). Embryological changes induced by weak, extremely low frequency electromagnetic fields. *J. Anat.* 134:533–551.

DODGE, C.H. (1969). Clinical and hygienic aspects of exposure to electromagnetic fields. *In*: Cleary, S. (ed.). Biological effects and health implications of microwave radiation, Symposium Proceedings, BRH/DBE 70–2, PB 193–898, Washington, D.C., NTIS, pp. 140–149.

DODGE, C.H., AND GLASER, Z.R. (1977). Trends in nonionizing electromagnetic radiation bio-effects research and related occupational health aspects. *J. Microwave Power* 12:319–334.

EDELMAN, G.M. (1984). Cell-adhesion molecules: a molecular basis for animal form. *Sci. Am.* 250:118–129.

EDWARDS, M.J., AND WANNER, R.A. (1977). Extremes of temperature. *In*: Wilson, J.G., and Fraser, F.C. (eds.). Handbook of teratology, Vol. 1. New York, Plenum Publishing Corp., pp. 421–444.

FROLEN, H., SVEDENSTAL, B.M., BIERKE, P., AND FELLNER-FELDEGG, H. (1987). Repetition of a study of the effect of pulsed magnetic fields on the development of fetuses in mice. Concluding report for National Institute of Radiation Protection, SSI Project No. 346,86, Sweden.

GRAVES, H.B., CARTER, J.H., KELLMEL, D., AND COOPER, L. (1979). Perceptibility and electrophysiological response of small birds to intense 60-Hz electric fields. *IEEE Trans. Power Apparat. Syst.* 97:1070–1073.

GUY, A.W., WALLACE, J., AND McDOUGALL, J.A. (1979). Circularly polarized 2450-MHz waveguide system for chronic exposure of small animals to microwaves. *Radio Sci.* 14:63–74.

HAMBURGER, V., AND HAMILTON, H.L. (1951). A series of normal stages in the development of the chick embryo. *J. Morphol.* 88:49–92.

JENSH, R.P. (1984a). Studies of the teratogenic potential of exposure of rats to

6000-MHz radiation. I. Morphologic analysis at term. *Radiat. Res. 97:*272–281.

JENSH, R.P. (1984b). Studies of the teratogenic potential of exposure of rats to 6000-MHz microwave radiation. II. Postnatal psychophysiologic evaluations. *Radiat. Res. 97:*282–301.

JENSH, R.P., WEINBERG, I., AND BRENT, R.L. (1983a). An evaluation of the teratogenic potential of protracted exposure of pregnant rats to 2450-MHz microwave radiation. I. Morphologic analysis at term. *J. Toxicol. Environ. Health 11:*23–35.

JENSH, R.P., VOGEL, W.H., AND BRENT, R.L. (1983b). An evaluation of the teratogenic potential of protracted exposure of pregnant rats to 2450-MHz microwave radiation. II. Postnatal psychophysiologic analysis. *J. Toxicol. Environ. Health 11:*37–59.

JOHNSON, R.B., MIZUMORI, S., AND LOVELY, R.H. (1977). Adult behavioral deficit in rats exposed prenatally to 918-MHz microwaves. *In:* Developmental toxicology of energy related pollutants. DOE Symposium Series 47, Hanford Life Symposium, Richland, Wash., pp. 281–289.

JUUTILAINEN, J. (1986). Effects of low frequency magnetic fields on chick embryos: dependence on incubation temperature and storage of the eggs. *Z. Naturforsch 41c:*1111–1115.

JUUTILAINEN, J., LAARA, E., AND SAALI, K. (1987). Relationship between field strength and abnormal development in chick embryos exposed to 50 Hz magnetic fields. *Int. J. Radiat. Biol. 5:*787–793.

JUUTILAINEN, J., HARRI, M., SAALI, K., AND LAHTINEN, T. (1986). Effects of 100-Hz magnetic fields with various waveforms on the development of chick embryos. *Radiat. Environ. Biophys. 25:*65–74.

JUUTILAINEN, J., AND SAALI, K. (1986). Development of chick embryos in 1 Hz to 100 Hz magnetic fields. *Radiat. Environ. Biophys. 25:*135–140

KNICKERBOCKER, G.G., KOUWENHOVEN, W.B., AND BARNES, H.C. (1967). Exposure of mice to strong AC electric field: an experimental study. *IEEE Trans. Power Apparat. Syst. 86:*498–505.

KRUEGER, W.F., GIAROLA, A.J., BRADLEY, J.W., AND SHREKENHANER, A. (1975). Effects of electromagnetic fields on fecundity in the chicken. *Ann. N.Y. Acad. Sci. 247:*391–398.

LARY, J.M., CONOVER, D.L., FOLEY, E.D., AND HANSER, P.L. (1982a). Teratogenic effects of 27.12 HMz radiofrequency radiation in rats. *Teratology 26:*299–309.

LARY, J.M., CONOVER, D.L., FOLEY, E.D., AND HANSER, P.L. (1982b). Thermal threshold for teratogenesis in rats exposed to 27.12 MHz radiofrequency radiation. *Teratology 23:*49A.

LARY, J.M., CONOVER, D.L., JOHNSON, P.H., AND BURG, J.R. (1983). Teratogenicity of 27.12-HMz radiation in rats is related to duration of hyperthermic exposure. *Bioelectromagnetics 4:*249–255.

LEAL, J., TRILLO, M.A., UBEDA, A., ABRAIRA, V., SHAMSAIFAR, K., AND CHACON, L. (1986). Magnetic environment and embryonic development: a role of the earth's field. *IRCS Med. Sci. 14:*1145–1146.

LOVELY, R.H., MIZUMORI, S.J.Y., JOHNSON, R.B., AND GUY, A.W. (1983). Subtle consequences of exposure to weak microwave fields: are there non-thermal effects? *In*: Adair, E.R. (ed.). Microwaves and thermoregulation. New York, Academic Press.

MAFFEO, S., MILLER, M.W., AND CARSTENSEN, E.L. (1984). Lack of effect of weak low frequency electromagnetic fields on chick embryogenesis. *J. Anat. 139*:613–618.

MARINO, A.A., BERGER, T.J., AUSTIN, B.P., AND BECKER, R.O. (1976). Evaluation of electrochemical information transfer system. I. Effect of electric fields on living organisms. *J. Electrochem. Soc. 123*:1199–1200.

NCRP (1986). National Council on Radiation Protection and Measurements. Biological effects and exposure criteria for radiofrequency electromagnetic fields. Bethesda, Md., NCRP.

O'CONNOR, M.E. (1980). Mammalian teratogenesis and radio-frequency fields. *Proc. IEEE 68*:56–60.

O'CONNOR, M.E. (1985). Effects of radiofrequency radiation during development: the prenatal period as a model system. *In*: Monahan, J., and D'Andrea, J. (eds.). Behavioral effects of microwave radiation absorption. HHS Publication No. FDA 85–8238, Washington, D.C., U.S. Government Printing Office, pp. 102–109.

O'CONNOR, M.E. (1988). Prenatal microwave exposure and behavior. *In*: O'Connor, M.E., and Lovely, R.H. (eds.). Electromagnetic fields and neurobehavioral function. New York, Alan R. Liss, pp. 265–288.

O'CONNOR, M.E., AND STRATTAN, R.A. (1985). Project summary: teratogenic effects of microwave radiation. EPA/600/S1–85/007, Springfield, Va., NTIS.

O'CONNOR, M.E., AND STRATTAN, R.A. (In press). Project summary: behavioral effects of microwaves: relationship of total dose and dose rate. EPA No. 68–02–4120, Springfield, Va., NTIS.

ROMMEREIM, D.N., KAUNE, W.T., BUSCHBOM, R.L., PHILLIPS, R.D., AND SIKOV, M.R. (1987). Reproduction and development in rats chronologically exposed to 60-Hz electric fields. *Bioelectromagnetics 8*:243–258.

RUGH, R., GINNS, E.I., HO, H.S., AND LEACH, W.M. (1974). Are microwaves teratogenic? *In*: Biological effects and health hazards of microwave radiation: proceedings of the International Symposium. Warsaw, Polish Medical Publishers, pp. 98–107.

SETO, Y.J., MAJEAU-CHARGOIS, D., LYMANGROVER, J.R., DUNLAP, W.P., WALKER, C.F., AND HSIEH, S.T. (1984). Investigation of fertility and in utero effects in rats chronically exposed to a high intensity 60-Hz electric field. *IEEE Trans. Biomed. Eng. 31*:693–700.

SIKOV, M.R., MONTGOMERY L.D., SMITH, L.G., AND PHILLIPS, R.D. (1984). Studies on prenatal and postnatal development in rats exposed to 60-Hz electric fields. *Bioelectromagnetics 5*:101–112.

SIKOV, M.R., ROMMEREIM, D.N., BEAMER, J.L., BUSCHBOM, R.L., KAUNE, W.T., AND PHILLIPS, R.D. (1987). Developmental studies of Hanford miniature swine exposed to 60-Hz electric fields. *Bioelectromagnetics 8*:229–242.

TRIBUKAIT, B., CEKAN, E., AND PAULSSON, L.E. (1987). Effects of pulsed magnetic fields on embryonic development in mice. *In*: Knave, B., and Wideback, P. (eds.). Work with display units 86. Amsterdam, Elsevier Science Publisher, pp. 129–134.

UBEDA, A., LEAL, J., TRILLO, M.A., JIMENEZ, M.A., AND DELGADO, J.M.R. (1983). Pulse shape of magnetic fields influences chick embryogenesis. *J. Anat. 137*:513–536.

UBEDA, A., LEAL, J., TRILLO, M.A., JIMENEZ, M.A., AND DELGADO, J.M.R. (1985). Pulse shape of magnetic fields influences chick embryogenesis: author's correction to data. *J. Anat. 140*:721.

16

Biological Effects of Millimeter-Wave Radiation

SHIRLEY M. MOTZKIN

Although high power levels of nonionizing radiation are known to destroy human tissue and cause heat-related health effects at selected frequencies, intensities, and periods of irradiation, we still do not know whether electromagnetic (EM) fields at low levels are harmless or hold a threat yet to be demonstrated. This is true particularly at high frequencies at which reported biological effects in organisms do not appear to be solely attributable to thermal conditions and evidence of simple cause-effect relationships is not readily available.

Evidence has been mounting that some biological effects are unrelated to thermal characteristics and that exogenous EM fields can modulate both in vivo and in vitro cell behavior. To understand the biological role of electrical currents, researchers have directed their attention to the cellular effects of EM fields.

After the development of millimeter band generators, few investigations were initiated because the low energy of millimeter waves (10^4 times less than the energy of chemical bonds) was thought to be too weak to break chemical bonds or produce irreversible damage to atoms and molecules. Subsequently, interest was aroused by Frohlich's calculated estimates of absorbed energy (1968) and his predictions that coherent vibrations play an important role in biological activity. He suggested that the imposition of external microwaves could act as a trigger of frequency-dependent effects for chemically oscillating biological molecules. These coherent excitations, which could occur when high-frequency millimeter energy exceeds a critical value, would be supplemented by small conformational changes and by selective long-range cooperative interactions to provide a multicausal process typical of biological events. Although Frohlich's hypothesis stimulated much interest in the frequency dependence of interactions, it has not enabled us to identify or predict the frequencies or powers most likely to produce bioeffects.

Studies initiated in the Soviet Union and Eastern Europe in 1965 and reported in the 1970s, in which a myriad of organisms were exposed to low-level millimeter wave energy, indicated sharp frequency dependencies suggestive of resonance for almost all biological components examined. These experiments, carried out primarily on microbial organisms, cultured cells, viruses, tumors, blood-forming organs, and biopolymers

(Devyatkov, 1974; Devyatkov et al., 1981, 1983), exhibited nonthermal frequency dependence without gross injury. An extensive search for biological effects at millimeter-wave frequencies was initiated. Unfortunately, this research has been plagued by widely divergent results and a lack of reproducibility. Differences observed may be attributed largely to variations in the experimental and technical design of the research. The use of different species, different periods within biological cycles and varying lengths of exposure, coupled with the enormity of frequency and power combinations made it unlikely that individual investigators would produce comparable data. This extensive variability has frequently led to conclusions that are diametrically opposed and that have prevented resolution of the major questions concerning the mechanisms of bioeffects.

An understanding of ways in which EM waves act on biological objects is of utmost importance to their applications in biology and medicine.

This chapter, which reviews investigations of the bioeffects of high-frequency EM fields in the millimeter range, also indicates the use of innumerable living systems under widely divergent experimental conditions. The research presented here used engineering technology and biophysical concepts applied to biological systems to elucidate the molecular basis of EM field bioeffects.

EXPERIMENTAL APPROACHES

EM fields at millimeter wavelengths interact with living systems at a molecular and cellular level, affecting physicochemical mechanisms, metabolism, and multiplication rates. Because of minimum depth of penetration, maximum energy absorption occurs at the surface and decreases with depth, implying that effects are limited to superficial cells and molecules. Identification of EM field effects and the sites and mechanisms of interaction depends on the demonstration of frequency dependence, which may be visualized by absorption and Raman spectra.

Experimental observations of frequency-specific biological effects suggestive of resonance, and sharp resonances associated with millimeter wave absorption spectra, support Frohlich's coherent oscillation hypothesis (Frohlich, 1968, 1970, 1972, 1973, 1975a,b, 1978, 1980), which can explain resonance phenomena. Other investigators have not been able to corroborate these findings by identifying frequency specificities or distinct resonances in absorption spectra.

Absorption Spectra

Ultraviolet–visible.   Comparative spectral analyses of *Escherichia coli* cells, water, protein, RNA, and DNA, irradiated at frequencies from

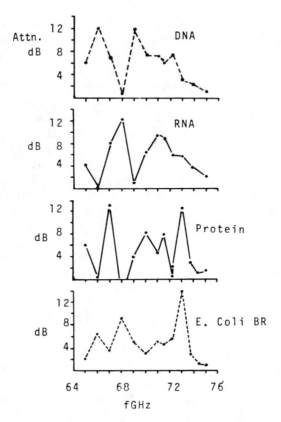

Figure 16-1   Absorption spectra of cells and molecules demonstrate frequency specificity. (From Webb, S.J., and Booth, A.D. [1969]. *Nature* 222:1199–1200.)

65 to 75 GHz (Webb and Dodds, 1968) (Figure 16-1) indicated that the fairly uniformly spaced absorption peaks of cellular spectra corresponded with frequencies that had a maximum effect on growth. Frequencies that decreased growth, 66, 71, and 73 GHz, matched the absorption maxima of DNA, RNA, and protein, respectively, indicating that bacterial cells may absorb specific frequencies that alter their metabolic processes and growth. If the growth pattern of these irradiated cells was affected by increased temperature, growth enhancement would have been expected. However, since the growth declined, it appears that temperature was not a contributory factor (Webb and Dodds, 1968; Lee, 1977).

Others have reported the existence of sharp millimeter-wave absorption peaks in a variety of biological components, including normal and diseased tissue (Dardanoni et al., 1976; Lee, 1977; Lee and Webb, 1977). Differences in normal and mouse virus–transformed BHK cells (Webb and Booth, 1971) and in normal and cancerous mammary glands indicated that viability and growth were unaffected by exposure to millimeter waves at frequencies between 50 and 90 GHz, but that tumor-producing capability was inhibited (Webb and Dodds, 1968; Webb et al., 1977). Stamm et al. (1974, 1975) apparently demonstrated marked absorption differences in normal and tumorous human tissues. If valid, these observations could have significant diagnostic and therapeutic implications (Frohlich, 1978; Webb and Booth, 1971; Stamm et al., 1974, 1975; Lee and Webb, 1977).

Devyatkov's examination of millimeter wave–induced intermolecular interactions in aqueous electrolyte solutions, as a consequence of pH and concentration, led to the conclusion that altered absorption was due to the rotational mobility of water molecules in solution reflecting the influence of the solute on the solvent's structure (Devyatkov et al., 1983).

In contrast to the preceding studies, Gandhi, with a swept-frequency measurement system, sampled a wide variety of biological and biochemical components, including water, RNA, DNA, BHK-21/C13 cells, *Candida albicans*, *Candida krusei*, and *E. coli*, at 900 frequencies from 26.5 to 90 GHz (Gandhi et al., 1980; Gandhi and Riazi, 1986). Samples at various combinations of cell concentration, dwell time, and incident power level, with and without modulation, in different media and in fresh and frozen states, were compared. To resolve the questions raised by the studies of Grundler and Keilmann and their co-workers (1977, 1978, 1981a,b, 1982, 1983, 1985), more extensive evaluation was targeted to the narrow frequency range. They used 41.200 to 41.794 GHz, in which frequency-specific bioeffects were reported. Unlike the observations of Webb and Booth (1969) and others who reported both frequency specificity and absorption spectral resonances, Gandhi's sweep width spectra were similar for all preparations (Figure 16-2) (Gandhi et al., 1980). None of his specimens exhibited sharp resonance peaks in the 26.5 to 90 GHz range, and no biological effects ascribable to millimeter-wave irradiation were observed for any power density up to 300 mW/cm^2.

Although reports of absorption have been used as proof of coherent phenomena in living cells, it is unlikely that specific absorbance differences can be detected in biological entities whose predominant component is water.

Raman spectra.   Since Raman scattering can provide information on the chemical and structural composition of molecules and organisms and their immediate environments, several investigators have used this physical technique to determine the effects of millimeter waves on living systems.

Microbial and mammalian cells are purported to absorb specific frequencies in the 50 to 150 GHz range, which might alter metabolic events. Webb et al. (1968, 1971, 1975, 1977) attempted to ascertain in

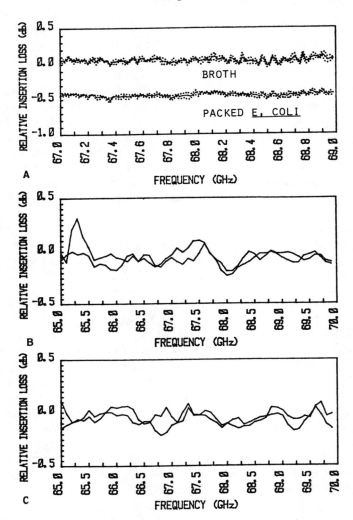

Figure 16-2 Absorption spectra of *Escherichia coli* cells demonstrate no absorption other than that related to water. **A,** Dotted curves are ± standard deviation. **B,** Low millimeter-wave power (1 to 4 μW) with no modulation; broth versus broth. **C,** Low millimeter-wave power (1 to 4 μW) with no modulation; *E. coli* versus broth. (From Gandhi, O.P., et al. [1980]. *Bioelectromagnetics 1*:285–298.)

vivo energy states, by laser Raman spectroscopy, of *E. coli*, *Bacillus megaterium* (Figure 16-3), and *Saccharomyces cerevisiae* cells in both living and dried states. They reported that molecular resonances, observed between 7.5×10^{10} and 5×10^{12} Hz, occur in living, actively metabolizing, synchronized bacterial cells, not in resting cells or in homogenates. Ear-

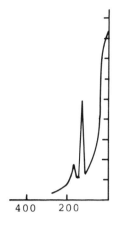

Figure 16-3 Raman spectrum of *Bacillus megaterium*. (From Webb, S.J., and Stoneham, M.E. [1977]. *Phys. Lett.* *60A*:267–268.)

lier, frequencies corresponding to these spectra were shown to affect microbial metabolism. The spectra produced were highly species specific and reflected the in vivo molecular organization essential to life. Spectra of the various organisms differed from one another and were not reproducible from scan to scan. The authors postulated that, because the existence of excited energy states was required to produce the time-varying lines of the spectra, these states might exist for only specific short periods during the cell cycle. Thus the presence and intensity of Raman shift lines were attributed to the energy state of a cell population at the particular frequency in the scans. To observe the Raman shift lines at 1835 cm^{-1}, activation of the respiratory chain in *B. megaterium* was initiated. It was the only energy state seen at set times and precise intervals during the lifetime of the cell. Webb's experimental findings supported Frohlich's theoretical predictions that coherent vibrations in the 10^{11} to 10^{12} Hz frequency regions are excited by metabolic processes and influence biological action.

Furia and Gandhi (1984, 1985) repeated Webb's experiments with *B. megaterium* at various stages of the cell cycle, at temperatures of 21° to 23° and 35° C under both nonflow (used by Webb) and flow conditions. Lines were not detected in the spectral regions between 20 and 300 cm^{-1} of specimens exposed for 10 minutes to 2½ hours. The random lines visible under flow conditions were attributed to the medium alone or to clumps of cells or fluorescent particles passing through the laser beam. That the strong spectral lines from metabolically synchronized cell suspensions of Webb et al. (1977) (Figure 16-3), which were attributed to the excited vibrations of macromolecules, are probably artifactual was demonstrated by Cooper and Amer (1983). These authors showed that Mie scattering and cell density fluctuations produce spurious Raman lines, whereas strongly vibrating molecules result in sharply distinct spectra. Therefore, if Cooper's observations are correct, Webb's experiments do not support theories of coherent vibrations or solitons.

Measurement of the intensity ratios of Stokes/anti-Stokes Raman lines offers a straightforward method for determining thermal excitation because nonthermal vibrational states lead to anti-Stokes scattering. Drissler's studies (1978, 1983) of *Chlorella pyrenoidosa* and *E. coli*, designed to clarify the role of vibrational states in biological membranes, demonstrated enhanced anti-Stokes scattering. Synchronized populations were required for optimal visualization. Resonances attributable to other sources were not ruled out. Subsequently, these results could not be reproduced.

Furia et al. (1986b) (Figure 16-4) also used this technique to determine conformational changes of phospholipids in liposomes above and below phase transition temperatures. The specific frequency selected, 41.65 GHz, was the one at which frequency-specific effects were reported by Grundler. Spectral lines indicating sites of interaction were not identified.

Frequency-Specific Effects

Growth. The effects of millimeter waves on growth rate have been monitored in a variety of prokaryotic and eukaryotic organisms. Mitotic activity and nucleic acid synthesis in yeast (*Rhodotorula rubra*) exposed to frequencies from 7.16 to 7.19 mm (Devyatkov, 1974) demonstrated growth increases of 30% at 41.783 GHz (7.18 mm) and decreases of 40% at 41.725 GHz (7.19 mm), which suggests a resonance-like frequency dependence.

Stimulated by Frohlich's predictions of frequency specificity and by the results of Devyatkov, Grundler (1981a,b, 1985; Grundler et al., 1977, 1982, 1983, 1983a; Grundler and Keilmann, 1978) and Keilmann (1982a, Keilmann and Grundler, 1984) investigated the growth rate of yeast (*S. cerevisiae*). Using antennas of two different shapes (fork and tube) (Figure 16-5), they photometrically examined growth characteristics of yeast exposed to low-level microwaves at frequencies from 41.65 to 41.80 and 83.55 to 83.77 GHz, at temperatures of 30.5° to 34° C, and at power levels of 1.2 to 2.7 mW/cm^2. Their results, which demonstrated 15% stimulation and 13% inhibition at power levels from 5 to 40 mW, suggested a frequency-selective, resonant growth rate response, with widely divergent excursions of stimulation and depression within 8 MHz. Results with both experimental systems were similar, but a nonzero frequency shift of +11 MHz was required to achieve cross-correlation. Subsequently, single yeast cells irradiated near 42 and 84 GHz were locally fixed to a medium enabling visualization of microcolonies and mitosis. The distribution of generation time was defined, and the relation-

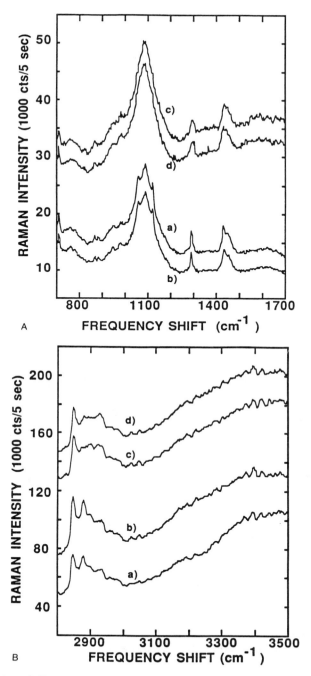

Figure 16-4 A, Raman spectra of dipyrenylpropane vesicles in conformational region with and without millimeter waves at 41.65 GHz: a, 25° C, nonirradiated; b, 25° C, irradiated; c, 45° C, nonirradiated, d, 45° C, irradiated. **B,** Raman spectra of dipyrenylpropane vesicles in C-14 stretching region with and without millimeter waves: a, 25° C, nonirradiated; b, 25° C, irradiated; c, 45° C, nonirradiated; d, 45° C, irradiated. (From Furia, L. et al. [1986]. *J. Appl. Phys. 60*:2991–2994.)

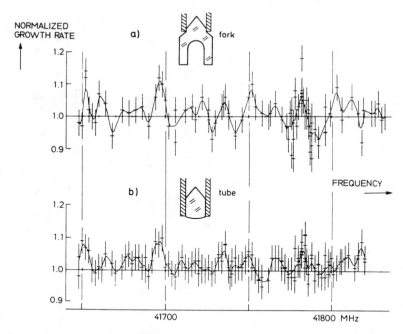

Figure 16-5 Normalized growth rate of yeast cultures at various millimeter-wave frequencies using, *a*, fork-shaped or, *b*, tubular antennas. Curves were obtained by single three-point smoothing. (From Grundler, W., and Keilmann, F. [1983]. *Phys. Rev. Lett. 51*:1214–1216.)

ship between millimeter waves and the different phases of the cell cycle was examined. The observed multipeaked distribution (Figure 16-6), attributed to frequency-dependent differences in cell population and generation time, resembles earlier results. Grundler et al. (1983) suggested that the small relative growth rate and the failure to identify the factor determining behavior militates against reproducibility.

Grundler (1985) demonstrated that millimeter effects were not unique to *S. cerevisiae* but could be produced in mammalian cells. In in vitro studies of Ehrlich ascites tumor cells, he showed that stimulation and inhibition were frequency dependent with maximum enhancement at 83568 MHz, twice that defined earlier microscopically. He concluded that the higher harmonics also influence growth in biological systems other than yeast.

Grundler and his colleagues continue to affirm their strong commitment to the concept of frequency-dependent effects of millimeter waves on biological systems. Based upon their yeast experiments they reassert the existence of frequency specific effects. The low intensity, limited depth of penetration, sharp frequency dependence, narrow line width, and nonhomogeneous irradiation field are thought to support a nonthermal effect.

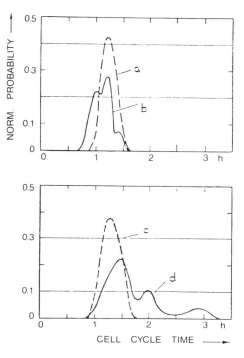

Figure 16-6 Multipeaked distribution of cell cycle times of growing single *Saccharomyces cerevisiae* cells showing generation time and frequency-dependent differences in cell populations: *a*, nonirradiated cells; *b*, cells irradiated at 41784 ± 1 MHz; *c*, cells irradiated at 83842 ± 2 MHz; *d*, cells irradiated at 83835 ± 2 MHz. (From Grundler, W. [1985]. Frequency-dependent biological effects on low intensity microwaves. *In*: Chiabrera, A., Niccolini, C., and Schwan, H.P. [eds.]. Interactions between electromagnetic fields and cells, pp. 459–481.)

Although these results confirm those of Devyatkov, they are not universally accepted. Nevertheless, their exquisite frequency sensitivity has stimulated a search for similar bioeffects phenomena that would permit a definition of the mechanisms of interaction.

Furia et al. (1986a) (Figure 16-7) repeated the Grundler experiments with *S. cerevisiae* exposed to millimeter waves at 13 frequencies between 41.650 and 41.798 GHz for 4 hours with an absorbed power of 20 ± 0.5 mW. An absence of detectable effects greater than ±4% on either viability or growth at any frequency indicated that the results were not significant.

The diametrically opposed conclusions of these yeast experiments are indicative of the unresolved controversies in millimeter-wave bioelectromagnetics research. Inherent technological difficulties at millimeter frequencies leave considerable room for error. In this case both groups have cautiously designed and carried out experiments to define frequency-dependent effects. Their instrumentation is of equivalent stability, precision, and accuracy. Both the positive and the negative results show small differences that fall within or close to normal biological variation. Grundler has attributed these different behavioral sensitivities to the two *S. cerevisiae* strains. This is difficult to accept, particularly because he supports his findings with those of Devyatkov, who also used a different yeast species (*R. rubra*). Using a laser-nephelometric system, Keilmann

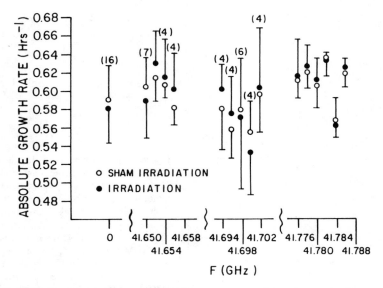

Figure 16-7 Experiments with *Saccharomyces cerevisiae* demonstrating no detectable effect. Each point and bar represent average ± standard deviation experiments at each frequency. Unless otherwise indicated, three experiments were performed at each frequency. (From Furia, L., et al. [1986]. Effects of millimeter waves on growth of *Saccharomyces cerevisiae*. *IEEE Trans. Biomed. Eng. 33*:993–999. © 1986 IEEE.)

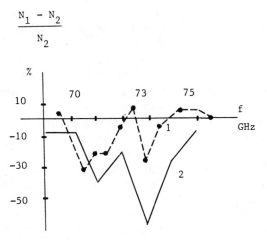

Figure 16-8 Growth rate of *Escherichia coli* as function of frequency. (From Berteaud, A.J., et al. [1975]. *C.R. Acad. Sci. [D] [Paris] 281*:843–846.)

(Grundler's coauthor) (1982b) was unable to repeat the reported yeast effects (Keilmann, 1982, personal communication). The absence of reproducibility, which would result in a consensus of frequency specifity, requires that independent confirmation be sought from other laboratories.

Other reported frequency-dependent effects on growth include inhibition of actively replicating synchronous *E. coli* at millimeter frequencies (65 to 75 and 136 GHz) and 7 μW power levels. The effect was found to depend on the cell cycle phase (Webb and Dodds, 1968). Altered growth rates were obtained in *C. albicans* (Dardanoni et al., 1979) with pulsed fields but not with continuous millimeter wave irradiation. The growth rate of *E. coli* exposed to 71.5 and 73 GHz was strongly inhibited, but no effect on survival or induction of mutations was seen (Berteaud et al., 1975) (Figure 16-8). The effect at 73 GHz was one-third that seen by Webb.

In contrast to the preceding observations, frequency-specific correlations were not noted in studies involving growth of *E. coli* exposed to 136 GHz (Blackman, et al., 1975), in the extensive studies by Gandhi and his colleagues involving a wide variety of systems, or in Webb's efforts to confirm his earlier results (Keilmann, 1982, personal communication).

Genetic systems

Colicin induction.   Most of the early evidence that biological systems could be altered by low-intensity EM fields was available below 30 GHz. Studies from the Soviet Union indicated that frequency-dependent effects suggestive of resonance existed above 30 GHz. Millimeter-wave effects on the genetic system that regulates the induction and lethal synthesis of colicin by *E. coli* were reported by Smolyanskaya and Vilenskaya (1973). Colicin is an antibiotic synthesized by bacterial strains harboring the plasmid-borne colicinogenic factor Col E1. If these cells are incubated at temperatures above 43° C, treated with mitomycin C, or exposed to ultraviolet light, active colicin synthesis and replication of DNA molecules that code for Col E1 occur. Normally, minute quantities of colicin are produced. Colicin is active against related strains in low concentrations and against the original strain in high concentrations. A careful analysis of cell proliferation at 11 closely spaced millimeter wavelengths, in the 6.50 to 6.59 mm range (45.5 to 46.1 GHz) and at 5.8 and 7.1 mm, revealed marked stimulation of growth, and increased colicin synthesis by as much as 300%. The effects were frequency dependent and almost insensitive to power density over two orders of magnitude, from 0.01 mW/cm^2 (Figure 16-9). These experiments support the contentions of others that resonant excitation of intrinsic systems is not produced by the weak energy of microwaves. The results suggest that millimeter waves influence the regulation of cellular function by affecting genetic elements. The Col

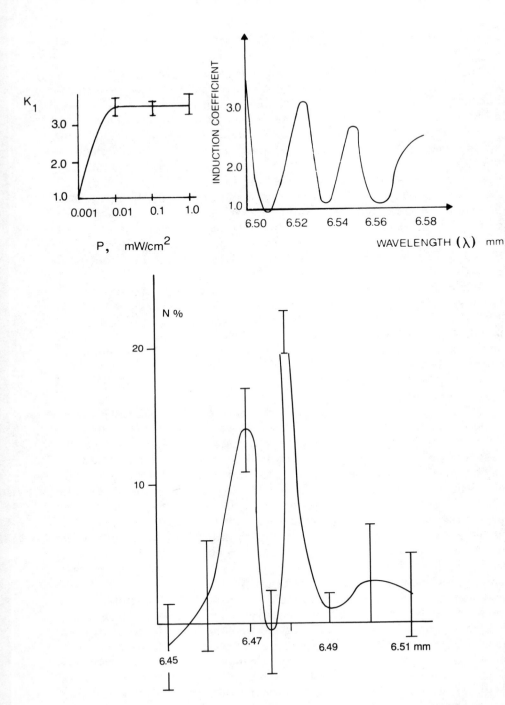

Figure 16-9 Colicin synthesis as function of power density and wavelength. (From Smolyanskaya, A.Z., and Vilenskaya, R.L. [1973]. *Usp. Fiziol. Nauk* *110*:458–460.)

E1 plasmid, which appears to be sensitive to certain wavelengths in the millimeter range, is derepressed, resulting in enhanced colicin synthesis.

Classically, mitomycin C and ultraviolet irradiation induce colicin production and interfere with chromosomal DNA synthesis by rupturing the chemical bonds of the molecule. Millimeter waves do not affect the functional cell by producing mutations or grossly altering DNA, but rather, may produce a conformational change without bond destruction.

Attempts by Swicord et al. (1978) to verify the existence of resonance in colicin induction at 46.1 to 47.7 GHz (6.50 to 6.59 mm) met with initial success. However, subsequent attempts at replication proved unsuccessful, since no differences between sham and experimental exposures were noted. In our laboratories, extensive efforts were mounted to understand the colicin induction phenomenon. Using continuous millimeter-wave exposures, we irradiated specimens at discrete wavelengths between 50 and 60 GHz (5 to 6 mm), at 35 GHz and at 40 to 50 GHz (6.50 to 6.59 mm), for 1 hour at 37° C in log phase of the cell cycle and at power levels of 5, 0.5, and 0.05 mW/cm^2. The results showed extensive variability and did not demonstrate frequency-related colicin stimulation or inhibition (Motzkin et al., 1983, 1984c). Occasional indications of significance at a 95% confidence level appeared in isolated instances at various frequencies. These were subsequently negated by pooled data analysis. To determine the role of cell cycle phase, temperature, and the duration of exposure in the induction of bioeffects, we also irradiated cells at lag or stationary phase (Figure 16-10) for 2 hours at 20° C, parameters reported by Smolyanskaya et al. (1981, 1983) to maximize colicin production. Synergistic interactions of subthreshold mitomycin C and EM fields also were investigated. None of the various combinations meaningfully affected the frequency specificity of colicin production.

To determine whether a millimeter-wave treatment effect could be correlated with some cell cycle event, we used cell synchronization to provide biological magnification capable of maximizing the effects of the applied field (Motzkin et al., 1986a) (Figure 16-11). Short-term synchrony was achieved through size selection by double filtration. Six frequencies and two power levels were examined in 120 experiments, each with 10 replications of 10 subsamples. Casual inspection of the log ratio data, plotted as the average of all replications for a power at each frequency, revealed peaks of stimulation and inhibition (Figure 16-12) reminiscent of Grundler's and Smolyanskaya's resonance figures. However, rigorous analysis of the data indicated that a conclusion of resonance was not statistically defensible. Synchronized E. coli Col E1 cells in lag, log, and stationary phases, exposed to low-power continuous millimeter waves for up to 2 hours at 20° C, did not demonstrate altered colicin production.

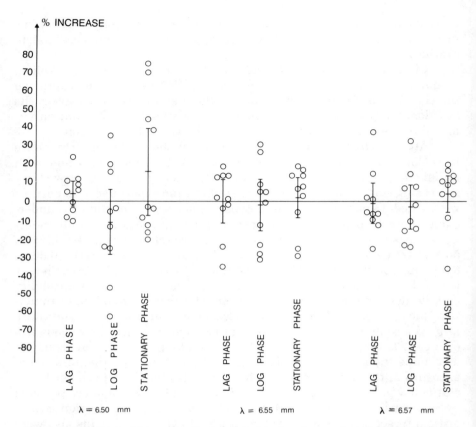

Figure 16-10 *Escherichia coli* cells irradiated in lag, log, and stationary phases to determine role of cell cycle phase.

Protocols and subcultures of our strains were provided to Santo (1983) in an attempt to resolve the question of reproducibility. Results of 60 experiments in the 50 to 60 GHz range confirmed our observations that there was no evidence of frequency-dependent effects in the induction of colicin.

Lambda phage. Since the biochemical pathways that cause colicin induction are believed to be similar to those of viral induction, several groups carried out experiments to elucidate the effects of millimeter waves on lambda phage induction in populations of *E. coli*. Webb (1979) reported that millimeter waves at 70.4 and 71 GHz at power densities of 10 μW/cm² enhanced phage induction. These observations were confirmed in

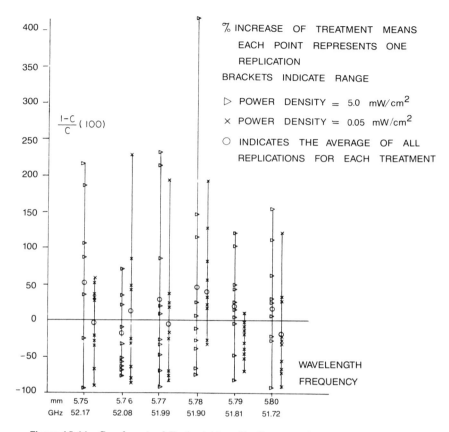

Figure 16-11   Synchronized *Escherichia coli* cells exposed to frequencies 51.72 to 52.17 GHz at 5 and 0.5 mW/cm² for 1 hour at 37° C. Results are not significant.

lysogenic *Staphylococcus aureus* (Makhov, 1979). Suslov described a 2.2-fold increase in phage particles after irradiation at 45.79 GHz. However, Athey and Krop's (1979, 1980) attempts to alter phage induction by exposure to 45.6 and 46.1 GHz frequencies for 40 and 90 minutes showed no treatment effect. The frequencies selected were purported by Smolyanskaya to affect colicin induction at power levels of 10 to 100 μW/cm². Enhancement of lambda phage activity was not evident in wild-type or temperature-sensitive lysogenic *E. coli* exposed at 42 to 48 and 65 to 75 GHz in 0.5 GHz increments for 30 minutes (Gandhi et al., 1982; Gandhi, 1983; Hill et al., 1983). Smolyanskaya (1983) contends that Athey and Krop's attempts to determine phage production from the presence of lactomase, rather than by the conventional plaque method, are errone-

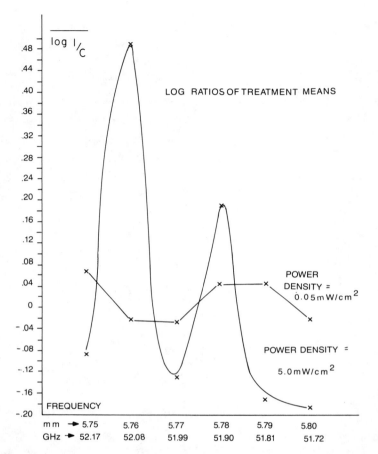

Figure 16-12 Log ratios of treatment means, which provide curves similar to those of Grundler and Smolyanskaya. Statistical analysis indicates nonsignificance.

ous because they assume that the two genes are transformed together. Furthermore, she takes exception to the assumption that the mechanisms for colicin and phage induction are alike. The assumption is based on the fact that ultraviolet radiation and mitomycin C induce both phage and colicin. These inductions are probably effected through the destruction of DNA. Smolyanskaya contends that, since millimeter waves do not appear to damage DNA, they must effect repression by some other mechanism.

Other genetic effects. A wide variety of genetic parameters have been examined to determine the effects of millimeter waves on survival, mutation, and repair. Demonstrable evidence of mutagenesis with resonant-like frequency specificity is unavailable. Back-mutation rates of the Hiŝ mutant *Salmonella typhimurium* were not affected by exposure to the 42 to 48 and 65 to 75 GHz frequency ranges (Gandhi, 1983). Comparative studies of millimeter wave–exposed wild-type and repair-deficient mutants of *E. coli* and *S. cerevisiae*, which were sensitive to radiation-induced DNA lesions, examined nuclear reversion, mitotic recombination, yeast sporulation, and formation of petite colonies (Dardalhon et al., 1980, 1981, 1985). Appreciable effects on cell survival of populations exposed to 70 to 75 GHz at power levels of about 60 mW/cm^2 were not evident, even in repair-deficient mutants. The reported absence of effects on DNA is contrary to the changes of DNA structure known to be caused by conventional heating. Even prolonged exposures to microwaves did not induce formation of cytoplasmic petite colonies, changes in ascospore production, or increased mortality. These results support those of others who have been unable to produce evidence of lethal or mutagenic effects. Temperature-sensitive yeast zygote formation (Dardalhon et al., 1985), used to monitor sample temperature during exposure to 73 GHz at power densities of 1 to 60 mW/cm^2, showed no differences between the control and sham groups. An increase in zygote production at 17GHz, 2 to 3 times higher than at other frequencies, was attributed to the dielectric absorption of microwaves by free or loosely bound water molecules in the cytoplasm, affecting the relaxation of the water molecules. If microwaves effect cellular alterations secondarily, the changes might be due to modifications of enzymes and membranes that cause a destabilization of molecular and intracellular equilibrium, since DNA is unaffected.

These observations agree with the conclusions of Smolyanskaya that millimeter waves do not destroy DNA but rather change the conformation of some functioning molecules. This effect corresponds to that of an equivalent increase of 3° C. Smolyanskaya believes that a much greater temperature increase would be needed to achieve corresponding physiological effects.

Microwaves do not appear to induce significant genetic effects, even at powers capable of increasing the temperature as seen in yeast zygote formation.

Salivary chromosomes of *Acricotopus lucidus* were exposed to swept millimeter-wave frequencies in the 64.1 to 69.1 GHz range at a power density of less than 5 mW/cm^2 (Kremer et al., 1983). Examination of the Balbiani rings indicated a reduction in puffing of specific rings (sites of active secretory protein synthesis), most prominently at 67.2 and 68.2 GHz. These results were significantly different from both sham and conventionally heated samples. Such experiments support the theory that externally applied EM fields may influence the excitation of biological systems.

Cellular and subcellular effects

Cellular effects.   Cytological effects of microwave radiation at sub-millimeter frequencies have been implicated in alterations of cellular structure and function, such as permeability of the erythrocyte membrane and of the nervous system microvasculature. An extensive study of milli-meter frequency effects has been carried out on monolayer cultures of mammalian BHK 21/C-13 cells to determine the effects of temperature and frequency on ultrastructure (Stensaas et al., 1981) and on protein and RNA synthesis (Partlow et al., 1981). Cells exposed to 41.8 and 74 GHz at average power densities of 320 or 450 mW/cm^2 for 1 hour, with and without temperature stabilization, were monitored during and after irradiation (Partlow et al., 1981). The results demonstrated that irradia-tion at high-power densities, at frequencies of 41.8 and 74 GHz, caused no discernible ultrastructural changes in the BHK 21/C-13 monolayers for cells maintained at constant temperatures below 44.5° C. However, increased temperature was shown to cause severe cytological damage. RNA and protein synthesis likewise were unaffected by millimeter-wave irradiation. Since examination was monitored during and after exposure, if present, transient and persistent effects would have been identified. Macromolecular synthesis was markedly altered by microwave-induced heat effects (Partlow et al., 1981). In addition, protein synthesis evaluated in cultures irradiated for 15 minutes at 202 closely spaced frequencies from 38 to 48 and 65 to 75 GHz in 0.1 GHz increments at average power densities of 292 and 177 mW/cm^2 failed to reveal changes suggesting resonant frequency dependence (Bush et al., 1981).

As the incident power varies along the waveguide aperture in the form of a sine wave, the power density changes from zero to twice the average at the center of the waveguide, exposing the sample to a variety of power densities. Because an intensity series, which incorporates this energy distribution, is provided in the experimental design, Stensaas et al. (1981) propose these experiments do not support the existence of power windows.

Other alleged cytological effects of millimeter-wave radiation re-ported include suppression of induced synthesis, but not activity, of peni-cillinase in *Staphylococcus aureus* (Smolyanskaya, 1983), a 60% decrease in the survival rates of various microorganisms irradiated at 6.5 mm, including *E. coli*, *Staphylococcus*, and *Streptococcus*, increased sensitivity to antibiotics, and modified antigenic properties (Zalyubovskaya, 1973). Also, damage to the cell membrane, including alteration of the hemolytic stability of red blood cells, and a decrease in the infectivity of adenovirus, vesicular stomatitis virus, and measles virus resulted from exposure to 6.5 mm radiation (Kiselev and Zalyubovskaya, 1973).

An incorporated fluorescent dye molecule, used to visualize microcy-toplasmic viscosity alterations, revealed an increase in microviscosity

and a decrease in enzymatic activity after conventional heating or exposure to microwaves (More et al., 1980). The exposure of rapidly proliferat-
ing roots of cress seedlings to millimeter waves at 43 and 56 GHz and
power densities from 0.1 to 110 mW/cm^2 resulted in a 30% reduction of
the rate of root growth at 56 GHz and 2 mW/cm^2 (Poglitsch, 1984, personal
communication). Similar results were not achieved at 43 GHz. The observed effects were strongly dependent on the polarization of the millimeter waves; effects were greater when the E vector of the microwave field
was parallel to the long axis of the roots. The radiation-induced temperature increase of 0.2° C is not believed to be responsible for the effect,
which instead is attributed to frequency and polarization dependence.

Subcellular effects

MITOCHONDRIA.   The effects of continuous wave millimeter irradiation on oxidative phosphorylation and Ca^{++} transport in freshly prepared
rat liver mitochondria have been examined in our laboratories at 35
GHz (8.58 mm) and at 41 discrete wavelengths between 5 and 6 mm
(50 to 60 GHz). Changes in respiratory control ratios observed at 250,
500, and 1000 mW/cm^2 at 30° C indicated membrane damage, which
was attributed to energy absorption and heat production. At 25° C respiratory control ratios were maintained at higher exposure levels, and at 4°
C some coupling in the mitochondria was maintained even at 1000 mW/
cm^2. No difference in adenosine triphosphate (ATP) synthesis was observed when mitochondria were irradiated at 25° C for 2 minutes at
34.92 GHz from 0.01 to 1000 mW/cm^2 or at 50 to 60 GHz at 5 mW/cm^2.
Mitochondrial suspensions irradiated at 25° C, 34.95 GHz, and 50 to 60
GHz at power densities of 1 to 1000 and 5 mW/cm^2, respectively, demonstrated no changes in ^{45}Ca^{++} uptake after 15 minutes , or efflux after 5
minutes of irradiation below 100 mW/cm^2. Above that power density,
decreased uptake and increased efflux were correlated with membrane
damage from thermal changes. No changes in the membrane processes
examined previously could be attributed, at low levels of power density,
to a specific frequency effect. The results of oxidative phosphorylation
bear a remarkable similarity to those of Ca^{++} uptake and efflux. The
results suggest that the ability of the mitochondrial membrane to maintain an electrochemical gradient was impaired at 500 and 1000 mW/
cm^2 because of measurable heating of the samples. That the effects are
a function of power density is further substantiated by evidence that
respiratory controls are not equivalent for equal time-dose exposures
(that is, 150 minutes at 100 mW/cm^2 and 15 minutes at 1000 mW/cm^2).
At the specific millimeter-wave frequencies employed, nonionizing radiation had no apparent effect on mitochondrial oxidative phosphorylation
and Ca^{++} transport other than those attributable to thermal change
(Motzkin et al., 1980).

MEMBRANES.   As the initial and primary structure encountered, the cell membrane appears to be the critical target of EM field–induced structural and functional alterations. Biological membranes are extremely complex structures composed of interactive lipid, protein, and carbohydrate components. Their functional properties are influenced by the fluidity of the lipid bilayer. The heterogeneity of the lipid packing results in regions of fluidity and stiffness that can be further altered by lipoprotein associations.

Since the complexity of membranes confounds our ability to understand their interactive mechanisms, it seems more appropriate to use simple, well-defined models that can be sequentially modified to more closely simulate natural membranes. Fluorescent dyes, which have sensitive spectroscopic properties that probe the characteristics of the environment in which they are located, are incorporated into natural and model synthetic membranes to enhance understanding of the interactive mechanisms of high-frequency, low-power EM fields and biological membranes. For the probe dipyrenylpropane (DPP), increased viscosity causes enhancement of the excimer and decrease of the monomer peak in the emission spectra. In our laboratories, lipid vesicles were irradiated at seven discrete frequencies from 50.90 to 52.17 GHz and at two power levels from 0.043 to 0.75 mW/cm^2 (Figures 16-13 and 16-14). Continuous millimeter-wave exposures did not alter the conformation or increase the fluidity of irradiated liposomes. Cholesterol-enriched vesicles also were examined. No significant alteration in the excimer/monomer ratio was ascertained, which indicates that no conformational alterations occurred (Motzkin et al., 1984a,b, 1986b,c, 1987).

In experiments by Furia et al. (1986b), sonicated liposomes irradiated with millimeter waves at 41.65 GHz were examined with Raman spectroscopy during the irradiation process to determine whether millimeter waves alter the conformation of phospholipids in vesicles above or below the transition temperature. Spectra were collected near the conformational shift region, 700 to 1700 cm^{-1}, and C-H stretching region, 280 to 350 cm^{-1}, at 25° and 45° C, below and above the phase transition temperature (41° C), to analyze effects in both the gel and the liquid crystalline phases. Changes in either location or relative intensities of Raman peaks were not detected above or below the phospholipid phase transition, indicating that the conformation of the model membrane was unaffected. In other studies, Raman spectra of phase transitions in the lipid bilayer have been reported to occur over a narrower temperature range during exposure to a low EM field irradiation than in its absence. It has been suggested that differential thermal gradients may be induced by EM fields (Sheridan et al., 1977).

Relatively few studies have been directed toward evaluating the effects of EM fields on membranes. Frohlich (1980) has suggested that

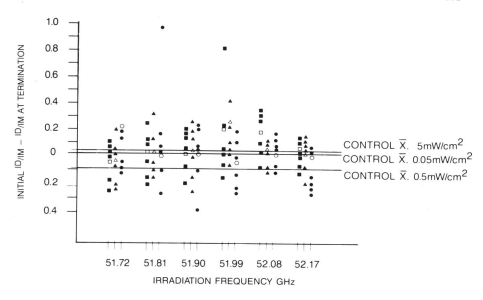

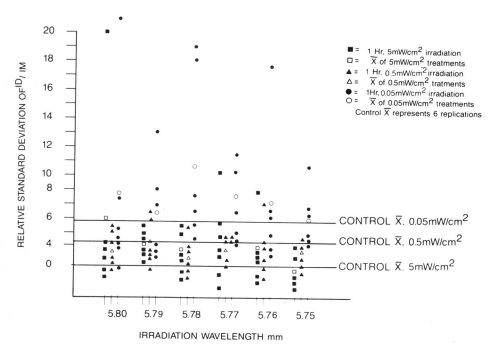

Figure 16-13 Effect of 1-hour continuous wave irradiation at 0.5 and 5 mW/cm² on fluorescence of dipyrenylpropane in dimyristoyl phosphatidylcholine vesicles.

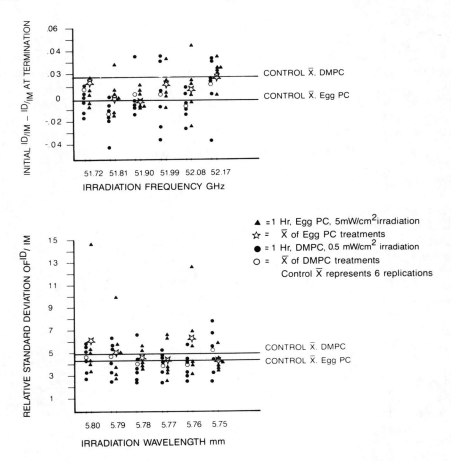

Figure 16-14 Effect of 1 hour continuous wave irradiation on fluorescence of cholesterol-enriched lipid vesicles. Dimyristoyl phosphatidylcholine cholesterol ratio 3:1 at 0.5 mW/cm^2; egg phosphatidylcholine/cholesterol ratio 1:1 at 5 mW/cm^2.

millimeter waves probably interact with membranes. Barnes and Hu (1977) have proposed that, because the membrane provides an opportunity for possible orientation of long-chain molecules and shifts of ion concentrations, it may serve as a model for nonthermal effects. It is conceivable that the exposure of such a model to pulsed microwaves could significantly change cell behavior. Barnes and Hu have further suggested that membrane stability depends on the intermolecular environment and field interactions with yet unidentified molecules.

Molecular effects

Biopolymers.   Millimeter-wave spectroscopy has been used to study various biological macromolecules. Absorption measurements in the 40 to 170 GHz range have been reported over a range of temperatures from liquid helium to room temperature for lyophilized hemoglobin, lysozyme, keratin, and poly-L-alanine (Genzel et al., 1983). The absorption coefficient of dried lysozyme exposed to three frequencies exhibited a nearly exponential increase, with temperatures from 50° to 300° K. In the region of exponential increase the absorption coefficient was almost linear in frequency (f) (Figure 16-15), whereas at low temperatures it was proportional to f^2. This frequency and temperature dependence could be explained by relaxation processes. At temperatures above 150° K, hydration results in a nearly frequency-independent contribution to the absorption. This indicates that the relaxation rates for bound water are small compared with the millimeter wave frequencies, enabling differentiation between the fast intrinsic process and the contribution of the bound water. Decreased absorption at low temperatures between 40 and 110 GHz presumably may be caused by bound and vicinal water absorbed at the macromolecule. Genzel et al. (1983) suggest that these picosecond relax-

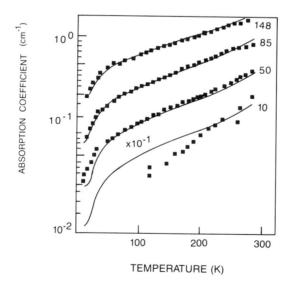

Figure 16-15   Absorption coefficient versus temperature of hemoglobin for frequencies 10, 50, 85, and 148 GHz. (From Genzel, L. [1983]. Millimeter-wave and far-infrared spectroscopy of biological macromolecules. *In*: Frohlich, H., and Kremer, F. [eds.]. Coherent excitations in biological systems. New York, Springer-Verlag, pp. 58–70.)

ations may be attributed to the NH::OC hydrogen bond of the peptide backbone. Genzel represented the dielectric behavior of hemoglobin by a three-fold relaxation process. A temperature increase is induced in specimens exposed to nonionizing radiation because surface molecules are forced to oscillate with the incident field, causing dielectric rotational losses.

These studies indicate a temperature and frequency dependence of the millimeter absorption coefficient, which is similar for various biomolecules. Of the mechanisms considered, only dielectric relaxation effects could explain this observation. In contrast to these reports, exposure of the enzyme alcohol dehydrogenase to swept frequencies between 40 and 115 GHz did not alter the rate at which NAD^{++} and acetaldehyde are formed from NAD^+ and ethanol (Tuegler et al., 1978).

Multicellular effects.   The limited depth of penetration of millimeter EM fields has stimulated research primarily of cellular and subcellular components rather than multicellular organisms.

Drosophila.   Nevertheless, some organismal studies have been carried out, particularly with *Drosophila*. Zalyubovskaya et al. (1974) studied the influence of millimeter waves on survival rates, ability to reproduce, and first- and second-generation offspring. Irradiation at 4.5 to 8 mm for 15 to 60 minutes resulted in fewer normal offspring. Fertility depended on both frequency and exposure time. At 44.12 GHz fertility was decreased by 40%. Prolonged exposure (3 to 5 hours) caused significant changes in the first and second generations. Male offspring of irradiated parents were less viable, and females did not produce eggs. *Drosophila* eggs, irradiated at 17 and 73 GHz and power densities up to 100 mW/cm² for 2 hours, did not exhibit detectable changes in hatching or development when irradiated at 73 GHz (Dardalhon et al., 1979). The increase in fertility at 17 GHz was attributed to microwave absorption by water molecules. Heating is achieved by dielectric absorption by free and loosely bound water molecules in the cytoplasm (Dardalhon et al., 1981).

Nimtz (1983a,b), in experiments on pupae exposed for 120 hours to 40 GHz at 10 μW/cm², examined the offspring of two generations. He concluded that the fertility of the parental generation was strongly enhanced in exposed insects but not in their offspring. The fertility of the F_2 generation decreased by about 10%. After two similar experiments, he subjected all of his data to a rigorous reanalysis and found that millimeter waves had no apparent effect.

Bone marrow.   Bone marrow of irradiated mice has been examined to determine the synergistic effects of millimeter waves and x-rays (Sevast'yanova, 1983). Treatments applied independently and in alternate sequential combinations (Figure 16-16) indicate that the combined action of x-rays and millimeter waves either protects or sensitizes the marrow cells to other agents by activating or suppressing biological processes; that is, cells of the erythroid and myeloid series are shielded from x-ray damage by microwave exposure, but cells of the lymphoid series are not protected. Similar studies were carried out on tumors (Sevast'yanova et al., 1983). The combined exposures significantly decreased the volume of sarcoma-45 cells when compared with the effects of x-rays alone (Figure 16-17). Changing the sequence of exposure so that microwaves preceded x-rays did not influence the amount of damage the x-rays caused. Millimeter waves also alleviated harmful affects of x-rays on bone marrow cells. Altered functional activity and retardation of tumor growth at 7.1 mm was attributed to the sensitization of tissues. Millimeter waves do not appear to cause gross damage to animals and do not stimulate tumor growth.

Ocular effects. Evidence that high-intensity exposures to EM fields induce cataracts stimulated special interest in the eye. The lens is a biconvex tissue encased in a thin, transparent membrane with anterior and posterior capsules. Opacification resulting from microwave irradiation is usually localized in the posterior portion of the lens capsule, but opacities caused by irradiation at higher frequencies are localized in the anterior portion.

Experiments performed in 1948 and 1950, in which dogs (Daily et al., 1948, 1950) and rabbits (Richardson et al., 1948) were exposed to microwave frequencies, first led to reports of induction of cataract formation. Subsequently, a report of lens opacity in a microwave generator technician was supported by numerous documented cases of microwave-induced cataracts in humans (Hirsch and Parker, 1952; Shimkovich and Shilyaev, 1959) and animals (Richardson et al., 1951). Early experiments involving short-term, high-intensity exposures to microwave radiation in the 0.8 to 10 GHz range, consistently demonstrated a high dose-response relationship in the production of lens abnormalities. Research focused on the establishment of quantitative threshold levels (Williams et al., 1955; Carpenter et al., 1960; Carpenter, 1962; Carpenter and Van Ummerson, 1968) related to radiation intensity (power) and to the duration of exposure. By subjecting the eyes of rabbits to frequencies up to 40 mW/cm^2 at 0.8 and 6.3 GHz for up to 60 minutes, Birenbaum et al. (1969) were able to plot a threshold curve for cataract induction. Curves at different frequencies were similar to each other and demonstrated that higher frequencies were more effective in cataractogenesis than lower ones. This appeared to be due to the deeper penetration of lower-frequency beams being "used to heat up an increasingly larger volume of the eye" (Birenbaum, 1969). Although cataracts were not produced by single 60-minute exposures to 80 mW/cm^2, repetitive exposures on each of 10 consecutive days did result in their formation (Carpenter, 1962). This result of multiple exposures suggests a cumulative effect based on some equilib-

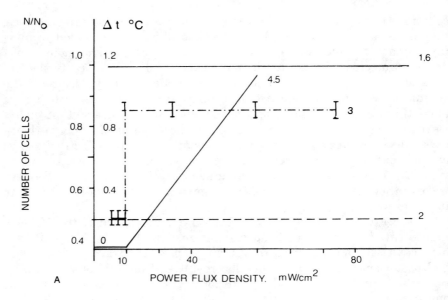

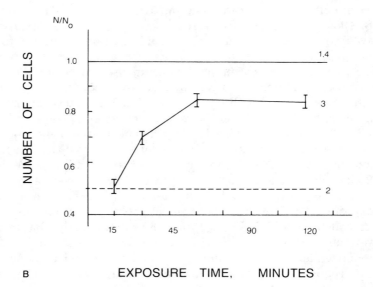

Figure 16-16 A, Influence of power density on change in number of bone marrow cells (N/N_0). *1*, Control. *2*, X-rays. *3*, Microwaves and x-rays. *4*, Skin temperature—microwaves and x-rays. *5*, Skin temperature—microwaves. *6*, Change in number of bone marrow cells with microwaves. **B,** Change in number of bone marrow cells as function of time. *1*, Control. *2*, X-rays. *3*, Microwave irradiation and x-rays. *4*, Microwave irradiation.

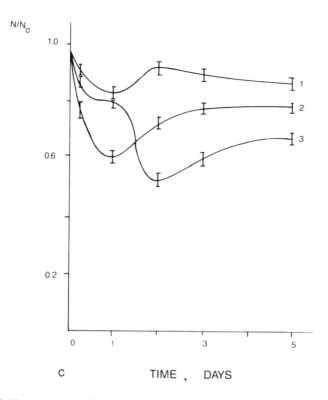

Figure 16-16, cont'd   C, Changes in number of bone marrow cells in various combinations of x-rays and microwaves. *1*, Microwaves and x-rays. *2*, X-rays. *3*, X-rays and microwaves. (From Sevast'yanova, L.A. [1983]. Specification of millimeter radio waves on biological systems. *In*: Devyatkov, N.D. [ed.]. Nonthermal effects of millimeter radiation. Moscow, U.S.S.R. Academy of Sciences, p. 54.)

rium between duration and absorbed power. In contrast, since neither a critical temperature nor an appreciable temperature elevation has been identified, the effect appears not to be temperature dependent. Comparing the effectiveness of continuous wave and pulsed power did not exhibit any significant detectable threshold differences but demonstrated that the average rather than the peak power results in opacification of the lens, thus implying a thermal insult as the causative factor.

As indicated, most of the early microwave eye research was carried out in the lower frequency range of the microwave spectrum, where the limited depth of penetration caused the conversion of microwave energy into heat near the posterior surface of the cornea.

With the development of radar installations it was noted that employee eyesight was susceptible to special wavelengths absorbed by the eye. Since progressive lenticular senescence normally occurs in humans

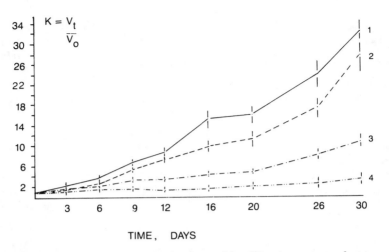

Figure 16-17 Change in volume of tumors with millimeter waves and x-rays. *1*, Control. *2*, Millimeter waves. *3*, X-rays. *4*, X-rays and millimeter waves. (From Sevast'yanova, L.A. [1983]. Specification of millimeter radio waves on biological systems. *In*: Devyatkov, N.D. [ed]. Nonthermal effects of millimeter radiation. Moscow, U.S.S.R. Academy of Sciences, p. 54.)

with aging, it appears that prolonged exposure to small doses of microwaves may facilitate the development of aging changes.

Relatively little eye research has been carried out in the millimeter range. Balutina (1965) demonstrated that corneal damage developed in the rabbit eye after free-field exposures to continuous wave, 30 GHz, at a power density of 120 mW/cm^2.

Irradiation of anesthetized rabbit eyes at 70 GHz for 30 or more minutes at power densities above 0.5 mW/cm^2 produced injuries to the cornea, conjunctiva, iris, and lens. Severity of the injury from acute exposures at 610 mW and others close to 600 mW was greatest at the corneal-air interface and decreased with depth. Yet at 570 mW no effect was evident. These studies suggested that the corneal stroma can serve as an indicator of threshold effects (Birenbaum et al., 1969). Subsequent studies at 35 and 107 GHz for 15 to 80 minutes and at powers up to 50 mW were designed to determine the threshold of acute radiation injury, to compare experimental results at these frequencies, and to determine which of the ocular tissues was the most sensitive indicator of injury for these frequencies. Although similar levels of injury were observable at both frequencies immediately after irradiation, damage at 35 GHz lasted longer. At 107 GHz the threshold near 15 mW was the more effective in causing immediate stromal damage, which usually disappeared by the next day. In contrast, at 35 GHz the threshold was higher (about 25 mW), but only slight improvement was noted the following day. Eyes exposed to these frequencies showed different radiation effects: injury of the corneal epithelium and the corneal stroma. Stromal injury accompanied by extensive epithelial damage observed at 35 GHz does not occur at 107 GHz (Rosenthal et al., 1977).

Damage levels were reassessed to ascertain the sites and compare the insult of continuous and pulsed microwaves at various power densities and specific absorption rates. The results indicated that increasing dose and dose-rate resulted in progressive corneal damage. The threshold for damage by continuous wave exposure (550 W/kg) was approximately 17 times higher than that for pulsed irradiations (22.6 W/kg). In each type of irradiation, damage increased with increasing dose (Trevithick, et al., 1987; Creighton, et al., 1988).

Results described in the preceding discussion refer to acute exposures. Little is known about the effects of chronic exposures, such as low-level, wider-beam, and repetitive exposures, or combinations of these.

Clearly a relationship exists between microwave exposure and the formation of cataracts, yet many questions require resolution before the mechanism of lens opacification can be defined. Is the temperature elevation of microwave radiation solely responsible for alterations in the crystalline lens? What other factors are involved? Is the action of radiofrequency energy on the lens fibers directly responsible for the opacity, or are the lens fibers affected secondarily by biochemical changes that alter metabolism in the lens?

Excitable tissues.   Reported effects of microwave exposure have implicated the brain and other excitable tissues. Significant effects have been demonstrated in experiments at lower frequencies, but comparable data are unavailable in the millimeter range. Preliminary electrical and fluorescence examination of in vitro rat flexor digitorum brevis muscle and cultured L6 myoblasts exposed to frequencies at 51.72 and 51.81 GHz and 5 mW/cm^2 for 10-minute intervals did not affect the resting potentials, or the frequency, amplitude, rise, or decay time of miniature end plate potentials (Motzkin et al., 1988a,b).

THEORETICAL APPROACHES

Knowledge indicative only of the existence of bioeffects is inadequate. If we are to fully comprehend the underlying mechanisms of interaction of living matter and EM fields, we need to understand the physicochemical properties of biological materials and how they are affected by extrinsic low-intensity fields.

Frohlich's theory of coherent excitations (1968, 1970, 1972, 1973, 1978, 1980), supported by model calculations, suggests that the interactions require an energy threshold and a frequency dependence for the onset of an effect. It has further been suggested that these oscillations may affect ionic distribution, resulting in cooperative interactions, as in the transport of molecules, the transfer of energy between molecular components, or the opening and closing of membrane protein channels. Based on the membrane thickness (10 nm) and the speed of sound, Frohlich proposed that oscillations in the 10^{10} to 10^{12} Hz range may be excited in the cell membrane, affecting DNA and enzyme-substrate complexes. It is possible that weak cooperative interaction between lipids and proteins helps stabilize membrane structure and that long-range interactions with EM fields can actually modify the system's equilibrium to produce bioeffects. The high electric field in the membrane is expected to raise proteins to a highly polar metastable state. This state, which could represent the active state of the enzyme, can store energy, reduce activation energies, and transfer energy from protein to protein. Two excitations may serve as an on-off switch to activate and deactivate chemical processes. Some oscillations may result in long-range, frequency-selective interactions between systems with comparable excitation frequencies, which may be required for cell communication and cell division as in cancer (Frohlich, 1980). Frequency selection may also initiate short-range chemical interaction by bringing relevant control systems together.

This theory has served as a mechanistic model of nonthermal effects that could produce significant biologic changes. It enables many conformations with different energies for bipolymers whose stability would depend on the intermolecular environment and field interactions. Lipoprotein complexes would then be susceptible to structural disturbance by EM fields, since they are susceptible to localized phase transitions.

Other proposed mechanisms involve critical phases (Bond, 1986; Bond and Wyeth, 1986), limit cycles (Kaiser, 1983), surface compartmental models (Blank and Britten, 1978), solitons (Scott, 1985), and the ubiquitous presence of bound, structural, or bulk water that may affect the rotational freedom of molecular components. Theoretical consideration has been given to the concept of deterministic chaos (Kaiser, 1984), which may influence biological systems.

CONCLUSION

Questions raised by the significant advances in microwave technology and the burgeoning of millimeter-wave applications stimulated numerous research endeavors to define the interactions of biological systems with higher frequencies. Although evidence that weak fields at lower frequencies affect living things is mounting, in the millimeter range the results are inconclusive. Reports of bioeffects, particularly on a cellular and subcellular level, are ambiguous, inconsistent, and contradictory. Research to confirm bioeffects has either been fruitless or met with limited success. Some promising results remain unsubstantiated. In fact, it is uncertain whether some of these observed effects are real or artifactual. Attempts to repeat experiments that have demonstrated nonthermal, resonant, frequency-dependent effects have been unsuccessful. Extrapolation from the more consistent evidence at lower frequencies to imply effects at higher frequencies is unacceptable, nor can one extrapolate information from one species to another or from in vitro to in vivo experiments.

The definition of bioeffects is hampered by limitations in basic knowledge of molecular interactions and mechanisms. Temperature, thermal gradients, hot spots, and nonhomogeneous energy absorption have been implicated in the production of effects. In vitro studies, often used because of the limited depth of penetration of millimeter waves, eliminate normal in vivo temperature controls and, frequently, tissue architecture. Reports of experimental results have often inadequately detailed monitoring systems. In an area replete with technological difficulties, the precision and accuracy of the instrumentation and design are essential to enable replication. The use of simple model systems that can readily be evaluated will net results.

Many attractive mechanisms have been proposed, but the evidence does not unequivocally support them or prove them wrong.

It is generally accepted that millimeter irradiation at high power levels interferes with living structure and function. The available data do not conclusively define low-level millimeter waves as a biological hazard. Reports of nonthermal frequency-dependent effects on cell division and membrane function have led to predictions that millimeter waves may prove helpful in the diagnosis or treatment of pathological states such as cancer. The available evidence does not support this hypothesis. The question of harmful or beneficial effects is unresolved.

The controversy remains, the debate continues.

ACKNOWLEDGMENT

I am pleased to acknowledge the invaluable editorial support of my Research Associate, Julie Feinstein. This chapter has benefitted immeasurably from her meticulous care in the preparation of the manuscript. Thanks also to Kim Beck for her dedicated secretarial assistance.

REFERENCES

ATHEY, T.W., AND KROP, B.A. (1979). Millimeter-wave radiation fails to induce lambda phage expression. In: Abstracts of USNC/URSI/BEMS International Symposium, June 18–22, Seattle, Wash.

ATHEY, T.W., AND KROP, B.A. (1980). Millimeter induction of lambda prophage—dependent on growth medium? *Bioelectromagnetics* 1:241.

BALUTINA, A.P. (1965). Experimental injury to the eye with ultra-high-frequency electromagnetic field. *Bull. Exp. 'noy. Biologii i Meditsiny* 60:1241–1243.

BARNES, F.S., AND HU, C.L. (1977). Model for some nonthermal effects of radio and microwave fields on biological membranes. *IEEE Trans. Microwave Theory Tech.* 25:742–746.

BERTEAUD, A.J., DARDALHON, M., REBEYROTTE, N., AVERBECK, D. (1975). Action d'un rayonnement electromagnetique a longueur d'onde millimetrique sur la croissance bacterienne. *C. R. Acad. Sci. [D] (Paris)* 281:843–846.

BIRENBAUM, L., KAPLAN, I.T., METLAY, W., ROSENTHAL, S.W., SCHMIDT, H., AND ZARET, M.M. (1969). Effect of microwaves on the rabbit eye. *J. Microwave Power* 44:232–242.

BLACKMAN, C.F., BENANE, S.G., WEIL, C.M., AND ALI, J.S. (1975). Effects of nonionizing electromagnetic radiation on single-cell biological systems. *In*: Tyler, P.E. (ed.). Biological effects of nonionizing radiation. New York, Academy of Science, pp. 352–366. Also *in Ann. N.Y. Acad. Sci.* 247.

BLANK, M., AND BRITTEN, J.S. (1978). The surface compartment model of the steady state excitable membrane. *Bioelectrochem. Bioenergetics.* 5:535–547.

BOND, J.D. (1986): Electromagnetic field effects in membranes: role of phase transitions and critical phenomena. Workshop on Critical Phenomena and Phase Transitions in Biomembranes. Bethesda, Md., National Institutes of Health.

BOND, J.D., AND WYETH, N.C. (1986). Are membrane microwave effects related to a critical phase transition? *J. Chem. Phys.* 85:7377–7379.

BUSH, L.G., HILL, D.W., RIAZI, A., STENSAAS, L.J., PARTLOW, L.M., AND GANDHI, O.P. (1981). Effects of millimeter wave radiation on monolayer cell cultures. III. A search for frequency-specific athermal biological effects on protein synthesis. *Bioelectromagnetics* 2:151–159.

CARPENTER, R.L. (1962). An experimental study of the biological effects of microwave radiation in relation to the eye. Tufts University Report. RADC-TDR-62-131 (Contract AF 41 [657]-86 for Rome Air Development Center).

CARPENTER, R.L., BIDDLE, D.K., AND VAN UMMERSEN, C.A. (1960). Opacities in the lens of the eye experimentally induced by exposure to microwave radiation. *IRE Trans. Med. Electron.* 7:152–157.

CARPENTER, R.L., AND VAN UMMERSEN, C.A. (1968). The action of microwave radiation on the eye. *J. Microwave Power* 3:3–19.

COOPER, M.S., AND AMER, N.M. (1983). The absence of coherent vibrations in the Raman spectra of living cells. *Phys. Lett.* 98A:138.

CREIGHTON, M.O., TREVITHICK, J.R., DZIALOSZYNSKI, T., SANWAL, M., BROWN, D.O., AND BASSEN, H.I. (1988). Comparison of histopathological effects of pulsed and continuous millimeter waves on rabbit corneas. *In*: Proceedings of the 10th Annual Meeting of the Bioelectromagnetics Society, June 19–24, Stamford, Conn., Frederick, Md., Bioelectromagnetics Society.

DAILY, L., WAKIM, K.G., HERRICK, J.F., AND PARKHILL, E.M. (1948). The effects of microwave diathermy on the eye. *Am. J. Physiol.* 155:432.

DAILY, L., WAKIM, K.G., HERRICK, J.F., PARKHILL, E., AND BENEDICT, W.L. (1950). The effects of microwave diathermy on the eye. *Am. J. Ophthalmol.* 33:1241–1245.

DARDALHON, M., AVERBECK, D., AND BERTEAUD, A.J. (1979a). Determination of a thermal equivalent of millimeter microwaves in living cells. *J. Microwave Power* 14:307–312.

DARDALHON, M., BERTEAUD, A.J., AND AVERBECK, D. (1979b). Microwave effects in *Drosophila melanogaster*. *Radioprotection* 14:145–159.

DARDALHON, M., AVERBECK, D., AND BERTEAUD, A.J. (1980). Action des ondes centimetriques seules ou combinees avec les rayons ultraviolets sur les cellules eucaryotiques. *In*: Berteaud, A.J., and Servantie, B. (eds.). Proceedings of an International Symposium Ondes Electromagnetiques et Biologie, Paris (URSI, CNFRS) Jouy en Josas, June 30–July 4, 1980, Paris, pp. 17–24.

DARDALHON, M., AVERBECK, D., AND BERTEAUD, A.J. (1981). Studies on possible genetic effects of microwaves in procaryotic and eucaryotic cells. *Radiat. Environ. Biophys.* 20:37–51.

DARDALHON, M., AVERBECK, D., BERTEAUD, A.J., AND RAVARY, V. (1985). Thermal aspect of biological effects of microwave in *Saccharomyces cerevisiae*. *Int. J. Radiat. Biol.* 48:987–996.

DARDANONI, L., TORREGROSSA, V., TAMBURELLO, C., AND ZANFORLIN, L. (1979). Sensitivity of *C. albicans* cells to frequency of modulation in 72–74 GHz band. Presented at the USNC/URSI meeting, June 18–22, Seattle, Wash.

DARDANONI, L., TORREGROSSA, V., TAMBURELLO, C., ZANFORLIN, L., AND SPALLA, M. (1976). Biological effects of millimeter waves at spectral singularities. *In*: Proceedings of the 3rd Wroclaw Symposium on Electromagnetic Compatability, Wroclaw, Poland, Wydawnictwo Politechniki, pp. 308–313.

DEVYATKOV, N.D. (1973). Influence of millimeter-band electromagnetic radiation on biological objects. *Usp. Fiziol. Nauk* 110:452–455. (Translated in English in *Sov. Phys. Usp.* 16:568–569, 1974.)

DEVYATKOV, N.D., BETSKIY, O.V., GEL'VICH, E.A., et al. Effects on biological systems of electromagnetic oscillations in the millimeter range of wavelengths. *Radiobiologica* 21:163.

DEVYATKOV, N.D., KHURGIN, Y.I., VETSKIY, O.V., KUDRYASHOVA, V.A., AND ZAVIZION, V.A. (1983). Using millimeter spectroscopy to study intermolecular interactions in solutions. *In*: Devyatkov, N.D. (ed.). Effects of nonionizing electromagnetic radiation: nonthermal effects of millimeter radiation. USSR Report, Life Sciences. (English translation in U.S. Joint Publications Research Service No. L/11770.)

DRISSLER, F., AND MacFARLANE, R.M. (1978). Enhanced anti-Stokes Raman scattering from living cells of *Chlorella pyrenoidosa*. *Phys. Lett.* 69A:65–67.

DRISSLER, F., AND SANTO, L. (1983). Coherent excitations and Raman effects. *In*: Frohlich, H., and Kremer, F. (eds.). Coherent excitations in biological systems. Berlin, Springer-Verlag, p. 6.

FROHLICH, H. (1968). Long-range coherence and energy storage in biological systems. *Int. J. Quantum Chem.* 2:64.

FROHLICH, H. (1970). Long-range coherence and the action of enzymes. *Nature* 228:1093.

FROHLICH, H. (1972). Selective long range dispersion forces between large systems. *Phys. Lett. 29A:*153–154.

FROHLICH, H. (1973). Collective behavior of non-linearly coupled oscillating fields, with application to biological systems. *J. Collective Phenomena 1:*101.

FROHLICH, H. (1975a). The extraordinary dielectric properties of biological materials and the action of enzymes. *Proc. Natl. Acad. Sci. U.S.A.* 72:4211–4215.

FROHLICH, H. (1975b). Evidence for Bose condensation-like excitation of coherent modes in biological systems. *Phys. Lett. 51A:*21–22.

FROHLICH, H. (1978). Coherent electric vibrations in biological systems and the cancer problem. *IEEE Trans. Microwave Theory Tech.* 26:613–617.

FROHLICH, H. (1980). Biological effects of millimeter waves and related questions. *In:* Advances in Electronics and Electron Physics *53:*85–152.

FURIA, L., AND GANDHI, O.P. (1984). Absence of biologically related Raman lines in cultures of *Bacillus megaterium. Phys. Lett. 102A:*380–382.

FURIA, L., AND GANDHI, O.P. (1985). Absence of lines in Raman spectra of living cells. *Phys. Lett. 111:*376–377.

FURIA, L., GANDHI, O.P., BENNER, R.E., AND HILL, D.W. (1986b). Raman spectroscopy of liposomes exposed to millimeter waves. *J. Appl. Phys.* 60:2991–2994.

FURIA, L., HILL, D.W., AND GANDHI, O.P. (1986a). Effects of millimeter waves on growth of *Saccharomyces cerevisiae. IEEE Trans. Biomed. Eng.* 33:993–999.

GANDHI, O.P. (1983). Some biological properties of biological tissues for potential biomedical applications of millimeter waves. *J. Microwave Power 18:*295–304.

GANDHI, O.P., HAGMANN, M.J., HILL, D.W., PARTLOW, L.M., AND BUSH, L. (1980). Millimeter wave absorption spectra of biological samples. *Bioelectromagnetics* 1:285–298.

GANDHI, O.P., HILL, D.W., RIAZI, A., WAHID, P., WANG, C.H., AND ISKANDER, M.F. (1982). Biological effects of millimeter wave irradiation. Report No. USAFAM-TR-82-49. Brooks Air Force Base, San Antonio, Tex.

GANDHI, O.P., AND RIAZI, A. (1986). Absorption of millimeter waves by human beings and its biological implications. *IEEE Trans. Microwave Theory Tech.* 34:228–235.

GENZEL, L., KREMER, F., POGLITSCH, A., AND BECHTOLD, G. (1983). Millimeter-wave and far-infrared spectroscopy of biological macromolecules. *In:* Frohlich, H., and Kremer, F. (eds.). Coherent excitations in biological systems. Berlin, Springer-Verlag, pp. 58–70.

GRUNDLER, W. (1981a). Biological effects of RF and MW energy at molecular and cellular level. *In:* Michaelson, S., Grandolfo, M., and Rindi, A. (eds.). Proceedings of the NATO Advanced Study Institute. Advances in biological effects and dosimetry of low energy electromagnetic fields, Erice, Sicily, Italy. New York, Plenum Publishing Corp.

GRUNDLER, W. (1981b). Recent results of experiments on nonthermal effects of millimeter microwaves on yeast growth. *J. Coll. Phenom. 3*:181–186.

GRUNDLER, W. (1985). Frequency-dependent biological effects on low intensity microwaves. *In*: Chiabrera, A., Niccolini, C., and Schwan, H.P. (eds.). Interactions between electromagnetic fields and cells. New York, Plenum Publishing Corp., pp. 459–481.

GRUNDLER, W., AND KEILMANN, F. (1978). Nonthermal effects of millimeter microwaves on yeast growth. *Z. Naturforsch 33C*:15–22.

GRUNDLER, W., AND KEILMANN, F. (1983). Sharp resonances in yeast growth prove nonthermal sensitivity to microwaves. *Phys. Rev. Lett. 51*:1214–1216.

GRUNDLER, W., KEILMANN, F., AND FROHLICH, H. (1977). Resonant growth rate response of yeast cells irradiated by weak microwaves. *Phys. Lett. 62A*:463–466.

GRUNDLER, W., KEILMANN, F., PUTTERLIK, V., AND STRUBE, D. (1982). Resonant-like dependence of yeast growth rate on microwave frequencies. *Br. J. Cancer Suppl. V*:206–208.

GRUNDLER, W., KEILMANN, F., PUTTERLIK, V., SANTO, L., STRUBE, D., AND ZIMMERMANN, I. (1983). Nonthermal resonant effects of 42 GHz microwaves on the growth of yeast cultures. *In*: Frohlich, H., and Kremer, F. (eds.). Coherent excitations in biological systems. Springer-Verlag, Berlin, pp. 21–37.

HILL, D.W., FURIA, L., TRACY, K., RIAZI, A., AND GANDHI, O.P. (1983). Lack of mutagenic effects of millimeter waves on *Salmonella typhimurium* and on induction of lambda phage. Presented at International Symposium on Techniques in Studies of Biological Effects of Low-Level Millimeter Waves, Sept. 4–6, Herrsching, West Germany.

HIRSCH, F.G., AND PARKER, J.T. (1952). Bilateral lenticular opacities occurring in a technician operating a microwave generator. *Am. Med. Assoc. Arch. Ind. Hyg. 6*:512–517.

KAISER, F. (1983). Specific effects in externally driven self-sustained oscillating biophysical model systems. *In*: Frohlich, H., and Kremer, F. (eds.). Coherent excitations in biological systems. Berlin, Springer-Verlag.

KAISER, F. (1984). Entrainment-quasiperiodicity-chaos-collapse, bifurcation routes of externally driven self-sustained oscillating systems. *In*: Adey, W.R., and Lawrence, A.F. (eds.). Nonlinear electrodynamics in biology. New York, Plenum Publishing Corp., pp. 393–412.

KEILMANN, F. (1982a). Experimental RF and microwave resonant nonthermal effects. *In*: Michaelson, S., Grandolfo, M., and Rindi, A. (eds.). Biological effects and dosimetry of nonionizing radiation. New York, Plenum Publishing Corp., pp. 299–318.

KEILMANN, F., AND GRUNDLER, W. (1984). Nonthermal resonant action of millimeter microwaves on yeast growth. *In*: Adey, W.R., and Lawrence, A.F., (eds.). Nonlinear electrodynamics in biology. New York, Plenum Publishing Corp., pp. 59–64.

KISELEV, R.I., AND ZALYUBOVSKAYA, N.P. (1973). Effects of millimeter-band electromagnetic waves in the cell and certain elements of the cell. *Usp. Fiziol. Nauk* *110*:465–466. (Translated in English in *Sov. Phys. Usp. 16*:576–577, 1974.)

KREMER, F., KOSCHNITZKE, C., SANTO, L., QUICK, P., AND POGLITSCH, A. (1983). The nonthermal effect of millimeter wave radiation on the puffing of giant chromosomes. *In*: Frohlich, H., and Kremer, F. (eds.). Coherent excitations in biological systems. Berlin, Springer-Verlag, pp. 10–20.

LEE, R.A. (1977). The absorption of millimeter microwaves by, and its effects on, bacterial, normal, and tumor cells. M.A. Thesis, Dept. of Physics, University of South Florida.

LEE, R.A., AND WEBB, S.J. (1977). Possible detection of *in vivo* viruses by fine-structure millimeter microwave spectroscopy between 68 and 76 GHz. *IRCS Med. Sci. 5*:222.

MAKHOV, A.M. (1979). Doklad na tret'yen vsesoyuznom soveshchanii po primene-niyu mm islucheniya v biologii. Khimii i meditsine. Moscow, pp. 28–38.

MORE, C., DARDALHON, M., BERTEAUD, A.J., AVERBECK, D. (1980). Detection de l'action des microndes sur le cytoplasme cellulaire par polarisation de fluores-cence. *In*: Berteaud, A.J., and Servantie, B. (eds.). Proceedings of an International Symposium Ondes Electromagnetiques et Biologie, Paris (URSI, CNFRS) Jouy en Josas, France, June 30–July 4, 1980, pp. 25–29.

MOTZKIN, S.M., BENES, L., BIRENBAUM, L., CHU, A., AND ROSENTHAL, S. (1984a). Excimer fluorescence as a probe of mechanisms by which electromagnetic fields may affect simulated membranes. *In*: International symposium on interactions of electromagnetic fields with biological systems, Florence, Italy, Aug. 28–Sept. 5, USNC/URSI/BEMS.

MOTZKIN, S.M., BENES, L., BIRENBAUM, L., CHU, A., AND ROSENTHAL, S. (1984b). Fluorescence as an indicator of millimeter wave effects. *In*: Proceedings of the 6th Annual Meeting of the Bioelectromagnetics Society. Gaithersburg, Md., Bioelectromagnetics Society.

MOTZKIN, S.M., BENES, L., BLOCK, N., et al. (1983). Effects of low-level millimeter-waves on cellular and subcellular systems. *In*: Frohlich, H., and Kremer, F. (eds.). Coherent excitations in biological systems. Berlin, Springer-Verlag, pp. 47–57.

MOTZKIN, S.M., FEINSTEIN, J., AND LU, Z. (1987). Do continuous low-level millimeter waves alter excimer fluorescence in natural and model membranes? *In*: Proceedings of the 9th Annual Meeting of the Bioelectromagnetics Society. Frederick, Md., Bioelectromagnetics Society.

MOTZKIN, S.M., FEINSTEIN, J., MARTUSCIELLO-FIRESTONE, M., AND ROSENTHAL S. (1986a). Effects of millimeter waves on colicin induction in synchronized *E. coli* cultures. *In*: Proceedings of the 8th Annual Meeting of the Bioelectromagnetics Society. Frederick, Md., Bioelectromagnetics Society.

MOTZKIN, S.M., FEINSTEIN, J., AND ZENG, J. (1988a). A system for determining the effects of millimeter waves on membrane potentials of rat muscle cells. *In*: Proceedings of the 10th Annual Meeting of the Bioelectromagnetics Society. Frederick, Md., Bioelectromagnetics Society.

MOTZKIN, S.M., FIRESTONE, M., FEINSTEIN, J., ROSENTHAL, S. (1986b). Alterations of simulated and living membranes with incorporated fluorescent probes in an electromagnetic field. Electromagnetic Society Extended Abstracts. *1*:688.

MOTZKIN, S.M., MARTUSCIELLO-FIRESTONE, M., FEINSTEIN, J., AND ROSENTHAL, S. (1986c). Molecular alterations in liposomes exposed to electromagnetic fields as visualized by fluorescence. *In*: Proceedings of the 8th Annual Meeting of the Bioelectromagnetics Society. Frederick, Md., Bioelectromagnetics Society.

MOTZKIN, S.M., MELNICK, R.H., RUBENSTEIN, C., ROSENTHAL, S., AND BIRENBAUM, L. (1980). Effects of CW millimeter wave irradiation on mitochondrial oxidative phosphorylation and Ca^{++} transport. *In*: Berteaud, A.J., and Servantie, B. (eds.). Proceedings of an International Symposium Ondes Electromagnetiques et Biologie, Paris (URSI, CNFRS) Jouy en Josas, France, June 30–July 4, 1980.

MOTZKIN, S.M., MOJTABAI, Z., BIRENBAUM, L., AND ROSENTHAL, S. (1984c). Effect of low-level millimeter waves on colicin induction. *In*: Technical report, Environmental Protection Agency. Research Triangle Park, N.C.

MOTZKIN, S.M., ZENG, J., CHEN, D., AND FEINSTEIN, J. (1988b). Visualization of millimeter wave effects on membrane potentials of nerve-muscle preparations. *In*: Proceedings of the 10th Annual Meeting of the Bioelectromagnetics Society. Frederick, Md., Bioelectromagnetics Society.

NIMTZ, G. (1983a). Effects of millimeter-wave radiation on *Drosophila melanogaster*. Presented at International Symposium on Techniques in Studies of Biological Effects of Low-Level Millimeter Waves, Sept. 4–6, Herrsching, West Germany.

NIMTZ, G. (1983b). On microwave response to *Drosophila Melanogaster*. *In*: Frohlich, H., and Kremer, F. (eds.). Coherent excitations in biological systems. Berlin, Springer-Verlag, pp. 38–46.

PARTLOW, L.M., BUSH, L.G., STENSAAS, L.J., HILL, D.W., RIAZI, A., AND GANDHI, O.P. (1981). Effects of millimeter wave radiation on monolayer cell cultures. I. Design and validation of a novel exposure system. *Bioelectromagnetics 2*:123–140.

RICHARDSON, A.W., DUANE, T.D., AND HINES, H.M. (1948). Experimental lenticular opacities produced by microwave irradiations. *Arch. Phys. Med. 29*:765–769.

RICHARDSON, A.W., DUANE, T.D., AND HINES, H.M. (1951). Experimental cataract produced by three centimeter pulsed microwave irradiations. *Arch. Ophthalmol. 45*:382–386.

ROSENTHAL, S.W., BIRENBAUM, L., KAPLAN, I.T., METLAY, W., SNYDER, W.Z., AND ZARET, M.M. (1977). Effects of 35 and 107 GHz CW microwaves on the rabbit eye. *In*: Biological effects of electromagnetic waves. Vol. 1, HEW Pub. No. (FDA) 77-8010. Rockville, Md., pp. 110–128.

SANTO, L. (1983). *E. coli* induction by millimeter waves. Presented at International Symposium on Techniques in Studies of Biological Effects of Low-Level Millimeter Waves, Sept. 4–6, Herrsching, West Germany.

SCOTT, A.C. (1985). Solitons in biological molecules. *Comments Mol. Cell Biophys. 3*:15.

SEVAST'YANOVA, L.A. (1983). Specification of millimeter radio waves on biological systems. *In*: Devyatkov, N.D., (ed.). Nonthermal effects of millimeter radiation. Moscow, U.S.S.R. Academy of Sciences, p. 54.

SEVAT'YANOVA, L.A., BORODKINA, A.G., GOLANT, M.B., AND REBROVA, T.B. (1983). Influence of millimeter radiowaves on tumor growth in experimental animals. *In*: Devyatkov, N.D. (ed.). Non-thermal effects of millimeter radiation. Moscow, U.S.S.R. Academy of Sciences, p. 89.

SHERIDAN, J.P., PRIEST, R., SCHOEN, P., AND SCHNUR, J.M. (1977). Molecular level effects of microwaves on natural and model membranes: A Raman spectroscopic investigation. *In*: Taylor, L.S., and Cheung, A.Y. (eds.). The mechanisms of microwave biological effects. College Park, Md., University of Maryland, p. 155.

SHIMKOVICH, I.S., AND SHILYAEV, V.G. (1959). Cataract of both eyes which developed as a result of repeated short exposures to an electromagnetic field of high intensity. *Vestn. Ophthalmol.* 72:12–16.

SMOLYANSKAYA, A.Z. (1983). Action of millimeter electromagnetic waves on fat cells. *In*: Devyatkov, N.D. (ed.). Nonthermal effects of millimeter radiation. Moscow, U.S.S.R. Academy of Sciences.

SMOLYANSKAYA, A.Z., MAKHOV, A.M., GEL'VICH, E.A., AND GOLANT, M.B. (1981). Influence of electromagnetic waves in the millimeter band on inductoproteins synthesis of penicillinase by *Staphylococcus aureus*. *Biol. Nauki* 5:24–48.

SMOLYANSKAYA, A.Z., AND VILENSKAYA, R.L. (1973). Effects of millimeter band electromagnetic radiation on the functional activity of certain elements of bacterial cells. *Usp. Fiziol. Nauk* 110:458–460. (Translated in English in *Sov. Phys. Usp.* 16:571–572, 1974.)

STAMM, M.E., WARREN, S.L., RAND, R.W., et al. (1975). Microwave therapy experiments with B-16 murine melanoma. *IRCS Med. Sci.* 3:392–393.

STAMM, M.E., WINTERS, W.D., MORTON, D.L., AND WARREN, S.L. (1974). Microwave characteristics of human tumor cells. *Oncology* 29:294–301.

STENSAAS, L.J., PARTLOW, L.M., BUSH, L.F., et al. (1981). Effects of millimeter-wave radiation on monolayer cell cultures. II. Scanning and transmission electron microscopy. *Bioelectromagnetics* 2:141–150.

SWICORD, M.L., ATHEY, T.W., BUCHTA, F.L., AND KROP, B.A. (1978). Colicin induction by exposure to millimeter-wave radiation (Abstract). *In*: Open Symposium on Biological Effects of Electromagnetic Waves, USRI 19th General Assembly, Helsinki.

TREVITHICK, J.R., CREIGHTON, M.O., SANWAL, M., BROWN, D.O., AND BASSEN, H.T. (1987). Histopathological studies of rabbit cornea exposed to millimeter waves. *In*: Conference Proceedings, IEEE Engineering in Medicine and Biology.

TUEGLER, P., KEILMANN, F., AND GENZEL, L. (1978). Search for millimeter microwaves effects on enzyme or protein functions. *Z. Naturforsch* 34:60–63.

WEBB, S.J. (1979). Factors affecting the induction of lambda prophages by millimeter microwaves. *Phys. Lett.* 73A:145–148.

WEBB, S.J., AND BOOTH, A.D. (1969). Absorption of microwaves by microorganisms. *Nature* 222:1199–1200.

WEBB, S.J., AND BOOTH, A.D. (1971). Microwave absorption by normal and tumor cells. *Science 174*:72–74.

WEBB, S.J., AND DODDS, D.D. (1968). Inhibition of bacterial cell growth by 136 GHz microwave. *Nature 218*:374–375.

WEBB, S.J., LEE, R.E., AND STONEHAM, M.E. (1977). Possible viral involvement in human mammary carcinoma: a microwave and laser-Raman study. *Int. J. Quantum Chem. 4*:277–284.

WEBB, S.J., AND STONEHAM, M.E. (1975). The display of *in vivo* energy states by laser-Raman spectroscopy. *Int. J. Quantum Chem. Quantum Biol. Symp. 2*:339–343.

WEBB, S.J., AND STONEHAM, M.E. (1977). Resonances between 10^{11} and 10^{12} Hz in active bacterial cells as seen by Raman spectroscopy. *Phys. Lett. 60A*:267–268.

WILLIAMS, D.B., MONAHAN, J.P., NICHOLSON, W.J., AND ALDRICH, J.J. (1955). Biologic effects studies on microwave radiation. *Arch. Ophthalmol. 54*:863–874.

ZALYUBOVSKAYA, N.P. (1973). Reactions of living organisms to exposure to millimeter-band electromagnetic waves. *Usp. Fiziol. Nauk 110*:460–462. (Translated in English in *Sov. Phys. Usp. 16*:574–576, 1974.)

ZALYUBOVSKAYA, N.P., GORDIYENKO, O.I., AND KISELEV, P.I. (1974). Action of electromagnetic fields of superhigh frequency on erythrocytes preserved at low temperature. *Probl. Gemalol. Perelivaniya Krovi 20*:31.

17

Epidemiological Studies of Cancer and Electromagnetic Fields

CHARLOTTE SILVERMAN

Cancer was not an end point of interest in human studies of the biological effects of electromagnetic (EM) radiation (up to 300 GHz) until quite recently. There have been case reports and occasional references to the presence or absence of malignancies in investigations of other effects of nonionizing radiation. Reports of clusters of tumor cases in industrial EM environments have not been validated, nor have geographical associations between cancer and proximity to military air bases or other high-power sources of EM energy. Systematic studies of cancer mortality or morbidity have been few in number (WHO, 1981, 1984, 1987; Elder and Cahill 1984; Silverman, 1985).

A large occupational cohort study of U.S. Navy enlisted men who were in technical job classifications (Robinette et al., 1980) found no consistent excess cancer mortality or acute morbidity that could be attributed to microwave (radar) occupational exposure. Another cohort study involved employees of the U.S. Embassy in Moscow who were exposed to very low levels of microwaves (5 to 18 μW/cm^2) during a long period of irradiation of the embassy building. In this case, too, no excess of cancer cases or deaths could be attributed to the microwave radiation (Lilienfeld et al., 1978).

Interest in human cancer as a consequence of EM field exposure was stimulated by a study report (Wertheimer and Leeper, 1979) of a positive correlation between childhood cancer and exposure to extremely low-frequency (ELF) fields from residential overhead power lines (60 Hz). The report, which hypothesized that the alternating magnetic field component of the EM field might be a cancer promoter, soon led to other studies of residential ELF exposures. A suggestion in the same publication that frequent exposure to alternating current (AC) magnetic fields in an occupational setting might also be associated with cancer excess was followed by a series of occupational studies and analyses involving workers in "electric or electronic" occupations (Milham, 1982). This chapter assesses recent residential and occupational studies that have investigated cancer as an outcome of exposure to EM fields.

RESIDENTIAL EXPOSURE TO ELECTRICAL POWER LINES

The 1979 Wertheimer and Leeper study was prompted by their earlier field investigation of possible environmental factors in childhood cancer, which suggested that the homes of children with cancer were often near high-current wiring configurations. Publication of this case-control study was followed by considerable journal commentary and criticism and several attempted replications. Case-control studies on cancer in individuals with residential exposure to very weak, alternating magnetic fields from high-voltage power lines (60 Hz in North America and 50 Hz elsewhere) are presented in Table 17-1.

The Wertheimer and Leeper study included persons who had died of cancer before age 19 in Colorado during the period 1950 to 1973 and who also had a Colorado birth certificate and Denver area address. The study group consisted of 344 cancer deaths (from death certificates) and 344 control subjects, matched for date and county of birth (from birth certificate files). The 491 residences of the cancer patients were compared with the 472 control addresses. Potential exposure to power frequency magnetic fields was estimated on the basis of various wiring configurations carrying high and low current (classified visually according to thickness of the wires, proximity to transformers, and number of multiple wires) and their distance from the homes of the study subjects within 40 m. Field measurements of magnetic fields around power wires were made, but no measurements were taken at the homes of cancer patients or controls, nor were records obtained from local utility companies.

Magnetic flux density was measured around various elements of the electrical power supply system. Median values varied from 0.09 μT (0.9 mG) to 0.33 μT (3.3 mG); the maximum value was 3.5 μT (35 mG).* High-current configurations (HCCs) were found significantly more often near the homes of cancer patients than the homes of control subjects. The most striking difference was seen between the homes of the 109 cases and 128 control subjects who had only one address from birth to death ($X^2 = 14.4, p < 0.0001$). A twofold to threefold excess of leukemia, lymphoma, and nervous system tumors was found among those living near HCCs compared with those in control homes near low-current configurations (LCCs); no excess of other tumors was found.

Several features of the design and conduct of this study limit the conclusions that can be drawn from the reported associations. The use of outside wiring configurations near the home in the 1970s as a surrogate for magnetic field exposure in the home two or more decades earlier when the disease was diagnosed had not been determined to be a valid indicator of exposure at the time of the study. Moreover, assignment of

* 1 T (tesla) = 10^4 gauss; 1 gauss = 0.1 mT = 100 μT.

TABLE 17-1 Selected Case-Control Studies of Cancer in Persons with Residential Exposure to Electrical Power Lines

Investigators	Geographical area	Case ascertainment	No. of cases/ controls	Findings
Wertheimer and Leeper (1979)	Denver, Colo.	Childhood cancer deaths 1950–1973; death and birth certificates	344/344	2- to 3-fold excess leukemia, lymphoma, nervous system tumors near high-current wiring
Fulton et al. (1980)	Rhode Island	Childhood leukemia deaths 1964–1978; death and birth certificates	119/240	No relationship between leukemia and electrical power lines
Wertheimer and Leeper (1982)	Denver, Colo.	Adult cancer deaths and cases 1967–1979; death certificates, cancer registry	1179/1179	Significant increase in cancer of nervous system, uterus, breast, lymphoma near high-current wires
Tomenius (1986)	Stockholm County, Sweden	Childhood cancer cases, national cancer registry, 1958–1978	716/716	2- to 3-fold increase total and nervous system tumors near high-current wires
Savitz (1987)	Denver, Colo.	Childhood cancer cases, 1976–1983, cancer registry	125/189	Some increase in total cancer, especially leukemia: odds ratio = 2
Stevens et al. (1987)	Three counties, Washington	Adult leukemia cases, regional cancer registry, 1981–1984	164/204	No association between leukemia and power lines

exposure status (HCC or LCC) to the residences was done with knowledge of the case or control status of the occupants. There are several additional potential sources of bias concerning case and control selection, tracing procedures, and analysis, such as the use of two different birth files for selection of control subjects, one for controls of children who died of leukemia and lymphoma (the original case group) and the other for children with other cancers who were added later (Crocetti, 1983); the lack of detailed residence information between birth and death of both cases and controls; and the inclusion in the analysis of some cases and controls for whom only birth or death addresses were available. Data were available to investigate a limited number of possible confounding factors that may have led to the observed associations.

In 1980 Fulton et al. reported on their attempt to repeat the substance of the Wertheimer and Leeper study in Rhode Island, with attention only to leukemia cases with onset up to 20 years of age during the period 1964–1978. From the files of the Rhode Island Hospital, which routinely maintained records and complete address histories on these patients, 119 patients were chosen and their 209 addresses noted. For each patient two control subjects of the same birth year were selected from the state birth certificate file and 240 control addresses were obtained. The 209 addresses of leukemia patients and 240 control addresses were studied by mapping power lines within about 50 m of each residence, and a summary exposure value was produced following the Wertheimer and Leeper procedure. No relationship was found with childhood leukemia, in contrast to the earlier study.

Wertheimer and Leeper (1980) speculated that differences in classifying certain wires and in matching control subjects between the two studies accounted for the negative findings in Rhode Island. They reworked the Rhode Island data, which Fulton et al. made available to them, and found a weak association between childhood leukemia and HCCs ($p = 0.05$). Many of the shortcomings of the Wertheimer and Leeper investigation are found in the Fulton et al. study, which has the additional handicap of a small study group.

To investigate further the association of cancer with high-current electrical wires near the home, Wertheimer and Leeper (1982) conducted a case-control study of adult cancers. Estimates of exposure were based on electrical wire configurations as in the childhood cancer study, with some modifications: four categories of wiring configuration were used instead of the original two, readings were taken just outside some representative houses that were accessible, and measurements were made inside 20 homes. The study group was composed of 1179 adult cancer subjects and 1179 matched control subjects identified in four samples from four areas of greater Denver for the period 1967–1979. In contrast to the childhood study, some living cancer patients (275) were included in the total study population. Cancer deaths were selected from death certificates; cancer patients were selected from the Colorado cancer registry and their control subjects were chosen from a telephone survey. A significant increase in four types of cancer—nervous system, uterus, breast, and lymphoma—was observed in those under 55 years of age who lived near HCCs. However, the association was considerably weaker than that observed for childhood cancer.

There are serious questions of bias in the methods of selection of control subjects, which were nonuniform and varied among the four geographical areas. The criteria for inclusion of the living cancer "survivors" (having a life-threatening form of cancer diagnosed 5 or more years previously, without recurrence in 1979) were sometimes difficult to meet and questionable in their usefulness. The same uncertainties about exposure estimates are apparent in this study as in the childhood studies. The unavailability of information about the many risk factors known to affect adult health, including occupational exposures and tobacco use, is an important weakness.

Tomenius (1986) undertook to replicate in Sweden the Colorado childhood case-control study, using all reported tumors. Individuals up to 18 years of age were drawn from the Swedish Cancer Registry from the county of Stockholm for the period 1958–1973, and control subjects were selected from parish and county birth registers matched for sex and birth date. The study was restricted to the 716 patients and an equal number of control subjects who where born in the county and still lived there at the time of diagnosis, and their 2098 dwellings. Tomenius noted wiring configurations within 150 m of the homes and measured AC magnetic fields outside the entrance doors of individual dwellings. Visible 200 kV wires were noted at 45 homes and twice as frequently at homes of cancer patients as at control dwellings. Magnetic fields of 3 mG (0.3 μT) or more were measured at 48 dwellings and were also twice as frequent at case residences as at control homes. The range of magnetic field measurements at residences was 0.004 to 19 mG (mean 0.69 mG), and the field was highest at dwellings with visible 200 kV wires (2.25 mG). There was no relationship between tumors and distance of dwellings from 200 kV lines within the 150 m limit of observation, that is, no "dose-response" relationship as postulated by Wertheimer and Leeper (1979, 1982) and challenged by Miller (1980). More extensive and systematic field measurements were made in this study than in the earlier ones, but uncertainty remains about the exposure experienced by the study subjects. The twofold excess of all tumor cases and the increase in nervous system neoplasms is in accord with the Wertheimer and Leeper findings; the absence of a leukemia and lymphoma excess is not, nor is the preponderance of female cases.

In the United States, as part of the New York State Power Lines

Project, multidisciplinary research programs were carried out on the biological effects of electric and magnetic fields associated with high-voltage transmission lines (Ahlbom et al., 1987). Two of the 16 research projects were epidemiological studies designed to replicate but improve on the Wertheimer and Leeper Denver studies. Considerable attention and resources were given to the construction of exposure facilities and to dosimetry, in order to provide a more accurate definition of the actual magnetic and electric fields.

A case-control study of childhood cancer was conducted in other sections of the Denver area, involving a final group of 125 cases out of 356 eligible cases reported to the cancer registry during the period 1976–1983, a randomly drawn, matched, child control group, and a residence control group (Savitz, 1987). Two approaches were used for exposure assessments: direct point-in-time measurements of electric and magnetic fields within the homes, and coding of external wires and other transmission facilities. Assessments were made without knowledge of case or control status of the homes. A third major data source was a lengthy household interview questionnaire covering residential history, family health history, medications, x-ray exposures, and other possible risk factors and confounders for childhood cancer.

Wiring configuration outside the home was found to correlate with direct measurements inside the home, and the major factor contributing to magnetic fields was found to be the distribution system and the power supply to the homes (Kaune et al., 1987). A positive association between wiring configuration and increased cancer risk was found for all cancers, particularly for the leukemias and less so for brain tumors; for the highest-exposed group the relative risk was more than twice as great. There was a suggestive dose-response relationship. No confounders were identified in the questionnaire response data. The principal and serious flaw in this study is the limited response rate of study subjects or surrogates. Among the patients eligible for study, just 71% were interviewed; only 62% of the child control subjects were interviewed, and the residence control group had to be excluded from analysis because of a response rate of only 39%.

The second epidemiological study was a case-control study of adult acute leukemia (nonlymphocytic) in a three-county area that includes the cities of Seattle, Tacoma, and Everett, Washington (Stevens, 1987). During the period 1961–1984, 164 cases and 204 control subjects were identified. Study procedures were similar to those in the childhood cancer study, and the response rates were also surprisingly low: only 70% of the cases and 65% of the control group. Even more extensive and detailed measurements of magnetic and electric fields were performed in this study (Kaune et al., 1987). Residential magnetic fields were found correlated with the external distribution wiring as characterized by the wiring code of Wertheimer and Leeper. In addition, obvious sources of magnetic fields such as lights and appliances were found not to be major contributors to residential fields away from the appliances. Both this study and the Savitz childhood study support the original hypothesis of Wertheimer and Leeper (1979) that return loop ground currents are an important source of residential magnetic fields. No association between adult acute leukemia and magnetic field exposure was found in this study.

The two epidemiological studies (Savitz, 1987; Stevens, 1987) of the New York State Power Lines Project are population based, well designed, and the most advanced in characterization and measurement of exposures, as well as identification of possible confounders. The major and serious shortcoming of each is the low participation rate, which results in small study populations and unanticipated biases. Several factors appear to be involved in this unusual situation: the reluctance of physicians to allow next-of-kin contact for deceased patients who constituted a large proportion of the cases, the high refusal rate of control subjects, and the long duration of the questionnaire-interview (1½ to 2 hours). Some of the problems associated with selection of controls have been discussed by Savitz and Pearce (1988) and Gordis (1982).

In the United Kingdom, Myers et al. (1985) conducted a case-control study of childhood cancer involving 376 cases diagnosed during the period 1970–1979 in the Yorkshire Health Region and 591 control subjects identified by birth certificate. Magnetic fields at all birth addresses within 100 m of an overhead line were estimated from actual load currents provided by the electricity boards. Only a small proportion of patients and control subjects lived near overhead lines. No significant relationship between cancer risk and exposure was found. Coleman et al. (1985) are engaged in a case-control study of all cases of leukemia registered in the Thames Cancer Registry from four London boroughs in 1965–1980 (769 cases). Two control subjects per case have been randomly selected from all registered solid tumors (excluding lymphoma) matched on age, sex, year of diagnosis, and borough of residence. Relative risks are being computed within 100 m of overhead lines, but less than 1% of the patients lived within that distance at diagnosis. A mortality study of persons living in the vicinity of electricity transmission facilities in the East Anglia region failed to support an association of EM field exposure with acute leukemia or other lymphatic cancers (McDowall, 1986). In the United Kingdom studies, calculated fields based on distance from a power line were used to assess exposure (Coleman and Beral, 1988). Such criteria are not comparable to those used in the U.S. and Swedish studies and may possibly account for differences in findings.

OCCUPATIONAL EXPOSURE TO ELECTROMAGNETIC FIELDS

In their 1979 paper on residential exposure and childhood cancer, Wertheimer and Leeper mentioned a brief attempt to explore occupational exposure to AC magnetic fields. They analyzed data on occupation by cause of death in the United States for 1950 (Guralnick, 1963). All occupational categories that seemed likely to include frequent exposure to AC magnetic fields were found to have, as a group, a cancer mortality rate significantly higher than that of the total population. The "exposed" categories included power station (switchyard) operators and engineers; telephone, telegraph, and power linemen and servicemen; street, subway, and elevated railway motormen; electricians; and welders and flame cutters. The standard mortality ratio (SMR) for total cancer for the group was 115, a significant increase over the ratio of 100 for all occupations; for other causes of death the SMR was a nonsignificant 102. This appeared to serve as a stimulus for the occupational studies that followed.

One of the first was by Milham (1982), who, in the course of updating a study of occupational mortality, noted that men whose occupations required them to work in electric or magnetic fields had more leukemia deaths than would be expected. In a continuing study of mortality records by occupational class in the state of Washington (Milham, 1983), all deaths of resident white men 20 years of age or older were coded to occupation for the 30-year period 1950–1979. Proportionate mortality ratios (PMRs) standardized by age and year of death were computed for 158 cause-of-death groups in each of 218 occupational classes. In all, 438,000 deaths were analyzed. Expected values were based on proportionate mortality for Washington State white men.

The 11 selected occupations with presumed exposure to electric or magnetic fields as listed by Milham (1982) in a letter to the editor were electronic technicians, radio and telegraph operators, electricians, linemen (power and telephone), television and radio repairmen, power station operators, aluminum workers, welders and flame cutters, motion picture projectionists, electrical engineers, and streetcar and subway motormen. PMRs were elevated for all leukemia in 10 of the 11 occupational groups (not for welders and flame cutters) and were significantly elevated above 100 in three, electricians (138), power station operators (259), and aluminum workers (189). PMRs for acute leukemia were elevated in eight of the occupational groups and significantly so for electricians (178), television and radio repairmen (291), and aluminum workers (258). The total number of leukemia deaths in the 11 occupational groups was 136, and the number of acute leukemia deaths was 60.

Since 1980 nearly 20 occupational studies have been published about the same or similar "electrical" or "exposed" occupations and associations with cancer mortality or incidence. They include proportionate mortality or incidence ratios, case-control studies, and retrospective cohort studies in the United States (Milham, 1982; Wright et al., 1982; Lin et al., 1985; Calle and Savitz, 1985; Thomas et al., 1987), the United Kingdom (Coleman et al., 1983; McDowall, 1983; Swerdlow, 1983), Sweden (Wiklund et al., 1981; Vagero and Olin, 1983; Olin et al., 1985; Vagero et al., 1985; Flodin et al., 1986; Tornqvist et al., 1986; McLaughlin et al., 1987), and New Zealand (Pearce et al., 1985 and 1989). Selected occupational studies are shown in Table 17–2 to illustrate the variety of findings.

In the United States, Wright et al. (1982) used the 10 occupations listed in the Milham mortality report to examine the 1972–1979 experience of the Los Angeles County Cancer Registry and found a significant increase in proportional incidence ratio (PIR) for acute leukemia in power and telephone linemen. Calle and Savitz (1985), on the other hand, found no excess leukemia mortality in the same occupational groups in Wisconsin.

In Britain, McDowall (1983) analyzed national leukemia mortality statistics for the electrical occupations in England and Wales for the years 1970 to 1972 and found a significantly increased PMR for acute myeloid leukemia for electrical engineers, telegraph and radio operators, and electronic engineers. In a follow-up case-control examination of national mortality statistics by occupation for only acute myeloid leukemia during 1973, an increased relative risk (RR) was found for all electrical occupations (RR = 2.3) with the highest for telecommunications engineers (RR = 4.0) and post office and telephone engineers (RR = 3.0). Coleman et al. (1983) used the same electrical occupations as McDowall and analyzed the cancer registry experience during 1961–1979 in southeastern England. For all 10 occupations taken together, the proportional incidence ratio showed a small significant excess for all leukemia, particularly in telegraph operators and electrical fitters. Radio and radar mechanics had a deficit of all leukemias.

In Sweden, Vagero and Olin (1983) used the newly created Swedish Cancer Environment Registry, formed by linkage of the Swedish Cancer Registry 1961–1973 to the 1960 population census, to assess the excess risk of cancer for those working in the electronics and electrical manufacturing industry. Comparison was made with the general working population for the period 1961–1973. A slight but significant excess of cancer occurred in all sites among men and women in the electronics industry as a whole. Noteworthy was a doubling of the relative risk for pharyngeal cancers in blue-collar workers (RR = 2.03, confidence limits 1.3 to 3.6), a raised relative risk for nasopharyngeal cancers in men in the radio and television industry, and an elevated risk for cancer of the nasal cavities for other electronic workers. No excess of any form of leukemia was found. A later study (Vagero et al., 1985) of the cancer morbidity experience of a cohort of telecommunications workers during the years

TABLE 17-2 Selected Studies of Cancer and Occupational Exposure to Electromagnetic Fields

Investigators	Geographical area	Data sources	Findings
Milham (1982)	Washington	Mortality statistics, males, by occupational class and cause of death, 1950–1979	Increased leukemia mortality in 10 "exposed" occupations, particularly aluminum workers, electricians, power station operators
Wright et al. (1982)	Los Angeles County, California	Cancer registry, males, electrical occupations, 1972–1979	Increased acute leukemia incidence in power and telephone linemen
McDowall (1983)	England and Wales	National leukemia mortality statistics, males, electrical occupations, 1970–1972	Increased acute myeloid leukemia mortality in electrical engineers, telegraph radio operators, and electronics engineers
Vagero and Olin (1983)	Sweden	National cancer registry, males and females, 1961–1973	Increased incidence of total and pharynx cancer in electronics industries; no excess leukemia
Swerdlow (1983)	England and Wales	National registry for eye cancer, males, 1968–1975	Increased incidence of eye cancer in electrical and electronic workers
Lin et al. (1985)	Maryland	Brain tumor deaths, males, by occupation, death certificates, 1969–1982	Excess central nervous system tumor deaths in electrical occupations
Pearce et al. (1985)	New Zealand	Cancer registry, leukemia, males, electrical occupations, 1979–1983	Excess leukemia in electronic equipment assemblers, radio and television repairmen
Vagero et al. (1985)	Stockholm, Sweden	Cancer registry, male and female workers in a telecommunications company, 1958–1979	Excess malignant melanoma of skin in soldering department workers
Tornqvist et al.	Sweden	Cancer registry, males, electric	No excess incidence of leukemia or

1958 to 1979 failed to reveal an excess of total cancer or pharyngeal cancers, in contrast to their earlier findings. However, there was an excess risk of malignant melanoma of the skin, especially where soldering was done. A second Swedish study reported excess malignant melanoma of the skin (Olin et al., 1985) in a cohort study of electrical engineering graduates from the Royal Institute of Technology in Stockholm (but not in architecture graduates).

From New Zealand, Pearce et al. (1985) noted in a letter the results of a national case-control study of leukemia and occupation. The study involved 546 adult male leukemia patients registered from 1979 to 1983 and 2184 control subjects from the cancer registry, with four control subjects per case matched for age and year of registration. In the "electrical" occupations a significant excess of total leukemia was found among those who were electronic equipment assemblers and radio and television repairmen. In a later report (Pearce et al., 1989) the highest RRs were for chronic lymphatic leukemia.

Swerdlow (1983), using the national cancer registration system, studied the epidemiology of eye cancer in England and Wales. For men in three occupational classes—administrators and managers; professional and technical workers and artists; and electrical and electronics workers—proportional incidence ratios for eye cancer (especially malignant melanoma) were substantially elevated during the years 1968 to 1975. The high ratios for the first two occupational classes were consistent with their upper social class standing and a reflection of social class gradient for eye cancer in England and Wales. The high ratios for electrical and electronics workers, on the other hand, were unexpected because eye cancer is less frequent among manual workers.

Lin et al. (1985) conducted a case-control study in Maryland to explore the association between occupation and brain tumor mortality. The death certificates of 951 adult white men who died of brain tumors during 1969–1982 were compared with those of 951 control subjects matched for age and date of death who died of nonmalignant causes. A significantly higher proportion of persons with primary brain tumors was found to have been employed in electrical occupations such as electrician, electrical or electronic engineer, and utility company serviceman. The occupations of cancer patients and control subjects were then grouped according to level of potential job exposure to EM fields (definite, probable, possible, no exposure), and an increase in the odds ratio for brain tumor was reported associated with potential exposure levels. Milham (1988) determined standardized mortality ratios (SMRs) for male members of the American Radio Relay League (amateur radio operators) and found significantly elevated SMRs for myeloid leukemia and multiple myeloma. An ongoing study in the United States (Matanoski and Obrams, 1984) is concerned with determining the risk of leukemia in telephone linemen, who are exposed to a wide variety of EM environments. Through the use of the Bell System employee records, about 160 deaths from acute myeloid leukemia that occurred in 1975 through 1980 and appropriate control subjects are under investigation.

DISCUSSION

Considerations that should affect the weight given to epidemiological evidence for the hypothesis that an environmental factor is an etiological agent of a chronic disease have been discussed by Sartwell (1960), Hill (1965), and others more recently (OTA, 1989). The principal elements are the strength of the association, its confirmation by additional studies, demonstration of a dose-response relationship, temporal relationships, and compatibility with other types of evidence, including biological reasonableness.

1. Strength of the association. This important element concerns the ratio of rates in the study and control groups. When the ratio is large, as in the 10- to 30-fold difference between cigarette smokers and nonsmokers concerning death rates from lung cancer, the hypothesis is greatly strengthened. Actual rates may be small, but the difference between exposed and nonexposed is the significant element. That many cases of a disease (cancer) occur without known exposure to the environmental factor (EM fields) does not invalidate the hypothesis, since the disease may have multiple causes, but it weakens it. On the other hand, the presence of EM fields in the absence of disease does not necessarily weaken the hypothesis because there are factors affecting susceptibility that are not well understood (not all persons exposed to ionizing radiation develop cancer).

In the studies reviewed here, RR estimates rarely exceed 3 and are more often around 1.2 to 2 for all cancers or for specific types such as leukemia and nervous system tumors. A weak association in itself, however, is not sufficient reason to reject a causal hypothesis (Wynder, 1987).

2. Confirmation by additional studies. Replication studies have been carried out by different investigators in different population groups, at different sites, with inconsistent findings. For residential exposures of the general population to nearby power transmission lines, all investigations have used the case-control method, which is appropriate and useful, especially when individuals rather than groups are studied. In the case of occupational exposures, proportionate mortality or morbidity ratios

have been computed for "electrical and electronic" occupations in about half the studies; limited case-control designs and retrospective cohort approaches have been used in the others. Proportionate ratios serve as a quick and economical way to use available statistics for preliminary test of a hypothesis before undertaking case-control and longitudinal studies. They are not useful for validation purposes.

The original report of a positive correlation between residential exposure to overhead transmission lines and childhood cancer in Denver has been followed by six other completed case-control studies of individuals. Four are studies of children, two of which confirm some of the findings of increased risk of nervous system cancer, lymphoma, and leukemia and two of which are negative for leukemia. Of two adult studies, one found excesses of several forms of cancer, but not leukemia, and the other was also negative for leukemia. The original method of estimating magnetic field exposure by outside wire configurations was validated by direct measurement.

Numerous studies of the "electrical and electronic" occupations have appeared since Milham's 1982 report of elevated proportional mortality ratios for leukemia in occupations with presumed exposure to electric and magnetic fields. Excess leukemia, of all types or of acute forms, has been found in the majority of studies that included leukemia as an end point, in the United States, United Kingdom, and New Zealand. Four retrospective cohort studies, which provide more reliable information, have failed to reveal any leukemia excess in Sweden but have found increases in other types of malignancies such as pharyngeal cancer and malignant melanoma.

Other occupational investigations, unrelated to replication efforts, have failed to establish an association between electrical occupations and cancer. A survey of cancer in relation to occupation in the United States (Decoufle et al., 1977) revealed no excess leukemia among linemen and servicemen for telegraph, telephone, and power lines. In a study of leukemia incidence by occupation in an entire metropolitan area in Canada, significant excess leukemia risks were found for 14 male and eight female occupational categories but none included electricians or electronic occupations or welders (Morton and Marjanovic, 1984). A study of cohorts of Navy enlisted men in technical occupational classifications related to the maintenance and operation of radar equipment (Robinette et al., 1980) could not establish consistent patterns of cancers related to presumed high and low exposure to radiofrequency (microwave) radiation.

Interest in reports of a possible connection between EM fields and cancer led several other investigators to speculate about such an explanation for their findings. An unexplained excess of oral or pharyngeal cancer in white women in North Carolina was thought possibly related to their work in the manufacture of electrical and electronic equipment (Winn et al., 1982). In a report of a cluster of endodermal sinus tumors, a rare tumor in children, among five black girls aged 1½ to 18 years in Jacksonville, Florida, it was noted that high-voltage power lines were in the area. Estimated exposures were said to be considerably higher (0.04 to 1.69 G) than observed values in the residential studies (Aldrich et al., 1984). Excess mortality risk of chronic lymphocytic leukemia in U.S. underground coal miners with long-term employment has been associated with power frequency electric and magnetic fields from overhead power distribution lines and other electrical sources in the mines (Gilman et al., 1985).

3. Demonstration of a dose-response relationship. The quantitative relationship between exposure (duration and intensity) and frequency of cancer cannot be determined from data available at this time. Duration of exposure is presumed prolonged in the residential and the occupational studies, but estimates of potential exposure level ("dose") are uncertain. In addition, it is not clear that the quantities used for the assessment of exposure are the most appropriate and relevant for dosimetric considerations (Czerski, 1988). In the original residential exposure studies in Denver a gradient of effect related to distance from high-power wire configurations was reported, but no evidence for this was found in a similar study in Sweden. A study in another section of Denver by another investigator reported a suggestive gradient (Savitz, 1987). The suggested gradient of effect of occupational exposure on brain tumor mortality was based on estimates of potential exposure according to job classification, an indicator of doubtful precision (Lin et al., 1985). The use of miniature personal dosimeters in future residential and occupational studies may improve monitoring of ELF field exposures (Tenforde, 1989).

4. Temporal relationships. Chronologic relationships must be such that exposure precedes disease, but this is often difficult to assess in the residential studies and cannot be assessed in the reported occupational studies. Suggestive evidence comes from the first childhood study (Wertheimer and Leeper, 1979), in which the most striking difference between cases and control subjects was found for the small group of children who had the same home address from birth to death. Latent periods could not be determined; they were arbitrarily assigned in some of the studies.

5. Biological reasonableness of the association. At this time there is no other published human evidence that alternating or static magnetic fields or electric fields, of any intensity, are implicated in carcinogenesis. The estimated AC magnetic fields of 0.1 to 0.7 μT in the homes of the

cancer patients are exceedingly weak, and Tenforde (1985) has compared them to the levels to which humans are generally exposed in nature. These alternating magnetic fields do not occur in nature, however, and as a by-product of industrial activity may have an added effect. Very weak magnetic fields may be biologically active, according to experimental reports of effects on reproductive processes (Delgado et al., 1982) and on cells including enhanced growth of tumor cells (Winters and Phillips, 1984), and electric fields are being used increasingly in bone and wound healing in humans and animals (Bassett et al., 1977). Studies from two laboratories have reported that 2.45 GHz microwave exposure may act as a cocarcinogen or a copromoter (Szmigielski et al., 1982; Balcer-Kubiczek and Harrison, 1989).

As far as occupational exposure is concerned, many types and levels of exposure are involved in "electrical and electronic occupations," including exposure to a variety of chemical and other physical agents that may be carcinogenic. An increase in cancer was not evident in a cohort study of cyclotron and bubble chamber workers exposed to high-intensity static magnetic fields for long periods of time (Budinger et al., 1984). Mortality studies of aluminum reduction plant workers, who are exposed to chemicals as well as strong magnetic fields, revealed an excess of pancreatic cancer, lymphoma, and leukemia, but the leukemia excess was negatively associated with the duration of employment (Rockette and Arena, 1983).

Although compatibility with other types of evidence must be considered in assessing possible causal relationships, it has its limitations because of the limitations of knowledge at any given time. An instructive illustration is provided from the infectious disease field (Sartwell, 1960). In 1861 Cheever, warning against attaching any significance to "nonsense correlations," wrote, "It could be no more ridiculous for the stranger who passed the night in the steerage of an emigrant ship to ascribe the typhus, which he there contracted, to the vermin with which bodies of the sick might be infested. An adequate cause, one reasonable in itself, must correct the coincidences of simple experience." It was learned later that this was indeed the way typhus was contracted.

To date the epidemiological evidence is weak for an etiological role of EM fields (up to 300 GHz) in the development of malignant neoplasms. Easterly (1981) proposed that magnetic fields may function as weak promoters in the initiation-promotion, two-step concept of carcinogenesis, a commonly used model of cancer induction. A hypothesis that use of electric power may increase the risk of breast cancer has been presented (Stevens, 1987a); this is based on the effect of light and ELF fields on pineal melatonin production and on the relationship of melatonin to mammary carcinogenesis. A biological basis or mechanism of action for possible carcinogenic effects has not yet been established. Cancers appear to be a heterogeneous group with a variety of causes and risk factors.

CONCLUSION

The possible association between exposure to magnetic, electric, or EM fields and the development of human cancer has been the subject of numerous epidemiological studies since the 1979 Wertheimer and Leeper study proposing low magnetic fields as a cancer promoter. Two lines of investigation have been followed: the role of residential exposure of the general population to ELF fields from power transmission lines and the effect of exposure at work to fields encountered in "electrical and electronic" occupations.

In the residential studies it was postulated that the significant exposure was to magnetic fields generated by the electrical wiring near the residences. Two objections were raised almost immediately: first, that the method of estimating magnetic fields by configurations of electrical wires outside the residences was unreliable, and second, that the estimated magnetic fields were so weak, on the order of 0.1 to 0.7 µT, that biological effects were unlikely. The first issue has been settled now that wiring configurations have been found to be a valid predictor of magnetic fields inside the homes (Kaune et al., 1987); the second remains under investigation. The association between residential exposure to power lines and cancer mortality or incidence has been investigated through case-control studies of children and adults in the United States, United Kingdom, and Sweden. A modest excess of leukemia and nervous system tumors has been found in several studies of children, but there are also negative reports. Among adults, nervous system tumors and nonleukemic cancers have been reported in one study; other studies of leukemia alone have had negative results. Excess leukemia has not been a feature of this type of exposure in adults.

In the electrical occupational studies the presence or characteristics of electric, magnetic, or EM field exposures have rarely been determined; analysis has been by job titles or classes, not by investigation of actual exposure situations. The studies of occupational exposure are numerous and geographically varied but rather limited in their contributions. The original designation of "electrical and electronic" occupations, useful as a first step in establishing some statistically significant associations, has been continued in nearly 20 studies, of which about half yield proportionate mortality or incidence ratios. With a few exceptions the studies have found a statistically significant excess of mortality or morbidity from some (but not necessarily the same) type of cancer, including acute leukemia, acute myeloid leukemia, pharyngeal cancer, brain tumor, malignant melanoma of the skin and eye, and total cancer. Excess acute leukemia or acute myeloid leukemia was the most frequent finding in the proportionate analyses and in some case-control studies. Swedish retrospective cohort studies reported no excess leukemia, contradictory findings of increased pharyngeal cancer, and excess malignant melanoma of the skin in two studies. Possible confounding by exposure to chemical or other physical work place carcinogens is mentioned with respect to classes of occupations but rarely investigated. Other occupational studies, not related to replication efforts, have failed to establish an association between electrical occupations and malignancies.

Five issues that affect the weight given to epidemiological evidence for a causal relationship have been reviewed: the strength of the association, its confirmation by additional studies, demonstration of a dose-response relationship, temporal relationships, and compatibility with other types of evidence. A modest positive association, with estimated relative risks of 1.2 to 3, has been found for total cancer and some specific types. There has been variable consistency in demonstrating the same associations in different population groups and geographical areas by different investigtors. A gradient of effect has been reported in several studies but needs confirmation. Some evidence exists for appropriate chronological relationships, that is, exposure *before* the effect, in children. Support of the association in terms of biological compatibility is not yet available; the cancer-promoting properties of very low time-varying magnetic fields are being investigated. Epidemiological evidence for a causal relationship can be considered inconclusive at this time.

Additional improved, *concurrent* replication studies of childhood cancer and residential exposure to ELF fields from power transmission lines are needed. The strongest associations have been found with young children in stable residences, but the study groups have been small. Particular attention should be given to adequate sample size, careful choice of control groups, and vigilant study management. With regard to occupational studies, little has been done to advance them beyond ill-defined groups of "electric and electronic" workers. At some point case-control studies of individuals should be considered and further attempts made to characterize the exposures and the confounders. Acute leukemia, acute myeloid leukemia, or malignant melanoma may warrant further exploration. The possibility of an indirect carcinogenic effect of magnetic, electric, or EM fields merits further investigation because of the near-universal exposure of general populations to power frequency fields and widespread occupational exposures to EM sources.

REFERENCES

AHLBOM, A., ALBERT, E.N., FRASER-SMITH, A.C., et al. (1987). Biological effects of power line fields, Panel's final report, Albany, N.Y., New York Power Lines Project.

ALDRICH, T.E., GLORIEUX, A., AND CASTRO, S. (1984). Florida cluster of five children with endodermal sinus tumors: possible environmental risk. *Oncology 41*:233–238.

BALCER-KUBICZEK, E.K., AND HARRISON, G.H. (1989). Induction of neoplastic transformation in C3H/I0T½ cells by 2.45 GHz microwaves and phorbol ester. *Radiation Research 117*:531–537.

BASSETT, C.A.L., PILLA, A.A., AND PAWLUK, E.J. (1977). A non-operative salvage of surgically-resistant pseudarthroses and non-unions by pulsing electromagnetic fields. *Clin. Orthop. 124*:128–143.

BUDINGER, T.F., BRISTOL, K.S., AND BUNCHER, T. (1984). Epidemiological survey of disease prevalence in 792 subjects exposed to static magnetic fields and 792 matched controls. Berkeley, Calif., Lawrence Berkeley Laboratory Report.

CALLE, E.E., AND SAVITZ, D.A. (1985). Leukemia in occupational groups with presumed exposure to electrical and magnetic fields (Letter). *N. Engl. J. Med. 313*:1476–1477.

CHEEVER, D.W. (1861). The value and fallacy of statistics in the observation of disease. *Boston Med. Surg. J. 63*:449–450.

COLEMAN, M., BELL, J., AND SKEET, R. (1983). Leukemia incidence in electrical workers. *Lancet 1*:982–983.

COLEMAN, M., BELL, C.M.J., TAYLOR H.-L., AND THORNTON-JONES, H. (1985). Leukemia and electromagnetic fields: a case-control study. Presented at International Conference on Electric and Magnetic Fields in Medicine and Biology, London, Dec. 4–5, 1985.

COLEMAN, M., AND BERAL, V. (1988). A review of epidemiological studies of the health effects of living near or working with electricity generation and transmission equipment. *Int. J. Epidemiol. 17*:1–13.

CROCETTI, A. (1983). Final report on Wertheimer and Leeper Denver studies to Power Lines Project, New York State Department of Health. Unpublished.

CZERSKI, P. (1988). Extremely low frequency magnetic fields: biological effects and health risk assessment. *In*: Repacholi, M.H. (ed.). Non-ionizing radiations. Proceedings of International Non-Ionizing Radiation Workshop, Melbourne, Apr. 5–9, 1988. Australian Radiation Laboratory, Yallambie, Victoria, pp. 291–302.

DECOUFLE, P., STANISLAWCZYK, K., HOUTEN, L., BROSS, I.D.J., AND VIADANA, E. (1977). A retrospective survey of cancer in relation to occupation. U.S. DHEW Center for Disease Control, NIOSH HSN 99–73–5, National Institute of Occupational Safety and Health.

DELGADO, J.M.R., MONTEAGUDO, J.L., GARCIA, M.G., AND LEAL, J. (1982). Embryological changes induced by extremely low frequency electromagnetic fields. *J. Anat. 134*:533–551.

EASTERLY, C.E. (1981). Cancer link to magnetic field exposure: a hypothesis. *Am. J. Epidemiol. 114*:169–174.

ELDER, J.A., AND CAHILL, D.F. (eds.). Biological effects of radiofrequency radiation, Research Triangle Park, N.C., U.S. Environmental Protection Agency. (EPA-600/8–83–026F).

FLODIN, U., FREDRICKSSON, M., AXELSON, O., PERSSON, B., AND BARDELL, L. (1986). Background radiation, electrical work and some other exposures associated with acute myeloid leukemia in a case-referent study. *Arch. Environ. Health 41*:77–84.

FULTON, J.P., COBB, S., PREBLE, L., LEONE, L. AND FORMAN, E. (1980). Electrical wiring configurations and childhood leukemia in Rhode Island. *Am. J. Epidemiol. 111*:292–296.

GILMAN, F.A., AMES, R.G., AND MCCAWLEY, M.A. (1985). Leukemia risk among U.S. white male coal miners. *J. Occup. Med. 27*:669–671.

GORDIS, L. (1982). Should dead cases be matched to dead controls? *Am. J. Epidemiol. 115*:1–5.

GREENBERG, R.S., AND SHUSTER, J.L. (1985). Epidemiology of cancer in children. *Epidemiol. Rev. 7*:22–48.

GURALNICK, L. (1963). Mortality by occupation and cause of death among men 20 to 64 years of age: United States, 1950. Vital Statistics Special Reports 53, No. 3.

HILL, A.B. (1965). The environment and disease: association or causation? *Proc. R. Soc. Med. 58*:295–300.

KAUNE, W.T., STEVENS, R.G., CALLAHAN, N.J., SEVERSON, R.K., AND THOMAS, D.B. (1987). Residential magnetic and electric fields. *Bioelectromagnetics 8*:315–335.

LILIENFELD, A.M., TONASCIA, J., TONASCIA, S., LIBAUER, C.A., AND CAUTHEN, G.M. (1978). Foreign service health status study—evaluation of health status of foreign service and other employees from selected Eastern European posts, Final Report, Contract No. 6025–6190973 (NTIS PB-288163), Department of State, Washington, D.C.

LIN, R.S., DISCHINGER, P.C., CONDE, J., AND FARRELL, K.P. (1985). Occupational exposure to electromagnetic fields and the occurrence of brain tumors. *J. Occup. Med. 27*:413–419.

MATANOSKI, G.M., AND OBRAMS, G.I. (1984). Feasibility study to determine risk of leukemia in telephone linemen (Abstract). *In*: Biological effects from electric and magnetic fields associated with high voltage transmission lines. Contractors Review, U.S. Department of Energy, Electric Power Research Institute, and State of New York. Department of Health, Nov. 4–7, St. Louis, Mo.

MCDOWALL, M.E. (1983). Leukemia mortality in electrical workers in England and in Wales. *Lancet 1*:246.

MCDOWALL, M.E. (1986). Mortality of persons resident in the vicinity of electricity transmission facilities. *Br. J. Cancer 53*:272–279.

MCLAUGHLIN, J.K., WALKER, H.S.R., BLOT, W.J., et al. (1987). Occupational risks for intracranial gliomas in Sweden. *J. Natl. Cancer Inst. 78*:253–257.

MILHAM, S., JR. (1982). Mortality from leukemia in workers exposed to electrical and magnetic fields (Letter). *N. Engl. J. Med. 307*:249.

MILHAM, S., JR. (1983). Occupational mortality in Washington State 1950–1979. HHS (NIOSH) Pub. No. 83–116, Cincinnati, Ohio, National Institute of Occupational Safety and Health.

MILHAM, S., JR. (1988). Increased mortality in amateur radio operators due to lymphatic and hematopoietic malignancies. *Am. J. Epidemiol. 127*:50–54.

MILLER, M.W. (1980). Electrical wiring configurations and childhood cancer (Letter). *Am. J. Epidemiol. 112*:165–167.

MORTON, W., AND MARJANOVIC, D. (1984). Leukemia incidence by occupation in Portland-Vancouver metropolitan area. *Am. J. Ind. Med. 6*:185–205.

MYERS, A., CARTWRIGHT, R.A., BONNELL, J.A., MALE, J.C., AND CARTWRIGHT, S.C. (1985). Overhead power lines and childhood cancer. Presented at International Conference on Electric and Magnetic Fields in Medicine and Biology, London, Dec. 4–5, 1985.

OLIN, R., VAGERO, D., AND AHLBOM, A. (1985). Mortality experience of electrical engineers. *Br. J. Ind. Med. 42*:211–212.

OTA (Office of Technology Assessment, U.S. Congress). (1989). Biological effects of power frequency electric and magnetic fields. *OTA-BP-E-53*, Washington, D.C.: U.S. Government Printing Office.

PEARCE, N., REIF, J., AND FRASER, J. (1989). Case-control studies of cancer in New Zealand electrical workers. *Int. J. Epidemiol. 18*:55–59.

PEARCE, N.E., SHEPPARD, R.A., HOWARD, J.K., FRASER, J., AND LILLEY, B.M. (1985). Leukemia in electrical workers in New Zealand (Letter). *Lancet 1*:811–812.

ROBINETTE, C.D., SILVERMAN, C., AND JABLON, S. (1980). Effects upon health of occupational exposure to microwave radiation (radar). *Am. J. Epidemiol. 112*:39–53.

ROCKETTE, H.E., AND ARENA, V.C. (1983). Mortality studies of aluminum reduction plant workers; potroom and carbon department. *J. Occup. Med. 25*:549–557.

SARTWELL, P.E. (1960). On the methodology of investigations of etiologic factors in chronic diseases. *J. Chron. Dis. 11*:61–63.

SAVITZ, D.A., AND PEARCE, N. (1988). Control selection with incomplete case ascertainment. *Am. J. Epidemiol. 127*:1109–1117.

SAVITZ, D.A. (1987). Case-control study of childhood cancer and residential exposure to electric and magnetic fields. Contractor's Final Report Contract No. 218217. Albany, N.Y., New York State Power Lines Project.

SILVERMAN, C. (1985). Epidemiology of microwave radiation effects in humans. *In*: Castellani, A. (ed.). Epidemiology and quantitation of environmental risk in humans from radiation and other agents, New York, Plenum Publishing Corp., pp. 433–458.

STEVENS, R.G. (1987). Epidemiological studies of cancer and residential exposure to electromagnetic fields. Contractor's Final Report, Contract No. 218218. Albany, N.Y., New York State Power Lines Project.

STEVENS, R.G. (1987a). Electric power use and breast cancer: a hypothesis. *Am. J. Epidemiol. 125*:556–561.

SWERDLOW, A.J. (1983). Epidemiology of eye cancer in adults in England and Wales, 1962–1977. *Am. J. Epidemiol. 118*:294–300.

SZMIGIELSKI, S., SZUDZINSKI, A., PIETRASZEK, A., BIELEC, M., JANIAK, M., AND WREMBEL, J.K. (1982). Accelerated development of spontaneous and benzopyrene-induced skin cancer in mice exposed to 2450 MHz microwave radiation. *Bioelectromagnetics 3*:179–191.

TENFORDE, T.S. (1985). Biological effects of ELF magnetic fields. *In*: American Institute of Biological Sciences: biological and human health effects of extremely low frequency electromagnetic fields. Post-1977 literature review, Arlington, Va., pp. 79–127.

TENFORDE, T.S. (1989). Applications, dosimetry and biological interactions of static and time-varying magnetic fields. *In*: ICRU News 1/89, pp. 17–20, International Commission on Radiation Units and Measurements, Bethesda, Maryland.

TOMENIUS, L. (1986). 50-Hz electromagnetic environment and the incidence of childhood tumors in Stockholm County. *Bioelectromagnetics 7*:191–207.

THOMAS, T.L., STOLLEY, P.D., STEMHAGEN, A., FONTHAM, E.T.H., BLECKER, M.L., STEWART, P.A., AND HOOVER, R.N. (1987). Brain tumor mortality risk among men with electrical and electronics jobs: a case-control study. *J. Natl. Cancer Inst. 79*:233–238.

TORNQVIST, S., NORELL, S., AHLBOM, A., AND KNAVE, B. (1986). Cancer in the electric power industry. *Br J. Ind. Med. 43*:212–213.

VAGERO, D., AHLBOM, A., OLIN, R., AND SAHLSTEN, S. (1985). Cancer morbidity among workers in the telecommunications industry. *Br. J. Ind. Med. 42*:191–195.

VAGERO, D., AND OLIN, R. (1983). Incidence of cancer in the electronics industry: using the new Swedish Cancer Environment Registry as a screening instrument. *Br. J. Ind. Med. 40*:188–192.

WERTHEIMER, N., AND LEEPER, E. (1979). Electrical wiring configurations and childhood cancer. *Am. J. Epidemiol. 109*:273–284.

WERTHEIMER, N., AND LEEPER, E. (1980). Electrical wiring configurations and childhood leukemia in Rhode Island (Letter). *Am. J. Epidemiol. 111*:461–462.

WERTHEIMER, N., AND LEEPER, E. (1982). Adult cancer related to electrical wiring near the home. *Int. J. Epidemiol. 11*:345–355.

WHO (1981). World Health Organization. Environmental Health Criteria 16. Radiofrequency and microwaves, Geneva, Switzerland, WHO.

WHO (1984). World Health Organization. Environmental Health Criteria 35. Extremely low frequency (ELF) fields, Geneva, Switzerland, WHO.

WHO (1987). World Health Organization. Environmental Health Criteria 69. Magnetic fields, Geneva, Switzerland, WHO.

WIKLUND, K., EINHORN, J., AND EKLUND, J. (1981). An application of the Swedish Cancer Environment Registry: Leukemia among telephone operators at the telecommunications administration in Sweden. *Int. J. Epidemiol. 10*:373–376.

WINN, D.M., BLOT, W.J., SHY, C.M., AND FRAUMENI, J.F. (1982). Occupation and oral cancer among women in the South. *Am. J. Ind. Med. 3*:161–167.

WINTERS, W.D.D., AND PHILLIPS, J.L. (1984). Electromagnetic field induced bioeffects in human cells in vitro. Presented at 23rd Hanford Life Sciences Symposium on Interaction of Biological Systems with Static and ELF Electric and Magnetic Fields, Oct. 2–4, 1984, Richland, Wash.

WRIGHT, W.E., PETERS, J.M., MACK, T.M. (1982). Leukemia in workers exposed to electrical and magnetic fields. *Lancet* 2:1160–1161.

WYNDER, E.L. (ed.). (1987). Workshop on guidelines to the epidemiology of weak associations. *Prev. Med.* 16:139–212.

Part 4

MEDICAL APPLICATIONS

18

Hyperthermia for Cancer Therapy

CARL H. DURNEY
DOUGLAS A. CHRISTENSEN

OVERVIEW OF HYPERTHERMIA THERAPY

The use of heat to treat cancerous tumors dates back almost 100 years (Coley, 1893). In the early days, patient temperature was increased by deliberately causing a bacterial infection or injecting toxins. In the past 20 years, primarily because of improved heat generation methods and thermometry, a renewed interest has arisen in hyperthermia as a possible cancer therapy. The motivation behind the search for a better cancer treatment is clear: the American Cancer Society estimates that cancer is diagnosed in about 1 million Americans each year and that each person has approximately a 30% chance of having cancer in his or her lifetime (American Cancer Society, 1988).

Hyperthermia has been investigated alone, in combination with drugs, and in combination with ionizing radiation. At present, most clinical attention is being given to thermal treatments preceded or followed by radiation. Several clinical studies have indicated that this hyperthermia-radiation combination is effective by producing complete or partial regression of many tumor types. Considering regression and palliation effects, hyperthermia shows promise as an adjuvant to traditional therapy modalities.

Heat therapy can be classified into three general categories depending on the extent of the volume heated.

1. *Whole-body* hyperthermia raises the entire body temperature to approximately 42° C, near the maximum that can be tolerated systemically. This whole-body heating is accomplished by surrounding the patient with a heated environment such as hot wax, by trapping metabolic heat, or by perfusing the patient with extracorporeally heated blood. As might be expected, patient discomfort is higher with whole-body hyperthermia, and careful patient monitoring is essential during treatment.

2. *Regional* hyperthermia is characterized by energy deposition over substantial regions of the body, such as the abdomen, pelvis, or thorax. The rest of the body is kept as close to normal temperature as possible. The rationale for regional heating is to raise the affected site to a temperature higher than whole-body heating will allow (to 43° to 44° C if possible), including large fringe areas of possible involvement around the tumor, and to spare the remainder of the body's normal tissues. Deep-seated tumors near or within major body organs are candidates for regional hyperthermia. Electromagnetic (EM) applicators, generally in the radio-frequency (RF) range below 450 MHz, and ultrasonic applicators at or below 1 MHz are currently being evaluated clinically for deep-heating use. As explained later, regional hyperthermia for deep-seated lesions remains one of the most challenging goals in applicator design.

3. *Localized* hyperthermia heats only the immediate volume containing the tumor (and perhaps a moderate margin). Temperatures near 44° C are desired. Tumors near the surface of the body, where EM or ultrasonic access is easier, are prime candidates for this type of treatment. EM and ultrasonic applicators at higher frequencies give the localization needed. Because of their higher frequencies and smaller aperture sizes, these applicators are lighter and generally more convenient to position than the large regional heaters. Invasive techniques, such as implanted electrodes or microwave antennas, give good control over power deposition, but at the expense of invasion of the body.

The biological basis for hyperthermia is still not entirely known. It has been suggested that heat is effective in killing hypoxic, low pH, and S-phase tumor cells (which tend to be resistant to radiation therapy) (Perez, 1984). Also, compromised blood circulation in tumors may reduce the dissipation of deposited energy, causing higher tumor temperatures than in normal tissue. Many research groups are active in studies to elucidate the biological actions of hyperthermia.

ENGINEERING CHALLENGES

Depositing heat in a carefully controlled manner in tumors of widely varying sizes and locations found in the body is an engineering and physics challenge. Especially perplexing is the goal of heating deep-seated tumors to adequate therapeutic temperatures without overheating tissues on the body surface. The basic laws of physics dictate necessary trade-offs here. Inhomogeneities in the body's tissues (variations in EM, ultrasonic, and blood profusion properties, for example) add to the difficulty of the task.

In addition to the challenges presented to an optimum heating pattern by the limitations of wave physics, other practical factors must be considered in clinical use of applicators, such as sensitivity to patient movement and irregular body surfaces, applicator weight and size, ease of frequency tuning, and convenience of any coupling medium that might be required. Each applicator design has advantages and disadvantages in these regards, as explained in this chapter.

Accurate thermometry is essential to the efficacious use of heat therapy. Too little temperature rise in the cancerous tissue means inadequate treatment; too much temperature increase in normal tissue leads to unwanted damage and premature termination of the treatment by patient pain. Spatial profiles of tissue temperature, which are possible only with multiple-point measurements, are necessary to ensure that therapeutic values are reached throughout the entire volume of the target tumor. Animal experiments performed by Dewhurst et al. (1984) show that tumor response is closely related to the *minimum* temperature achieved within the tumor volume. This places increased emphasis on thorough and accurate spatial monitoring.

Temperature probes for EM heating pose a particular problem. The metallic components found in conventional thermal sensors (thermocouples and thermistors) cause erroneous temperature readings when immersed in the EM fields (Christensen and Durney, 1981). Several styles of noninteracting probes, including fiber-optic and high-resistance lead styles, have been developed for use in EM hyperthermia. Ultrasonic heating does not exhibit this problem, but care must be taken to avoid the use of catheter or sheathing materials that preferentially heat in the ultrasonic fields, as discussed later in the chapter.

In this chapter we explore the fundamental mechanisms of heat generation by both EM and ultrasonic fields, relate the characteristics of each type of energy to the design trade-offs necessary for successful applicator development (including the interaction between focusing, penetration, and frequency), and review the various categories of applicators that have been developed to date. Special attention is paid to the difficulty of heating deep tumors in the presence of an overlying surface layer of fat. Thermometry techniques for nonperturbing monitoring in both EM and ultrasonic fields are discussed.

FUNDAMENTALS

This section describes the fundamental principles underlying generation of tissue hyperthermia.

Basic Mechanisms of Tissue Heating

Electromagnetic heating.   Heat is generated in materials by energy transferred from the electric field to the charges in the material. This transfer of energy occurs through three basic mechanisms of interaction between the EM fields and the charges: orientation of electric dipoles that already exist in the atoms and molecules in the tissue, polarization of atoms and molecules to produce dipole moments, and displacement (drift) of conduction ("free") electrons and ions in the tissue. In the orientation of electric dipoles and in polarization, heat is generated by the "friction" associated with the movement of the atoms and molecules in response to a time-varying electric field. In the displacement of conduction electrons and ions, heat is generated by collisions of the conduction charges with immobile atoms and molecules of the tissue structure.

Heat is generated in tissue by the *internal* electric field, that is, the electric field inside the tissue. The internal magnetic field does not transfer any net energy to tissue charges and therefore does not produce heat. Since the internal electric field is produced by both the incident electric field and the incident magnetic field of an EM applicator, both incident fields are important to the generation of heat, but it is only the internal electric field that actually produces the heat. As explained later, the internal E field in tissue placed in the incident fields of a given EM applicator depends on the frequency, the size and shape of the tissue body, and the nature of the applicator fields. Thus the generation of heat in a biological body is a complex interaction involving many parameters.

These three basic mechanisms of interaction of EM fields with material charges are described by a macroscopic model of materials called *permittivity*, often designated by the symbol ϵ, with units of farads per meter. For sinusoidal steady-state fields, the permittivity is a complex number with real and imaginary parts given by $\epsilon = \epsilon_0(\epsilon' - j\epsilon'')$, where ϵ_0 is the permittivity of free space (units of farads per meter), ϵ' is the real part of the *relative* permittivity (unitless), and ϵ'' is the imaginary part of the relative permittivity (unitless).

The relative permittivity ϵ/ϵ_0 is also called the *dielectric constant*. The ϵ' is a measure of the generation of electric dipoles in the material by the internal electric field either by orientation or by polarization. The ϵ'' is a measure of the energy transferred from the internal electric field to the material (loss). A lossy material is one that has a large ϵ''. The quantity ϵ''/ϵ' is called the *loss tangent*, since it is a measure of the lossiness of the material. The loss tangent is often designated by tan δ. The energy transfer to the material is also frequently represented by another parameter called the *effective conductivity* of the material, which is usually designated by the symbol σ. ϵ'' and σ are related by $\sigma = \omega\epsilon_0\epsilon''$. Some tables of material properties list ϵ' and ϵ'', some list ϵ' and tan δ, and some list ϵ' and σ. For tissue, both ϵ' and ϵ'' are strong functions of frequency. Extensive measurements of the permittivity of tissue have been made and tabulated. Table 18-1 gives some representative values pertinent to generating heat in tissue.

For sinusoidal steady-state fields, the time-averaged power trans-

TABLE 18-1   Typical Values of Tissue Permittivity

Frequency (MHz)	Muscle		Fat	
	ϵ'_m	ϵ''_m	ϵ'_f	ϵ''_f
10	160.0	1123.98		
27.12	113.0	405.82	20.0	7.23–28.65
40.68	97.3	306.36	14.6	5.57–23.34
433	53.0	59.39	5.6	1.57–4.90
915	51.0	31.45	5.6	1.09–2.89
2450	47.0	16.22	5.5	0.71–1.56

Data from Johnson, C.C., and Guy, A.W. (1972). *Proc. IEEE* 60:692–718.

ferred to tissue per unit volume at a given point in the tissue is given by

$$P = \sigma \mathbf{E} \cdot \mathbf{E}^* \quad \text{W/m}^3 \tag{1}$$

where σ is the effective conductivity in siemens per meter and $\mathbf{E}$ is the RMS value of the *internal* electric field at that point in volts per meter. The total time-averaged power transferred from an electric field to an object is given by

$$P_T = \int_V \sigma \mathbf{E} \cdot \mathbf{E}^* dV \quad \text{W} \tag{2}$$

where the integral is carried out over the volume of the object. In the literature, particularly that related to EM safety, P is often called the *specific absorption rate* (SAR).

It is important to remember that the internal electric field is strongly affected by the frequency and the properties of the absorber. A rough idea of how P depends on frequency in biological bodies is given by the set of curves in Figure 18-1. These curves are for a dielectric half-space irradiated by an EM plane wave. Although a half-space is not a representative model of a human body and a plane wave is often not a very good representation of the EM fields produced by a hyperthermia applicator, the curves do indicate the general dependence of power absorption on frequency, which is more superficial with higher frequencies. For example, at 2450 MHz the relative power absorbed at 5 cm compared with that at the surface is practically zero, whereas at 10 MHz it is more than 60%. This occurs because the plane wave is attenuated as it propagates into the tissue by an exponential factor that increases with σ, and as shown in Table 18-1, σ increases with frequency. Thus, at higher frequencies, power is transferred rapidly near the surface, attenuating the wave

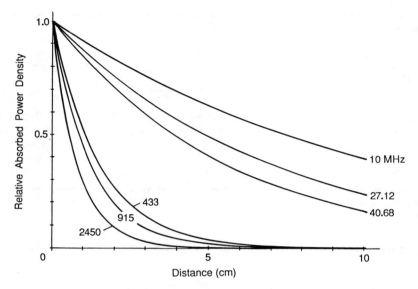

Figure 18-1   Absorption characteristics of dielectric half-space with permittivity of muscle tissue irradiated by electromagnetic plane wave. $P_n = P/P_o$ where P is given by Eq. 1 and P_o is the value of P at surface.

as power is taken out of it. Since the wave is highly attenuated deeper into the tissue, there is practically no energy left to extract from it.

The shallow penetration of EM fields shown in Figure 18-1 for plane waves is generally true of all EM fields, plane wave or not. Such shallow penetration at higher frequencies results in a fundamental problem in EM hyperthermia: how to heat deeper tissues without overheating the surface. Since the penetration is so shallow at higher frequencies (for example, at 2450 MHz), there seems to be no alternative to using lower frequencies to heat deep tissue. As explained later in the chapter, however, other problems at lower frequencies also make it difficult to heat deep tissue without overheating the surface. The depth of penetration is also a strong function of the applicator's aperture size compared to wavelength. At lower frequencies, physical limitations usually restrict apertures to sizes small compared to wavelength, which makes the penetration depth much less than the plane-wave penetration shown in Figure 18-1. Furthermore, since the wavelength is large at the lower frequencies, EM heating cannot be localized to restricted regions like a small tumor.

Because of the trade-off between frequency and depth of penetration, it appears that deep heating with EM applicators must include heating a relatively large region. Thus heating deep tissue without overheating the surface is a problem that has not yet been completely solved.

Ultrasonic heating.   Ultrasonic energy is carried into the body tissues in the form of vibrating waves—the organized motion of the atoms or molecules composing the tissue. When the frequency of the oscillation is above the frequency of human hearing (above 20 kHz), the waves are classified as ultrasound. Such waves are routinely used at low power levels in the clinic for imaging body organs by reflections, especially for obstetrical and cardiac scans. For imaging, in which the spatial resolution (limited to the wavelength of the incident radiation) must be as small as possible, high frequencies between 2 and 10 MHz are normally used. For hyperthermia applications in which pinpoint focusing is not so important as penetration depth, lower frequencies between 250 kHz and 3 MHz are generally employed.

Some of the propagating ultrasound energy is absorbed as it passes through the tissues. Although this absorption is a disadvantage in imaging, it is the mechanism by which ultrasound heats tissue. The physical basis for the loss of energy in the propagating ultrasound beam is still not thoroughly understood. It appears to be a complex combination of various relaxation phenomena (Herzfeld and Litovitz, 1959). Relaxation effects are molecular responses that accompany the ultrasonic vibrations of the tissue particles but have a finite time of response. They lag behind the primary vibratory wave, and the out-of-phase component takes power out of the incident wave, leading to a local rise in tissue temperature. Since the degree of phase lag increases with increasing frequency, one would expect that absorption increases with frequency, and indeed this has been experimentally observed.

Fluid viscosity is a simple model of an effect that produces absorption. In this phenomenon the neighboring layers of fluid particles are viscously coupled together. When an ultrasound wave passes through the medium, a force is required to overcome the viscosity of the medium. This force is out of phase with the inertial forces in the material and subtracts from the forces propagating the wave. Absorption losses proportional to the viscosity coefficient are thus encountered (Christensen, 1988b).

In actual tissue the simple viscosity model is not complete, since it predicts an absorption coefficient that varies as the square of the frequency, whereas experimental data for most soft tissues reveal an absorption coefficient that rises approximately linearly with frequency. The model becomes more correct, however, when viscosity relaxation effects are taken into account, and the model does give qualitative insight into the nature of absorptive tissue losses. Also, absorption is not the only cause of attenuation of an ultrasound wave; scattering can also reduce the forward propagating energy. For typical body tissues other than lungs, scattering is small and can be ignored when calculating the absorption losses in hyperthermia.

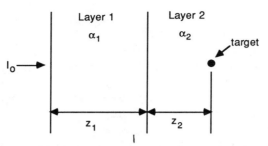

Figure 18-2 Model of ultrasound beam passing through overlying layer *1* of absorption α_1 before reaching target in layer *2* of absorption α_2.

If α is defined as the amplitude absorption coefficient, the power density (intensity) of a propagating plane wave with an initial intensity I_0 has the form

$$I(z) = I_0 e^{-2\alpha z} \tag{3}$$

Table 18-2 lists typical values of attenuation coefficients for various tissue types. These experimental values include scattering, but since scattering is usually small for hyperthermia purposes, α in Table 18-2 may be considered the amplitude absorption coefficient.

If the wave first passes through a layer of thickness z_1 with an absorption coefficient α_1 before penetrating a distance z_2 into a layer with absorption coefficient α_2, as shown in Figure 18-2, the intensity at point z_2 (neglecting the small reflection at the interface) is given by

$$I(z_2) = I_0 e^{-2\alpha_1 z_1} e^{-2\alpha_2 z_2} \tag{4}$$

The power absorbed per unit volume of tissue at point z_2 can be found by differentiating Eq. 4:

$$P = dI(z_2)/dz_2 = -2\alpha_2 I_0 e^{-2\alpha_1 z_1} e^{-2\alpha_2 z_2} \tag{5}$$

Examination of Eq. 5 reveals an interesting trade-off in the power deposited versus absorption coefficient, since α_2 enters Eq. 5 in two places. The first occurrence of α_2 shows an increase in power absorption as α_2 increases (as expected from the cause of power deposition). The exponential terms show that the power remaining in the beam will decrease if absorption in the path increases.

There is thus an optimum absorption condition that maximizes power deposition at a given depth; the absorption coefficients, being approximately linear with frequency, can be adjusted to their optimum values by choosing the appropriate frequency. Let

$$\alpha_1 = a_1 \cdot f \tag{6}$$

and

$$\alpha_2 = a_2 \cdot f$$

to explicitly express their frequency dependence; a_1 and a_2 are absorption values (in cm^{-1} MHz^{-1}) normalized to 1 MHz, and f is frequency (in MHz). Putting Eq. 6 into Eq. 5 and differentiating with respect to frequency, then setting the result to zero yields the optimum frequency f_0:

$$f_0 = \frac{1}{2\,a_1 z_1 + 2\,a_2 z_2} \qquad (7)$$

For example, if the beam passes through a 2 cm layer of fat ($a_1 = 0.07$) to a target location 5 cm deeper in kidney ($a_1 = 0.09$), Eq. 7 predicts an optimum frequency of

$$f_0 \approx 850 \text{ kHz} \qquad (8)$$

Shorter paths or paths through more fat or blood will raise this value of frequency; travel through muscle will lower the value.

Table 18-2 also lists the acoustic impedance Z for several tissues and for air. These values are important in determining the reflection from interfaces between tissues of different types, since the fraction of power reflected as a beam passes from a medium of impedance Z_1 into a medium of impedance Z_2 is given by Wells (1969) as

$$r = [(Z_1 - Z_2)/(Z_1 + Z_2)]^2 \qquad (9)$$

assuming normal incidence. Calculations using Eq. 9 show that the fraction of beam power reflected at each interface between soft tissues is not large (0.009 for a fat-muscle interface, for example), so unless many

TABLE 18-2   Ultrasound Parameters for Selected Tissue

Tissue type	Attenuation* (cm^{-1})	Acoustic impedance $(\times 10^5$ g/s-cm$^2)$	Remarks
Brain, fresh	0.06	1.50	
Fat	0.07 ± 0.02	1.39	Measurements at 37° C
Kidney	0.09	1.63	
Liver, fresh	0.149	1.67	
Muscle, striated	0.15	1.68	Attenuation perpendicular to fibers
Whole blood, fresh	0.034 at $f = 2$ MHz	1.67	Attenuation dependence approx $f^{1.25}$
Bone, skull	1.5	4.81	Attenuation dependence approx. $f^{1.7}$
Air	—	0.00034	

f, Frequency.
* At frequency of 1 MHz.

interfaces are encountered in the path of a hyperthermia beam as it travels to its desired deposition site, reflections are not a major source of power loss. However, when air or bone is encountered, the large impedance differences between those media and soft tissues mean that a great deal of the incident beam power will be reflected at even one interface between soft tissue and bone or air, limiting the areas of ultrasonic access within the body.

Electromagnetic Applicator Techniques

Since the beginning of EM hyperthermia studies, a variety of applicators have been used to introduce EM energy into the human body (Guy, 1984). Although different in form, all of these applicators can be classified into several groups. Since restricted space does not allow a detailed description of all applicators here, only the general characteristics of applicators are explained in this section. A brief description of some representative applicators is given later in the chapter.

Classification of applicators. All EM applicators can be classified approximately into the groups and subgroups shown in Table 18-3. Although this classification is imperfect, it does serve to indicate the interrelated characteristics of EM applicators. These basic characteristics are described in some detail in this section.

Noninvasive applicator characteristics

Radiative applicators. Radiative applicators include all those that couple energy into tissue primarily by propagating waves, such as horns and open-ended waveguides. These propagating waves consist of both E and H fields. For efficient coupling of energy from the applicator to the tissue, at least one dimension of the applicator must be on the order of $\lambda/2$, where λ is the wavelength in tissue. Turner and Lalit (1982) show that the depth of penetration is strongly dependent on aperture size. Applicators with apertures small compared with $\lambda/2$ produce a depth of penetration that is significantly less than the plane-wave penetration shown in Figure 18-1. The wavelength in tissue is given by $\lambda = c/(f)$ $Re\sqrt{\epsilon' - j\epsilon''}$, where f is frequency, Re means the real part, and $\epsilon' - j\epsilon''$ is the relative permittivity of the tissue (Table 18-1). At 10 MHz, $\lambda = 1.18$ m, which means that a 10 MHz applicator must be about 60 cm in at least one dimension to produce deep penetration. This is too large compared with body size for local heating, and it is often too large to be practical. Consequently, radiative applicators seem to be best suited for superficial heating at higher frequencies.

Efficient coupling from radiative applicators also requires that the

TABLE 18-3   Classification of Electromagnetic Applicators

Group	Definition
Noninvasive applicators	Applicators do not penetrate body tissue and are not placed in a body cavity.
Radiative	Coupling of energy into tissue is based primarily on radiation, in which both E and H are important.
E Field	Applicators generate primarily an electric field that is dominant in coupling energy into tissue. Magnetic field that always accompanies RF E field is weak and does not play important role in heating.
H Field	Applicators generate primarily magnetic fields that are dominant in heating. RF magnetic field generates electric field in tissue that heats it.
Invasive applicators	Applicators or part of them penetrate body tissue or are placed in body cavity.
Conductive	Currents produced by potential differences between pairs of electrodes generate heat.
Radiative	Radiation by implanted antennas generates heat.
Magnetic induction	Implanted particles are heated by magnetic induction. Thermal conduction from particles heats tissue.

wave impedance E/H be matched between the applicator and the tissue. Since $E/H = \sqrt{\mu/\epsilon}$ for a plane wave, the E/H in tissue is generally much lower than that in air. An air gap between the applicator and the body therefore causes a large impedance mismatch, high reflection from the body, and poor transmission into the body. Some sort of water bolus is usually employed to provide impedance matching between the applicator and the body. The applicator usually cannot be placed directly on the body because the strong near fields at the applicator aperture often burn the skin.

E-field applicators.   E-field applicators are those that generate primarily an electric field. All RF electric fields are accompanied by magnetic fields, but at low frequencies this magnetic field can be very weak, as it is in E-field applicators. Maxwell's equations show that, at higher frequencies, stronger coupling exists between E and H, and the H cannot be negligible. Thus E-field applicators are low-frequency devices.

The familiar capacitor-plate applicator illustrated in Figure 18-3 is a good example of an E-field applicator. An RF voltage applied between the plates produces the E field. The plates are sometimes made of different

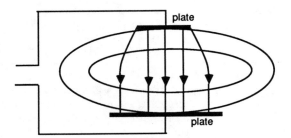

Figure 18-3 Capacitor-plate E-field applicator.

sizes to help shape the E field, and sometimes a water bolus is used between one or both plates to prevent surface burns near the edges of the plates.

A serious problem with any applicator that produces an electric field perpendicular to the fat-muscle interface is that the fat often becomes overheated. This restricts such applicators to use in very thin patients. The basic reason that the fat heats more than the muscle was explained by Guy et al. (1974). It can be explained in terms of the infinite parallel-plate capacitor model shown in Figure 18-4, in which the E fields are constant in the fat and in the muscle. The boundary conditions at the fat-muscle interface require that

$$\epsilon_f E_f = \epsilon_m E_m \qquad (10)$$

where ϵ_f and ϵ_m are the relative complex permittivities of fat and muscle, respectively. Since E_f and E_m are constant throughout the respective materials, Eq. 10 is also valid for the fields at any point, not just on the boundary. From Eq. 1, the power absorbed per unit volume, respectively, is

$$P_f = \frac{1}{2} \sigma_f |E_f|^2$$

$$P_m = \frac{1}{2} \sigma_m |E_m|^2$$

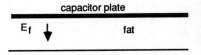

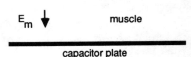

Figure 18-4 Infinite parallel-plate capacitor model used to explain why fat often overheats when E field is perpendicular to fat-muscle interface.

The ratio of the two is

$$\frac{P_f}{P_m} = \frac{\sigma_f |E_f|^2}{\sigma_m |E_m|^2} \tag{11}$$

and from Eq. 10,

$$\frac{|E_f|^2}{|E_m|^2} = \frac{|\epsilon_m|^2}{|\epsilon_f|^2} \tag{12}$$

Some typical values of σ and ϵ from Table 18-1 illustrate why the fat can overheat. At 27.12 MHz, $\sigma_f/\sigma_m = 0.02$, which means that the fat is much less lossy than the muscle. The ratio $|E_f|^2/|E_m|^2 = |\epsilon_m|^2/|\epsilon_f|^2 = |113 - j405.82|^2/|20 - j7.23|^2 = 392$, however, shows that the E field in the fat is much stronger than that in the muscle. Since the absorption goes as E^2, the heating in the fat is greater, as indicated by $P_f/P_m \approx 8$. Thus, even though the fat is less lossy than the muscle, it heats more because E_f is stronger than E_m.

Since boundary conditions require parallel components of E to be continuous at a dielectric interface, these results show that it is desirable to have the E field parallel to fat-muscle interfaces. If it is not, special precautions must be taken to prevent burning of the fat.

Coupling of energy from E-field applicators to the body is usually quite sensitive to position of the applicators because the presence of a dielectric material has a strong effect on the E field. Thus such factors as patient movement and perspiration sometimes make it difficult to keep an applicator tuned for efficient coupling.

H-field applicators.   H-field applicators are those that generate primarily a magnetic field. Any RF magnetic field must be accompanied by an electric field, but at low frequencies the accompanying electric field can be weak, which is characteristic of H-field applicators. H-field applicators, like E-field applicators, are low-frequency devices.

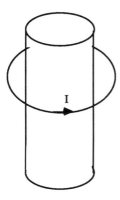

Figure 18-5   Single current loop H-field applicator.

The induction heater, which in simplest form is a single coaxial loop of current as shown in Figure 18-5, is a good example of an H-field applicator. The current I produces an H that is mostly axial and nearly uniform in the central part of the loop. This time-changing H induces an E inside the absorber that produces current that heats. These induced currents are usually called eddy currents.

H-field applicators seem to have the advantage that they are not very sensitive to position of the body. Since the body is essentially nonmagnetic, it does not strongly perturb the H field generated by the applicator, and since the applicator E field is very weak, the permittivity of the body does not affect the coupling much. Thus tuning of an H-field applicator is not highly sensitive to body position.

A disadvantage of H-field applicators is that the induced eddy currents must always flow in closed loops around the magnetic field lines. This means that the eddy currents are zero at some point that is a center of symmetry, and the heating is zero there. The magnitude of the eddy currents also increases approximately with distance from that center, which produces a very nonuniform heating pattern. For example, for the circular cylinder in Figure 18-6, the heating would be zero in the center and maximum at the surface, varying as the square of the distance from the center of the cylinder (current varies as distance, heating as the square of the current).

Basic problems in noninvasive applicator design. The principal desirable features of a noninvasive EM applicator for deep regional heating can be summarized as follows:

1. Produces an E field that is parallel to the fat-muscle interface
2. Produces an E field that is strong in the central part of the body
3. Requires no water bolus
4. Is relatively insensitive to body position (is easy to tune)
5. Does not produce strong fields outside the region of the body to be heated

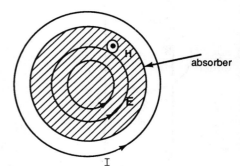

Figure 18-6 Eddy-current pattern induced by H field of current loop in Figure 18-5.

As far as we know, no existing applicator has all these features. Some of the fundamental limitations that make design of the ideal applicators difficult can be explained in terms of the equations for the E field generated by currents and charges. The following description is approximate and qualitative, especially since it is based on the E field produced by the applicator in empty space, not the E field inside the body. Calculation of the E field inside the body is too complicated to be used in a simplified explanation.

Maxwell's equations for sinusoidal steady-state EM fields that vary as $e^{j\omega t}$ are

$$\nabla \times \mathbf{E} = -j\omega\mu\mathbf{H} \tag{13}$$

$$\nabla \times \mathbf{H} = \mathbf{J} + j\omega\epsilon\mathbf{E} \tag{14}$$

$$\nabla \cdot \epsilon\mathbf{E} = \rho \tag{15}$$

$$\nabla \cdot \mu\mathbf{H} = 0 \tag{16}$$

where $\mathbf{E}$ is electric field strength, $\mathbf{H}$ is magnetic field strength, $\mathbf{J}$ is current density, ρ is charge density, ϵ is permittivity, and μ is permeability. As described in most textbooks on electromagnetics, a solution to Maxwell's equation is:

$$\mathbf{E} = -\nabla\Phi - j\omega\mathbf{A} \tag{17}$$

where the scalar potential function Φ and the vector potential function $\mathbf{A}$ are given by

$$\Phi(x,y,z) = \frac{1}{4\pi\epsilon} \int_V \rho(x',y',z') \frac{e^{-jkR}}{R} dV' \tag{18}$$

$$\mathbf{A}(x,y,z) = \frac{\mu}{4\pi} \int_V \mathbf{J}(x',y',z') \frac{e^{-jkR}}{R} dV' \tag{19}$$

where $k = \omega\sqrt{\mu\epsilon}$, V is a volume including all charge and current, and R is the distance from the source point (x',y',z'), where charge and current exist, to the field point (x,y,z) at which $\mathbf{E}$ is being evaluated, as shown in Figure 18-7. The integration is carried out over all charge density ρ and current density $\mathbf{J}$, which are the sources of the fields.

Substituting Eqs. 18 and 19 into Eq. 17 gives

$$\mathbf{E}(x,y,z) = -\frac{1}{4\pi\epsilon} \int_V \rho(x',y',z') \nabla\left(\frac{e^{-jkR}}{R}\right) dV'$$
$$-\frac{j\omega\mu}{4\pi} \int_V \mathbf{J}(x',y',z') \frac{e^{-jkR}}{R} dV' \tag{20}$$

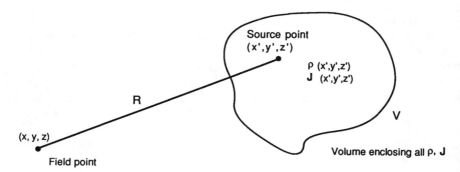

Figure 18-7   Geometry for Eqs. 18 and 19.

where the ∇ operator has been taken inside the integral because it operates only on (x,y,z), not on (x',y',z'). From the continuity equation

$$\nabla \cdot \mathbf{J} = -j\omega\rho \tag{21}$$

Solving for ρ from Eq. 21 and substituting into Eq. 20 gives

$$\mathbf{E}(x,y,z) = -\frac{j}{4\pi\epsilon\omega} \int_V \nabla' \cdot \mathbf{J}(x',y',z') \, \nabla \left(\frac{e^{-jkR}}{R}\right)$$

$$dV' - \frac{j\omega\mu}{4\pi} \int_V \mathbf{J}(x',y',z') \frac{e^{-jkR}}{R} dV' \tag{22}$$

Eq. 22 is an expression for $\mathbf{E}$ at the point (x,y,z) produced by the current density $\mathbf{J}(x',y',z')$. The second term on the right represents the electric field generated by a time-varying $\mathbf{H}$, which is produced by $\mathbf{J}$. It is usually called the magnetic induction term. The first term on the right is the electric field produced by charges. In some configurations one or the other of these terms is dominant. For example, the $\mathbf{E}$ produced by the charge in a parallel-plate capacitor is described mostly by the first term; the second term is usually negligible in comparison because $\mathbf{J}$ is almost zero. On the other hand, the $\mathbf{E}$ produced by a simple small closed loop of current is described almost entirely by the second term because the charge density is negligible.

Thus E-field applicators are described primarily by the first term, and H-field applicators primarily by the second term. In E-field applicators the E begins and ends on charges. In H-field applicators the E-field lines form closed loops, since $\nabla' \cdot \mathbf{J} \approx 0$ and there is no charge for the field lines to begin and end on. Since E-field applicators generate a strong E and a weak H, the impedance E/H is high for E-field applicators. For H-field applicators E/H is low. This may have some relevance for coupling to tissue, since E/H for a plane wave in tissue is much lower than for a plane wave in free space. Eq. 22 also describes radiative applicators, but not conveniently, since the charges and currents in radiative applica-

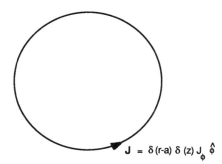

$$\mathbf{J} = \delta(r\text{-}a)\,\delta(z)\,J_\phi\,\hat{\phi}$$ **Figure 18-8**   Filamentary current loop.

tors are not usually easy to visualize. A similar equation in terms of integrals over aperture fields is usually used to describe radiative applicators.

A simple example that illustrates the use of Eq. 22 is the filamentary current loop shown in Figure 18-8. Eq. 22 is solved for two cases: (1) $J_\phi = J_0$; (2) $J_\phi = J_0 \sin\phi$. The first case corresponds to magnetic induction, since $\nabla' \cdot \mathbf{J} = 0$ and there is no charge present. Figure 18-9, A shows the E-field pattern for this case. For $r < a$, E varies directly as r, being zero in the center and increasing to a maximum at the loop. The second case includes both terms, since $\nabla' \cdot \mathbf{J} = \dfrac{\delta(r-a)\delta(z)\cos\phi}{r}$. The magnitude of the charge is maximum at $\phi = 0$ and $\phi = \pi$, so field lines begin and end on charge as shown. Although both terms in Eq. 22 contribute to the E-field pattern, the first term is dominant. The first term often seems to dominate. The pattern in Figure 18-9, A, has the obvious disadvantage that the E field is zero in the center. The one in Figure 18-9, B, has the disadvantage that the E field would be perpendicular to the fat-muscle

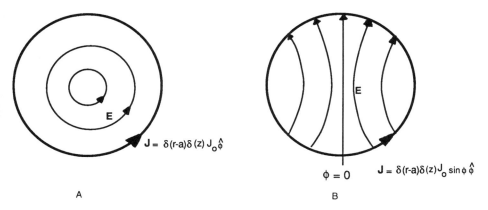

A   B

Figure 18-9   A, E produced by constant-current loop. **B,** E produced by current that has sin φ variation around loop.

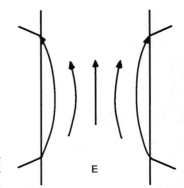

Figure 18-10 Possible E-field configuration for E both strong in center and
mostly parallel to fat-muscle interface.

interface. Apparently the current loop in Figure 18-9, *B*, is more like
an E-field applicator than an H-field applicator, at least in the sense
that the E-field lines begin and end on charges instead of forming closed
loops. The E field inside a body placed inside the current loop would of
course be modified from that shown in Figure 18-9, but the empty-space
patterns show the basic characteristics of the device.

For a low-frequency applicator to produce an E field that is both
parallel to the fat-muscle interface and strong in the center, the field
pattern must be something like that shown in Figure 18-10. Here the
E field is mostly parallel to the fat-muscle interface, but not completely.
However, if the perpendicular component is spread out over the circumference of the body, it will be small compared to the axial component in
the center. In the pattern of Figure 18-10, the E-field lines must either
terminate on charge or bend around in closed loops. The first would be
an E-field applicator, and the second would be an H-field applicator.
Since an H-field applicator would tend to have lower impedance, it might
couple better to the body, but this is not entirely clear because wave
impedance is a characteristic of wave propagation, and H-field applicators
are not radiative in nature. For either an E- or H-field applicator to
produce the pattern shown in Figure 18-10, the presence of the body
would probably affect the tuning, since the high permittivity would bend
the E-field lines significantly.

The design of an ideal applicator is indeed challenging. Consideration
of the fundamental principles emphasizes the difficulty of embodying
all five features of the ideal applicator in one device. An array of radiative
apertures at lower frequencies could perhaps satisfy all the requirements
except the third (not requiring a water bolus). H-field applicators probably
do not satisfy requirement two (strong central E field), and E-field applicators usually do not satisfy requirement one (E field parallel to fat-muscle
interface).

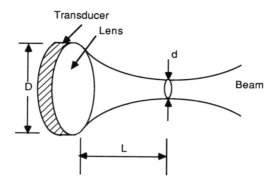

Figure 18-11   Beam shape from focused ultrasound transducer.

There are many practical problems in applicator design in addition to the fundamental ones just described. The irregular geometry of the human body makes it difficult to design applicators that will couple efficiently. Any change in parameters, such as body position and perspiration, can make it difficult to maintain constant coupling of the EM fields from an applicator to the body.

Ultrasonic Applicator Techniques

Focusing of ultrasonic beams.   Ultrasound waves are generated by transducers that transform electrical excitation into vibrational waves, which are then coupled into the tissue via an applied coupling medium such as gel or water. Piezoelectric crystals are by far the most common transducers used for generating high-power beams. The frequency and focusing characteristics of the transducer have a profound effect on the beam shape and penetration depth.

Figure 18-11 shows the beam shape from a focused round transducer. A focused beam is obtained when a lens is added to the transducer face or the transducer surface is formed into a concave curvature. At the focal point of the beam the beam diameter d is given approximately by (Christensen, 1988b):

$$d = 2.44 \, L\lambda/D \tag{23}$$

where λ is the wavelength of the ultrasound wave, L is the focal length of the focusing element, and D is the diameter of the transducer. In turn, the wavelength is related to frequency in the same manner as for EM waves:

$$\lambda = c/f \tag{24}$$

where c is now the speed of sound in tissue. The speed of sound in most soft tissues is similar (within $\pm 5\%$) to that in water, or

$$c \approx 1.5 \times 10^5 \text{cm/s} \tag{25}$$

At a typical hyperthermia frequency of 750 kHz, Eq. 24 gives a wavelength of 2 mm, very short compared with EM waves used in hyperthermia. Substituting this value into Eq. 23 shows that for focal lengths a few times (for example, 4 ×) the diameter of the transducer, the focused spot size is small, less than 2 cm.

Comparison of ultrasound with electromagnetic techniques. At the operating frequency chosen in the preceding example, 750 kHz, the ultrasound penetration depth is still quite deep, approximately 9 cm to the e^{-2} power point in muscle, and even deeper for fat and kidney. This deep penetration holds for a beam that can be concurrently focused. Therefore, ultrasound has the advantage over EM energy in that its focusing ability (because of its short wavelength) is much better at frequencies that will still penetrate appreciably into the body. In fact, with ultrasound, focusing is rarely a limiting factor. The beam divergence is so low that unfocused transducers are often used to completely cover the volume being treated.

The disadvantage of ultrasound compared with EM is that its use is restricted to body regions with no air spaces or bony regions in the path of the beam to the desired site. This eliminates regions in the skull, the lungs, behind or near skeletal bones, and regions blocked by an air-filled intestine (unless pressure is applied to force out the air, or fluid is introduced into the intestine to facilitate the ultrasound passage).

Another potential problem has arisen in clinical experience: sometimes when ultrasound is focused on a tumor in front of nearby bone, the patient reports limiting pain (Meyer et al., 1985). It has been suggested that, as the high-power beam strikes the bone, much of its compressional wave energy is converted to shear waves that damp very quickly at the bone's surface, disturbing the periosteum and related nerves. This has excluded the use of ultrasound in certain regions that are in front of large masses of bone, particularly near the jaw and clavicle.

ELECTROMAGNETIC APPLICATORS

The literature includes descriptions of many applicators that have been used over the years to produce hyperthermia in body tissues. This section gives a brief description of some of these applicators and their basic characteristics.

Electromagnetic Applicators for Noninvasive Superficial Heating

High-frequency applicators.   At the higher frequencies, where the waveguide is of reasonable physical size, open-ended waveguides or horns can be used as applicators. Open-ended waveguides are usually filled with dielectric material with about the same permittivity as water to provide a good impedance match between the waveguide and the tissue. This has the added advantage of reducing the size of the waveguide. Horns of various kinds have also been used, but they are large and bulky.

The aperture size has a significant effect on the heating pattern of radiative applicators. Calculations by Guy (1971) of the fields in a two-layer semi-infinite tissue model irradiated by a transverse electric TE_{10}-mode rectangular aperture showed the effects of aperture dimensions and thickness of the equivalent fat layer. For some combinations of parameters, the TE_{10} fields of the direct-contact aperture provided deeper heating of the muscle than a plane wave. On the basis of his results Guy concluded that the ISM frequency of 915 MHz produced a better ratio of muscle/fat heating than the more commonly used ISM frequency of 2450 MHz, and Guy et al. (1978) designed a $13 \times 13 \times 13$ cm applicator to operate at 915 MHz that allowed air cooling of the skin. The applicator has been found to work well for heating muscle tissue to a depth of about 4 cm.

Chueng et al. (1977) designed an open-ended waveguide applicator based on a quasi–transverse electromagnetic (TEM) mode to make the transverse heating pattern more uniform. The waveguide cross section is shown in Figure 18-12. Dielectric strips along the side walls are used to produce a quasi-TEM mode in the central region. The waveguide was matched to body tissue with a quarter-wave transformer.

Waveguides at lower frequencies, where penetration is greater, are large and awkward. One way to reduce the size of a waveguide for a given frequency is to add a ridge to the top or bottom (or both) of the waveguide. These ridged waveguides have been used as hyperthermia applicators, but they have the disadvantage that the EM fields are mostly concentrated directly between the ridges, producing a small, localized region of heating.

A microstrip transmission line is more compact than a waveguide, so hyperthermia applicators based on a microstrip transmission line are more compact than waveguide applicators. These microstrip applicators consist of some kind of radiating element, such as a patch or a loop, on a microstrip transmission line. A diagram of a rectangular patch radiator on a microstrip transmission line is shown in Figure 18-13.

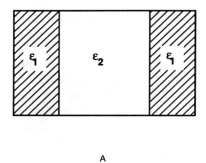

A

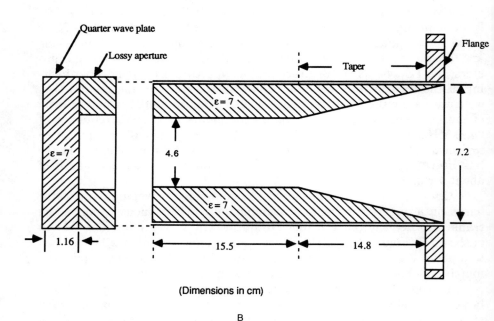

(Dimensions in cm)

B

Figure 18-12 A, Cross section of waveguide loaded with dielectric strips (ϵ_1) to produce
quasi–transverse electromagnetic (TEM) mode in central region. **B,** Top sectional view
of TEM-mode applicator and quarter-wave transformer designed by Cheung et al. (1977).

Design procedures that can be used for microstrip patch radiators
for heating tissue are given by Bahl and Stuchly (1980) and for microstrip
loop radiators by Bahl et al. (1982). Microstrip slot antennas consisting
of a slot in the groundplane of a microstrip transmission line have been
developed by Bahl et al. (1980). They used a reflector on the side opposite
the groundplane to confine the radiation to the half-space adjacent to
the slot.

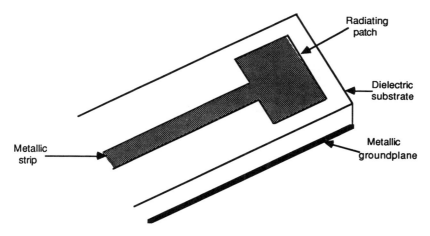

Figure 18-13   Rectangular patch radiator on microstrip transmission line.

Johnson et al. (1984) have designed and tested microstrip hyperthermia applicators operating at frequencies ranging from 120 to 915 MHz. They also extended the design of microstrip applicators to include permeable material in combination with dielectric material to reduce the size of the applicator for a given frequency of operation and to maximize the depth of heating.

Microstrip hyperthermia applicators are relatively easy to design and fabricate and are mechanically convenient because they are flat, compact, and lightweight. They tend to be narrow band, and they produce some leakage radiation. They have been useful for heating superficial tumors, typically at frequencies of 433, 915, or 2450 MHz.

Low-frequency applicators.   The most commonly used low-frequency applicators, other than those described in the next section under deep-heating applicators, are the E-field capacitor-paddle applicator and the H-field pancake-coil applicator, both of which were developed for diathermy.

The capacitor paddles are placed on the body as illustrated in Figure 18-14. As explained by Guy et al. (1974), the E fields produced by the paddles are mostly perpendicular to the fat-muscle interface and therefore often overheat the fat, for the reasons explained previously.

The pancake-coil applicator is a helical coil placed on the body surface. The magnetic field it produces heats by eddy currents, as explained by Guy et al. (1974) and illustrated in Figure 18-15, which is taken from their paper. A pancake coil operating at 27.12 MHz can heat to a depth of about 4 cm (depth at which power absorption is e^{-2} times the maximum), and it does not overheat the fat, since the generated E field

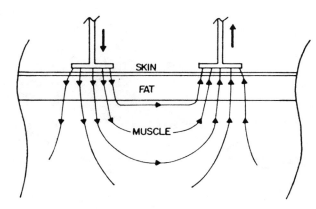

Figure 18-14 E fields produced by capacitor paddles. (From Guy, A.W., et al. [1974]. *Proc. IEEE 62*:55–75.)

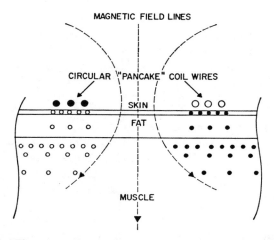

Figure 18-15 Electromagnetic fields produced by pancake-coil applicator. Dark dots represent current into paper, and open circles current out of paper. (From Guy, A.W., et al. [1974]. *Proc. IEEE 62*:55–75.)

is mostly parallel to the fat-muscle interface. The heating pattern is torroidal in nature.

Another type of inductive applicator has been designed and tested by Bach Andersen et al. (1984). It is based on a current loop placed next to the tissue, as illustrated in Figure 18-16. Theoretical work by Morita and Bach Andersen (1982) showed that good heating patterns could be obtained by a distribution of electrical currents parallel to the surface. Since a return current must always be present, this configuration cannot be practically achieved. The current loop shown in Figure 18-16

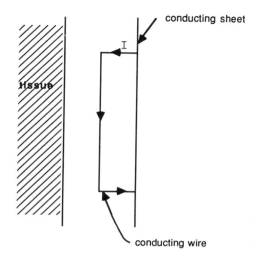

conducting sheet

I

tissue

conducting wire

Figure 18-16   Diagram of inductive applicator designed by Bach Andersen et al. (1984).

is a practical realization of the idealized parallel-current configuration. The device includes a coaxial feed line tapped into the loop near one end and a series capacitance for tuning.

Applicators for Noninvasive Deep Heating

Capacitor-plate E-field applicators have been used for deep heating, but they require special precautions to avoid burning the fat, for the reasons explained previously. Bini et al. (1985) have designed and built an applicator with a water bolus and a combination of a smaller capacitor plate and a larger one to optimize the heating pattern. Capacitor-plate applicators do not work well in patients with thick fat layers, but good results can be obtained in patients with thin layers of fat.

An H-field applicator consisting essentially of a current loop made of an aluminum band tuned with series capacitance at 13.57 MHz has been designed and used by Storm et al. (1982). This device, called a Magnetrode, has the basic characteristics of the simple current loop described previously. Although the power deposition produced by the Magnetrode is generally low in the center and higher near the surface, the penetration depth compares favorably with that of some E-field applicators, depending on aperture size (Harrison et al., 1985). The Magnetrode requires no water bolus, is easy to operate, and produces an E field that is mostly parallel to the fat-muscle interface.

A radiative applicator called the annular-phased array (APA) has been designed by Turner (1984b). The APA consists of two side-by-side arrays of eight dielectrically loaded apertures. Each aperture is a 20 × 23 cm, horn-shaped radiator that radiates an approximately TEM field.

The TEM waves radiated by the 16 apertures tend to converge toward the axis of the array. The patient is placed inside the array, and water-filled bags fill the space between the patient and the apertures. The APA operates at frequencies from 55 to 110 MHz. The APA is capable of central heating, but the heating pattern is affected by the shape of the body and by its dielectric inhomogeneities. Extensive measurements of internal electric field patterns in mannequins have been made (Turner, 1984a). More uniform central heating is obtained at 55 to 70 MHz, and more centrally focused heating at higher frequencies.

Turner recently designed a second-generation APA called the Sigma-60. It operates over a frequency range of 60 to 120 MHz. The radiators are eight electric dipoles, which are electrically isolated into four pairs. The four pairs can be excited with controlled phasing and amplitude to focus and steer the absorbed energy pattern.

Another kind of radiative applicator consisting of an open-ended ridged waveguide loaded with deionized water and operating at 27 MHz has been designed by Sterzer et al. (1980). Since the waveguide cross section is rather large, even with the ridge and dielectric loading, the patient usually sits or lies on the open end of the waveguide, which stands vertically on the floor. Operation at 27 MHz is an advantage of this applicator because penetration is greater at the lower frequencies.

Ruggera and Kantor (1984) have investigated use of the helical coil as a hyperthermia applicator. Chute and Vermeulen (1981) showed that the axial electric field inside a helix operating at frequencies where the wavelength is long compared to the helix is approximately uniform across the cross section of the coil. The measurements of Ruggera and Kantor (1984) in 3 and 12 cm diameter phantoms (physical replicas with electromagnetic properties approximating tissue) heated by helical coils demonstrated uniform cross-sectional heating within about 10% and 20%, respectively. They obtained the best results when the total length of the wire in the helix was equal either to one-half wavelength or one wavelength. For these two conditions the driving-point impedance was purely resistive. For the first case a coil length-to-diameter ratio of 2 was needed for approximately uniform heating. In the other case a ratio of 4 was needed. These results indicate that helical coils could be used to heat arms and thighs satisfactorily, but apparently the practicality of using a helical coil to heat torsos has not yet been established.

Tsai et al. (1984) have made calculations showing that a coplanar three-element phased array of dipoles at 27 MHz in a water bolus on the body would produce deeper heating than a plane wave along a line directly under the center element of the array. Destructive interference under the center element reduces the heating near the surface, allowing the deeper tissue to be heated more than the surface tissue. Surface cooling would probably be needed directly under the two outside elements.

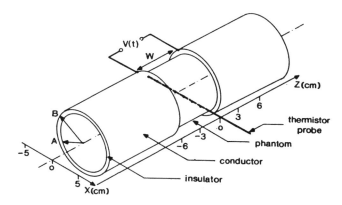

Figure 18-17   Applicator designed by Raskmark and Bach Anderson (1984b).

Calculations also showed that an array on each side of the body would produce good central heating. Experimental results for such arrays have not been published yet.

Raskmark and Bach Andersen (1984b) have designed an applicator consisting of a cylindrical tube with a gap in it (Figure 18-17). An RF voltage is applied across the gap. By choosing the proper combination of frequency, gap width, and cylinder diameter, they achieved focused heating in a 10 cm diameter phantom. The frequency was chosen so that the radius of the cylindrical phantom was about equal to the focal spot size in the lossy medium. The frequency (100 MHz) was low enough to minimize exponential decay effects but high enough to provide constructive interference near the center. Their calculations showed that the gap width w should be larger than about a quarter-wavelength in the lossy medium.

Raskmark and Bach Andersen (1984a) also split the cylindrical applicator into four sections and showed that the heating pattern could be steered by proper adjustment of the gap voltage phases and amplitudes in each of the four sections. They arrived at these voltages by placing a small probe at the point in the phantom where the maximum temperature was desired, exciting the probe, and measuring the voltages induced on each section of the applicator. Then they removed the probe and excited the applicator with the conjugate of the induced voltages. According to the reciprocity theorem, this excitation should produce a local maximum around the probe position. According to the authors' measurements, the local maximum was close to the probe position. Apparently they have not tried to extend their technique to larger phantoms.

A TEM deep-heating applicator designed by Lagendijk (1983) consists of a slot in a large coaxial applicator, as shown in Figure 18-18.

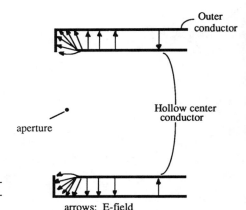

Figure 18-18 Cross section of transverse electromagnetic applicator designed by Lagendijk (1983).

arrows: E-field

An analysis based on rings of dipole sources to simulate the aperture fields gave calculated results that agreed well with measurements in a 20 cm diameter phantom irradiated by a prototype applicator at 434 MHz. Calculations at 27 MHz showed that good central heating would occur in a 40 cm diameter phantom.

Invasive Heating Devices

The commonly used invasive heating techniques can be classified into three main groups: conductive RF current electrodes, radiating implanted antennas, and implanted ferrite seeds heated by magnetic induction. Invasive heating techniques have the advantage of highly controllable heating patterns and the disadvantage of requiring insertion of part of the device into the tissue.

Conductive radiofrequency implanted electrodes.   Highly controllable heating patterns can be generated by inserting RF needle electrodes into the tissue so that RF conduction current flows between them. Pairs or arrays of needles can be used to direct the current through the tissue to be heated (Doss and McCabe, 1976). Cetas et al. (1980) combined RF heating with interstitial radiation therapy by using the hollow needles filled with radioactive material that provide conventional radiation therapy also as RF electrodes to produce heating. They call this technique interstitial thermoradiotherapy.

Implanted antennas.   Implanted radiating antennas have the advantage that two electrodes are not required to heat the tissue. This is especially an advantage when the tumor is located in a hollow organ that can be reached through a body orifice, in which case an antenna can be inserted into the orifice to heat the tumor. Strohbehn et al. (1979) stated and Taylor (1980) showed that the heating patterns produced by implanted antennas are better than those of hot probes such as resistance heaters.

The implanted antennas used to heat tissue usually consist of a radiator excited by coaxial cable. Several kinds of radiators have been used. Bigu-del-Blanco and Romero-Sierra (1977) used a monopole with a flange for a groundplane. This configuration limits the depth of insertion to the length of the needle. Frequently the center conductor of the coaxial cable is extended to act as a radiator. Sometimes it is coated with a dielectric sleeve to extend propagation along it, and sometimes a quarter-wavelength choke is added to reduce transmission back toward the generator along the coaxial cable. The various techniques have been reviewed by Taylor (1980).

Instead of extending the center conductor, Samaras (1984) short-circuited the end of the coaxial cable and excited the end section of it by a gap in the outer conductor, which then acted like a dipole antenna. Somewhat directional radiation patterns have been created by adding semicylindrical metallic reflectors or dielectric bulbs around the radiator (Mendecki et al., 1978, 1980). Arrays of implanted antennas have also been used to increase the volume of heating and to control the heating pattern (Trembly et al., 1982, 1988).

Hyperthermic treatment of brain tumors has been studied by Samaras (1984) and by Lyons et al. (1984).

Implanted ferrite seeds.   Highly controlled internal heating patterns can be produced by implanting ferromagnetic particles in the tissue and then heating these through magnetic induction with an externally applied RF magnetic field (Moidel et al., 1976; Stauffer et al., 1982). In some cases an array of ferromagnetic particles, such as an array of small ferrite cylinders, can be implanted and left in the tissue for repeated hyperthermic treatments.

Atkinson et al. (1984) calculated the heating produced by magnetic induction in implanted ferromagnetic particles. They recommended that frequencies less than about 200 kHz be used for the heating.

Stauffer et al. (1984) described the design of coils to produce the magnetic fields needed for the induction heating and the results of anecdotal clinical trials in animals. They showed that a maximum frequency of 500 kHz should be used in heating seeds in large body volumes, such as the human abdomen, and a maximum frequency of 1.9 MHz for heating in smaller volumes, such as the human brain. Higher frequencies produce too much unwanted heating of the tissue, particularly surface tissue, outside of the heating produced by the implanted seeds. They concluded from these studies that useful focused heating may be obtainable in human patients by these techniques.

ULTRASOUND APPLICATORS

The ultrasound applicators are most conveniently classified according to the number and arrangement of the transducer elements employed. Frequencies range from less than 500 kHz for deep heating to more than 3 MHz for surface tumors.

Single-Transducer Applicators

The simplest configuration consists of a single (usually round) transducer that is coupled to the body by a degassed water bath or bag. Figure

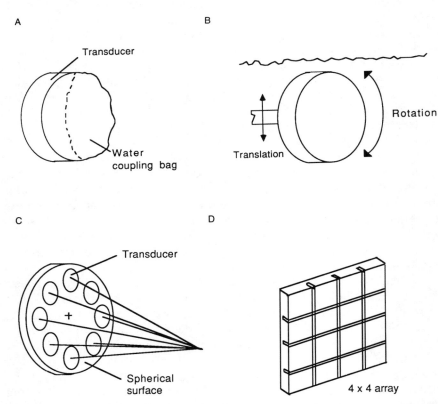

Figure 18-19 Some styles of ultrasonic hyperthermia applicators. **A,** Single transducer. **B,** Mechanically swept transducer. **C,** Array of transducers aimed at common point. **D,** Square array of individually controlled elements.

18-19, A, shows such an arrangement. If focusing is desired for very small, deep tumors, the face of the transducer may be concave, or for more flexibility in matching varying target depths, various focal length lenses may be attached to the transducer. Often with these manually positioned applicators no focusing is used. This is because little divergence takes place during beam propagation (owing to the short ultrasound wavelength compared to transducer diameter), so even an unfocused ultrasound beam is usually not much larger, if at all, than the desired heating volume at depth. Typical single transducer diameters range from 3 to 12 cm. Transmitted power densities are approximately 1 to 5 W/cm^2.

Swept-Transducer Applicators

Since the ultrasound beam shape is generally narrow, coverage of larger tumor volumes may be accomplished by mechanically or electronically sweeping the beam around the target volume to achieve a very flexible heating pattern. Irregularly shaped tumors or irregular blood flow may be accommodated by this technique. Figure 18-19, B, indicates a transducer that is simultaneously translated and rotated.

Sweeping may be done manually or under computer control (Lele, 1983). Temperature probes guide the trajectory and velocity of the beam sweeping. Advanced electronic beam steering techniques that use phased arrays are also being investigated (Ocheltree et al., 1985).

Multiple-Transducer Applicators

For high-power, deep-lying treatments, the confined beam size emanating from a relatively small, single ultrasound transducer may cause too high a concentration of power at the beam's entrance into the body, leading to overheating of surface tissues. This problem is alleviated with multiple transducers arranged in a contour around the body but aimed at a common target. In some designs the transducers are fixed rigidly to a substrate, as in Figure 18-19, C, whereas in other instruments each transducer can be aimed and focused at a unique location during treatment, giving a great variety in the radiation pattern.

Figure 18-19, D, shows a square array of transducer elements. In this approach each element is excited individually and incoherently with its own power amplifier. The overall pattern is shaped by computer-controlling the amount of average power emanating from each element by controlling the element's duty cycle. The elements are unfocused, so coverage can be as large as the overall array size or as small as the area of one element.

In many of these multiple-transducer applicators, a separate ultrasound imaging element is affixed to give echo-mode images of the tissue region being treated, thereby locating the heating beam with respect to anatomical features determined from a pretreatment computerized tomographic scan.

THERMOMETRY

Thermometry for Electromagnetic Hyperthermia

Difficulties with metallic probes.   Conventional temperature probes such as thermistors or thermocouples have certain advantages (Coremans, 1988; Welch and Pearce, 1988): they are small, inexpensive, and accurate enough for clinical hyperthermia monitoring. However, because they possess metallic lead wires, their use in EM fields can cause significant temperature errors. The source of these errors can be traced to induced internal currents flowing in the metal wires.

Figure 18-20 shows how these internal currents are generated. When the metallic component is immersed in the E fields, boundary conditions require that the component of the external electric field tangential to the metal (E_t) be matched by an equal E_t field inside the wire at its surface. This internal E_t field in turn causes a current to flow whose density J is proportional to both the magnitude of E_t and the conductivity σ of the wire:

$$J = \sigma E_t \tag{26}$$

This current is associated with three sources of measurement error (Christensen, 1988a): it causes ohmic heating in the wire itself, an especially troublesome problem because the heat is produced so close to the

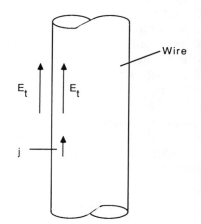

Figure 18-20   Internal currents set up inside metallic temperature probe wire when placed in tangential electric field E_t, leading to perturbations of temperature readings.

temperature sensor; it can perturb the incident EM fields by reradiation; and it can couple EM noise to the sensitive analog and digital electronics of the readout device, if unfiltered.

Noninterfering probes.   A direct way to avoid the measurement errors caused by the presence of metallic lead wires is to reduce (or even eliminate) the electrical conductivity σ of these components, thereby decreasing the induced currents. Two approaches have been employed to accomplish this: high-resistance leads and fiber-optic leads.

High-resistance leads.   Bowman (1976) pioneered the use of high-resistance (low σ) leads attached to a small thermistor. The leads were carbon-impregnated plastic. Because of the special nature of the lead wires, their diameter is relatively large and the maximum probe length is limited. The advantage of this technique is that stable thermistor sensors and standard electronics are used.

Fiber-optic probes.   Several groups have developed optical temperature sensors connected to the readout module with glass or plastic fibers. Since the electrical conductivity of the optical fibers is zero, there are no induced currents and accompanying perturbation. The liquid crystal sensor (Johnson et al., 1975) was one of the first styles developed. Later versions of the optical sensor include a birefringent crystal sensor that rotates polarization (Cetas, 1976), a gallium arsenide sensor that changes optical absorption as a function of temperature (Vaguine et al., 1984), and a fluorescent tip whose emission dynamics depend on temperature (Wickersheim and Alves, 1979; Samulski and Shrivastava, 1980).

Some styles of fiber-optic probes have been refined recently to include multiple-sensor linear arrays (four to six sensors per probe). This development allows faster acquisition of temperature profile data during treatment, which is especially important considering the vast amount of data required to determine thermal mapping. An advantage of the fiber-optic probes is their very low thermal smearing of temperature gradients because of the small thermal conductivity possessed by the glass or plastic fiber leads. Long-term stability and accuracy are improved in later versions of these optical monitors.

Thermometry for Ultrasound Hyperthermia

The problems mentioned previously in connection with the use of metallic components in an EM environment do not exist in ultrasound fields. Therefore standard thermocouples or thermistors may be used for tissue temperature monitoring in ultrasound hyperthermia and yield stable, accurate results.

One pitfall to avoid with ultrasound exposure, however, is the use

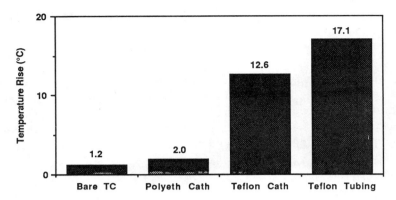

Figure 18-21 Ultrasonic heating trials of different sheathing materials surrounding thermocouple. Beam power 100 W; beam diameter 5.2 cm.

of certain highly absorbing plastic materials to sheath the temperature probes. Kuhn and Christensen (1986) found experimentally that some common sheathing materials absorb incident ultrasound waves to a much greater extent than tissue does, and their use surrounding temperature probes will lead to large measurement errors in typical ultrasound hyperthermia fields. Figure 18-21 shows the temperature rise encountered in a high-power ultrasound beam (100 W, 5.2 cm diameter) when several different types of tubing and catheters were used to surround a standard thermocouple in a water bath test. As shown, there is severe heating of the Teflon, which is a popular material for probe sheathing because of its low friction and biocompatibility properties. Teflon should be avoided as a probe covering in ultrasound fields. Stainless-steel hypodermic needle tubing works well as an ultrasound probe protection and stiffening sheath. With a sharpened tip and surrounding a small thermocouple, stainless-steel tubing facilitates probe placement in the tissue. Multiple-sensor thermocouple arrays are available.

Temperature Mapping Requirements and Thermal Dose

The number of temperature data points required for thorough monitoring of a hyperthermia treatment is very large. For example, assuming that a spatial sampling resolution of 1 cm between points is needed for full characterization of the volume temperature distribution and that measurements must be taken at least once every minute of a 30-minute treatment, a total of 15,720 points must be accessed, measured, stored, and analyzed to cover a 10 cm diameter treatment volume. Of course, it is not practical to access all these points throughout the volume with invasive probes, but even with less frequent spatial sampling, the number of data points is still cumbersome to collect and analyze. Multiple-sensor probes or pull-back techniques help reduce the data acquisition time somewhat, but display and analysis remain a challenge.

Perez and Sapareto (1984) proposed definitions of effective "thermal dose" that integrate weighted temperature data over time, resulting in a single expression at each spatial point per treatment. This reduces the amount of data considerably. More clinical studies are needed, however, to ascertain which thermal dose definition has the best correlation to the treatment outcome.

CONCLUSION

Some fundamental problems must be solved before truly practical applicators are available for routine clinical use. In particular, heating deep-lying tumors in a patient without overheating the surface tissue or the fat tissue remains a significant challenge to the designer of hyperthermia applicators. The heating pattern produced by many applicators varies with the patient's internal geometry, and adjusting the heating pattern in an individual patient may prove difficult. In addition to the fundamental limitations on focused deep heating, many practical problems must be solved before routine clinical hyperthermia treatment can be provided. Progress in developing applicators, both EM and ultrasonic, has been made, but much work remains.

Heating a given tumor in a highly controlled fashion to a desired temperature range for a desired period appears more difficult than was first anticipated. This has hindered the evaluation of hyperthermia as therapy because the evaluation cannot be conducted without heating the tumors well enough to study the response. The effectiveness of hyperthermia as a practical clinical modality will probably not be fully known until better heating methods and more thorough thermometry are developed so better studies can be conducted. From the data available, however, hyperthermia does seem to be an effective therapy in at least some cases, and it is worth pursuing to determine just how effective it might be.

Because tumors vary so much in location, size, shape, and other characteristics such as degree of vascularization, a wide variety of hyperthermia applicators are required for general treatment. Furthermore, hyperthermia treatments require significantly more time and effort by clinical staff than do other kinds of treatment. Unless some methods for reducing the costs are developed, hyperthermia may not become a widely used method of therapy. On the other hand, if hyperthermia therapy can be used to treat tumors that do not respond to other methods, it will probably be used even if it is expensive.

Future efforts in developing applicators will likely center on finding better methods of adjusting heating patterns with use of feedback from improved temperature measurements. This will require advanced methods for handling the enormous amount of data collected by thermometry systems and using it effectively.

REFERENCES

American Cancer Society (1988). Cancer facts & figures—1988. New York, The Society.

ATKINSON, W.J., BREZOVITCH, I.A., AND CHAKRABORTY, D.P. (1984). Usable frequencies in hyperthermia with thermal seeds. *IEEE Trans. Biomed. Eng. 31:*70–75.

BACH ANDERSEN, J., BAUN, A. HARMARK, K., HEINZL, L., RASKMARK, P., AND OVERGAARD, J. (1984). A hyperthermia system using a new type of inductive applicator. *IEEE Trans. Biomed. Eng. 31:*21–27.

BAHL, I.J., AND STUCHLY, S.S. (1980). Analysis of a microstrip covered with a lossy dielectric. *IEEE Trans. Microwave Theory Tech. 28:*104–109.

BAHL, I.J., STUCHLY, S.S., LAGENDIJK, J.J.W., AND STUCHLY, M.A. (1982). Microstrip loop radiators for medical applications. *IEEE Trans. Microwave Theory Tech. 30:*1090–1093.

BAHL, I.J., STUCHLY, S.S., AND STUCHLY, M.A. (1980). New microstrip slot radiator for medical applications. *Electronics Lett. 16:*731–732.

BIGU-DEL-BLANCO, J., AND ROMERO-SIERRA, C. (1977). The design of a monopole radiator to investigate the effect of microwave radiation in biological systems. *J. Bioengineering 1:*181–184.

BINI, M., IGNESTI, A., MILLANTA, L., OLMI, R., RUBINO, N., AND VANNI, R. (1985). An unbalanced electric applicator for RF hyperthermia. *IEEE Trans. Biomed. Eng. 32:*638–641.

BOWMAN, R.R. (1976). A probe for measuring temperature in radio-frequency-heated material. *IEEE Trans. Microwave Theory Tech. 24:*43–45.

CETAS, T.C. (1976). A birefringent crystal optical thermometer for measurements in electromagnetically induced heating. *In:* Johnson, C.C., and Shore, J.L. (eds.). Proceedings of the 1975 USNC/URSI Symposium. Bureau of Radiological Health, Rockville, Md.

CETAS, T.C., HEVEZI, J.M., MANNING, M.R., AND OZIMEK, E.J. (1980). Dosimetry of interstitial thermoradiotherapy. Paper Te5 presented at the 3rd International Symposium: Cancer Therapy by Hyperthermia, Drugs, and Radiation, Fort Collins, Colo., June 22–26, 1980.

CHEUNG, A.Y., DAO, T., AND ROBINSON, J.E. (1977). Dual-beam TEM applicator for direct-contact heating of dielectrically encapsulated malignant mouse tumor. *Radio Sci. 12:*81–85.

CHRISTENSEN, D.A. (1988a). Thermometry. *In:* Webster, J.G. (ed.). Encyclopedia of medical devices and instrumentation. New York, John Wiley & Sons, pp. 2759–2765.

CHRISTENSEN, D.A. (1988b). Ultrasonic bioinstrumentation. New York, John Wiley & Sons.

CHRISTENSEN, D.A., AND DURNEY, C.H. (1981). Hyperthermia production for cancer therapy: a review of fundamentals and methods. *J. Microwave Power 16*:89–105.

CHUTE, F.S., AND VERMEULEN, F.E. (1981). A visual demonstration of the electric field of a coil carrying a time-varying current. *IEEE Trans. Educ. 24*:278–283.

COLEY, W.B. (1893). The treatment of malignant tumors by repeated inoculations of erysipelas. *Am. J. Med. Sci. 105*:487.

COREMANS, J. (1988). Thermistors. *In*: Webster, J.G. (ed.). Encyclopedia of medical devices and instrumentation. New York, John Wiley & Sons, pp. 2730–2738.

DEWHURST, M.A., SIM, D.A., SAPARETO, S.A., AND CONNOR, W.G. (1984). Importance of minimum tumor temperature in determining early and long-term responses of spontaneous pet animal tumors to heat and radiation. *Cancer Res. 44*:43–60.

DOSS, J.D. AND McCABE, C.W. (1976). A technique for localized heating in tissue: an adjunct to tumor therapy. *Med. Instrument. 10*:16–21.

GUY, A.W. (1971). Electromagnetic fields and relative heating patterns due to a rectangular aperture source in direct contact with bilayered biological tissue. *IEEE Trans. Microwave Theory Tech. 19*:214–223.

GUY, A.W. (1984). History of biological effects and medical applications of microwave energy. *IEEE Trans. Microwave Theory Tech. 32*:1182–1120.

GUY, A.W., LEHMANN, J.F., AND STONEBRIDGE, J.B. (1974). Therapeutic applications of electromagnetic power. *Proc. IEEE 62*:55–75.

GUY, A.W., LEHMANN, J.F., STONEBRIDGE, J.B., AND SORENSON, C.C. (1978). Development of a 915 MHz direct-contact applicator for therapeutic heating of tissues. *IEEE Trans. Microwave Theory Tech. 26*:550–556.

HARRISON, W.H., STORM, F.K., ELLIOTT, R.S., AND MORTON, D.L. (1985). A comparison of deep-heating electrode concepts for hyperthermia. *J. Microwave Power 20*:1–8.

HERZFELD, K.F., AND LITOVITZ, T.A. (1959). Absorption and dispersion of ultrasonic waves. New York, Academic Press.

JOHNSON, C.C., GANDHI, O.P., AND ROZZELL, T.C. (1975). A prototype liquid crystal fiberoptic probe for temperature and power measurements in RF fields. *Microwave J. 18*:55–59.

JOHNSON, R.H., JAMES, J.R., HAND, J.W., HOPEWELL, J.W., DUNLOP, P.R.C., AND DICKINSON, R.J. (1984). New low-profile applicators for local heating of tissues. *IEEE Trans. Biomed. Eng. 31*:28–37.

KUHN, P.K. AND CHRISTENSEN, D.A. (1986). Influence of temperature probe sheathing materials during ultrasonic heating. *IEEE Trans. Biomed. Eng. 33*:536–538.

LAGENDIJK, J.J.W. (1983). A new coaxial TEM radiofrequency/microwave applicator for noninvasive deep-body hyperthermia. *J. Microwave Power 18*:367–376.

LELE, P.P. (1983). Physical aspects and clinical studies with ultrasonic hyperthermia. *In*: Storm, F.K. (ed.). Hyperthermia in cancer therapy. Boston, G.K. Hall Medical Publishers, pp. 333–367.

LYONS, B.E., BRITT, R.H., AND STROHBEHN, J.W. (1984). Localized hyperthermia in the treatment of malignant brain tumors using an interstitial microwave antenna array. *IEEE Trans. Biomed. Eng. 31*:53–62.

MENDECKI, J., FRIEDENTHAL, E., BOTSTEIN, C., PAGLIONE, R., AND STERZER, F. (1980). Microwave applicators for localized hyperthermia treatment of cancer of the prostate. *Int. J. Radiat. Oncol. Biol. Phys. 8*:1583–1588.

MENDECKI, J., FRIEDENTHAL, E., BOTSTEIN, C., ET AL. (1978). Microwave induced hyperthermia in cancer treatment: apparatus and preliminary result. *Int. J. Radiat. Oncol. Biol. Phys. 4*:1095–1103.

MEYER, J., SAMULSKI, T., LEE, E., ET AL. (1985). Therapeutic impact of symptoms induced during ultrasound hyperthermia. Abstract Cd-17, Annual Meeting of the Radiation Research Society, Los Angeles, May 5–9, 1985.

MOIDEL, R.A., WOLFSON, S.K., JR., SELKER, R.G., AND WEINER, S.B. (1976). Materials for selective tissue heating in an RFEM field for combined chemothermal treatment of brain tumors. *J. Biomed. Materials Res. 10*:327–334.

MORITA, N., AND BACH ANDERSEN, J. (1982). Near-field absorption in a circular cylinder from electric and magnetic line sources. *Bioelectromagnetics 3*:253–274.

OCHELTREE, K.B., BENKESER, P.J., FRIZZELL, L.A., AND CAIN, C.A. (1985). Comparison of heating deposition patterns for stacked linear phased array and fixed focus ultrasonic hyperthermia applicators. Abstract Ad-26, Annual Meeting of Radiation Research Society, Los Angeles, May 5–9, 1985.

PEREZ, C.A. (1984). Clinical hyperthermia: mirage or reality? *Int. J. Radiat. Oncol. Biol. Phys. 10*:935–937.

PEREZ, C.A., AND SAPARETO, S.A. (1984). Thermal dose expression in clinical hyperthermia and correlation with tumor response/control. *Cancer Res. 44*:4818s–4825s.

RASKMARK, P., AND BACH ANDERSEN, J. (1984a). Electronically steered heating of a cylinder. *In*: Overgaard, J. (ed.). Proceedings of the 4th International Symposium on Hyperthermic Oncology. London, Taylor & Francis, pp. 617–620.

RASKMARK, P., AND BACH ANDERSEN, J. (1984b). Focused electromagnetic heating of muscle tissue. *IEEE Trans. Microwave Theory Tech. 32*:887–888.

RUGGERA, P.S., AND KANTOR, G. (1984). Development of a family of RF helical coil applicators which produce transversely uniform, axially distributed heating in cylindrical fat-muscle phantoms. *IEEE Trans. Biomed. Eng. 31*:98–106.

SAMARAS, G.M. (1984). Intracranial microwave hyperthermia: heat induction and temperature control. *IEEE Trans. Biomed. Eng. 31*:63–69.

SAMULSKI, T., AND SHRIVASTAVA, P.N. (1980). Photoluminescent thermometer probes: temperature measurements in microwave fields. *Science 208*:193–194.

STAUFFER, P.R., CETAS, T.C., FLETCHER, A.M., ET AL. (1984). Observations in the use of ferromagnetic implants for inducing hyperthermia. *IEEE Trans. Biomed. Eng. 31*:76–90.

STAUFFER, P.R., CETAS, T.C., AND JONES, R.C. (1982). System for producing localized hyperthermia in tumors through magnetic induction heating of ferromagnetic implants. *Natl. Cancer Inst. Monogr. 61*:483–488.

STERZER, F., PAGLIONE, R.W., MENDECKI, J., FRIEDENTHAL, E., AND BOTSTEIN, C. (1980). RF therapy for malignancy. *IEEE Spectrum 17*:32–37.

STORM, F.K., ELLIOTT, R.S., HARRISON, W.H., AND MORTON, D.L. (1982). Clinical RF hyperthermia by magnetic-loop induction: a new approach to human cancer therapy. *IEEE Trans. Microwave Theory Tech. 30*:1149–1158.

STROHBEHN, J.W., BOWERS, E.D., WALSH, J.E., AND DOUPLE, E.B. (1979). An invasive microwave antenna for locally induced hyperthermia for cancer therapy. *J. Microwave Power 14*:339–350.

TAYLOR, L.S. (1980). Implantable radiators for cancer therapy by microwave hyperthermia. *Proc. IEEE 68*:142–149.

TREMBLY, B.S., STROHBEHN, J.W., DE SIEYES, D.C., AND DOUPLE, E.B. (1982). Hyperthermia induction by an array of invasive microwave antennas. *Natl. Cancer Inst. Monogr. 61*:497–499.

TREMBLY, B.S., WILSON, A.H., HAVARD, J.M., SABATAKAKIS, K., AND STROHBEHN, J.W. (1988). Comparison of power deposition by in-phase 433 MHz and phase-modulated 915 MHz interstitial antenna array hyperthermia systems. *IEEE Trans. Microwave Theory Tech. 36*:908–916.

TSAI, C.T., DURNEY, C.H., AND CHRISTENSEN, D.A. (1984). Calculated power absorption patterns for hyperthermia applicators consisting of electric dipole arrays. *J. Microwave Power 19*:554–556.

TURNER, P.F. (1984a). Hyperthermia and inhomogeneous tissue effects using an annular-phased array. *IEEE Trans. Microwave Theory Tech. 32*:874–882.

TURNER, P.F. (1984b). Regional hyperthermia with an annular-phased array. *IEEE Trans. Biomed. Eng. 31*:106–114.

TURNER, P.F., AND LALIT, K. (1982). Computer solution for applicator heating patterns. *J. Natl. Cancer Inst. Monogr. 61*:521–523.

VAGUINE, V.A., CHRISTENSEN, D.A., LINDLEY, J.H., AND WALSTON, T.E. (1984). Multiple sensor optical thermometry system for application in clinical hyperthermia. *IEEE Trans. Biomed. Eng. 31*:168–172.

WELCH, A.J., AND PEARCE, J.A. (1988). Thermocouples. *In*: Webster, J.G. (ed.). Encyclopedia of medical devices and instrumentation. New York, John Wiley & Sons, pp. 2739–2746.

WELLS, P.N.T. (1969). Physical principles of ultrasonic diagnosis. New York, Academic Press.

WICKERSHEIM, K.A., AND ALVES, R.V. (1979). Recent advances in optical temperature measurement. *Ind. Res. Dev. 21*:82.

19

Potential Electromagnetic Techniques in Medical Applications

MAGDY F. ISKANDER

Some methods that use electromagnetic (EM) energy for medical diagnosis have been under investigation since early in this century, whereas others are still in their infancy. Advances and breakthroughs have been made in some techniques, which raises hopes for their final development into clinical tools, while others are still merely intriguing ideas. For example, the use of electrical bioimpedance to monitor the development of pulmonary edema goes back to 1926 when Lambert and Gremels first used these measurements to correlate the resistance across isolated cat lung to the change in its water content. Recently a symposium was totally devoted to exploring the various possible applications of the electrical bioimpedance method (Kanai, 1981). Also, although the basic idea of EM flowmeters was first introduced by Kolin (1936), efforts are still under way to use this idea for in vivo measurement of the blood flow (Salles-Cunha et al., 1980).

Many of the ideas involving the use of EM techniques for medical applications, on the other hand, have sprung from recent advances in the development of EM methods and devices. For example, the use of passive microwave methods (radiometers) for detecting cancer tumors was reported only in the early 1970s (Barrett and Myers, 1975). Other applications of the radiometer methods, such as for measuring changes in lung water or for the noninvasive determination of the temperature distribution in the human body, are still in their infancy, and much more work is required before these methods become clinically useful. The development of EM imaging techniques is also still in its preliminary stages. Serious questions remain regarding its accuracy, resolution, and general adequacy for clinical use. If nuclear magnetic resonance (NMR) imaging can be characterized as one of the EM methods, the rapid growth of this method and its recent development certainly indicate a bright future with extensive medical use.

Several other EM techniques have been under investigation for several years. These include, for example, the microwave method for measuring changes in lung water (Süsskind, 1973; Iskander et al., 1979b) and the use of microwaves for the fixation of brain tissue for neurochemical applications (Merritt and Frazer, 1977). Several advances have been made in the development of these methods, but their full clinical utilization awaits further studies to ensure their reliability, accuracy, and in some cases patient safety (Iskander and Durney, 1980a).

This chapter reviews the various EM methods and outlines the principles underlying their operation. These methods are broadly grouped into (1) active techniques that use external sources (radiation) of EM energy to achieve the measurement, (2) passive methods that use the EM radiation naturally emitted from the human body, and (3) EM imaging techniques. In each of these groups the methods are subgrouped according to the frequency of the EM radiation used. In all cases, experimental and numerical results illustrating the advantages and limitations of each method are presented and suggestions for future improvements are discussed.

Compiling all these methods in a single chapter and outlining the remaining problems in each, as well as the work needed to be done before these methods can be fully used clinically, may stimulate further research in this important area, which is directly related to the well-being of humankind.

FUNDAMENTAL DIFFERENCES BETWEEN LOW-FREQUENCY (KILOHERTZ) AND HIGH-FREQUENCY (MICROWAVES) MEASUREMENT METHODS

Before a discussion of the various EM methods for medical applications, some fundamental differences between the low- and high-frequency EM methods should be described. Although both methods use EM energy, the propagation characteristics of these energies actually depend on the ratio between the conduction and displacement currents (Johnk, 1975). At lower frequencies (such as the kilohertz range used in impedance plethysmography), the conduction current is almost an order of magnitude larger than the displacement current. At the microwave frequencies, on the other hand, the ratio of the displacement current to the conduction current is sufficiently high and hence the propagation phenomenon is dominated by radiation-type fields. This simply means that the signal is transmitted into the human body in the form of propagating waves rather than conduction currents.

Although at lower frequencies simple electrodes usually are used to terminate the currents and measure terminal voltage, specially designed antennas are used at microwave frequencies to efficiently couple and transmit these signals into the human body. Among the many important requirements of the antennas are these (Durney and Iskander, 1988):

1. Good impedance match to the human body, possibly over a rather broad frequency band

2. Compact size and light weight (particularly important when the antennas are used for continuous monitoring)
3. Minimum external leakage radiation (important to minimize artifacts in measurements and for the safety of the medical personnel)
4. Uniform heating pattern if the antenna or another EM device is to be used for heating purposes (thawing frozen organs)

The short-circuiting effects often occurring at the lower frequencies because of the highly conducting chest wall may be minimized if microwaves

---

TABLE 19-1   Fundamental Differences between High-Frequency (Radiation-Type) and Low-Frequency (Conduction Current–Dominated) Electromagnetic Procedures

High-frequency "radiation"	Low-frequency "conduction current"
1. Propagation-type phenomenon that involves transmission of electromagnetics waves into tissue (ratio M = displacement current/conduction current $>> 1$).	1. Lumped circuit–type phenomenon involving circulation of currents in closed circuit. Human body is considered part of circuit ($M << 1$).
2. Wave attenuates as it propagates inside tissue, hence term "depth of penetration."	2. Current circulation is described by circuit laws, and laws such as Kirchhoff's laws can be approximately applied. Short-circuiting effects occur because of large current density circulating in highly conducting chest wall.
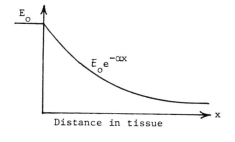	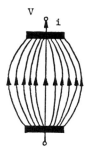
3. For efficient transmission, antenna size should be of order of $\lambda/2$.	3. Does not require any special applicator design, only electrodes or coil to provide closed path for current. Dimension of circuit element is small compared to wavelength.

are used instead of low-frequency signals. This is simply because microwave transmission is dominated by radiation-type fields, which minimizes the short-circuiting effects of any circulating conduction current in the chest wall. These and other differences are illustrated in Table 19-1.

ACTIVE ELECTROMAGNETIC METHODS FOR MEDICAL APPLICATIONS

Most of the techniques in this section are related to the use of external EM radiation to monitor various physiological parameters of interest. Others are related to the use of EM energy for thawing frozen organs, healing wounds, or possibly selectively heating cancer tumors at the millimeter-wave frequencies. All these active EM methods are classified according to the frequency of the EM radiation used. Therefore the first of the various medical applications presented are those of the electrical bioimpedance method, which uses frequencies in the kilohertz range. Next the EM methods for blood flow measurements and the various potential medical applications at microwave frequencies are described. No attempt is made to cover established microwave techniques that are routinely used clinically (such as microwave hyperthermia devices), since these methods are described in other chapters.

Potential Medical Applications of the Electrical Bioimpedance Method

Description of the method.   The electrical impedance (EI) method is the simplest and most extensively tested EM method in many medical diagnostic procedures (Kanai, 1981). In its basic form it involves applying a small signal (a fraction of a volt) in the frequency range from 20 to 100 kHz across a suitable location in the subject's body and measuring the resulting current. Frequencies in kilohertz range are commonly used in these measurements to avoid problems with electrode polarization and in particular a high impedance value at the electrode-skin interface (Nyboer, 1959). This basic design has found many useful applications, particularly those involving in vitro measurements. For example, as long ago as 1926 Lambert and Gremels used such a procedure to monitor the fluid accumulation in the lung by measuring the EI directly across the lungs of cats and dogs. However, the use of this method for in vivo measurements was limited owing to, among other reasons, excessive artifacts because of skin-electrode contact resistance, which obscured the desired variation in the impedance. To overcome this difficulty, investigators developed a four-electrode system for in vivo measurements (Kubicek et al., 1966; Kubicek et al., 1974; Bleicher et al., 1981). The four-electrode

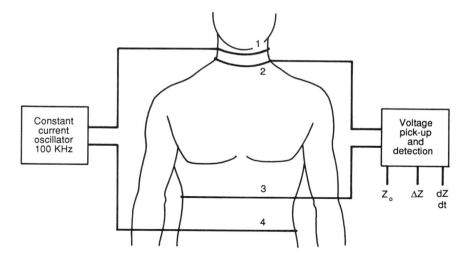

Figure 19-1 Schematic diagram illustrating use of four-electrode electrical impedance method in studying cardiac function. Electrodes *1* and *4* are current electrodes, and *2* and *3* are voltage electrodes.

arrangement in a typical clinical measurement is shown in Figure 19-1. Two conductive strip electrodes are placed around the neck, and two others around the abdomen. The outer two electrodes are connected to a constant current source that provides a few milliamperes, while the inner two electrodes are connected to a high-impedance voltmeter. A suitable detection circuit is used to determine the impedance between the two inner electrodes, Z_0, and the change as well as the rate of change of this impedance, ΔZ and dZ/dt. This information regarding the value of the impedance and its variation has been used extensively to measure physiological parameters such as stroke volume, cardiac output, blood flow, and arterial volume pressure characteristics. Specific examples of these measurements are given later in this section.

Despite the extensive clinical and laboratory evaluations of the EI method, some efforts are still being devoted to the development of the electrode system used in the method. For example, to eliminate problems associated with the relative inflexibility of the metallic electrodes, which impeded free respiration of patients, Sramek (1981) proposed an array of 12 standard electrocardiographic (ECG) spot disposal electrodes. Specifically it was found that four spot electrodes, properly placed, can replace each band on the lower thorax and two electrodes can replace each band on the neck, resulting in a total of 12 electrodes. It was also pointed out that the electrical quality of these electrodes is not so critical as in ECG applications, since the applied frequency is greater than 20 kHz,

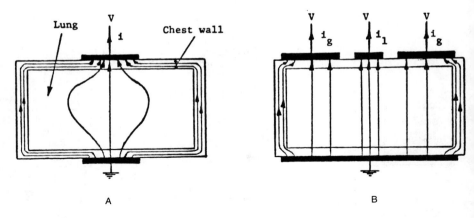

Figure 19-2 Electrical impedance method for measurng changes in lung water. **A,** With small unguarded electrodes, major part of measured current i passes through low impedance chest wall section of thorax. **B,** with guard electrode, most chest wall currents flow through guard ring. Current flowing through central electrode i_1 is largely directed through lung. (After Iskander, M. F., and Durney, C. H. [1980] *Proc. IEEE 68*:126–132.)

a frequency at which the skin-electrode interface is mostly capacitive (Sramek, 1981).

The four-electrode method and its variations, however, still were found inadequate to monitor physiological changes in an interior high-impedance region such as the lungs. This is simply because the lung region is surrounded by a highly conductive chest wall, and in a method such as the four-electrode procedure the current path in the chest wall is parallel to that in the lung, which causes short-circuiting of the impedance variation in the high-resistance region of the lung (Iskander and Durney, 1980a). Also, with the four-electrode system the volume involved in the measured impedance often includes more than the volume of prime interest (Graham, 1965). To facilitate "seeing" through the intact chest wall to obtain information about changes in lung impedance, Graham (1965) proposed the use of guard electrodes. The importance of guard electrodes is illustrated in Figure 19-2, where it is clear that with a small unguarded electrode the major part of the measured current i passes through the low-impedance chest wall. With the guard ring placed over the lateral chest wall, however, most of the chest wall current would flow through the guard ring if maintained at the same potential as the detection electrode. With this arrangement the current flowing through the central electrode is largely directed through the underlying lung. With a guard ring, it is possible not only to reduce the chest wall short-circuiting effect but also to limit the volume involved in the impedance measurement (Aoyagi et al., 1981). Figure 19-3 illustrates the differences

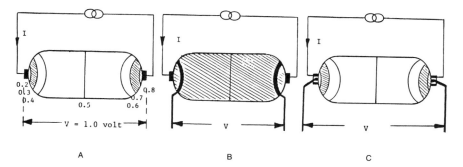

Figure 19-3 Schematic diagram illustrating impedance volumes (*shaded region*) measured by various electrodes arrangements. **A,** Single unguarded electrode. **B,** Four-electrode arrangements. **C,** Coaxial electrode arrangements. Although coaxial-electrode method is variation of four-electrode procedure, measured impedance is related mainly to tissue volume in neighborhood of electrodes (After Aoyagi, T., et al., [1981]. A study to assess pulmonary circulation by impedance method. *In*: Proceedings of the 5th International Conference on Electrical Bio-Impedance, Tokyo. Tokyo, Business Center for Academic Societies Japan pp. 401–404.)

in the volumes involved in the impedance measurements with the various methods. From Figure 19-3 it is clear that the use of guard ring methods limits the impedance measurement to principally the volume in the neighborhood of the electrodes.

The idea of the guard electrode was implemented by Cooley and Longini (1968) in an automatically balanced bridge detector system. They maintained the guard ring at the same potential as the central detection electrode and introduced a small electrode to detect the skin potential gradient lateral to the detector electrode. The potential gradient drove the guard ring to inject sufficient current into the chest virtually to eliminate this lateral gradient. This procedure not only minimized the lateral (chest wall) current flow from the active electrode, but also minimized artifacts arising from skin contact resistance in the guard ring. The sensitivity of this focusing electrode bridge was evaluated by conducting several experiments on dogs and comparing the results with those obtained through the double indicator-dilution technique. The reproducibility of the results obtained was encouraging.

In another attempt to optimize the EI meaurement procedure, Fuse et al. (1981) conducted experiments on animals and humans and examined the variation of the measurement with changes in the shape and location of electrodes. Specific shapes of the electrodes examined in Fuse's measurements are shown in Figure 19-4. These electrodes, unlike the four-band electrodes, are intended for obtaining local information. The experimental results showed that the optimum electrode shape is the coaxial

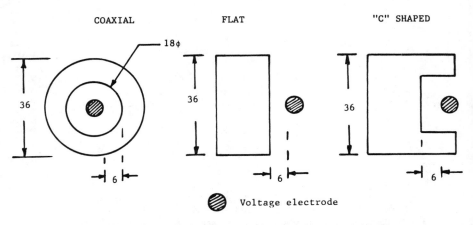

Figure 19-4 Various shapes of electrodes examined to improve performance of electrical bioimpedance method. Results indicated that coaxial electrode is optimum electrode shape. All dimensions are in millimeters. (After Fuse et al., 1981.)

one (that is, an inner voltage pickup electrode and an outer ring-shaped current electrode). Like the guarded electrodes described earlier, the coaxial electrodes are adequate for minimizing the short-circuiting effects and providing relatively local information. Representative examples of use of the EI method for monitoring various physiological parameters are given in the following section.

Examples of medical applications using the electrical impedance method. The use of the EI method as a means of measuring various physiological activities in the human body has been investigated for many years. A good record of the recent progress made was included in the *Proceedings of the Fifth International Conference on Electrical Bioimpedance*; the conference was held in Tokyo in August 1981. A few examples of these types of applications are presented with special emphasis on the type of results obtained and the remaining problems to be solved in each.

Measurement of cardiac function. The use of the transthoracic EI method for noninvasively determining stroke volume and cardiac output is extensively described in the literature. Two basic formulas have been derived to relate the measured change in the electrical impedance to the stroke volume. The first simply relates the stroke volume to the change in electrical impedance by

$$\text{Stroke volume (ml)} = \frac{\rho L^2}{Z_0^2} \Delta Z \qquad (1)$$

where ρ is the resistivity of blood (ohm meters), L is the distance between the sensing electrodes (centimeters), Z_0 is the base impedance level (ohms), and ΔZ is the pulsatile change of impedance (Nyboer, 1959). However, this expression did not fit all the experimental and clinical measurements, and instead a different formula was suggested (Kubicek et al., 1966, 1974):

$$\text{Stroke volume} = \frac{\rho L^2}{Z_0^2}\, T\, dZ/dt\, \Big|_{\text{max}} \qquad (2)$$

where T is the ventricular ejection time and dZ/dt is the rate of pulsatile impedance change.

The formula by Kubicek et al. (1966, 1974) was found to fit well the results obtained with use of other invasive techniques (Pate et al., 1975). A specific result is shown in Figure 19-5, where it is clear that the EI method does provide a noninvasive technique to monitor the cardiac output continuously during surgery and also is capable of measuring cardiac output postoperatively (Baker et al., 1971).

Measurement of changes in lung water.   Although the idea of using the EI method directly across the lungs to measure changes in lung

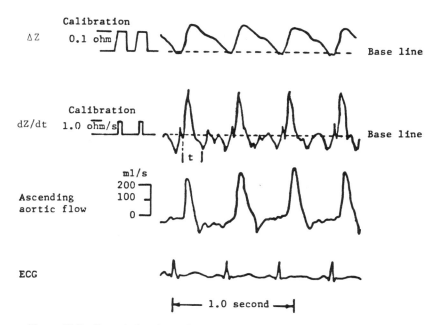

Figure 19-5   Record showing ΔZ, dZ/dt, aortic blood flow, and electrocardiogram in dog. Aortic flow was measured with electromagnetic flowmeter. (After Baker, L. E., et al. [1971]. *Cardiovasc. Res. Cent. Bull.* 9:135–145.)

water is an old one, efforts to develop similar measurements in vivo were unsuccessful because of the short-circuiting effects indicated earlier. Only after further developments (Graham, 1965; Cooley and Longini, 1968; Severinghaus et al., 1972), such as those involving the development of guard electrodes, was good correlation between the impedance measurements and the results of other invasive or more complicated but comprehensively tested techniques obtained. The reproducibility of the results (about ±5%) was good, but more work is needed to improve the sensitivity of the EI method.

Other applications. Obtaining cross-sectional images of the human body is yet another application of the EI method (Henderson and Webster, 1978). Some results based on simulated data are encouraging (Kim et al., 1983), but significant difficulties still have to be overcome before this method can be clinically useful. More detailed discussion of low-frequency EI imaging is included later in this chapter. Another application of the EI method is related to measurement of urinary bladder fullness (Waltz et al., 1971; Denniston and Baker, 1975; Abbey and Close, 1983). Abbey and Close (1983) concluded that, although baseline impedance depended on individual subjects, good correlation showing an impedance decrease with urinary bladder filling and an impedance increase on voiding was observed. The observations were moderated by the many questions they raised, particularly related to defining capacity residual and effect of the bladder shape. It was even indicated that EI measurements might require adaptation and modification for use with each subject (Abbey and Close, 1983).

Electromagnetic Methods for Blood Flow Measurements

Cardiovascular surgery is usually aimed at either the improvement of the heart as a pump or the improvement of the arteries in conducting blood. During such operations, blood flow measurements play an important role in evaluation of the effects of different procedures. Several techniques are available for making in vivo blood flow measurements, but none is in common use (Cappelen and Hall, 1967). Either they are too complicated or inaccurate, or they may involve a considerable risk to the patient.

Recently an EM device suitable for blood flow measurements has received renewed attention for its use in vivo in monitoring blood flow in humans (Salles-Cunha et al., 1980, 1981; Battocletti et al., 1983). The principle of operation which was first introduced by Kolin (1936), is based on Faraday's law of EM induction as illustrated in Figure 19-6.

If blood is flowing in a tube or blood vessel oriented at right angles

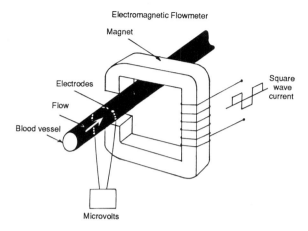

Figure 19-6   Schematic diagram illustrating basic principle of electromagnetic flowmeter. (After Cappelen, C., and Hall, K. V. [1967]. *Acta Chir. Scand. Suppl. 368*:3–37.)

to the magnetic field, the voltage generated across a diameter perpendicular to the magnetic field and to the direction of flow is given by Cappelen and Hall (1967) as

$$E = BLu \times 10^{-8} \tag{3}$$

where E is the potential difference in volts, B is the magnetic field strength in gauss, L is the length of the conductor in centimeters within the field, and u is the speed of blood flow in centimeters per second. An alternating magnetic field is desirable to prevent electrode polarization problems (Figure 19-6). In this case an extra term must be added to the right-hand side of the preceding equation to account for the electrodes and their leads acting as a one-turn transformer (Cappelen and Hall, 1967). From Faraday's law indicated previously, it is clear that by measuring the potential difference across the diameter of the blood vessel, one can calculate the mean velocity of blood flow. The induced voltage may be picked up from electrodes in contact with the outer surface of the vessel wall without opening the artery. Studies performed on flow models have demonstrated a linear relationship between the blood flow and the electrical signal, as well as excellent reproducibility (Cappelen and Hall, 1967).

Despite the wide use of the EM flowmeter in surgical applications, technical problems are sometimes encountered. These include electrocardiographic (ECG) pickup, particularly when the surgeon is working with vessels close to the heart, zero-point drift and instability, and some other minor artifacts resulting from vessel drying and varying vessel diameter.

Zero-point instability can be recognized easily by clamping the vessel and readjusting the instrument to zero. The problem of ECG signal interference can be recognized and accounted for. As mentioned previously, efforts in developing this method are being focused on its use in noninvasive monitoring of blood flow in humans (Salles-Cunha et al., 1981; Battocletti et al., 1983). In addition to the mathematical modeling, which is aimed at relating the pickup voltage at the body surface to the blood flow in arteries (Salles-Cunha et al., 1980), initial experimental and clinical results were encouraging (Salles-Cunha et al., 1981).

Several problems still exist in the EM flowmeter measurement procedure, and more work is needed before the method can be used clinically. Battocletti et al. (1983), for example, indicated that the most severe limitation of this method is related to the inadequacy of using steady magnetic fields in the measurement, since it results in voltage offset and drift at the electrode-skin interface. As in the case of invasive EM blood flow measurement, an alternating magnetic field would overcome this problem. For noninvasive measurements, however, the required high-intensity alternating magnetic field would generate eddy currents in the body, which could cause hazardous tissue heating. Another problem is the limited accuracy of the mathematical models developed for these measurements (Salles-Cunha et al., 1980, 1981). For example, simplified models of concentric cylinders, which assume homogeneous tissue surrounding the blood vessel and ignore the presence of bone, are often used. Based on experiments with humans, investigators have indicated that the primary difficulties of the method are movement of the subject and the care necessary when attaching the electrodes. Detailed descriptions of these difficulties, as well as an interesting comparison between EM flowmetry and blood flow measurement by NMR, are given by Battocletti et al. (1983).

Potential Microwave Methods for Medical Applications

In this section a variety of applications of EM techniques at microwave frequencies are described. They include the use of microwave methods for measuring changes in lung water content, thawing frozen organs, detecting heart dynamics, and repairing skin wounds. Microwave methods have also been used in a variety of other medical applications (Burdette et al., 1982; Lin and Clarke, 1982), but the following discussion is limited to sufficiently investigated methods and those considered to have potential.

Microwave method for measuring changes in lung water content. The importance of measuring changes in lung water content hardly needs justification, since most medical and surgical pulmonary abnormalities are associated with changes in lung water. The techniques available for making these measurements are either inadequate for continuous clinical use, since the measurement procedure is long and complicated, or simply insensititive to small and early changes in the lung water content. Therefore, a significant need exists for developing new techniques of making these measurements, particularly for detecting early and small changes and for making the measurements continuously.

As indicated earlier in the chapter, problems have been encountered in using the electrical impedance method for in vivo measurements of physiological parameters such as changes in lung water content. Using signals at microwave frequencies offers certain advantages, such as overcoming the chest wall short-circuiting problems. The microwave method of lung water measurement basically uses changes in the dielectric properties of lung tissue to determine the amount of water present. The method is based on a continuous monitoring of the reflection or the transmission coefficient, or both, to indicate changes in the permittivity of lung tissue. A feasibility study to explore further the potential usefulness of the microwave method for making these measurements was initiated several years ago at the University of Utah. The study was aimed at answering the following specific questions (Durney et al., 1978; Pedersen et al., 1978; Iskander and Durney, 1979):

1. Which of the scattering coefficients should be used in these measurements? The determining factor in answering this question is obviously related to the relative sensitivity of the reflection versus the transmission coefficient measurements as a function of changes in lung water.

2. What is the optimum frequency for these measurements?

3. What is the best antenna that can be used for coupling the EM energy into the body with minimum external leakage? Although the electrical impedance measurement does not require special applicator design but only simple metallic electrodes to terminate the conduction current, the microwave method depends on the development of a compact applicator that provides maximum coupling to tissue and minimum radiation leakage. The minimum external leakage is a critical requirement because the signal transmitted in the body is highly attenuated, and therefore leakage radiation could obscure information about changes in lung water content.

The feasibility study group initially answered these questions by developing a three-layer planar mathematical model (Pedersen, 1976; Pedersen, et al., 1978; Shoff, 1978) in which the three layers represented the front chest wall, the lung, and the back chest wall. Based on this model, the calculation of plane-wave reflection and transmission coefficients showed that the transmission coefficient (particularly the phase) should be used in these measurements to achieve adequate sensitivity (Iskander et al., 1979). Through the same analysis a trade-off between the sensitivity of the phase of the microwave-transmitted signal and the attenuation of this signal across the thorax was identified. At higher frequencies, the phase was found to be more sensitive to changes in lung water content, but at these higher frequencies the attenuation is greater. As a result of this trade-off, it was decided that the frequency band between 700 MHz and 1.5 GHz is the optimum one for measuring the transmission coefficient across the thorax. The upper frequency limit of this range is related to the maximum allowable attenuation, and the lower limit is related to the desired sensitivity of the phase of the microwave-transmitted signal to changes in the lung's water content. Since the frequency of 915 MHz, which is allocated by the Federal Communications Commission for medical and industrial applications, is within the identified optimum frequency range, this frequency has been used in all the reported experimental measurements.

The antenna used was a unique microwave applicator developed to couple the energy into the thorax with minimum radiation leakage around the body (Iskander and Durney, 1979; Iskander and Durney, 1980b). With the decision to measure transmission coefficients, the development of this applicator became particularly important because leakage radiation could obscure the information carried by the highly attenuated signal transmitted through the body.

Attempts to use radiation-type applicators such as dielectrically loaded waveguides have been unsuccessful because of the excessive external leakage radiation. The use of flanged waveguides, on the other hand, although minimizing the external radiation, makes the applicator large, heavy, and hence undesirable for clinical use (Yamaura, 1977). The unique applicator developed by Iskander and Durney (1980b) is a surface-strip transmission line (coplanar waveguide) applicator with the ground plane

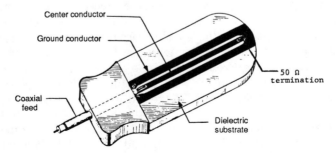

Figure 19-7 Open-strip transmission line applicator used for electromagnetic energy coupling. (After Iskander, M. F., and Durney, C. H. [1979]. *Proc. IEEE* 67:1463–1465.)

placed on both sides of the center strip conductor (Figure 19-7). This geometry allows the spread of the EM fields around the transmission line rather than confining them between the conductors. Since this guiding structure does not normally radiate in the absence of any discontinuities along the transmission line, the transmitted EM energy is confined in a limited space around the applicator. A discontinuity along the line, such as a contact with the thorax, sets up radiation fields at the region of contact, with the power mostly flowing into the discontinuity. This and other features of the new microwave applicator are described elsewhere (Iskander and Durney, 1979; Durney and Islander, 1988).

To verify the calculated results illustrating the superior sensitivity of the phase of the microwave-transmitted signal, researchers conducted many experiments on phantoms (physical replicas), anesthetized dogs, and several isolated dog lungs (Shoff, 1978; Iskander et al., 1979; Ovard, 1979; Iskander and Durney, 1980a). The experimental procedure routinely uses the microwave network analyzer system, described elsewhere (Iskander et al., 1979), and the results show good correlation between the change in the phase of the microwave-transmitted signal and the change in the water content. A typical experimental result from an in vivo dog experiment is shown in Figure 19-8 (Iskander and Durney, 1983), where it is clear that the change in the phase of the microwave-transmitted signal is extremely sensitive to early changes in lung water. Results from an isolated lung experiment in which the phase of the microwave-transmitted signal was compared with the absolute weight of an extracted dog's lung are shown in Figure 19-9. The excellent agreement of the results emphasizes the feasibility of using microwaves for measuring changes in lung water. Although we have studied the possibility of measuring absolute levels of water content by microwave methods (Iskander et al., 1981, 1982a), the microwave methods appear to be most useful for monitoring only changes in lung water content.

In summary, the sensitivity of the change in phase of the microwave transmission coefficient to small changes in lung water content has been illustrated experimentally and theoretically. The theoretical calculations included planar phantom models and a two-dimensional numerical simulation in which the method of moments was used (Iskander et al., 1981; Maini, 1981). The experimental measurements were made on phantoms, anesthetized dogs, and isolated dog lungs.

With the promising results from the feasibility study, the microwave method was tried experimentally on dialysis patients. The microwave-transmitted signal was correlated with the loss of patient's weight during the dialysis process. Two basic problems that had not been experienced with dogs were encountered with patients. First, since the patients were larger than dogs, the higher attenuation in patients caused the received signals to be so weak that the results were inconclusive. Second, the

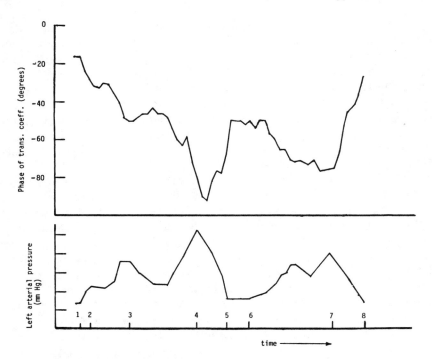

Figure 19-8 Results of dog experiment illustrating sensitivity of active microwave method (particularly phase of transmission coefficient) for measuring changes in lung water content. Numbers on time axis indicate various stages of experiment. *1*, Start of infusion; *2*, 100 ml of blood has been infused; *3*, 500 ml of blood has been infused; *4*, 1000 ml of blood has been infused, also bleeding has been started to reverse edema; *5*, 500 ml of blood has been withdrawn; *6*, start infusion; *7*, 500 ml of blood has been infused, and also start of withdrawing blood; and *8*, time at which 1000 ml of blood has been withdrawn. Between *3* and *4*, oscillation in left arterial pressure occurred while perfusion was continued. Changes in left arterial pressure are known to correlate well with changes in lung water. (After Iskander, M. F., and Durney, C. H. [1983]. *J. Microwave Power* 18:265–275.)

received signals were strongly affected by patient movement and probably magnified by the high attenuation of the signals. Some of these problems might have been solved by increasing the power level of the applied signals, but such an approach was avoided to rule out any possible hazard to the patients. Therefore, to overcome these problems and maintain the input power to the acceptably low value of 10 mW, investigators developed a suitable pulsed microwave system providing the high signal level required in certain measurements but at the same time maintaining a small average power density.

The problem of sensitivity of the measurements to patient movement was also traced back to the coupling characteristics of the strip transmis-

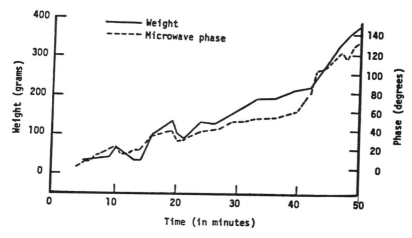

Figure 19-9 Results from isolated lung experiment illustrating good correlation between phase of microwave-transmitted signal and weight of isolated lung. (After Iskander, M. F., and Durney, C. H. [1980]. *Proc. IEEE* 68:126–132.)

sion line applicator described earlier. Some of the reflected radiation at the area of contact between the applicator and the patient was actually being guided on the outer conductor of the feeding cable. This problem was minimized by development of a new applicator that is 50 ohms when coupled to the body rather than 50 ohms when in free space (Iskander et al., 1982b). The new strip transmission line applicator is shown in Figure 19-10 together with a summary of its coupling characteristics (Iskander and Durney, 1983). In addition to minimizing the sensitivity of the measurement to cable movements, the new applicator significantly improves the transmission efficiency. With these new developments it is expected that the microwave method will perform far better in future trials on patients.

Application of microwave thawing to the recovery of deep-frozen cells and organs.   There is a significant need to store vital organs for transplantation, not only to allow time for transportation and the transplantation procedure, but also to allow physicians to find the full tissue match between donor and recipient required for success of the transplantation. The development of suitable systems for the uniform deep freezing and microwave thawing of whole organs, especially kidneys, has been reported (Rajotte et al., 1974; Voss et al., 1974; Burdette et al., 1978). The freezing procedures are described elsewhere; special emphasis is placed in this section on the design requirements of the microwave systems and the results of some experiments.

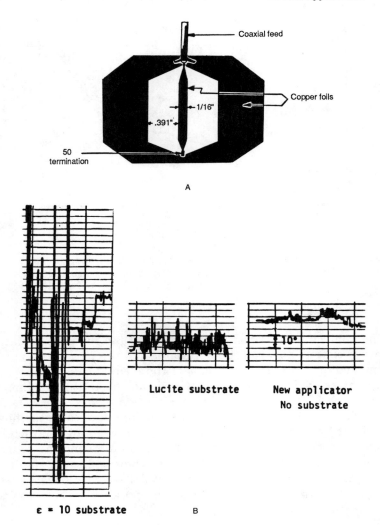

Figure 19-10 A, Schematic diagram of new transmission line applicator. This applicator has 50 ohms input impedance when coupled to human body. **B,** Sensitivity of phase measurement to movement of cables connected to applicator for three different versions of applicator. In all cases, results of maximum distortion are presented. (After Iskander, M. F., and Durney, C. H. [1983]. *J. Microwave Power 18*:265–275.)

In the design of a microwave system for thawing whole organs, often with irregular geometries, two major considerations are emphasized: uniformity of the resulting heating pattern and control of the rate of heating. Voss et al. (1974) developed resonant microwave cubic cavities for heating, with rotating as well as oscillating turntables to achieve a uniform heating pattern. The input microwave power was in the range of 1 to 2 kW at 2.45 GHz frequency. The perfused, frozen kidneys to be heated were immersed in a Teflon container filled with fluorocarbon, the material also used for perfusing the organ in the initial freezing stage. Cubic structures of the microwave cavities were chosen because they have the greatest number of modes of resonance and therefore improve the uniformity of the heating pattern. In the 10- and 17-inch cubic cavities used by Voss et al. (1974), an appreciable number of modes were coupled with a folded strip-line antenna.

With Voss's system it was possible to thaw kidneys from $-197°$ C to above zero at a heating rate of 100 to 200° C/min, while still maintaining uniformity to within $\pm 10°$ C. In the process of testing the uniformity of thawing, it became apparent that the kidney was uniformly thawed only when prefreezing perfusion had been uniform and complete. A summary of the experimental procedure is shown in Figure 19-11. After the kidneys were thawed, the data were analyzed by probing to determine temperature gradients in hemisected kidneys, performing histological studies on stained sections of thawed kidneys and comparing them with nonfrozen ones, and analyzing the preservation of the kidney's microcirculation. One of the frozen and thawed kidneys was implanted into the groin of a dog for 5 days (Rajotte et al., 1974). There was no evidence that the implanted kidney was functional at any time, and histological examination showed that some isolated areas were preserved whereas others were grossly damaged.

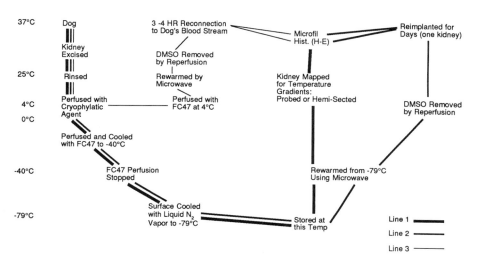

Figure 19-11   Diagram of experimental procedure used for freezing and microwave thawing of deep-frozen cells and organs. (After Voss, W. A. G., et al. [1974]. *J. Microwave Power* 9:181–194.)

Similar efforts were made to use microwaves for thawing tissue culture cells and fetal mouse hearts (Voss et al., 1974). In both cases the conclusion was that rapid absorption of microwave energy appears acceptable and that there is no significant difference between microwave and water bath thawing. In particular, the frozen-thawed implanted hearts continued to beat for up to 100 days with no detectable difference in the electrical activity between control implants and those that had survived the freeze-thawing process.

From the preceding discussion it is clear that the use of microwave energy for rapidly heating deep-frozen cells and organs is feasible and has clinical potential. Much more work needs to be done to optimize the design of microwave heating devices so that uniform heating, particularly of large organs, is ensured and the rate of heating is better controlled. A fairly complex heating system is needed to achieve uniformity and predictability of heating. Such a system could be a resonant device (for example, the cubical cavities used by Voss et al., 1974), the multifrequency thawing system developed by Burdette et al. (1978), a traveling-wave heating system (such as a waveguide applicator), or a flared horn applicator. Many theoretical and practical aspects of microwave heating should be studied before any of these systems is routinely used clinically.

Microwave fixation of brain tissue.   The determination of the distribution of neurochemicals is an important tool in neurobiological research. For example, this information is routinely used to evaluate the effect of drugs and hormones on the central nervous system. To measure the concentration of the various neurotransmitters as they exist in vivo, however, a procedure for rapidly halting enzymic processes is required. Enzymic activity is conventionally terminated by freezing the brain in liquid nitrogen or cooled Freon. Since this process does not immediately freeze the entire brain, considerable changes in the neurochemicals occur during the freezing period. Rapid freezing methods such as the freeze-blowing procedure (Veech et al., 1973), although offering the advantage of relatively fast inactivation times, have distinct drawbacks, including destruction of the brain anatomical structure. To overcome the slowness of freezing methods and other limitations in the other procedures available, Stavinoha et al. (1970) proposed the use of microwave irradiation as a fixative. Recent reports indicate that this technique is gaining acceptance as a true in vivo procedure for measuring neurochemicals.

In early experiments of applying microwave energy to brain fixation, the whole body of the animal was irradiated in a commercial microwave oven. But in these rather large exposure devices the microwave radiation was diffuse and unfocused, resulting in longer inactivation times (10 to 20 seconds) and the inevitable occurrence of postmortem changes (Schmidt et al., 1972).

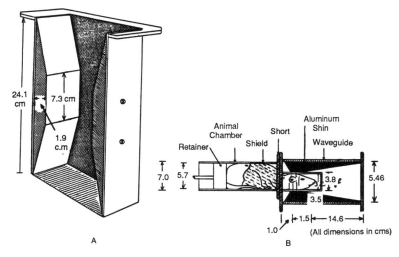

Figure 19-12 Schematic diagram of design of waveguide applicator suitable for rapid inactivation of brain enzymes. Generator is terminated in short-circuiting endplate with central 3.8 cm diameter hole. Hole diameter was just sufficient to allow protrusion of only rat head. Location of shorting plate helped maintain mode pattern in waveguide. **A,** Design modification of waveguide chamber of broadface microwave applicator. **B,** Shorting endplate microwave applicator. (After Lenox, R., et al. [1976]. *IEEE Trans. Microwave Theory Tech.* 24:58–61.)

Since then, several waveguide devices have been developed to focus microwave radiation on the head of the experimental animal (Guidotti et al., 1974; Butcher et al., 1976; Lenox et al., 1976). A typical design of these microwave applicators is shown in Figure 19-12 (Lenox et al., 1976). This applicator was found suitable for focusing the microwave energy on the animal's brain, thus reducing the inactivation time, and also for obtaining uniform field distribution over the 2.5 cm longitudinal extent of the rat brain. These features, as well as others such as minimizing the leakage radiation of the applicator, are described by Lenox et al. (1976). With the development of the applicators it was possible in milliseconds to heat animal heads to temperatures between 55° to 90° C. Thus the microwave fixation technique appears suitable for preventing postmortem changes in heat-stable, rapidly changing biochemicals.

Other miscellaneous applications of microwaves.   This section briefly summarizes some other reported medical applications of microwave methods, which are potentially useful but have not been completely evaluated.

Among the methods is the use of EM fields for stimulating and accelerating wound healing. In experiments to identify biological effects of EM radiation, Romero-Sierra et al. (1975) indicated the possible stimulation and enhancement of collagen production in tissue after its exposure to EM radiation. The same group investigated use of this enhancement to improve the rate and quality of wound healing. Evidence shows that wounds treated with EM fields at 27 MHz were at least 24 hours ahead of the control group in healing (Romero-Sierra et al., 1975). Tensile tests on skin specimens showed improvement in the healed strength of wounds treated with histamine and EM radiation. Although the exposure power density was not reported, irradiation times between 15 and 30 minutes were indicated (Romero-Sierra et al., 1975).

The demonstration of accelerating and improving the healing process with EM radiation is interesting. However, more evaluation of this effect is required. Studies to explore the effect of various radiation parameters such as the power density, frequency, and duration of exposure, must be conducted to validate the reported observation.

Another promising application of microwaves is for monitoring heart dynamics (Yamaura, 1978). In a preliminary study Yamaura (1979) presented a point-by-point mapping of the transmitted microwave power through the human thorax at 2 GHz. The transmitting antenna was an open-ended and flanged, S-band, standard waveguide with aperture dimensions of 10.9×5.5 cm^2, and the receiving antenna was a 2.3×1.0 cm^2, X-band waveguide dielectrically loaded with a material of $\epsilon_r = 15$ so that the waveguide could be used for receiving signals at 2 GHz. The incident power was 200 mW, and the power density at the transmitting aperture was estimated at 8 mW/m^2 (Yamaura, 1979). Yamaura mapped a 10×10 cm^2 area of the chest in 2 cm steps. The obtained microwave projection (attentuation) image of the human thorax suggested the position of the heart.

The presented data, however, did not provide a qualitative evaluation of the imaging procedure or an estimate of the diffraction and interference effects. A comprehensive evaluation of the microwave, as well as other imaging procedures, is given later in the chapter.

Potential Medical Applications at Millimeter Wavelengths

During the last decade a number of investigators have reported distinct resonance absorption by various biochemical and biological preparations in the millimeter-wave range (Webb and Booth, 1969, 1971; Stamm et al., 1974; Lee and Webb, 1977). It was suggested that this observed resonance absorption could be employed in diagnostic applications and for developing new forms of treating cancer (Stamm et al., 1974; Lu et al., 1977; Frolich, 1978; Swicord and Davis, 1982). As of this date, however, the existence of these enhanced and resonant absorption at millimeter wave is in question (Gandhi et al., 1980; Gandhi,

1983), and no clear mechanism of interaction between such radiation and the biological systems has been identified. To verify the presence of these effects, Gandhi et al. (1980) made extensive swept-frequency measurements in the Ka, U, and E frequency bands (26.5 to 40, 40 to 60, and 60 to 90 GHz) with a solid-state, computer-controlled system. They observed no frequency-specific absorption and concluded that this sharp resonant-type absorption does not exist, particularly because of the very high absorbence of water, which is an essential part of living tissues. They also suggested that the interpretations made by others who reported these effects are in error because of unsophisticated methodology, including interference in the measurement system (Gandhi, 1983).

POTENTIAL APPLICATION OF PASSIVE ELECTROMAGNETIC METHODS (RADIOMETRY) IN MEDICINE

Radiometry is based on the fact that all objects above absolute zero temperature emit energy in the form of EM radiation. Curves of brightness of a perfectly absorbing body (black body) are shown in Figure 19-13 as

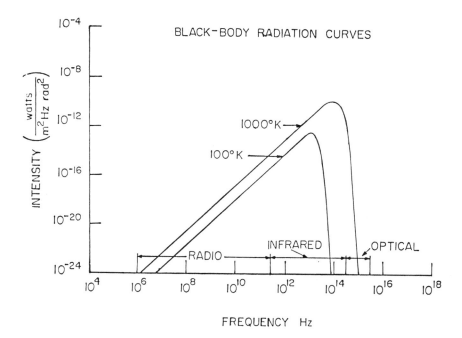

Figure 19-13 Specific intensity of black-body thermal radiation with frequency, for absolute temperatures 100° K and 1000° K. (After Myers, P. C., et al. [1979]. *J. Microwave Power* 14:105–114.)

a function of frequency (Kraus, 1966). From the figure it is clear that, although the emitted radiation is spread over a very wide frequency band, the frequency at which maximum radiation occurs from bodies at temperatures of practical interest ($T < 1000°$ K) is in the infrared region. This is why the emitted part of the spectrum has been detected and used for more than 30 years to obtain thermographic images.

The radiative properties of a practical object (not black body) vary according to the body's nature, temperature, orientation, composition, and surface conditions. The concept of gray bodies is therefore introduced to relate the radiation intensity to the specific properties of the object. The radiative properties of gray bodies are still described by the same physical laws governing the emission from a black body with the exception of introducing a new parameter called the emissivity. Generally, this radiation can be described according to Planck's law, which is given by Kraus (1966)

$$P(f) = \frac{2\pi h f^3}{c^2} e[\exp(hf/kT) - 1]^{-1} \qquad (4)$$

where e is the emissivity, h is Planck's constant (Joule second), k is Boltzmann's constant (Joule $°K^{-1}$), c is the velocity of light in air (cm$\cdot$s^{-1}), and T is the molecular temperature of the surface. For moderate temperatures and the frequency range for which $f << kT/h$ (for example, the microwave frequency range), Planck's distribution formula reduces to Rayleigh-Jean's expression (Kraus, 1966)

$$P(f) = e\,\frac{2\pi k T f^2}{c^2} \qquad (5)$$

which simply indicates that the power density of the emitted radiation is directly proportional to the body's temperature T as well as to its emissivity e. The emitted radiation at these frequencies also has a spectrum whose frequency distribution is proportional to the square of the frequency.

For many years microwave radiometry has been applied to a variety of problems, including radioastronomy, communications, and atmospheric and other remote sensing applications. Calculations based on the gray body theory, however, show that biological systems emit microwave radiation that may be detected by currently available microwave radiometers (Bigu-Del-Blanco and Romero-Sierra, 1975). The major advantage of using the emitted radiation at the microwave frequencies is simply the greater penetration depth compared with that obtained at infrared frequencies where higher radiation intensity is available. The increased depth of penetration permits measurements of microwave radiation from structures within the body. At these lower frequencies, however, coarser spatial resolution than that available with infrared thermography is only possible. The trade-off between the desired depth of penetration and the necessary resolution is an important consideration in determining the operating frequency range in a radiometer experiment. Therefore, depending on the application, measurements have been made in the frequency band between 0.6 and 1 GHz by Enander and Larson (1974) to monitor temperature changes inside the body, at 1.3, 3.3, and 6 GHz by Barrett et al. (1977) and Myers et al. (1979), and at 1.7 GHz by Porter and Miller (1978), both to detect breast cancer. Edrich (Edrich and Hardy, 1974; Edrich, 1979) obtained thermographic images of sections of the human body at 45 GHz, and Bigu-Del-Blanco et al. (1975) used an X-band radiometer at 9.2 GHz to explore possible means of neural communications in biological systems. Leroy (1982) used microwave radiometers operating at various frequencies to develop microwave thermography techniques suitable for application in medical problems. A dual-mode microwave system that combines the use of an active microwave transmitter to achieve heating and a passive microwave radiometer for detecting the presence of tumors has been developed by Nguyen et al. (1979, 1980) and by Carr et al. (1981). These and other recent developments on the use of microwave radiometery in medical applications are described in this section. It should be emphasized, however, that because the intensity of the emitted radiation (Eq. 5) is related to the temperature of the object T as well as to the emissivity e, measurement of this emitted radiation can be used to detect changes in physiological parameters associated with variation in temperature (such as tumor detection and monitoring of arthritis) or to monitor other changes associated with variation in the emissivity value such as changes in lung water content (Iskander et al., 1984). Although most of the medical applications reported in the literature are related to detection of cancer tumors, recent feasibility studies showed the adequacy of the radiometer procedure for measuring changes in lung water (Iskander and Durney, 1983). A more detailed description of the obtained results in various applications is described in the following subsections.

Radiometry Measurement Systems for Medical Applications

The detection and measurement of thermal radiation at microwave frequencies require different techniques from those commonly used for monitoring continuous wave signals of relatively high power levels. The power level of a radiometer signal is usually on the order of 10^{-15} to 10^{-20} W, and receivers of high sensitivity and stability are therefore required. In most of the medical applications described earlier, the Dicke-type radiometers operating at various frequencies were used (Myers et al., 1979). Typical sensitivity of this type of radiometer is 0.1° K, which is certainly adequate for medical applications. A schematic diagram of

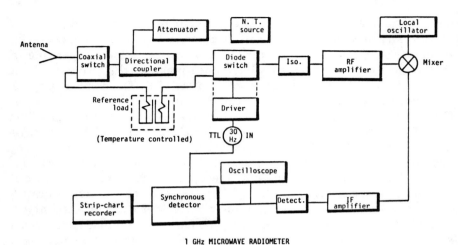

1 GHz MICROWAVE RADIOMETER

Figure 19-14   Schematic diagram of various components of 1 GHz Dicke radiometer. (After Myers, P. C. et al. [1979]. *J. Microwave Power* *14*:105–114.)

a Dicke receiver–type radiometer is shown in Figure 19-14. Although it uses a basic heterodyne method of detection, this radiometer reduces instability limitations by continuously switching the receiver input between the detection antenna and a comparison noise source at a frequency high enough to limit the variation in the system gain during each cycle (Dicke, 1946).

Mamouni et al. (1983) suggested the use of correlation microwave radiometers to improve the ability of localizing thermal gradients and for obtaining a better spatial resolution. A schematic diagram of this radiometer is shown in Figure 19-15. Analysis of the output signal shows that the radiometer output is proportional to the thermal emission of the overlapping volume of material v_i, which is coupled to both receiving probes P_1 and P_2. This simply means that the coupled signal to each antenna, which is related to its receiving pattern, does not directly contribute to the output signal (Mamouni et al., 1983). Such a performance certainly provides an improved resolution over other microwave radiometers, which are often limited by the receiving pattern of the used antenna. Other advantages of this correlation radiometer, including its sensitivity to only temperature gradient in the material covered by both probes, are described elsewhere (Mamouni et al., 1983).

Lüedeke et al. (1979, 1983) addressed some practical problems in using radiometer methods in medical applications. One of the problems they discussed (1979) is related to the variable impedance mismatch between the receiving antenna and the various spots on the surface of the subject under test. These impedance mismatches are the result of

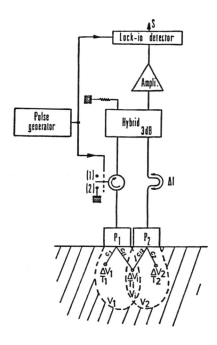

Figure 19-15 Schematic diagram of system of correlation microwave radiometer. (After Mamouni, A., et al. [1983]. *J. Microwave Power* 18:285–293.)

the variation in the thickness of the body tissues (fat, skin, muscle) in the various locations on the body. To overcome this problem, Lüedeke et al. (1979) proposed a system that uses noise injection by a quasilinearly controllable noise source to simulate elevated receiver temperatures electronically. A control loop automatically adjusts the receiver temperature to be equal to the body temperature, and therefore balance occurs. Other extensions in the radiometer techniques to enhance early detection of cancer tumors involve the use of dual systems for heating the tumor site by EM energy at a sufficiently different frequency, such as 27 MHz (Nguyen et al., 1979) or 1.6 GHz (Carr et al., 1981), from that used in the detection system with the radiometer. Although some promising results from this dual system have been reported, much more work is required to verify the usefulness of such a system. It is not clear what drawbacks may be suffered by nonuniformly heating the tumor site (that is, nonuniformities owing to depth of penetration and cross-sectional distributions of heating patterns) against taking advantage of the differential heating of the tumor resulting from the vascular insufficiency associated with it. In fact, Barrett and Myers (1975) reported only marginally positive results when they attempted to detect enhanced microwave emission by artificially inducing an inflammation in the thigh muscle of an anesthetized cat.

A variety of antennas were used in these radiometer measurements.

A straight section of a rectangular waveguide filled with dielectric to reduce its physical size was used in several experiments (Barrett et al., 1977), whereas others used receiving probes such as a small loop (Enander and Larson, 1974) or an elliptical dish antenna (Edrich, 1979). Carr et al. (1981) used a single-ridged waveguide that was dielectrically loaded to further reduce its size. A small (3 × 3 cm^2), double-ridged waveguide that was not dielectrically loaded was used by Iskander and Durney (1983) in measurements at 1 GHz. Achieving lower operating frequencies without dielectric loading is important, since a lower frequency makes it quite easy to control the physical temperature of the receiver (reduce thermal mass) so as to minimize the temperature gradient between the human body and the antenna. The impedance of this double-ridged waveguide is easy to match to the impedance of the human body by simple adjustment of the dimensions and the separation distance between the two ridges. Another broad-band receiver that may be used in these measurements is the transmission line–type receiver described earlier (Iskander and Durney, 1979). A common problem among all antennas used for microwave radiometry measurements is the broad-receiving beamwidth (Iskander and Durney, 1979). For such antennas, not only is the measurement resolution significantly reduced, but also the feasibility of using radiometer measurements for detecting relatively deep-seated and small tumors is seriously diminished. Efforts to develop more directive antennas are desirable.

Results of Experimental Measurements with Radiometers

As indicated earlier, radiometer measurements may be used to monitor physiological changes associated with temperature variations such as tumor detection, or for the measurement of other parameters such as the change in the water content of the lung. Although the first group of these applications is related to using the change in the intensity of the emitted radiation with variation in the temperature, the latter is based on measuring the effect of the variation in the emissivity (such as a result of changes in lung water) on the intensity of the emitted radiation from the body. It should be noted, however, that the success in using the radiometer measurement in one medical application or another is strongly related to the particular application and the specific problems encountered in making the measurement and analyzing the obtained results. For example, radiometry has been used with marginal success to detect breast tumors, especially small tumors. Although many factors have contributed to this conclusion, as will be described later in this section, an important problem was related to the broad radiation patterns of the antennas used, which resulted in averaging the temperature variation over a broad area and hence limiting the sensitivity and the resolution of the method. An analogous problem would not be expected in using radiometry to measure changes in lung water because such high spatial resolution is not required. Measurement of even an average change in lung water is significantly important and highly desirable (Staub, 1983). In the lung water application, on the other hand, it is extremely important to monitor the variation of the body's temperature accurately and continuously during the measurements. This is simply because the intensity of the emitted power is proportional to the emissivity, as well as to the temperature of the body. Therefore, for an accurate and reliable determination of the in-depth change in the lung water content, the variation in the surface temperature should be accurately monitored and accounted for. It is possible to use two or more radiometers operating at frequencies that are sufficiently different (by at least one octave) to monitor surface and at-depth changes separately. It is suggested that the high-frequency radiometer (for example, a millimeter-wave or an X-band radiometer) would measure the average temperature of the chest wall while the low-frequency (microwave) radiometer would provide information on the in-depth changes in lung water content. From this discussion it is clear that various types of problems are encountered in applying the radiometer measurements to different medical problems. In the following paragraphs, results illustrating the adequacy of using radiometry to detect cancer tumors and measure changes in lung water are given.

Microwave thermography for detecting cancerous tumors.   The feasibility of using microwave radiometry to detect breast cancer tumors has been demonstrated by conducting experiments on phantoms (Porter and Miller, 1978) and by clinically screening hundreds of patients (Myers et al., 1979). Results from clinical trials were generally marginal. For example, based on the true-positive (TP) and true-negative (TN) rates of data analysis (Myers et al., 1979), the x-ray procedure was clearly found to be superior in both TP and TN to that of either microwave or infrared techniques. In numerical terms, the microwave, infrared, and x-ray TP rates were 0.73, 0.77, and 0.89, respectively, while the TN rates were 0.73, 0.68, and 0.92, respectively. The hazardous effects associated with exposure to x-rays, as compared with the complete passivity of the microwave and infrared radiometer techniques, encourage further development in the radiometer systems to improve their performance. Another set of clinical data relating to use of the dual-mode microwave system was reported by Carr et al., (1981), who obtained thermograms of 11 women with biopsy-proven primary or current carcinomas of the breast and of four patients with lymphoma. From the results it is clear that temperature differentials $\Delta T > 0$ consistent with the known tumors were found in nine of the 11 breast carcinomas and all four of the lymphomas (Carr

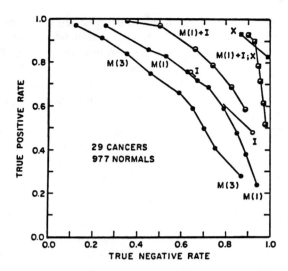

Figure 19-16 Breast cancer detection performance of various combinations of microwave thermography at 1 GHz ($M(1)$) and at 3 GHz ($M(3)$); of infrared thermography (I), and of zeromammography (X). True positive rate is fraction of cancers diagnosed correctly; true negative rate is fraction of normal individuals diagnosed correctly. For each method, family of points depends on choice of detection threshold. Curve labeled $M(1) + I$; X shows result of two-step examination in which 1 GHz and infrared tests are used in first step; x-ray examination is used for follow-up only if first-step test is positive. (After Myers, P. C., et al. [1979]. *J. Microwave Power* 14:105–114.)

et al., 1981). In addition to inconsistencies between the results obtained for some patients with microwave thermograms and xeromammograms, it was indicated that attempts to locate more deeply seated malignancies by microwave thermography have all met with failure.

Another important characteristic of the results may be identified by examining the data in Figure 19-16, which shows the TP and TN performance for approximately 1000 patients, some of them with cancer. Besides the indicated relative superiority of detection at 1 GHz as compared with 3 GHz, the 1 GHz and infrared results showed two definite characteristics (Myers et al., 1979). In particular, it was reported that among the 29 cancer patients examined, 12 (41%) had disagreement in their diagnoses by the microwave and infrared methods. This lack of correlation simply suggests the possibility of combining these two passive methods for clinical screening with no particular concern about the possible hazardous effects, since both methods are passive and hence completely safe. In Figure 19-16 the curve for combined microwave (1 GHz) and infrared thermography shows 10% improvement in the TP detection over either the microwave or the infrared curves alone.

It is clear from the preceding discussion that the conclusions regarding the adequacy of the passive radiometer method for detecting cancer tumors are tentative. More refined experiments should be conducted and better instrumentation developed, particularly for detecting deep-seated tumors. The idea of using correlation radiometers to improve the resolution of the thermographic scans is attractive, but more work is needed to explore its potential properly (Mamouni et al., 1983). Also, more effort should be directed to developing antennas with reduced receiving patterns to help improve the resolution in directly detecting radiometers such as the Dicke receiver types. Recently, successful use of radiometer measurements to image temperature distribution in tumors was reported (Leroy et al., 1987).

Microwave radiometry for measuring changes in lung water content. Because of the occasionally expressed concern regarding the possible hazards of using microwave radiation to measure changes in lung water (see earlier discussion), particularly by continuous monitoring, use of microwave radiometry for making these measurements was described (Iskander et al., 1984a,b). Although, in the active microwave method, incident microwave radiation far below the safety standard was used (Durney et al., 1978), whether long-term effects occur when critically ill patients are monitored on a continuous or long-term basis is unknown. Microwave radiometry, on the other hand, uses the EM radiation emitted naturally from the human body; hence it is passive, unconditionally safe, and suitable for continuous monitoring. Another advantage of microwave radiometry is the need for only one applicator (receiver), which means that a specific microwave path through the thorax does not have to be identified and maintained during the course of measurement. Because the radiometer does not use active signals, it is expected to be free from the problems caused by patient movements that have been associated with the active microwave method.

Recognizing the advantages of using the radiometer for measuring lung water, we pursued two tasks to explore the feasibility of the method (Iskander et al., 1983, 1984). First the change in the brightness temperature (which is proportional to the intensity of the emitted radiation) was calculated as a function of changes in water content in a simplified planar model of the lung. By examining the various components of the lung and identifying the complex permittivity of each, we calculated the change in the emissivity with changes in lung water content (Iskander and Durney, 1983). These changes were then used to calculate variations in the brightness temperature as measured by the radiometer. The results are shown in Figure 19-17, where it is clear that changes in lung water content significantly change the calculated emissivity and hence the brightness temperature as measured by the radiometer. Although these

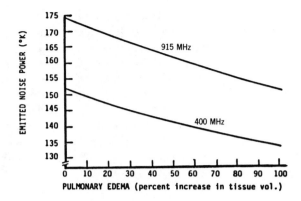

Figure 19-17 Calculated noise power radiated by half space representing lung region as function of degree of pulmonary edema. (After Iskander, M. F., and Durney, C. H. [1983]. *Proc. IEEE 68*:126–132.)

results show that a 1% change in lung water content corresponds to a 0.26° K change in T_B, which is well within the detection capability of currently used radiometers (usually 0.1° K), such optimistic estimations should be moderated by the effect of reflections at the lung-muscle (chest wall) interface and the wave attenuation through the 2 to 3 cm layer of the high-conductivity chest wall. If a planar model of the thorax consisting of three layers, including the lung, a 2 to 3 cm thick layer of high-conductivity chest wall, and skin, is considered, the change in brightness temperature received by the radiometer antenna will be different from the true contribution originating in the lung region. According to the radiative transfer equation (Chandrasekhar, 1950), the two quantities are related by the power transmission coefficients at the interfaces between the various layers and the attenuation in each conductive layer (Edrich, 1979). Assuming an EM field reflection coefficient Γ of 0.5 between the lung and chest wall tissues (Johnson and Guy, 1972), and 60% to 70% attenuation in the chest wall layer in the frequency range from 400 MHz to 1 GHz, currently available radiometers would still be capable of detecting changes in lung water content as small as 3% to 4%, even in a conservative estimate (Iskander and Durney, 1983). Recently an actual multilayer tissue calculation performed with the procedure described by Bardati and Solimini (1984) confirmed these estimates.

The preceding theoretical finding is certainly significant, particularly because it confirms the feasibility of using the passive and safe radiometer technique for measuring early and small changes in lung water content.

To verify the theoretical calculations, Iskander et al. (1984) constructed a standard 1 GHz Dicke receiver–type radiometer and used it to conduct experiments on phantoms. The receiving antenna used in

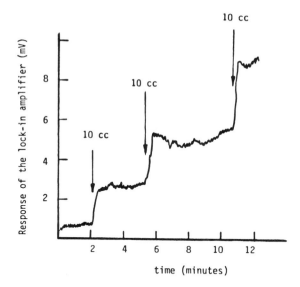

Figure 19-18   Changes in signal received by 1 GHz radiometer as result of injecting water into lung phantom. (After Iskander, M. F., and Durney, C. H. [1983]. *Proc. IEEE 68*:126–132.)

this 1 GHz radiometer was a 3×3 cm^2, open-ended, ridged, waveguide receiver. The results are shown in Figure 19-18, which shows that the radiometer response to changes in water content is definite and immediate. Another important observation is related to the fact that the output signal tends to reach a new steady-state level, which is different from the initial value, after each injection. The peak that occurred after each injection was due to the initial burst of water, which slowly diffused into the sponges, simulating the lung tissue.

In summary therefore the preliminary theoretical and experimental work described in the previous sections clearly shows that microwave radiometry may be used for detecting early and small changes in lung water content. Before this technique can be adopted for clinical use, however, some problems need to be solved. The following fundamental question should be answered first: can in-depth radiation from the lung be satisfactorily detected in the presence of strong emission from the body surface? The idea of using two or more precision radiometers with operating frequencies separated by at least one octave (that is, a millimeter-wave radiometer to measure average chest wall temperature and a low-frequency microwave radiometer that, when properly calibrated, would provide accurate information on the in-depth changes in lung water content) is intriguing and deserves exploration.

ELECTROMAGNETIC IMAGING TECHNIQUES

With the significant advances in developing x-ray and ultrasound imaging techniques, including improving the resolution and reducing the data collection time, investigation is being directed to other imaging methods. EM imaging is particularly attractive, since it provides a complex permittivity image that is different from the information available from the other types of images. EM methods might also help in imaging organs such as the lung, where the use of x-ray or ultrasound imaging is insensitive and generally difficult. Based on a rough estimate of the level of EM radiation required for imaging, the EM imaging procedure should provide an alternative to the excessive exposure to x-ray radiation in certain medical applications.

Spectacular advances have been made in nuclear magnetic resonance (NMR) imaging since it was conceived 15 years ago. Since Paul Lauterbur published the first image in 1973, numerous scan systems and data generation and collection procedures have been developed (Lauterbur, 1973; Mansfield et al., 1976; Hinshaw et al., 1978). Unlike the other EM techniques, NMR imaging has produced true pictures of anatomical sections of the human body (Foster, 1984; Foster and Hutchison, 1987). In addition to the excellent resolution obtained, which in many ways is comparable to that of computerized tomographic (CT) scans, NMR imaging may provide valuable information about the functional and physiological state of internal organs and further distinguish between healthy and diseased tissue (Coles, 1976; Damadian et al., 1976). Recent efforts include the development and practically realization of fast-imaging techniques (Haacke, 1988; Van Der Meulen et al., 1988), improvement in the quality of NMR images, and expression of the biological and clinical significance of the obtained images (Podo, 1988).

Since NMR imaging is strictly an extension of the NMR spectroscopy and has been developed mostly by chemists and physicists who previously worked in this area, it is debatable whether such a technique should be included among potential EM methods. NMR imaging has achieved tremendous success, and fortunately for those of us who work in the EM area, interesting EM problems are associated with the use of RF energy in this imaging method. Among these problems are realistic evaluation of the biological hazards associated with the use of RF fields, study of the effect of EM attenuation and change in phase, particularly at higher frequencies, on the quality of the produced images, and use of multifrequency selective RF pulses for multislice NMR imaging (Müller, 1988).

In the following discussion, brief descriptions of the EM imaging methods are given with special emphasis on the problems involved in each and the ongoing efforts to solve these problems.

Low-Frequency Electrical Impedance Imaging

As indicated previously, electrical impedance measurements have been used to monitor various physiological parameters, including cardiac output, stroke volume, lung water content, and many others. This section discusses the feasibility of using the impedance method to reconstruct the impedance distribution within the body from information measured at its surface. Although many attempts at imaging conductivity distributions have been made (Lytle and Dines, 1978; Schomberg, 1981; Kim et al., 1983), debate continues on the impossibility of obtaining these images (Bates et al., 1980). The basic problem centers on the nonstraight current streamlines between the imaging electrodes. In contrast to x-ray imaging, in electrical impedance imaging the path of the electric current depends on the conductivity distribution in the cross section being imaged and is not always a nearly straight line. Therefore the coordinates of these current paths are not known in advance and can be determined only after the spatial distribution of the complex permittivity (or the conductivity) of the body is identified.

As a result, the x-ray imaging problem is usually reduced to finding a solution for a linear system of equations in the form $[c][\mathbf{d}] = [P]$, where $[c]$ is a coefficient matrix, $[\mathbf{d}]$ is a vector representing the unknown densities, and $[P]$ is the measured attenuation factor. In EM imaging the resulting system of equations is of the form (Schomberg, 1981) $[c(d)][\mathbf{d}] = [P]$ where the coefficient matrix $c(d)$ depends on the solution d. The problem is therefore nonlinear, and the currently available algorithms cannot be applied directly in the case of EM imaging. Bates et al. (1980) showed that the straightforward impedance CT approach cannot be used to obtain a conductivity image from a measured finite number of projections. Instead, nonlinear and possibly iterative reconstruction procedures are required. Tasto and Schomberg (1978) suggested a simple extension of the well-known algebraic reconstruction technique (ART) for low-frequency conductivity imaging. The proposed extension involves determining the electric potential V interior to the object by solving Laplace's equation $\nabla \cdot (\sigma \nabla V) = 0$ numerically. An initial conductivity profile is first assumed, and the potential computation, subject to the given boundary conditions, is then performed by means of the finite-difference method. The current entering or leaving each electrode follows the gradient of the potential field. Once these streamlines are known, a line integral similar to that encountered in the x-ray reconstruction can be determined and the reconstruction procedure continues in a manner similar to the x-ray case.

In an iterative reconstruction procedure the calculation of the electric potential is performed after each iteration and the current streamlines are modified accordingly. Kim et al. (1983) employed a similar procedure to reconstruct images from simulated data on simple phantoms. In addition to solving Laplace's equation for every iteration, they used a back-projection algorithm to modify the impedance profile. Specifically they used eight projections, and instead of determining current paths, their reconstruction algorithm used a perturbation method to relate changes in the resistivity of one element to the change in the values of the current densities at all the sensing electrodes. This perturbation process forms what is called a sensitivity matrix for each projection. In the back-pro-

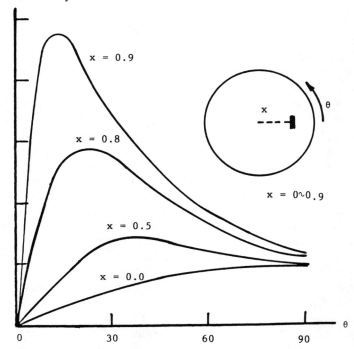

Figure 19-19 Relative sensitivity of electrical impedance measurement as function of location of impedance inhomogeneity. Coordinate (x, θ) shows position of inhomogeneity. It is shown that 1 cm × 1 cm inhomogeneity with 10% difference in conductivity would result in 10^{-5} potential difference measured at periphery of 13 cm radius homogeneous cylinder. This example illustrates difficulties in obtaining detailed cross section of conductivity image. (After Mochdizuke, A., et al. [1981]. Impedance computed tomography and the design of hyperthermia. Presented at the 5th International Conference on Electrical Bio-Impedance, Tokyo. Tokyo, Business Center for Academic Societies Japan.

jected algorithm therefore the modified value of each element's resistivity is related to its previous value by the equation (Kim et al., 1983)

$$r_i^n = r_i^{n-1} + k \frac{\sum\limits_{j=1}^{M} RC_j^n \, T_{ij}}{\sum\limits_{k=1}^{M} |T_{ik}|} - r_i^{n-1} \tag{6}$$

where r_i^n and r_i^{n-1} are the resistivity values of element i after n and $(n-1)$ iterations, k is a relaxation factor that sets the rate of convergence, T_{ij} and T_{ik} are the sensitivity matrix entries, and RC_j^n is the difference between calculated and measured current densities at the current sensing electrode j in the nth iteration. Although no attempt was made to reconstruct images of humans, the results from the data-simulated computer runs were encouraging. Depending on the initial assumption of the conductivity distribution, the solutions were found to converge after 30 to 150 iterations (Kim et al., 1983).

In a similar effort, Mochdizuki et al. (1981) pointed out interesting aspects regarding the sensitivity of the impedance-computed tomography. It was indicated that an inhomogeneous area of 1×1 cm^2 with 10% difference in conductivity from the surrounding medium, which is a homogeneous cylinder of 13 cm radius, produces only 10^{-5} in potential difference on the contour (Mochdizuki et al., 1981). Some of the obtained results are shown in Figure 19-19, where it is clear that inhomogeneity nearer to the surface is easier to detect. These sample calculations certainly illustrate some of the difficulties associated with electrical impedance tomography. Another difficulty associated with impedance tomography is related to the procedure's inadequacy to image a high-resistance region when surrounded by a highly conducting one. This is simply because of the preferred current path through the high-conductivity tissue. This difficulty is clearly illustrated in the set of images obtained by Lytle and Dines (1978) (Figure 19-20). These images were obtained with the straight-line ART algorithm and clearly illustrate the inability of the procedure even when simulated data are used to reconstruct the high-resistance region in the middle section of the object.

It is clear that, although some efforts were successful in obtaining adequate impedance images, other investigators are still pessimistic about the possibility of reconstructing these types of images. A special issue of the *Clinical Physics and Physiological Measurement Journal* titled "Electrical Impedance Tomography–Applied Potential Tomography" was published in 1987 (Brown et al., 1987). Articles in this issue addressed a wide range of topics varying from theoretical estimates of limitations to sensitivity and resolution in impedance imaging to the clinician's view

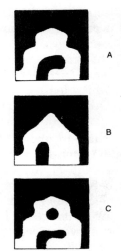

Figure 19-20 A, Conductivity profile with white and black colors representing conductivities of 0.015 and 0.005 S/m, respectively. **B,** Conductivity image obtained after one iteration. **C,** Image obtained after two iterations. In all cases it is not possible to image low-conductivity region when surrounded with high-conductivity one. (After Lytle, R. J., and Dines, K. A. [1978]. An impedance camera: a system for determining the spatial variation of electrical conductivity. Livermore, Calif., Lawrence Livermore Laboratories, No. UCRL-52413.)

of evaluating applied potential tomography. Some reconstruction algorithms were described and examples of potential application of this imaging technology in monitoring human breast temperature mapping in hyperthermia (Conway et al., 1985) and in localizing cardiac-related impedance changes in the thorax were presented.

High-Frequency Permittivity Imaging

Undoubtedly, low-frequency conductivity imaging is much simpler than complex permittivity imaging at higher frequencies. At lower frequencies the process is scalar, which simplifies the mathematics, and the measurements are also relatively easier. This explains the limited literature available on high-frequency EM imaging (Jacobi and Larsen, 1978, 1980; Larsen and Jacobi, 1978, 1980; Maini et al., 1981; Johnson et al., 1983; Ghodgaonkar et al., 1983; Slaney et al., 1984; Pichot et al., 1985). Imaging at higher frequencies, on the other hand, has certain advantages over the low-frequency impedance imaging procedure. For example, it is clear from the differences between these two techniques listed in Table 19-1 that a high-frequency imaging procedure would overcome the difficulty of imaging a low-conductivity region when surrounded by a high-conductivity one. The solution of this problem is particularly important in medical imaging, since the human thorax, including the lung region, is surrounded by a highly conducting chest wall. Certainly the introduction of an array of guarded electrodes would improve the procedure, but nevertheless a complex permittivity image is useful to have.

Among the few publications available on microwave imaging is the work by Maini et al. (1981) in which they used the method of moment computer program (Iskander et al., 1981) to evaluate the feasibility of the linear reconstruction technique for microwave imaging. The results were fairly encouraging in two-dimensional cross sections of the thorax, which led to the use of the ART to develop images of simple objects. Other numerical efforts include the estimation of the complex permittivities of three-dimensional inhomogeneous biological objects recently described by Ghodgaonkar et al. (1983). The process is based on an inverse solution of the method of moments computer program developed to calculate the EM power absorption pattern in block models of humans (Hagmann et al., 1979). Difficulties were encountered in this approach, particularly that the inverse problem was ill posed and unsolvable for a larger number of buried cells (Ghodgaonkar et al., 1983). Further improvement in the procedure, which is related to the use of more than one measurement of projection in the method of moments inverse program, was discussed later (Johnson et al., 1983)

Diffraction tomography appears suitable for providing good images of inhomogeneous objects (Pichot et al., 1985). When the object inhomogeneities become comparable to a wavelength, it is not appropriate to talk about propagation along lines or rays. Despite these difficulties, good images were obtained with techniques based on the Fourier diffrac-

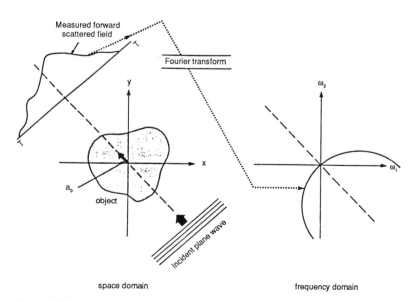

Figure 19-21   Fourier diffraction projection theorem. (After Slaney, M., et al. [1984]. *IEEE Trans. Microwave Theory Tech.* 32:860–874.)

tion projection theorem (Pan and Kak, 1983). This theorem states that, when an object is illuminated with a plane wave as shown in Figure 19-21, the Fourier transform of the forward scattered fields measured on a line perpendicular to the direction of propagation gives the values of the two-dimensional Fourier transform of the object along a circular arc, as shown in Figure 19-21. By combining the Fourier transforms of the forward scattered fields for incident waves propagating in different directions, one would have sufficient information in the frequency domain to obtain a tomographic image by taking the inverse transform (Pichot et al., 1985). Major limitations of this imaging procedure are that the Fourier diffraction theorem is valid only when the inhomogeneities in the object are weakly scattering (Slaney et al., 1984) and that the resulting images are for the induced polarization current distribution in the object rather than of the complex permittivity, which is the desirable quantity.

Regarding the experimental efforts to obtain microwave images, the reported experimental results have presented an optimistic picture of the feasibility of developing microwave images. Rao et al. (1980), for example, used x-ray CT scan algorithms to develop promising microwave images at 10.5 GHz. They moved the object along the middle line between the transmitting and receiving antennas and obtained the various projections by rotating the object after each traversal. The obtained resolution is about a wavelength in the liquid filling the scanning tank. Larsen and Jacobi (1978, 1980) reported several experimental possibilities of obtaining microwave images. Some of the measurements were based on scanning the transmission coefficient (insertion loss) through the object, whereas others were based on the use of difference in polarization between the incident microwave signal and the one transmitted through the object. Images of inhomogeneous bodies obtained with diffraction imaging were also reported (Pichot et al., 1985).

In conclusion, the importance of developing new procedures for medical imaging, such as microwave imaging, has been recognized. However, all reported efforts are still preliminary, and because of the difficulty of the problem, a significant advancement in this imaging procedure has not yet been made.

Nuclear Magnetic Resonance Imaging

Initial NMR imaging methods are based on extending the NMR spectroscopy procedure to obtain projections of the proton density distribution in the object (Lauterbur, 1973). In regular NMR spectroscopy it is important to use a static magnetic field that is uniform throughout the sample under test. In this way the measured NMR signal is expected to be in the form of a narrow peak that includes contributions from all nuclei of the same type. For molecules of complex structure, however, shifts in the resonance frequency of the NMR signals occur, and these "chemical shifts" are often used to study the molecular structure of the material under test. As indicated earlier, to relate these shifts to the chemical structure, the investigator must maintain uniform static magnetic fields. Lauterbur (1973) showed this by *intentionally* applying a density distribution in the sample under test integrated over planes perpendicular to the gradient directions. His procedure to obtain a two-dimensional image therefore consisted simply of rotating the object to obtain several of these projections and combining the projections by means of one of the available imaging algorithms (Brooks and Dichiro, 1976). This imaging procedure was then extended to improve the sensitivity and the resolution of the image, reduce the data collection time, or obtain on-line imaging (Kumar et al., 1975). The spatial resolution of an NMR image is unlike those obtained by different imaging systems because it does not depend on the frequency of the RF radiation used to construct the image. The resolution of an NMR image is basically related to the size of the region of interaction between the static magnetic and RF fields and the shift produced by the gradient of the magnetic field. Depending on the imaging procedure, the obtained images may display the density distribution of hydrogen or other nuclei, such as phosphorus, in the object (Pykett, 1982), the spin-spin relaxation time T_2, the spin lattice relaxation time T_1, or a combination of these (Damadian et al., 1976; Goldsmith et al., 1977). The preference in choosing to image one parameter rather than another depends on the sensitivity of the imaged parameter to the physiological (medical) function of interest. For example, reports have indicated differences in the relaxation times T_1 and T_2 between normal and tumor tissues (Coles, 1976). Therefore displaying these parameters in the images may simply lead to tumor detection by NMR. NMR imaging has come a long way (Foster and Hutchison, 1987). Several methods for selecting imaged slices have been developed, contrast agents are now available for clinical use, and fast imaging techniques have been practically realized.

A few interesting RF problems in NMR imaging require further study. The first is related to realistic evaluation of the hazardous effects associated with the RF radiation and fast-switching magnetic field gradients. Some studies have concluded that such imaging procedures are safe (Gadian and Robinson, 1979; Foster and Hutchison, 1987). Müller (1988) described a method for multislice imaging by means of pulses that contain a multifrequency excitation spectrum. This method, although attractive, requires spacing between adjacent slices and also requires higher levels of RF power. It is, however, an interesting RF problem, and more work to solve the remaining limitations is justified. A procedure to improve the signal-to-noise ratio in NMR imaging is by increasing the strength of the static magnetic field used. Higher RF frequencies are therefore required to maintain the same Larmor frequency of the proton nuclei. Orcutt and Gandhi (1988) analyzed the coupling of NMR-related RF fields with an anatomically based model of the human body and showed that fairly low rates of energy deposition (0.7 to 1 W/kg peak) are encountered (see Figure 6-2). These higher RF frequencies, however, may result in a further image distortion owing to the nonuniformity of the RF fields inside the human body because of the depth of penetration. Also, in this frequency range (10 to 60 MHz) the human object absorbs more RF power with the increase in the exposure frequency (Durney et al., 1978). A detailed evaluation of the trade-offs is needed to improve and elucidate the effects of NMR imaging.

CONCLUSION

A large variety of EM techniques that are potentially useful for medical applications are presented in this chapter. These methods use active and passive EM radiation for measuring various physiological activities in the human body. Imaging of the human body by means of either low-frequency electrical impedance cameras or microwave imaging techniques seems to be progressing steadily. More sophisticated numerical procedures for accounting for the current bending in the electrical impedance imaging methods are being developed (Brown et al., 1987), and reasonably accurate images are available. The use of Fourier diffraction methods in microwave imaging is promising, although serious research work is still needed to overcome the limitations of this imaging procedure. Among the remaining problems in this technique is the use of first-order Born and Rytov approximations, the inability to account for the high attenuation in biological systems, and the limitation of the analysis procedure to plane-wave incident excitation. Efforts to overcome some of these problems are under way in several institutions.

NMR imaging is a different matter. Beginning in the late 1970s, when the first recognizable images of the human brain were shown, major manufacturers of x-ray equipment intensified their efforts to improve the technique and produce commercial models. The property that makes NMR imaging so important is its ability to characterize human tissue by displaying the distribution and relaxation characteristics of water protons in the tomographic sections under examination. Thus the tissues and organs of the body can be characterized by properties that were not accessible to previous imaging systems, and additional clinical information can be expected. Magnetic resonance (MR) imaging has emerged as an established biomedical technique with widespread clinical use. Recent research trends include further developing fast-imaging procedures, improving the quality of MR images, and accurately relating the obtained images to pathophysiological information important to clinical treatments and biological studies. In other words, although research programs are being carried out in several medical centers to evaluate the applicability of MR imaging, technological and biomedical research is still needed for assessing the clinical value of tissue characterization by MR imaging. It is unlikely that the phenomenal commercialization of MR imaging will be met with similar developments in active and passive microwave imaging. Academic curiosity, however, is sustaining progress in this area.

REFERENCES

ABBEY, J.C., AND CLOSE, L. (1983). Electrical impedance measurement of urinary bladder fullness. *J. Microwave Power 18*:305–309.

AOYAGI, T., FUSE, M., YOSHINISA, T., HORIKAWA, M., SUGIYAMA, Y., AND KANEMOTO, N. (1981). A study to assess pulmonary circulation by impedance method. *In*: Proceedings of the 5th International Conference on Electrical Bio-Impedance, Tokyo. Tokyo, Business Center for Academic Societies Japan, pp. 401–404.

BAKER, L.E., JUDY, W.V., GEDDES, L.A., LANGLEY, F.M., AND HILL, D.W. (1971). The measurement of cardiac output by means of electrical impedance. *Cardiovasc. Res. Cent. Bull. 9*:135–145.

BARDATI, F., AND SOLIMINI, D. (1984). On the permissivity of layered materials. *IEEE Trans. Geosci. 22*:374–376.

BARRETT, A.H., AND MYERS, P.C. (1975). Subcutaneous temperature: a method of noninvasive sensing. *Science 190*:669–671.

BARRETT, A.E., MYERS, P.C., AND SADOWSKY, N.L. (1977). Detection of breast cancer by microwave radiometry. *Radio Sci. 12*:167s–171s.

BATES, R.H.T., MCKINNON, G.C., AND SEAGAR, A.D. (1980). A limitation on systems for imaging electrical conductivity distribution. *IEEE Trans. Biomed. Eng. 27*:418–420.

BATTOCLETTI, J.H., HALBACH, R.E., SALLES-CUNHA, S.X., AND SANCES, A. (1983). Nuclear magnetic resonance and transcutaneous electromagnetic blood-flow measurement. *J. Microwave Power 18*:221–232.

BIGU-DEL-BLANCO, J., ROMERO-SIERRA, C., AND WATTS, D.G. (1975). Microwave radiometry and its potential applications in biology and medicine: experimental studies. *Biotelemetry 2*:298–316.

BLEICHER, W., STEIL, E., FIDERER, F., WOLF, M., AND FAUST, U. (1981). Noninvasive monitoring of heart function with the aid of the automatically processed impedance cardiogram. *In*: Proceedings of the 5th International Conference on Electrical Bio-Impedance, Tokyo. Tokyo, Business Center for Academic Societies Japan, pp. 57–60.

BROOKS, R.A., AND DICHIRO, G. (1976). Principles of computer assisted tomography (CAT) in radiographic and radioisotopic imaging. *Phys. Med. Biol. 21*:689–732.

BROWN, B.H., BARBER, D.C., AND TARRASENKO, L. (eds.) (1987). Special issue of *Clin. Phys. Physiol. Measure. 8*(supp. A).

BURDETTE, E.C., KAROW, A.M., JR., AND JESKE, A.H. (1978). Design, development, and performance of an electromagnetic illumination system for thawing cryopreserved kidneys of rabbits and dogs. *Cryobiology 15*:152–167.

BURDETTE, E.C., PITAL, D.J., AND BURNS, M.A. (1982). Effect of hyperthermia on solid tumor dielectric properties and blood flow. Presented at the 4th Annual Bioelectromagnetics Society Meeting, June 28–July 2, 1982, Los Angeles.

BUTCHER, S., BUTCHER, L., HARMS, M., AND JENDEN, D. (1976). Fast fixation of brain *in situ* by high intensity microwave irradiation: application to neurochemical studies. *J. Microwave Power 11*:61–65.

CAPPELEN, C., JR., AND HALL, K.V. (1967). Electromagnetic blood flowmetry in clinical surgery. *Acta Chir. Scand. Suppl. 368*:3–37.

CARR, K.L., EL-MAHDI, A.M., AND SHAEFFER, J. (1981). Dual-mode microwave system to enhance early detection of cancer. *IEEE Trans. Microwave Theory Tech. 29*:256–260.

CHANDRASEKHAR, S. (1950). Radiative transfer. London, Oxford University Press.

COLES, B.A. (1976). Dual-frequency proton spin relaxation measurements on tissues from normal and tumor bearing mice. *J. Natl. Cancer Inst. 57*:389–393.

CONWAY, J., HAWLEY, M.S., SEAGAR, A.-D., BROWN, B.H., AND BARBER, D.C. (1985). Applied potential tomography (APT) for noninvasive thermal imaging during hyperthermia treatment. *Electron. Lett. 21*:836–838.

COOLEY, W.L., AND LONGINI, R.L. (1968). A new design for an impedance pneumograph. *J. Appl. Physiol. 25*:429–432.

DAMADIAN, R., MINKOFF, L., GOLDSMITH, J., STANFORD, M., AND KOUTCHER, J. (1976). Field focusing nuclear magnetic resonance (FONAR): visualization of a tumor in a live animal. *Science 194*:1430–1432.

DENNISTON, J.D., AND BAKER, L.E. (1975). Measurement of urinary bladder emptying using electrical impedance. *Med. Biol. Eng. 13*:305–330.

DICKE, R.H. (1946). The measurement of thermal radiation at microwave frequencies. *Rev. Sci. Instr. 17*:268–275.

DURNEY, C.H., AND ISKANDER, M.F. (1988). Antennas for medical application. *In*: Lo, Y.T., and Lee, S.W. (eds.). Antenna handbook: theory applications and design. New York, Van Nostrand Reinhold Co. Inc.

DURNEY, C.H., ISKANDER, M.F., AND BRAGG, D.G. (1978). Noninvasive microwave methods for measuring changes in lung water content. *Proc. IEEE Electro. 78*, Boston, session 30.

DURNEY, C.H., JOHNSON, C.C., BARBER, P.W., et al. (1978). Radiofrequency radiation dosimetry handbook, 2nd ed. USAF School of Aerospace Medicine, Brooks Air Force Base, Tex., Contract No. SAM-TR-78–22.

EDRICH, J. (1979). Centimeter- and millimeter-wave thermography—a survey on tumor detection. *J. Microwave Power 14*:95–104.

EDRICH, J., AND HARDEE, P.C. (1974). Thermography at millimeter-wavelength. *Proc. IEEE 62*:1391–1392.

ENANDER, B., AND LARSON, G. (1974). Microwave radiometric measurements of the temperature inside the body. *Electron. Lett. 10*:317.

FOSTER, M.A. (1984). Magnetic resonance in medicine and biology. Oxford, Eng., Pergamon Press.

FOSTER, M.A., AND HUTCHISON, J.M.S. (1987). Practical NMR imaging. Oxford, Eng., IRL Press.

FRÖHLICH, H. (1978). Coherent electric vibrations in biological systems and the cancer problem. *IEEE Trans. Microwave Theory Tech. 26*:613–617.

FUSE, M., YOSHINISA, T., SUGIYAMA, Y., AND OHTA, Y. (1981). Changes in electrical impedance due to the shapes and locations of the electrode by multi-impedance method. *In*: Proceedings of the 5th International Conference on Electrical Bioimpedance, Tokyo. Tokyo, Business Center for Academic Societies Japan, pp. 77–80.

GADIAN, D.G., AND ROBINSON, F.N.H. (1979). Radiofrequency losses in NMR experiments on electrically-conducting samples. *J. Magnet. Reson. 34*:449–455.

GANDHI, O.P. (1983). Some basic properties of biological tissues for potential biomedical applications of millimeter waves. *J. Microwave Power 18*:295–304.

GANDHI, O.P., HAGMANN, M.J., HILL, D.W., PARTLOW, L.M., AND BUSH, L. (1980). Millimeter-wave absorption spectra of biological samples. *Bioelectromagnetics 1*:285–298.

GHODGAONKAR, D.K., GANDHI, O.P., AND HAGMANN, M.J. (1983). Estimation of complex permittivities of three-dimensional inhomogeneous biological models. *IEEE Trans. Microwave Theory Tech. 31*:442–446.

GOLDSMITH, M., KOUTCHER, J.A., AND DAMADIAN, R. (1977). Nuclear magnetic resonance in cancer. XII. Application of NMR malignancy index to human lung tumors. *Br. J. Cancer 36*:235–242.

GRAHAM, M. (1965). Guard ring use in physiological measurements. *IEEE Trans. Biomed. Eng. 12*:197–198.

GUIDOTTI, A., CHENEY, D., TRABUCHHI, M., WANG, C., AND HAWKINS, R. (1974). Focused microwave radiation: a technique to miminize postmortem changes of cyclic nucleotides, dopa, and choline and to preserve brain morphology. *Neuropharmacology 13*:1115–1122.

HAACKE, E.M. (1988). *Magn. Reson. Imaging. 6*(4):353–354.

HAGMANN, M.J., GANDHI, O.P., AND DURNEY, C.H. (1979). Numerical calculation of electromagnetic energy deposition for a realistic model of man. *IEEE Trans. Microwave Theory Tech. 27*:804–809.

HENDERSON, R.P., AND WEBSTER, J.G. (1978). An impedance camera for specific measurements of the thorax. *IEEE Trans. Biomed. Eng. 25*:250–254.

HINSHAW, W.S., ANDREW, E.R., BOTTOMLEY, P.A., HOLLAND, G.N., AND MOORE, W.S. (1978). Display of cross-sectional anatomy by nuclear magnetic resonance imaging. *Br. J. Radiol. 51*:273–280.

ISKANDER, M.F. (1984). Apparatus and method for measuring lung water content. U.S. Patent No. 4,488,559.

ISKANDER, M.F., AND DURNEY, C.H. (1979). An electromagnetic energy coupler for medical applications. *Proc. IEEE 67*:1463–1465.

ISKANDER, M.F., AND DURNEY, C.H. (1980a). Electromagnetic techniques for medical diagnosis: a review. *Proc. IEEE 68*:126–132.

ISKANDER, M.F., AND DURNEY,C.H. (1980b). Electromagnetic energy coupler/receiver apparatus and method. U.S. Patent No. 4,240,445.

ISKANDER, M.F., AND DURNEY, C.H. (1983). Microwave methods for measuring changes in lung water. *J. Microwave Power 18*:265–275.

ISKANDER, M.F., DURNEY, C.H., BRAGG, D.G., AND OVARD, B.H. (1982a). A microwave method for estimating absolute value of average lung water. *Radio Sci. 17*:111s–117s.

ISKANDER, M.F., DURNEY, C.H., GRANGE, T., AND SMITH, C.S. (1984). A microwave radiometer for measuring changes in lung water content. *IEEE Trans. Microwave Theory Tech. 32*:554–556.

ISKANDER, M.F., DURNEY, C.H., AND JONES, S.S. (1982b). An improved microwave method for measuring changes in lung water content. Presented at the 4th Annual Meeting of the Bioelectromagnetics Society, June 28–July 2, 1982, Los Angeles.

ISKANDER, M.F., DURNEY, C.H., SHOFF, D.J., AND BRAGG, D.G. (1979). Diagnosis of pulmonary edema by a surgically noninvasive microwave technique. *Radio Sci. 14*:265–269.

ISKANDER, M.F., MAINI, R., DURNEY, C.H., AND BRAGG, D.G. (1981). A microwave method for measuring changes in lung water content: numerical simulation. *IEEE Trans. Biomed. Eng. 28*:797–804.

JACOBI, J.H., AND LARSEN, L.E. (1978). Microwave interrogation of dielectric targets. II. By microwave time delay spectroscopy. *Med. Phys. 5*:509–513.

JACOBI, J.H., AND LARSEN, L.E. (1980). Microwave time delay spectroscopic dimagery of isolated canine kidney. *Med. Phys. 7*:1–7.

JOHNK, C.T.A. (1975). Engineering electromagnetic fields and waves. New York, John Wiley & Sons.

JOHNSON, C.C., AND GUY, A.W. (1972). Nonionizing electromagnetic wave effects in biological materials and systems. *Proc. IEEE 60*:692–718.

JOHNSON, S.A., YOON, T.-H., AND RA, J.-W. (1983). Inverse scattering solutions of the scalar Helmholtz wave equation by a multiple source, moment method. *Electron. Lett. 19*:130.

KANAI, H. (ed.) (1981). *In*: Proceedings of 5th International Conference on Electrical Bio-Impedance, Aug. 24–26, Tokyo. Tokyo, Business Center for Academic Societies Japan.

KIM, Y., WEBSTER, J.G., AND TOMPKINS, W.J. (1983). Electrical impedance imaging of the thorax. *J. Microwave Power 18*:245–257.

KOLIN, A. (1936). Electromagnetic flowmeter: principle of method and its application to blood flow measurements. *Proc. Soc. Exp. Biol. Med. 35*:53–56.

KRAUS, J.D. (1966). Radio astronomy. New York, McGraw-Hill Book Co.

KUBICEK, W.G., KARNEGIS, J.N., PATTERSON, R.P., WITSOE, D.A., AND MATTSON, R.H. (1966). Development and evaluation of an impedance cardiac output system. *Aerospace Med. 37*:1208–1212.

KUBICEK, W.G., KOTTKE, F.J., RAMOS, M.U. et al. (1974). The Minnesota impedance cardiography—theory and applications. *IEEE Trans. Biomed. Eng. 9*:410–416.

KUMAR, A., WELTI, D., AND ERNST, R.R. (1975). NMR Fourier zeugmatography. *J. Magnet. Reson. 18*:69–83.

LAMBERT, R.K., AND GREMELS, H. (1926). On the factors concerned in the production of pulmonary edema. *J. Physiol. 61*:98–112.

LARSEN, L.E., AND JACOBI, J.H. (1978). Microwave interrogation of dielectric targets 1. By scattering parameters. *Med. Phys. 5*:500–508.

LARSEN, L.E., AND JACOBI, J.H. (1980). The use of orthogonal polarizations in microwave imagery of isolated canine kidney. *IEEE Trans. Nucl. Sci. 27*:1184–1191.

LAUTERBUR, P.C. (1973). Image formation by induced local interactions: examples employing nuclear magnetic resonance. *Nature 242*:190–191.

LEE, R.A., AND WEBB, S.J. (1977). Possible detection of *in vivo* viruses by fine-structure millimeter-wave spectroscopy between 68 and 76 GHz. *IRCS Med. Sci. 174*:72–74.

LENOX, R., GANDHI, O.P., MEYERHOFF, J., AND GROVE, M. (1976). A microwave applicator for *in vivo* rapid inactivation of enzymes in the central nervous system. *IEEE Trans. Microwave Theory Tech. 24*:58–61.

LEROY, Y. (1982). Microwave thermography for biomedical applications. Presented at the 12th European Microwave Conference, September, Helsinki, Finland.

LEROY, Y., MAMOUNI, A., VAN DE VELDE, J.C., BOCQUET, B., AND DUJARDIN, B. (1987). Microwave radiometry for noninvasive thermometry. *Automedica 8*:181–202.

LIN, J.C., AND CLARKE, M.J. (1982). Microwave imaging of cerebral edema. *Proc. IEEE 70*:523–524.

LU, K.C., PROHOFSKY, E.W., AND VAN ZANDT, L.L. (1977). Vibrational modes of A-DNA, B-DNA, and A-RNA backbones: an application of a Green function refinement procedure. *Biopolymers 16*:2491–2506.

LÜEDEKE, K.M., KOHLER, J., AND KANZENBACH, J. (1979). A new radiation balance microwave thermography for simultaneous and independent temperature and emissivity measurements. *J. Microwave Power 14*:117–121.

LÜEDEKE, K.M., KOHLER, J. (1983). Microwave radiometric system for biomedical "true temperature" and emissivity measurements. *J. Microwave Power 18*:277–283.

LYTLE, R.J., AND DINES, K.A. (1978). An impedance camera: a system for determining the spatial variation of electrical conductivity. Livermore, Calif., Lawrence Livermore Laboratories, No. UCRL-52413.

MAINI, R. (1981). A microwave method of lung water measurements. M.S. Thesis, Dept. Electrical Engineering, University of Utah, Salt Lake City.

MAINI, R., ISKANDER, M.F., AND DURNEY, C.H. (1981). On the electromagnetic imaging using linear reconstruction techniques. *Proc. IEEE 68*:1550–1552.

MAMOUNI, A., LEROY, Y., VANDEVELDE, D., AND BALLARBI, L. (1983). Introduction to correlation thermography. *J. Microwave Power 18*:285–293.

MANSFIELD, P., MAUDSLEY, A.A., AND BAINES, T. (1976). Fast scan proton density imaging by NMR. *J. Phys. E. Sci. Instrum. 9*:271–278.

MERRITT, J.H., AND FRAZER, J.W. (1977). Microwave fixation of brain tissue as a neurochemical technique—a review. *J. Microwave Power* 12:133–139.

MOCHDIZUKI, A., TAKADA, H., AND SAITO, M. (1981). Impedance computed tomography and the design of hyperthermia. *In*: Proceedings of the 5th International Conference on Electrical Bio-Impedance, Aug. 24–26, Tokyo. Tokyo, Business Centers for Academic Societies Japan.

MÜLLER, S. (1988). Multifrequency selective RF pulses for multislice MR imaging. *Magnet. Reson. Med.* 6:364–371.

MYERS, P.C., SADOWSKY, N.L., AND BARRETT, A.H. (1979). Microwave thermography: principles, methods and clinical applications. *J. Microwave Power* 14:105–114.

NGUYEN, D.D., CHIVE, M., LEROY, Y., AND CONSTANT, E. (1980). Combination of local heating and radiometry by microwaves. *IEEE Trans. Instrument. Measure.* 29:143–144.

NGUYEN, D.D., MAMOUNI, A., LEROY, Y., AND CONSTANT, E. (1979). Simultaneous microwave local heating and microwave thermography: possible clinical applications. *J. Microwave Power* 14:135–137.

NYBOER, J. (1959). Electrical impedance plethysmography. Springfield, Ill., Charles C Thomas, Publisher.

ORCUTT, N., AND GANDHI, O.P. (1988). A 3-D impedance method to calculate power deposition in biological bodies subjected to time-varying magnetic fields. *IEEE Trans. Biomed. Eng.* 35:577–583.

OVARD, B.H. (1979). A microwave transmission method for measuring fluid accumulation in the lung. M.S. Thesis, Dept. of Electrical Engineering, University of Utah, Salt Lake City.

PAN, S.X., AND KAK, A.C. (1983). A computational study of reconstruction algorithms for diffraction tomography: interpolation vs. filtered back propagation. *IEEE Trans. Acoust. Speech Signal Processing* vol. ASSP-31, pp. 1262–1275.

PATE, T.D., BAKER, L.E., AND ROSBOROUGH, J.P. (1975). The simultaneous comparison of electrical impedance method of measuring stroke volume and cardiac output with four other methods. *Cardiovasc. Res. Cent. Bull.* 14:39.

PEDERSEN, P.C. (1976). Diagnostic application of microwave radiation. Ph.D. Dissertation, Dept. of Bioengineering, University of Utah, Salt Lake City.

PEDERSEN, P.C., JOHNSON, C.C., DURNEY, C.H., AND BRAGG, D.G. (1978). Microwave reflection and transmission measurements for pulmonary diagnosis and monitoring. *IEEE Trans. Biomed. Eng.* 25:40–48.

PICHOT, C., JOFRE, L., PERSONNET, G., AND BOLOMEY, J.-CH. (1985). Active microwave imaging of inhomogeneous bodies. *IEEE Trans. Antennas Prop.* 33:416–425.

PODO, F. (1988). Tissue characterization by MRI: a multidisciplinary and multicenter challenge today. *Magnet. Reson. Imag.* 6:173–174.

PORTER, R.A., AND MILLER, H.H. (1978). Microwave radiometric detection and location of breast cancer. *Proc. IEEE Electro/78*, session 30, Boston.

PYKETT, I.L. (1982). NMR imaging in medicine. *Sci. Am.* 246:78–88.

RAJOTTE, R.V., DOSSETOR, J.B., VOSS, G.W.A., AND STILLER, C.R. (1974). Preservation studies on canine kidneys recovered from the deep frozen state by microwave thawing. *Proc. IEEE 62*:76–85.

RAO, P.S., SANTOSH, K., AND GREGG, E.C. (1980). Computed tomography with microwaves. *Radiology 135*: 769–770.

ROMERO-SIERRA, C., HALTER, S., TANNER, J.A., ROOMI, M.W., AND CRABTREE, D. (1975). Electromagnetic fields and skin wound repair. *J. Microwave Power 10*:59–70.

SALLES-CUNHA, S.X., BATTOCLETTI, J.H., AND SANCES, A., JR. (1980). Steady magnetic fields in noninvasive electromagnetic flowmetry. *Proc. IEEE 68*:149–155.

SALLES-CUNHA, S.X., BATTOCLETTI, J.H., SANCES, A., JR., BERNHARD, V.M., AND TOWNE, J.B. (1981). Transcutaneous electromagnetic flowmetry: concentric vessel, three media cylindrical model. *J. Clin. Eng. 6*:283–292.

SCHMIDT, M., SCHMIDT, D., AND ROBISON, G. (1972). Cyclic AMP in rat brain: microwave irradiation as a means of tissue fixation. *Adv. Cyclic Nucleotide Res. 1*:425–434.

SCHOMBERG, H. (1981). Nonlinear image reconstruction from projections of ultrasonic travel times and electric current density. *In*: Herman, G.T., and Natterer, F. (eds.). Mathematical aspects of computerized tomography. New York, Springer-Verlag.

SEVERINGHAUS, J.W., CATRON, C., AND NOBLE, W. (1972). A focusing electrode bridge for unilateral lung resistance. *J. Appl. Physiol. 32*:526–530.

SHOFF, D.J. (1978). Noninvasive microwave methods for measuring tissue volume in normal dogs after whole blood infusion. M.S. Thesis, Dept. of Electrical Engineering, University of Utah, Salt Lake City.

SLANEY, M., KAK, A.C., AND LARSEN, L.E. (1984). Limitations of imaging with first-order diffraction tomography. *IEEE Trans. Microwave Theory Tech. 32*:860–874.

SRAMEK, B.B. (1981). Noninvasive technique for measurement of cardiac output by means of electrical impedance. *In*: Proceedings of the 5th International Conference on Electrical Bio-Impedance, Tokyo. Tokyo, Business Center for Academic Societies Japan, pp. 39–42.

STAMM, M.E., WINTER, W.D., MORTON, D.L., AND WARREN, S.L. (1974). Microwave characteristics of human tumor cells. *Oncology 29*:294–301.

STAUB, N.C. (1983). The measurement of lung water content. *J. Microwave Power 18*:259–263.

STAVINOHA, W., PEPELKO, B., AND SMITH, P. (1970). Microwave irradiation to inactivate cholinesterase in rat brain prior to analysis for acetylcholine. *Pharmacologist 12*:257.

SÜSSKIND, C. (1973). Possible use of microwaves in the management of lung disease. *Proc. IEEE 61*:673.

SWICORD, M.L., AND DAVIS, C.C. (1982). Microwave absorption of DNA between 8 and 12 GHz. *Biopolymers 21*:2453–2460.

TASTO, M., AND SCHOMBERG, H. (1978). Object reconstruction from projections and some nonlinear extensions. Presented at NATO Advanced Study Institute on Pattern Recognition and Signal Processing, June 25–July 4.

VAN DER MEULEN, P., GROEN, J.P., TINUS, A.M.C., AND BRUNTINK, G. (1988). Fast field echo imaging: an overview and contrast calculations. *Magnet. Reson. Imag.* 6:355–368.

VEECH, R., HARRIS, R., VELOS, D., AND VEECH, E. (1973). Freeze-blowing: a new technique for the study of brain *in vivo*. *J. Neurochem.* 20:183–188.

VOSS, W.A.G., RAJOTTE, R.V., AND DOSSETOR, J.B. (1974). Applications of microwave thawing to the recovery of deep-frozen cells and organs: a review. *J. Microwave Power* 9:181–194.

WALTZ, F.M., TIMM, G.W., AND BRADLEY, W.E. (1971). Bladder volume sensing by resistance measurement. *IEEE Trans. Biomed. Eng.* 18:42–46.

WEBB, S.J., AND BOOTH, A.D. (1969). Absorption of microwaves by micro-organisms. *Nature* 222:1199–1200.

WEBB, S.J., AND BOOTH, A.D. (1971). Microwave absorption by normal and tumor cells. *Science* 174:72–74.

YAMAURA, I. (1977). Measurements of 1.8–2.7 GHz microwave attenuation in human torso. *IEEE Trans. Microwave Theory Tech.* 25:707–710.

YAMAURA, I. (1978). Measurement of heart dynamics using microwaves—microwave stethoscope. *Inst. Electron. Commun. Eng. Japan* vol. TG-EMCJ78 15:9–14.

YAMAURA, I. (1979). Mapping of microwave power transmitted through the human thorax. *Proc. IEEE* 67:1170–1171.

Part 5

MISCELLANEOUS

20

Some Misconceptions about Electromagnetic Fields and Their Effects and Hazards

The subject of the bioeffects and health hazards of nonionizing electromagnetic radiation has evolved in a complex milieu of sociotechnical events that has so clouded the facts that the subject is now often described by such words as "murky," "loose," or "controversial." Not only has some sloppy research contributed to this state of affairs, but often profit, power, or personal vanity has led to dissemination of erroneous information. The history of diathermy in the first half of this century was plagued by extravagant, nonsensical claims about the effect of radiofrequency (RF) energy on the human body (Bierman, 1942; Schwan, 1981). Much of this was related to claims of low-level nonthermal effects—so-called specific effects. This led the medical community in the United States eventually to issue an ultimate challenge that has some relevance even today: "The burden of proof still lies on those who claim any biologic action of these currents other than heat" (Mortimer, 1935).

Research directed toward settling the debate about specific effects has contributed significantly to the fund of misconceptions, but to the degree that even today there is some doubt, such misconceptions are not dealt with here. Instead this chapter deals with more blatant misconceptions that live on even though they can be disproved. That myths are born from once-printed misconceptions was well illustrated by the great American journalist H. L. Mencken in his hoax on the history of the bathtub (Mencken, 1958). The relation between Mencken's example and the prevalence of myths in health-related environmental issues was pointed out by Davey (1983).

This chapter deals with two types of misconception or myth—those arising out of historical error and those arising out of technical or scientific error. The latter can be refuted convincingly by theoretical explanation or reference to ample experimental evidence. The former is more difficult, since it involves delving into difficult-to-obtain resource documents to establish whether a reported event really took place. In addition, we are often driven to technical arguments on the basis of plausibility. Whether the reader is convinced by all the rebuttals presented here is less important than the reader's acceptance of the reality of misconception or myth in this field and the need to deal with it by scholarly criticism and scientific studies.

HISTORICAL MYTHS

Radar Death

Most people who work with microwaves or radar have heard stories about the man who was "cooked" or "fried" to death when he accidentally stood in front of a high-power radar antenna for an unspecified time. No doubt many variations of this story are in circulation. In fact, only one historical report of such an incident exists, and there is good reason to believe it is not factual.

In 1957 McLaughlin published a case report of an unidentified 42-year-old white man who stood "within ten feet of the antenna. In a few seconds he had a sensation of heat in the abdomen. The heat became intolerable in less than a minute and he moved away from the antenna. Within 30 minutes he had acute abdominal pain and vomited," (McLaughlin, 1957). McLaughlin then went on to describe this patient's medical symptoms before, during, and after an operation and the subsequent death and autopsy. McLaughlin wrote that "the frequency and power factors of the microwave radiation to which the patient was exposed were unavailable because of security regulations. It was enough to cause a painful sensation of heat in the abdomen, however, and when heat can be felt, the tolerable level has been exceeded. Although the power factor is not known, it is known that the Armed Forces are using equipment emitting 2.5 megawatts peak power." McLaughlin claimed that the pathological findings were similar to those of Boysen (1953) in experimental animals exposed to 5 to 500 W of microwave (UHF) radiation.

Soon after, *Newsweek* reported the story and quoted McLaughlin as describing "a hole as big as a silver dollar burned in his [the victim's] small bowel" (Cooking, 1957). After concluding that the victim had been "cooked" by microwave radiation, the magazine quoted McLaughlin as stating that some radar is so powerful that no human is safe directly in front of it—not even if he is 10 miles away.

Within a short time the death was quoted as fact in a British journal (Radio-frequency, 1960), in the question and answer section of the *Journal of the American Medical Association* (1971), and elsewhere (Rose et al., 1969).

The report was accepted despite the open skepticism of most researchers and reviewers. For example, Quan (1960) wrote, "The validity of ascribing this fatality to microwaves has been vigorously protested. It has been denied that any exposure occurred, and further, that the case of death was an ordinary ruptured appendix accompanied by generalized peritonitis. At this time the McLaughlin findings are neither accepted nor rejected. . . ."

In 1971, Ely, one of the leading investigators during the Tri-Service Program (Michaelson, 1971), objected to any acceptance of McLaughlin's report and referred to a review by the Armed Forces Institute of Pathology that "thoroughly discounted" it. In fact, at the first Tri-Service meeting in 1957 it was stated that "further investigation revealed that this person died of other causes" (Cooking, 1957; Mumford, 1961).

Despite authorities' rejection of the radar death report, it continues to surface in the literature. For example, an article by a historian (Steneck, 1984) resurrected the radar death report and objected to the dismissal of the report by the contemporary authorities (Ely, 1971; Michaelson, 1973) on the grounds that, even though McLaughlin had not proved the radar-death connection, neither was it disproved. This led to a response from Ely (1985). In his last (to be hoped) commentary Ely pointed out that, when the alleged radar victim became ill, he was in a drafting room with "no radar equipment within several hundred feet." Furthermore, the nearest radar was at X band, and radiation at this frequency would definitely have injured the skin before damaging the internal organs. Ely's rebuttal was convincing then and now to knowledgeable professionals, even though no claim of absolute epistemological nature is made. In 1973 Michaelson wrote, "The case report of a microwave death has persisted in causing misunderstanding and confusion since its publication in 1957, and it continues to be revived and cited in spite of repeated repudiation."

In the view of the authorities of the day, McLaughlin's report of a "radar death" is invalid. Some further observations show the implausibility of such an occurrence in the 1950s.

An ample number of experimental studies have determined the lethality thresholds for various animals. As Czerski (1977) points out, they generally suggest that this threshold is associated with a critical rise of rectal temperature on the order of $4°$ to $10°$ C. Of course, the data refer to animals that are confined or restrained and that do not have the superior properties of human thermoregulation. Czerski (Baranski and Czerski, 1976) shows that a pessimistic estimate of lethal threshold for a 1-minute exposure of a man is about 5 W/cm^2. This means the absorption of tens of kilowatts by a man unless the radar beam diameter was much smaller than the area of the human body. Such exposure would be possible only if the frequency were much higher than 10 GHz. Since radar of tens of kilowatts average power did not exist in the early 1950s and since McLaughlin did not report intense skin burns that would be associated with a frequency greater than 10 GHz, the report by McLaughlin makes no physical sense.

Death Ray

A fiction similar to radar death is the microwave death ray story often attributed to anonymous military sources. In the 1930s British defense planners contemplated the idea, but Sir Watson Watt (1957) quickly rejected the feasibility of such a weapon by "a back-of-the-envelope calculation." The idea was resurrected from time to time as by the Japanese during World War II (Overy, 1980), but with no success. According to an unpublished report by McLaughlin (1953), Collins Radio, Company, in cooperation with researchers at the University of Iowa, was investigating a death ray, but nothing came of the effort. At that time the idea was no doubt conceivable after researchers witnessed the ability of a radar beam to pop flash bulbs at distances of 100 feet (Clark et al., 1949).

In the 1960s and 1970s rumors of a microwave death ray probably originated from a study by the U.S. Army (Frankfort Arsenal, 1957). The study was recently declassified. In 1957 an Army group predicted that "a flux of 10 W/cm^2 is indicated as being lethal for humans in an irradiation time of one second or less." The report discussed a weapon that could kill troops 5000 m away with a 1-second irradiation time at a total microwave power of 900 kW. The report was in gross error in arriving at the lethal threshold condition. After beginning with an out of context quotation from Schwan that "0.3 watts per cm^2 causes a 1° temperature rise per minute," the report applied the false premise that transient heating varies with square of power to calculate power density for a 13° C temperature rise. For very short transient periods of heating, temperature is proportional to power. Thus, while the Army report assumes that an absorbed power of the order of 50 to 100 kW is sufficient to kill in 1 second, the true required absorbed power is of the order of 3 MW, that is, an error factor of 30. This scheme becomes impractical.

Rumors of a microwave weapon continue to this day, encouraged partly by a report by the Defense Intelligence Agency that discussed potential "offensive weapons development" of "low-level biological effects of microwave radiation" (Adams et al., 1976). The report, however, referred only to speculation on low-level effects on the blood-brain barrier and the heart.

In recent years publicity has been given to a microwave weapon employing very high peak powers of the order of a gigawatt at very short pulses (nanoseconds) (Florig, 1988). This generally has been described not as an antipersonnel weapon but as a means of achieving "soft-kill" of missiles and other military systems through speculative radiofrequency interference (RFI) phenomena.

Microwave Oven

The preceding two examples of persistent misinformation, in the form of legends, or rumors, originated from invalid technical reports or scientific publication of *acute* microwave exposure effects. Before another example is discussed, a review of a simple rule of thumb for minimum threshold for acute damage is useful. If we accept Czerski's (1977) conservative value of 5° C as damaging temperature rise, regardless of duration, we can roughly estimate that 21 kJ/kg is required for thermal damage. This is equivalent to 21 kW/kg for 1 second, 2.1 kW/kg for 10 seconds, 210 W/kg for 100 seconds, and so on, until the applicable thermal time constant is exceeded. A large amount of power—many kilowatts—is required even in a small volume, for example, 1 kg, to inflict damage before a person has an evasive reaction. That level of power is unlikely except in the few superpower radar arrays or industrial heating systems. (The 5° C temperature rule is very conservative. For example, to cause a skin burn in 3 seconds requires a temperature rise of approximately 30° C [Moritz and Henriques, 1947].)

Despite this, acute damage from exposures of much smaller energy occasionally is reported. A recent example is that of Fleck (1983), who reported acute dermatological and neurological injury over an extensive area of the body of a woman alleged to have been exposed to the full power of a consumer microwave oven for 3 seconds. This report has been refuted by the manufacturer and independent experts who found no evidence of defective interlocks (Bronx County Supreme Court, 1981). But even if the interlocks were defective, a 3-second exposure would not produce acute thermal injury.

A person absorbs one third to one half of the total oven power as he puts his arm into an operating microwave oven. By withdrawing beyond 5 or 6 feet, the person lowers the power density of exposure well below 10 mW/cm^2. Thus the total energy absorbed by any part of the body during retrieval of an object from an oven is trivial compared with that absorbed in a diathermy treatment in which a power of about 100 W at the same frequency as the microwave oven is applied to a small part of the body for 15 to 20 minutes—for beneficial purposes!

My colleagues and I have experienced exposure analogous to that claimed by Fleck either inadvertently—during laboratory experiments when interlocks had been deliberately overridden—or deliberately, for example, in preparation for lawsuits involving allegations of such exposure (Arizona Superior Court, 1975). We experienced an immediate warming sensation in the abdomen (or chest depending on oven height) after the door was opened. Then the arms felt a transient warmth as they passed into and out of the oven. The experience is not shocking or dramatic, nor should one expect it to be comparable to the exposure with diathermy.

Cancer Connection

The mass media often make a loose connection between "microwave" exposure and cancer. Even more professional literature makes some link.

For example, a bulletin from the Carcinogen Information Program at Washington University, St. Louis, says, "NIR (nonionizing radiation) has been found to cause such adverse health effects in humans as cancer." (Center for the Biology of Natural Systems, 1980). In a recent issue of *Science Teacher* magazine a similar statement is made (McAllister, 1981). Both publications mention a World Health Organization (WHO) study that is reported to show a correlation between high incidence of cancer in Finland (North Karelia) and the presence of a nearby early-warning radar system in the Soviet Union. Both cases refer to a National Institute of Organizational Safety and Health (NIOSH) report (Dwyer and Leeper, 1978).

In fact, no such WHO study exists. The NIOSH report mistakenly interpreted a paper by Zaret (1976). This error has been admitted by NIOSH (Parr, 1981), has been refuted by Finnish health authorities (Finnish Institute of Radiation Protection, 1978), and has been pointed out by Kirk (1983) in an Environmental Protection Agency (EPA) review of the literature.

The connection between cancer in Finland and Soviet radar was a bald speculation by Zaret (1976). Although he mentioned a WHO study, he did it only as the source of a report of a high incidence of cancer. Zaret, not WHO, made the connection with Soviet radar.

Zaret later (1977) quoted his earlier paper in support of the possibility that NIR is carcinogenic. Then Becker (1977) applied Zaret's 1977 paper in support of a speculative link between NIR and cancer in the Syracuse, N.Y., region.

Despite the spreading reports of the microwave-cancer link, resembling the bathtub hoax of Mencken, no WHO study or other established scientific basis in the literature supports this link—especially regarding studies on humans.

In recent years, reports on animal experiments (Szmigielski, 1982; Guy, 1985) have suggested some promotion of cancer in rodents under chronic mild heating conditions. An independent biostatistical review, however, concluded after reviewing 32 recent publications on bioeffects of electromagnetic energy, including those suggesting cancer promotion in rodents, that there was "no conclusive evidence of harmful effects, except for laboratory studies where RFEM radiation produced substantial heating" (Selwyn, 1987). Many recent epidemiological studies have suggested a link between exposure to electromagnetic fields and cancer, but the evidence is weak and inconclusive (see Chapter 17 and Silverman, 1980).

Medical Opposition to Research

In the popular press (Brodeur, 1978), allegations of suppression of research on health hazards by the military-industrial-government complex have become popular. Recently, however, a historian has chosen to supplant this with the theory that medical proponents of microwave diathermy and its industrial supplier, Raytheon Company, opposed scientific research on microwave hazards (Steneck, 1980). Steneck (1980) states: "At the same time that such military contractors as Hughes Aircraft and Lockheed were anxious to have active research on biohazards begun, the Raytheon Company, which produced diathermy equipment, was reported to have attempted to persuade the military to terminate its sponsorship of the Iowa research on cataracts (9, p. 26)." The reference is to p. 26 of the 1953 report by McLaughlin cited earlier. Although unpublished copies of this report were supplied to Steneck (and to me), p. 26 is headlined "For distribution at Hughes Aircraft only," that is, this page was never distributed. On this page McLaughlin paraphrases suspicions that Raytheon may have pressured the U.S. Navy to discontinue work at Iowa.

The allegation that Raytheon Company tried to suppress such research reflects badly on Dr. Percy Spencer, (Yankee Genius, 1958) a talented inventor who supervised the work on microwaves at Raytheon. In fact, there is no evidence of such a conspiracy nor reports of such a conspiracy in the literature or among Tri-Service Program researchers or even co-workers (Osepchuk, 1981) at the University of Iowa and Collins Radio Company. No one has ever suggested that Spencer or Raytheon Company would hinder research on bioeffects. On the contrary, Raytheon has contributed equipment to researchers, beginning with donations of diathermy sources to researchers at Mayo Clinic, Tufts University, and the University of Iowa and various microwave tubes to researchers thereafter.

Moscow Embassy Story

In recent years the United States learned that the Soviet government was irradiating the upper floors of the U.S. Embassy in Moscow with low-level microwaves (up to 18 μW/cm^2). Soon rumors about health effects among employees of the U.S. Embassy began. These rumors have appeared not only in the general press but also in professional literature (Steneck, 1982). Less well publicized are the studies that have shown no ill effects among the employees. These include an extensive epidemiological study that found "no convincing evidence that would directly implicate the exposure to microwave radiation experienced by the employees at the Moscow Embassy in the causation of any adverse health effects as to the time of this analysis" (Lilienfeld, 1978). A rational explanation of the history of this affair was presented by Pollack (1977) to Congress, but despite this Pollack (1979) has deplored the media response. The epidemiological aspects of this and other studies are effectively summarized by Silverman (1980). If one is to ask why the irradiation occurred in the first place—if it was not health related—one is referred to a congressional report (Smich, 1980) where, after hearing a classified explanation, inquiring senators dropped the question.

TECHNICAL MISCONCEPTIONS

"Microwave" Bioeffect

How is a "microwave" bioeffect different from an RF or infrared bioeffect? What causes the popular media and even technical publications to impute a unique danger to microwaves, as reflected in a letter by a radio engineer to a newspaper: "For your article to infer that TV and FM broadcast radiation is in the same category as microwaves is very irresponsible"?

Is there a meaningful definition of microwaves? The original definition by engineers was related to the minimum frequency at which it was practical to use a pipe to conduct electromagnetic energy—about 1 GHz for a 6-inch pipe. Others (Baranski, 1976; GAO, 1978) typically define microwaves arbitrarily as RF frequencies above 100 or 300 MHz with upper limit set at 300 GHz. Baranski and Czerski (1976) suggest that the implicit definition in the United States is 10 MHz to 100 GHz because that was the range addressed by the American National Standards Institute (ANSI C95) standards in 1966 and 1974. None of these definitions has any useful meaning with regard to understanding the term "microwave bioeffect."

The scientific and engineering literature suggests that the meaningful definition of microwaves relates to that frequency range in which only a few modes are required to describe the electromagnetic field in the object or system under study, that is, the object size L is of the order of the wavelength λ. I have suggested that this is the basis for a meaningful definition of microwave bioeffect, that is, the type of bioeffect that occurs when an animal is exposed to radiation in or close to the resonance frequency range for that animal, which is where L is on the order of λ (Osepchuk, 1979).

On this basis 10 MHz to 100 GHz is not an unreasonable definition of microwaves because it includes the resonance frequency range for humans: 30 to 300 MHz (Gandhi, 1979). The possibility of resonance is the unique aspect of microwaves. Not only is the total body absorption a maximum at resonance (Gandhi, 1979), but the penetration of nonionizing radiation into most animals is also significant only in the resonance range for that animal. As I have pointed out (Osepchuk, 1979), the internal E field is comparable to the external E field for animals of macroscopic size only in the resonance range. At quasistatic frequencies, for instance, 60 Hz, or at frequencies above 10 GHz, the internal field in the center of a human body is predictably many orders of magnitude below the external field.

The popular media and even at times scientific and government reports say that the human body is transparent to low RF energy and therefore low RF energy is less harmful than the more absorbed microwave energy. On its face, such a statement presents a fallacy. If the body is transparent, the internal fields are as strong as external fields and presumably of concern whether absorption is strong or not. In fact, this statement is false technically. It can be shown (Schwan, 1981) that, for small spherical objects compared with a wavelength, the internal E field E_i is related to the external E field E_0 by the equation

$$E_i = \left(\frac{3j\omega\varepsilon_0}{(2j\omega\varepsilon_0) + \sigma + j\omega\varepsilon}\right) E_0 \tag{1}$$

where ε_0 is the dielectric permittivity of free space (8.86×10^{-12} F/m), ω is radian frequency, σ is conductivity in the body, and ε is the dielectric permittivity of the body. For high-water-content biological material at low frequencies, $\sigma \gg \omega\varepsilon$ crudely (Figure 20-1). If so, Eq. 1 shows that $E_i \lll E_0$, for example, by nearly six orders of magnitude at 60 Hz.

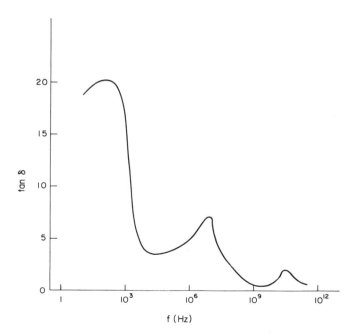

Figure 20-1   Loss tangent, tan δ, of muscle tissue as function of frequency.

This means the E field is shunted out of the body by the surface charges just as it would be for a pure conductor. This is not "transparency."

The misconception about transparency probably derives from some invalid conclusions drawn from the concept of skin depth, which in general for lossy media is given by

$$d_s = \cfrac{1}{\omega \sqrt{\dfrac{\mu \epsilon}{2}\left[\sqrt{1+\left(\dfrac{\sigma}{\omega\epsilon}\right)^2}-1\right]}} \tag{2}$$

where μ is the magnetic permeability. For "good" conductors $\sigma \gg \omega\epsilon$

$$d_s \approx \sqrt{\frac{2}{\omega\mu\sigma}} \tag{3}$$

which is the more familiar expression in microwave engineering. For low-loss dielectrics $\sigma \ll \omega\epsilon$, Eq. 2 becomes

$$d_s \approx \frac{2}{\sigma\sqrt{\dfrac{\mu}{\epsilon}}} = \frac{2\sqrt{\epsilon_r}}{120\pi\sigma} = \frac{\lambda}{\pi\sqrt{\epsilon_r}}\tan\delta \tag{4}$$

This again is a familiar expression to those involved in dielectric heating. One might think that, if a body's thickness is small compared with d_s, it is transparent. This is not necessarily true.

For a plane-parallel sheet of thickness s and infinite in the plane of the sheet, and upon which a plane wave with electric field E_{inc} impinges in a normal direction, one finds for $s \ll d_s$ and $\sigma \gg \omega\epsilon$

$$\frac{E_i}{E_{\text{inc}}} \approx \frac{1}{1+\dfrac{1}{\sqrt{2}}\left(\dfrac{377}{R}\right)} \tag{5}$$

where R is the resistance per square of the sheet in ohms, that is, $R = \frac{1}{\sigma s}$.

If $s \gg d_s$ and $\sigma \gg \omega\epsilon$

$$\frac{E_i}{E_{\text{inc}}} \approx \frac{1}{\sqrt{\dfrac{\sigma}{2\omega\epsilon}}} \tag{6}$$

Thus, even though $s \ll d_s$ according to Eq. 5, as long as $R \ll 377$, $E_i \ll E_{\text{inc}}$. This is the case for metals of reasonable thickness at low frequencies. For biological media such as muscle, Eq. 5 predicts a value of about 0.5 at 60 Hz for s on the order of 0.2 m.

The lessons to be drawn are (1) that at low frequencies biological media are not transparent in common subjects of small size ($<< \lambda$) and (2) that if such media were present in large sheets, they would be penetrated even at 60 Hz. The lack of penetration at low frequency depends therefore on substantial conductivity in biological media *and* the fact that small size prevents any substantial currents or wave propagation phenomena.

Of course, at low frequencies where objects are small compared with wavelength, the effects of electric and magnetic fields must be considered separately. Magnetic fields penetrate biological media, since biological media contain virtually no significant ferromagnetic material (Kirschvink, 1981). Thus, for biological objects, $B_{ext} = B_{int}$ and $H_{ext} = H_{int}$ and there are induced currents from H_{int} (Gandhi, 1979). Until recently no suggestion that such magnetic fields have a biological effect had been made.

It is a general precept that microwave bioeffects are a function of internal field E_i where $E_i = E_{ext} F(\omega/\omega_r)$ and $F(\omega/\omega_r)$ has a maximum value at the body resonance frequency ω_r. Assuming no molecular resonance or other reason for frequency specificity, extrapolation of animal experiments to humans should be based on an invariant value of ω/ω_r. This is the basis for use of the *Radiofrequency Radiation Dosimetry Handbook* (Durney et al., 1980).

A review of the several thousand reports of animal bioeffect experiments shows that the overwhelming majority have been done in the frequency range of 1 to 3 GHz, principally with rodents. In fact, in the United States a scan of the papers from the last 10 years shows that the great majority are at one frequency, 2450 MHz, presumably because of the ease and economy of work at this frequency.

On the basis for such scaling given in the *Radiofrequency Radiation Dosimetry Handbook*, one would conclude that most experimental results with animal microwave bioeffects apply to humans in their resonance frequency range, that is, 30 to 300 MHz or thereabouts. This practice is indeed implicit in the use of equivalent specific absorption rate (SAR) in the development of the latest ANSI C95 standard (Guy, 1979). Unfortunately, many retain a more rigid view of specific frequency effects; most of the results at 2450 MHz are publicized as significant because that is the frequency of exposure from microwave ovens.

In fact, extrapolation of animal experiments to humans should be based on normalized frequency (relative to resonance). It should also be recognized that resonance for humans has been found to be less dramatic than for animals (Gandhi, 1979). This in part reflects the fact that the loss tangent of biological tissue (muscle) is low only in the frequency band 1 to 10 GHz (Figure 20-1). Thus at the resonant frequency of mice (2450 MHz) tan δ is about 0.3, whereas at the resonance frequency of humans (80 MHz) tan δ is about 6. A more fundamental explanation relates to the scaling of SAR. For comparable shapes, that is, shapes identical except for changed dimensions, the power absorbed at resonance (from scaled Maxwell's equations) is proportional to absorption cross section that is proportional to the physical cross section and hence is smaller for smaller bodies. However, since the SAR is power absorbed for unit volume and volume decreases faster with the dimensions, the SAR increases for smaller bodies.

More work with a variety of animals and frequency is needed to confirm the scaling theory to the satisfaction of the public and the scientific community.

The final view of the uniqueness of microwave bioeffects is that internal fields determine bioeffects; body size and shape determine internal fields, and the latter are maximized in the resonance range of a given animal—which is the range of microwave bioeffects for that animal. For all animals of significant size the resonance range corresponds to the rough range of 10 MHz to 10 GHz. For convenience, study of nonresonant regimes is added to resonance ranges to set standards, and this corresponds to approximately 300 kHz to 100 GHz, the range covered by ANSI C95.1 (1982).

The property of maximum penetration is one reason for the special mystique surrounding microwave bioeffects and health hazards. To this can be added the factual observation that natural electromagnetic fields are minimum in the resonance range of humans and animals, that is, about 0.1 to 10 GHz. Other, less well-founded factors behind this mystique include the effects of historical myths and other misconceptions—particularly the property of focusing of microwave beams where action at a distance is conceivable, as with the "death ray."

The general presumption here is that bioeffects have no molecular basis; that is, there are no "specific" bioeffects. Recent work at millimeter waves, > 30 GHz, however, suggests the possibility that some type of macromolecular resonance properties can induce some frequency specificity (Frohlich, 1980; Grundler et al., 1983). This view is not well confirmed (see Chapter 16 and Bush et al., 1981). Often the effects are only a weak, quasiperiodic function of frequency. In addition, since penetration depth at such frequencies is well below 1 mm, whatever health hazards such frequencies pose would involve only the skin. There is no evidence of such frequency dependence below 30 GHz. Therefore the above view of what a microwave bioeffect is will probably prevail.

Natural "Microwave" Background

The popular press has carried loose statements that microwaves are unnatural. For example, Zaret (1973) suggested that leakage levels from microwave ovens were 10 million times that emitted by the sun.

In 1980 Ralph Nader reported that "many scientists believe we have already increased the level of microwave radiation over the natural background on earth by 100,000 percent."

The sun is a principal source of microwaves, as is any hot body, but of course the flux level by the time they arrive at earth is much weakened. A much larger source of microwaves on earth is the black-body radiation from the earth or any warm body on earth.

Black-body radiation is proportional to the fourth power of the absolute temperature. For a body at the temperature T_e of the living human body, the emission density of microwaves (base band) radiation, assuming an emissivity of 1, can be shown to be

$$S(f) = 0.3 \left(\frac{f}{300}\right)^3 \left(\frac{T_e}{300}\right)^4 \mu W/cm^2 \qquad (7)$$

where f is the maximum frequency in gigahertz and T_e is in degrees Kelvin.

Therefore, if microwaves are defined as bounded by 300 GHz on the high end, we find $S(f) = 0.3 \ \mu W/cm^2$. Despite Ralph Nader, the ambient man-made level is not 100,000% above this value. Even the value up to 30 GHz ($0.0003 \ \mu W/cm^2$) is significant compared with long-term man-made exposures.

In the literature the black-body radiation in the microwave range is often not discussed or is miscalculated. For example, a recent NRCP report (1981) stated that the radiation at "wavelengths $> 100 \ \mu m$ is below the mW/m^2 range." Actually, according to Eq. 7, the value is 300 $\mu W/cm^2$ up to 3000 GHz (100 μm) or 3000 mW/m^2. Therefore the validity of further remarks in the report is questionable, namely: "Man-made sources in the microwave and RF region have power outputs many orders of magnitude above background." It is not clear how one can assign a power value rather than power density to background.

Presman (1970) and Minin (1965) present discussions of solar noise in a plot of flux on earth ($\mu W/cm^2/Hz$) versus frequency. Flux values shown appear to contradict those discussed in accompanying texts. Furthermore, these authors claim that man-made sources are as much as 18 orders of magnitude higher than natural sources. They compare flux densities in very narrow spectral bands, on the order of 0.1 MHz. In general, comparison of total flux over a wide part of the spectrum would seem to be more meaningful.

More accurate estimates of solar fluxes in the microwave range can be reached by using the data of Sinton (1952) and Kundel (1965). Thus, below 30 GHz, flux from a quiet sun $\rightarrow 2 \cdot 10^{-7} \ \mu W/cm^2$ and bursts $\rightarrow 10^{-5} \ \mu W/cm^2$ for durations of minutes to hours. Below 300 GHz, flux from a quiet sun $\rightarrow 1.5 \cdot 10^{-5} \ \mu W/cm^2$.

These values, even though small, are significant compared with *median* broadcast levels, which are on the order of 10^{-3} μW/cm^2.

At low frequencies the peak E fields of sferics in the atmosphere can reach as high as 10 kV/m, and static fields can be higher during a storm. As I have pointed out (Osepchuk, 1979), the spectral region of minimum natural noise background is the microwave range. It is by chance that this is the resonance frequency range for humans and the range of most stringent standards.

Misconceptions about "Exposure"

The concept of "exposure" is badly treated in the press and often mishandled in professional literature, as witness statements such as "He was exposed to mind-boggling levels of microwaves" or "As many as 21 million workers are exposed to microwaves."

Definition of exposure.   To aid in the exposition of the many misconceptions about exposure, an exposure diagram is useful. Exposure is some specified combination of field intensity or power flux and duration of time during which an animal or a person is subjected to that field or power flux—presumably a "whole-body" exposure, that is, field averaged over the whole body, unless otherwise specified. Any biological effect is likely to have a threshold or threshold area as depicted in Figure 20-2, with allowance for biological variability and other factors. In general, for very short exposure time the threshold is assumed to follow a constant "dose" or "absorbed energy" line, that is, specific absorption (SA) (NCRP, 1981). For a very long exposure time the threshold is generally assumed to follow a constant "dose rate" or "specific absorption rate" (SAR) (NCRP, 1981) line that is horizontal, that is, a constant power flux. (We are neglecting extremes of time in which physical and epistemological questions can be raised.) The region connecting the two lines of constant SA and constant SAR defines the characteristic time or time constant T of the effect. The time constant T denotes the delay time after inception of energy input or biological insult or stress before a compensating process, such as energy loss or transfer, biological adjustment, or repair, comes into play and leads to a steady-state balance between stressing and relieving processes, a balance associated with constant SAR. The time constant T generally increases with volume, thickness, or other measure of size of the biological system being exposed. The absence of a constant SAR region implies $T \rightarrow \infty$, that is, no repair or compensation process in the biological system and a truly cumulative effect. Even if the threshold lines were constant SA lines, implicit in the idea of threshold is a boundary between safety and hazard. It is generally accepted even in Eastern Europe (Minin, 1965; Baranski, 1977) that bioeffects of RF radiation

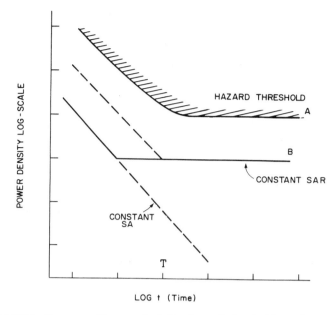

Figure 20-2 Exposure diagram depicting hazard threshold and hypothetical safety limit curves composed of lines of constant specific absorption rate or constant specific absorption or both.

exhibit thresholds. Furthermore, it is generally accepted that long-term exposure exhibits thresholds of constant SAR.

Scaling of exposure time.   Beyond the aforementioned general agreement lies confusion about the value of time constants for various bioeffects and animals and about how to extrapolate equivalent exposure from animal to human. The confusion is compounded when "standards," exposure limits related to these bioeffect thresholds, are derived.

Tell and Harlen (1979) point out that the thermal time constant for a human under near-resonance, whole-body exposure is about an hour. They recognize that much shorter time constants would apply for very high microwave frequency or localized or partial-body heating. They make no attempt to generalize. They discuss the question of scaling from animal to human in the steady-state regime but do not tackle the question of scaling in terms of time of exposure.

Tyazhelova and Tyazhelov (1980) neglect the existence of any time constants and assume that long-term exposure causes truly cumulative effects (constant SA). Thus they conclude that animal exposure experiments are scaled to humans with exposure time proportional to lifetime but that equivalent power densities for humans are *always* less than for animals; for example, at high microwave frequencies, effects with small animals (mice) are extrapolated to humans at lower power densities. This contradicts U.S. assumptions that equivalent long-term bioeffects occur at constant SAR (Guy, 1979). Furthermore, it contradicts the admission in the Soviet Union that there are thresholds of power density below which there is safety (Minin, 1965). It is clear that Tyazhelova is simply extrapolating an idea of constant dose threshold from the field of ionizing radiation. Very little discussion of the time-scaling problem exists elsewhere.

Safety limits: time dependence and safety factor.   In Figure 20-2 a safety limit can be derived as shown with a safety factor of 10 by simply lowering the bioeffects threshold curve by a factor of 10 in power density. This leads to a curve with the same time constant T. If we decrease T in the exposure limit curve, the safety factor for short times is increased, that is, a more conservative limit. This is essentially the procedure followed in ANSI C95 (Guy, 1979) in which a 6-minute time constant is used. Even though a written standard such as ANSI C95 does not explicitly describe a curve like curve A in Figure 20-2, it specifies an approximation curve, B, through the shorthand procedure of a long-term limit and an "averaging time," which is essentially T.

In the U.S. standard the time dependence is clear and so is the way to measure the exposure fields. In the absence of a subject they are measured with an instrument of known time constant and then extrapolated to the average value for 6 minutes.

In many other standards the time dependence and required measurement techniques are ambiguous. Until recently, Soviet standards exhibited discontinuous changes (factor of 10) in safety levels at time values of 0.33 and 2 hours with no apparent time constant, except that it is implied that the time is about 8 or 24 hours. This has no apparent relationship to a biological time constant in microwave experiments.

Recently, however, the Soviet Union has modified such standards to specify essentially a constant SA or dose line but with an implied time constant of 24 hours, since cumulative effect beyond 24 hours is not specified Savin (1983) (this contradicts Tyazhelova). For short periods of time, such as a minute, ANSI C95 and Soviet limits are essentially the same. Only for long-duration exposure (> 8 hours) does the oft-quoted discrepancy of 1000 seem to apply.

The new Soviet standard specifies a maximum microwave exposure limit of 200 $\mu W \cdot h/cm^2$ with an upper maximum of 1000 $\mu W/cm^2$ (Savin, 1983). This is ambiguous because no mention is made of averaging time or measurement technique. (In addition, no justification exists in the bioeffects research literature for such an arbitrary limit.)

In a late revision (1983) a long-standing ambiguity of Soviet standards is perpetuated: the different limits applied to cases of scanning. The above limit applies to nonscanning or continuous exposure. The limit for irradiation from scanning (for example, radar) systems is 2000 μW/cm²/hr. No measurement procedure is specified. Some readers have assumed therefore that Soviets permit *higher* exposure for scanning systems. Not so! The official document (GOST, 1976) in the Soviet Union, although hardly a model of clarity, seems to specify that a scanning source must be nonscanning while a power density measurement is made in the beam. Thus, if the scanning beam is narrow, the standard, in effect, implies a considerably lower value of the time-averaged exposure when the exposure is intermittent, as with the scanning radar. Higher exposure (time averaged over many seconds) is permitted if the exposure is continuously at one level. This does not make much sense, since intermittent exposure can arise in many ways, for example, if a person walks or rides through an ambient field, which typically shows hot and cold spots, or if a person is near a heat sealer that operates intermittently. In the main, real-life exposure consists of intermittent exposure.

In an attempt to deal with these ambiguities, Czerski (1977) relates how the Polish standard was developed. A careful reading reveals a residuum of ambiguities, for example, a formula $t = 32/p^2$ for short-term exposure, where p is power density.

In addition to ambiguities in time dependence, current safety standards show ambiguities in frequency dependence and partial-body exposure. Improvements, however, are being made. It is becoming universally recognized that frequency dependence and time dependence must be continuous functions (Guy, 1979). Past pleas that discontinuities allow "simple" rules are being discounted as it is becoming recognized that those responsible for applying such regulations are fully competent to make calculations and use sophisticated instrumentation. Although simple rules for partial-body limits do not exist yet it is generally recognized that exposure flux or field can be higher for smaller areas of exposure.

Emission standards. An "emission" standard specifies a limit on microwave flux or field at a specified distance from a leak or source. Because of the generally applicable inverse-square law, the flux numbers clearly cannot be compared with whole-body exposure limits. Unfortunately, this comparison exists even in professional literature. For the same exposure one can specify an almost infinite range of emission values simply by changing the measurement point from very near a leaking hole or crack to a great distance from the leak. Whereas the United States specifies an emission limit at 5 cm, the Soviets specify a limit at 50 cm from a microwave oven, which is exactly the limit derived by inverse-square law from the U.S. limit.

The fallacy of comparing emission versus exposure exists with sources of ionizing as well as nonionizing radiation (Osepchuk, 1978). The same misconception arises in both cases, namely, that the emission value is construed as an exposure value. Perhaps it would be more logical to specify a leakage limit in terms of total power radiated!

In the literature one still finds statements like a report that the subject device was emitting X mW/cm^2. This is of course meaningless, just as meaningless as stating that a radioactive stone was emitting X mR/hr of radiation. Recently a scientist cogently objected to the latter, saying: "Radiation sources emit gamma rays, beta particles etc., not mrems, which are a measure of radiation levels created at a specific point of measurement due to these emissions. The radiation levels given for the gemstones are meaningless without specifying the distance from the stone at which they were measured!" (Sorensen, 1983).

Similarly, microwave or RF devices emit RF radiation or fields, not milliwatts per square centimeter. An emission level must always specify the distance at which it was measured.

There are other cogent reasons for specifying leakage in terms of power rather than flux. Even though the same leakage emissions exist for a large aperture source (leak) as for a small source, the exposure values at a distance are quite different and more in proportion to total power radiated. Or the emission limit can be reduced by a significant factor by interposing a transparent plastic part to a device, thus effectively changing the measurement point. For the same actual leakage one might measure 1 mW/cm^2 near a microwave oven door but only 0.5 mW/cm^2 or lower if a plastic part is added to keep the probe 1 to 2 inches farther from the actual metallic leakage site.

Focusing and magnification. The unlikely potential that high-frequency microwaves can be focused to a small area, on the order of ($\lambda/2 \times \lambda/2$), was advanced as a reason for not allowing relaxation of exposure limits in ANSI C95 (1982) for partial-body exposure when $f > 1$ GHz (Guy, 1979). Below 1 GHz, if the total radiated power is less than 7 W, power densities higher than specified for whole-body exposure are permitted. Besides being ambiguous because of the arbitrary boundary at 1 GHz with discontinuity in outlook, it is misleading because energy can be concentrated in many ways besides radiative focusing. Thus, if the energy is coupled to a coaxial line and concentrated at a center conductor, one can readily produce pain and even burns in a small skin area that touches the open end of such a cable connector—at any frequency even below 1 GHz—with only a fraction of a watt (Osepchuk, 1983).

Similar concentration of RF energy exposure can be created (Gandhi et al., 1982) when touching large metal objects that act as antennas at low frequency. In principle, as has been pointed out in the general press, the possibility of almost infinite magnification of even weak fields is possible in the vicinity of sharp needles as in a hospital. Rather than suggesting that microwaves are generically more dangerous in a hospital because of the presence of needles, a more realistic assessment must be made of whether such localized exposures have any real effect despite the intense fields over a very small volume that a finger is exposed to for a very short time before the finger itself modifies the field by touching the point. In the end a measure of total available power will be a better measure of likely effect and hazard than field or flux measurements over small volumes, whether near a source or near the exposed person.

Radiofrequency interference hazards. In modern society where a wide variety of electronic systems and devices are used, RFI is a possibility and even a potential hazard if the device receiving interference is a cardiac pacemaker or a control circuit governing a critical chemical interaction. In the general press and even professional literature these possibilities are cited as further examples of potential "radiation" hazards or the penalties for electromagnetic "pollution." These pejorative terms are unsuitable in a scientific discussion of the question because legal and desirable electromagnetic radiations are not "pollution," whereas the fault for RFI incidents is often the inadequate design of devices like pacemakers. If the devices do not incorporate adequate filtering or shielding, they exhibit the defect of susceptibility or lack immunity.

The necessity of controls on receivers (or nonreceivers) if there is to be electromagnetic compatibility has slowly diffused from a purely military specification to general societal recognition. In 1981 Congress passed a law that gives the Federal Communications Commission the power to impose susceptibility limits on such home entertainment devices as radio, TV receivers, tape recorders, and hi-fi sets (Goldwater, 1981). In 1976, Congress had given the Food and Drug Administration the power to impose similar controls on medical equipment. In neither area have formal susceptibility standards been developed. Voluntary standards are likely to be developed first by ANSI (Committee C63).

Sometimes anecdotal reports of RFI incidents do not include a valid technical analysis. This leads to unfounded myths like the oft-repeated allegation that microwave ovens are particularly hazardous for pacemaker wearers because of microwave leakage. This rumor derived from a 1970 report of an interference incident involving a pacemaker wearer in a restaurant. However, that incident probably did not involve microwave (2450 MHz) radiation but spurious emission at around 200 MHz (Osepchuk, 1981), which Mitchell et al. (1976) have shown to be a far more likely source of RFI to implanted pacemakers than the 2450 MHz leakage.

Artifacts in Biological Experiments

The assumption that physical or engineering details are irrelevant or secondary to the biological data in an experiment often leads, especially in the Eastern European literature, to the exclusion of the key physical or technical details. This has led standards development groups in the United States to produce lists of key descriptors required in a paper if it is to be useful for developing quantitative safety limits (Guy, 1979). These lists include many presumably obvious requirements such as description of geometry of exposure system, radiated power, exposure parameters, and modulation parameters. Only a few of the less obvious but potential sources of artifacts are listed here. These cannot be neglected in evaluating today's research, which seems to yield results that are weak and sometimes difficult to reproduce.

Such a checklist would include:

1. Source—all spurious signals including harmonics and their levels emanating from the intentional output port and other extraneous radiators, for example, the high-voltage bushing of a crossed-field tube; secondary physical or chemical agents produced by the source and its microwave output, for example, ozone, air ions, incidental x-rays, and acoustic emissions

2. Exposure system—all temperature parameters, including air temperature and wall temperatures, which may incidentally be high as in anechoic chamber; all physical objects near the exposed animal that could contribute to specific coupling modes, that is, plastic and metal objects that could create focused or magnified fields

3. Instrumentation—the susceptibility properties of the equipment and incidental fields produced by the experiment at the site of such instruments

REFERENCES

Adams, R.L., and Williams, R.A. (1976). Biological effect of electromagnetic radiation (radiowaves and microwaves—Euroasian communist countries). Report No. DST-18103–074–76. Washington, D.C., Defense Intelligence Agency.

Arizona Superior Court (1975), Mayo v Raytheon Company (June 1975), Phoenix, Arizona.

Baranski, S., and Czerski, P. (1976). Biological effects of microwaves. Stroudsburg, Pa., Dowden, Hutchinson & Ross, pp. 11–15.

Becker, P.O. (1977). Microwave radiation. *N.Y. State J. Med.* 77:2172.

Bierman, W. (1942). The medical applications of the short-wave current. Baltimore, Williams & Wilkins Co.

BOYSEN, J.E. (1953). Hyperthermic and pathologic effects of electromagnetic radiation (350 Mc). *A.M.A. Arch. Indust. Hyg. Occup. Med.* 7:516.

BRODEUR, P. (1978). The zapping of America. New York, W. W. Norton.

Bronx County Supreme Court (1981): Farmakis *v* Tappan (Nov. 30, 1981). New York.

BUSH, L.G., et al. (1981). Effects of millimeter-wave radiation on monolayer cell cultures. *Bioelectromagnetics* 2:151–160.

Center for the Biology of Natural Systems (1980). CIP Bulletin No. 12 (July 1980). Microwaves and radiowaves. Carcinogen Information Program, Washington University, St. Louis, MO.

CLARK, J.W., HINES, H.M., AND SALISBURY, W.W. (May 1949). Exposure to microwaves. *Electronics* 22:66–67.

Cooking a man (1957). National Affairs Column, *Newsweek*, June 10, 1957.

CZERSKI, P. (1977). Overviews on nonionizing radiation. Paris, International Radiational Protection Association.

DAVEY, T. (1983). The menace of media myths. *Eng. Times* 17:2.

DURNEY, C.H., et al. (1980). Radiofrequency radiation dosimetry handbook. (3rd Ed.). Dept. of Bioengineering, University of Utah, Salt Lake City.

DWYER, M.J., AND LEEPER, D.B. (1978). A current literature report on the carcinogenic properties of ionizing and non-ionizing radiation. II. Microwave and radiofrequency radiation. DHEW (NIOSH) Pub. No. 78–134. Washington, D.C., National Institute of Occupational Safety and Health.

ELY, T.S. (1971). Microwave death. JAMA *217*:1394.

ELY, T.S. (1985), Science and standards (Letter). *J. Microwave Power* 20:137.

Finnish Institute of Radiation Protection (1978). Statement to Embassy of Finland in Washington, D.C., Nov. 22, 1978.

FLECK, H. (1983). Microwave oven burns. *Bull. N.Y. Acad. Med.* 59:3, 313.

FLORIG, H.K. (1988). The future battlefield: a blast of gigawatts. *IEEE Spectrum* 25:50–54.

Frankfort Arsenal (1957). Report No. TN-1097 (Dec. 13, 1957), Philadelphia, River Styx.

FROHLICH, H. (1980). The biological effects of microwaves and related questions. *Adv. Electron. Electron Phys.* 53:85–152.

GANDHI, O.P. (1979). Dosimetry—the absorption properties of man and experimental animals. *Bull. N.Y. Acad. Med.* 55:999–1017.

GANDHI, O.P., et al. (1982). Radiofrequency hazards in the VLF to MF band. *Proc. IEEE* 70:1462–1464.

General Accounting Office (1978). More protection from microwave radiation hazards needed. Report No. HRD-79–7. Washington, D.C., U.S. Government Printing Office.

GOLDWATER, B. (1981). Legislation sponsored by Sen. Barry Goldwater.

GOST (1976). U.S.S.R. State Committee on Standards. Standard 12.1.006–76 (Jan. 26, 1976). Occupational safety standards system, electromagnetic fields of radiofrequency, general safety requirements. Moscow, Standards Publishers.

GRUNDLER, W., et al. (1983). Sharp resonances in yeast growth prove nonthermal sensitivity to microwaves. *Phys. Rev. Lett. 51*:1214–1216.

GUY, A.W. (1979). Non ionizing radiation: dosimetry and interactions. *In*: Proceedings of the Non-Ionizing Radiation Symposium, Washington, D.C., American Conference on Government Industrial Hygienists.

GUY, A.W., et al. (1985). Effects of long-term low level radiofrequency radiation exposure on rats, Vol. 9. Summary, USAF Contract No., SAM-TR-85–64, Brooks Air Force Base, Tex.

JAMA *216*:1651 (June 7, 1971).

KIRK, W. (1983). Life span and carcinogenesis. *In*: Cahill, D.F., and Elder, J.F. (eds.). Biological effects of radiofrequency radiation. Sect. 5.9, Document No. EPA-600/8–83–026A.

KIRSCHVINK, J.L. (1981). Ferrimagnetic crystals (magnetite) in human tissue, *J. Exp. Biol. 92*:333–335.

KUNDEL, M. (1965). Solar radio astronomy. New York, Interscience Publishers.

LILIENFIELD, A.M., et al. (1978). Foreign-Service health status study—evaluations of health status of foreign service and other employees from selected Eastern European posts. Final Report (Contract No. 6025–6190731) to U.S. Dept. of State.

MCALLISTER, K. (1981). Microwave and radiowave radiation: how much is to much? *Sci. Teacher 48:* 25–27.

MCLAUGHLIN, J.T. (1953). A survey of possible health hazards from exposure to microwave radiation, unpublished report, Culver City, Calif., Hughes Aircraft Co., p. 26.

MCLAUGHLIN, J.T. (1957). Tissue destruction and death from microwave radiation radar. *Cal. Med. 86*:336–339.

MENCKEN, H.L. (1958). The bathtub hoax. New York, Alfred A. Knopf, pp. 3–24.

MICHAELSON, S.M. (1971). The Tri-Service Program—a Tribute to George M. Knauf, USAF (MC). *IEEE Trans. Microwave Theory Tech. 19*:131–146.

MICHAELSON, S.M. (1973). Testimony before U.S. Senate on P.L. 90–602; Washington, D.C., U.S. Government Printing Office, Serial No. 93–24, pp. 155–156.

Microwave exposure discussion (1957). *In*: Proceedings of the 1st Annual Tri-Service Conference on Biological Hazards of Microwave Radiation, Rome Air Development Center, Griffis Air Force Base, N.Y.

MININ, B.A. (1965). Microwaves and human safety. I. Translation from U.S. Joint Publications Research Service, JPRS 65506–1, U.S. Dept. of Commerce.

MITCHELL, J.C., AND HURT, W.D. (1976). The biological significance of radiofrequency radiation emission on cardiac pacemaker performance. Tech. Report 76–4, USAF School of Aerospace Medicine, Brooks Air Force Base, San Antonio, Tex.

MORITZ, A.R., AND HENRIQUES, F.C., JR. (1947). Studies of thermal injury. II. The relative importance of time and surface temperature in the causation of cutaneous burns. Am. J. Pathol. *23*:695–720.

MORTIMER, B., AND OSBORNE, S.L. (1935). JAMA *104*:1413.

MUMFORD, W.W. (1961). Some technical aspects of microwave radiation hazards. *Proc. IRE 49* (suppl. 461):427–447.

NADER, R. (1980). Microwaves: menace of future. New York, King Features Syndicate, Inc. (Aug. 10).

NCRP (1981). National Council on Radiation Protection and Management. Radiofrequency electromagnetic fields. Rep. No. 67, Washington, D.C., NCRP.

OSEPCHUK, J.M. (1978). A review of microwave oven safety. *J. Microwave Power* 13:13–26.

OSEPCHUK, J.M. (1979). Basic characteristics of microwaves. *Bull. N.Y. Acad. Med.* 55:976–998.

OSEPCHUK, J.M. (1981). Private communications: Professors Carpenter, Schwan, Michaelson, Ely, Mumford, Goldman, Imig, and McAfee, Dr. Salisbury, Messrs. Gurley, and Bucksbaum (formerly at Collins Radio Co.).

OSEPCHUK, J.M. (1981). Debunking a mythical hazard. *Microwave World* pp. 16–19.

OSEPCHUK, J.M. (1983). The microwave stimulus. *In*: Adair, E. (ed.). Microwaves and thermoregulation. New York, Academic Press, pp. 33–56.

OVERY, R.J. (1980). The air war 1939–1945. Briarcliff Manor, N.Y., Stein & Day, p. 195.

PARR, W.H. (1981). Personal communication (June 18, 1981).

POLLACK, H. (1977). Hearings before U.S. Senate on radiation health and safety, U.S. Government Publication, Serial No. 95–49, pp. 268–288.

POLLACK, H. (1979). The microwave syndrome. *Bull. N.Y. Acad. Med.* 55:1240–1244.

PRESMAN, A.S. (1970). *Electromagnetic fields and life* (translated from Russian). New York, Plenum Publishing Corp.

QUAN, K.C. (1960). Hazards of microwave radiations. *Ind. Med. Surg.* 30:315–318.

Radio-frequency radiation (1960). *Lancet*, 484–486 (Aug. 27, 1960).

ROSE, V.E., et al. (1969). Evaluation and control of exposures in repairing microwave ovens. *Am. Ind. Hyg. Assoc. J.* 30:137–142.

SAVIN, B.N., et al. (1983). New trends in the standardization of microwave electromagnetic radiation. *Gig. Tr. Prof. Zabol.* 3:1–4.

SCHWAN, H.P. (1981). History of the genesis and development of the study of effects of low energy electromagnetic fields. In Grandolfo, M., Michaelson, S. and Rindi, A. (eds.). Biological effects and dosimetry of non-ionizing radiation. New York, Plenum Publishing Corp., pp. 1–17.

SELWYN, M.R., ANDERSON, J., AND MALETSKOS, C. (1987). Biostatistical review of selected literature on the biological effects of radiofrequency electromagnetic (RFEM) energy. Washington, D.C., Electromagnetic Energy Policy Alliance.

SILVERMAN, C. (1980). Epidemiological studies of microwave effects. *Proc. IEEE* 68:78–83.

SINTON, W.M. (1952). Detection of millimeter-wave solar radiation. *Phys. Rev.* 86:424.

SMICH, E. (1980). Report on Moscow Embassy incident, U.S. Senate Commerce Committee.

SORENSON, J.A. (1983). Inaccurate, misleading. . . . *Ind. Res.* p. 194.

STENECK, N.H. (1980). The origins of U.S. safety standards for microwave radiation. *Science 208*:1230–1236.

STENECK, N.H. et al. (1982). *Risk/benefit analysis: the microwave case.* San Francisco, San Francisco Press, Inc., pp. 20–22.

STENECK, N.H. (1984). Science and standards: the case of ANSI C95.1–1982, *J. Microwave Power 19*:153–158.

SZMIGIELSKI, S., et al. (1982). Accelerated development of spontaneous and benzopyrene-induced skin cancer in mice exposed to 2450-MHz microwave radiation. *Bioelectromagnetics 3*:179–191.

TELL, R.A., AND HARLEN, F. (1979). A review of selected biological effects and dosimetric data useful for development of radio-frequency safety standards for hermia exposure. *J. Microwave Power 14*:405–424.

TYAZHELOVA, V.G., AND TYAZHELOV, V.V. (1980). Equivalent intensities of nonionizing radiation chronic exposure of different mammals. *In*: Proceedings of an International Symposium Ondes Electromagnetiques et Biologie, URSI/CNFRS, Jouy en Josas, France, June 30–July 4, 1980, pp. 53–57.

U.S. Congress (1976). Medical Device Act of 1976.

WATT, W. (1957). Three steps to victory. London, Odhams Press Limited.

YANKEE GENIUS (1958). *Reader's Digest.*

ZARET, M.M. (1973). Testimony before U.S. Senate Hearings on P.L. 90–602. U.S. Government Print. Office Document, Serial No. 93–24.

ZARET, M.M. (1976). Electronic smog as a potentiating factor in cardiovascular disease: a hypothesis of microwaves as an etiology for sudden death from heart attack in North Karelia. *Med. Res. Eng. 12*:13–16.

ZARET, M.M. (1977). Potential hazards of hertzian radiation and tumors. *N.Y. State J. Med. 77*:146–147.

Index

A

Absorption rate, specific; *see* Specific absorption rate

Acetylcholinesterase, serum levels of, ELF EM fields and, 210–211

Acoustic pressure, measurement of, 301–308, *303, 304, 305, 306, 307,* 308t

Action potential, model of initiation and propagation of, 104–105

Alternating current electrical generation, 49–50

AM; *see* Amplitude modulation

American Conference of Governmental and Industrial Hygienists (ACGIH), RF exposure standards of, 20

American National Standards Institute (ANSI), radiation protection guide of, 18–20, 19t

Amino acids, electrical properties of, 84

Amplitude modulation (AM), 3

Annular-phased arrays (APAs)
of aperture and dipole antennas for hyperthermia, SAR distributions for, 132, *133,* 134–136
for noninvasive deep heating, 463–464

ANSI; *see* American National Standards Institute

ANSI Radiofrequency Protection Guide, 28–74, 30t
biological basis of, 29
compared with previous ANSI guidelines, 44
compared with standards at other frequencies, 43–44
problems with, 29–31
suggested exposures for general public, 41–43, *42,* 42t
suggested occupational exposures of, 38–41, *39,* 39t

Antennas
far-field region of, 6

implanted, for deep heating, 466–467
television; *see* Television antennas

APAs; *see* Annular-phased arrays

Appliances, household; *see* Household appliances

Astrocytomas and 60 Hz electric fields, 249

Auditory effect, microwave; *see* Pulsed microwave radiation, auditory perception of

B

Bacteria, electrical properties of, 84

Behavior
descriptions of, 321–323
effects of electromagnetic fields on, 319–338; *see also* Microwave radiation, behavioral effects of
ELF EM fields and, 207–208
innate, 321–322
learned, 322–323
microwave radiation and
absorption characteristics and, 325–327
long-term exposure studies of, 327–333
thermal effects and, 324–325

Behavioral thermoregulation, 243–244

Bioeffects experiments
cavity exposure systems for, 148–149
corner reflector exposure devices for, 145, *145*
far-field, plane-wave, 144–145
free-field, 143–144
helical coil exposure system for, 149–150
in vitro exposure systems for, 143
in vivo and in vitro exposures, techniques for implementing, 143–146
in vivo exposure systems for, 143
irradiation systems for, 143–150
microwave aperture applicators exposure system for, 149

introduction of, 57
parallel-plate, SARs and induced
current distributions for leakage fields of, 129–132
radiation exposure from, 57–58
total power used for, 57
Dielectric spectroscopy, 78
α-Dispersion, 85
β-Dispersion, 85
DNA
ELF EM fields and, 218–219
millimeter-wave radiation and, 391
Doppler radar, 3
Dose, thermal, definitons of, 473
Dosimeters, personal radiofrequency,
153–154
Dosimetry
distributive, 191
experiments with, 190
experimental, simulated biological
tissues for, 165–169
RF; see Radiofrequency dosimetry
Down's syndrome, 358
Drills, electric, fields emitted from, 55
Drugs, psychoactive, interaction with
microwave radiation, 320

E

E fields, defining SAR in terms of, 155
EFIE; see Electric field integral equation
E-field applicators, 449–451
capacitor-plate, for deep heating,
463
E-field instruments, performance parameters for, 150–152
E-field probes, 152–153
errors near active radiator, 161
errors near reflecting objects, 160
implantable
calibration of, 164–165
for SAR measurement, 158
spurious responses of, 160
E-H field probe, 153
Electric drills, fields emitted from, 55
Electric field integral equation
(EFIE), 115

Electric fields; see also Electromagnetic fields; Magnetic fields
cancer induction and, 249–250
extremely low-frequency, human
sensitivity to, 250
high-intensity, interaction with biological substances, 102
increased background levels of, 197
natural background levels of, 197
power frequency, 50, 53
typical environments of, 54–55
Electric power; see also Transmission
lines
AC systems for generating, 49–50
Electric properties
macropic, 78–79
molecular, 79–81
Electric shavers, fields emitted from,
55
Electrical bioimpedance method
description of, 482–486
for measuring cardiac function,
486–487
for measuring changes in lung water, *484*, 487–488
medical applications of, 486–488
for obtaining cross-sectional images, 488
potential medical applications of,
482–488
in studying cardiac function, *483*
Electrical impedance imaging
high-frequency, medical applications of, 516–518
low-frequency, medical applications
of, 513–516
techniques for, 518–520
Electrical properties
of biological substances; see Biological substances, electrical properties of
experimental techniques for, 92–
100
low radiofrequency measurement
techniques for, 92–93
time-domain techniques for determining, 93–94